Confirmed and presumptive cases of **St. Louis encephalitis**, by county—Florida, as of October 17, 1990. (From Centers for Disease Control, Morbidity and Mortality Weekly Report, 39(42):757, 1990.)

Locations of three malaria outbreaks—northern San Diego County, California, August 1988 and July and August 1989. (From Centers for Disease Control, Morbidity and Mortality Weekly Report, 39(6):92, 1990.)

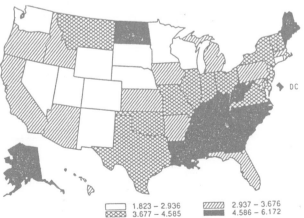

Mean annual age-adjusted cervical cancer mortality rates per 100,000 females, by quartile—United States, 1984–1986. (From Centers for Disease Control, Morbidity and Mortality Weekly Report, 38(38):652, 1989.)

These 2 maps show *A*, the distribution of **sickle cell disease**, and *B*, the **distribution of malaria**. One can superimpose maps *A* and *B* and identify the distribution of malaria and sickle cell disease in Africa. The sickle cell gene is not a significant part of the gene pool in Asia. Since the presence of the sickle cell trait (heterozygous) appears to confer some immunity to malaria, it is thought that the sickle cell trait is an evolutionary adaptation to malaria in the environment. (From Motulsky, A. G.: Metabolic polymorphisms and the role of infectious diseases in human evolution. Human Biol., 32:43, 1960.)

Boyd's
INTRODUCTION TO THE
STUDY OF DISEASE

Cover (Front and Back)

Top row (diapositive no. 1)

Left panel. Image of a plane of the living human brain obtained by positron emission tomography 60 minutes after injection of fluorine-18-labeled fluoro-dihydroxyphenylalanine [FDOPA], a radioactive precursor of dopamine. The image plane shows the accumulation of radioactive products of FDOPA in structures rich in dopa decarboxylase, the enzyme responsible for the synthesis of the neurotransmitter dopamine. These structures include the caudate nucleus and the putamen. The pseudocolor scale to the right of the image plane indicates radioactivity level.

Right panel. The radioactivity image of the left panel has been converted to an image of the activity of the enzyme dopa decarboxylase in a normal male volunteer, aged 42 years. The pseudocolor scale to the right of the image plane now indicates true enzyme activity in units per hour. Note the greater contrast between regions of the striatum and cerebral cortex.

Bottom row (diapositive no. 2)

Left panel. Enzyme activity image of the distribution of dopa decarboxylase in a 69 year old male with Parkinson's disease of Hoehn and Yahr stage 2.5. Note the moderate depletion of the enzyme in regions of the striatum, compared to the image of a normal volunteer shown above.

Right panel. Enzyme activity image of the distribution of dopa decarboxylase in a 47 year old male with advanced Parkinson's disease of Hoehn and Yahr stage 4.0. Note the severe depletion of the enzyme in regions of the striatum, compared to the image of the patient in Hoehn and Yahr stage 2.5 shown to the left.

(Gabriel Leger, BSc; Hiroto Kuwabara, MD, PhD; and Albert Gjedde, MD, Ph.D., McConnell Brain Imaging Center, Montreal Neurological Institute, McGill University, Montreal, Canada)

Boyd's
INTRODUCTION TO THE STUDY OF DISEASE

Huntington Sheldon, M.D., F.R.C.P.(C)

Professor of Pathology
McGill University, Montreal

Eleventh Edition

LEA & FEBIGER
1992

Philadelphia/London

Lea & Febiger
200 Chester Field Parkway
Box 3024
Malvern, Pennsylvania 19355
U.S.A.
1-800-882-8532

Manuscript Editor:
Lisa Stead

Production Manager:
Thomas Colaiezzi

First Edition, 1937   Reprinted 1938, 1939
Second Edition, 1941   Reprinted 1942, 1944
Third Edition, 1945   Reprinted 1945, 1947, 1948, 1949, 1950 (Twice)
Fourth Edition, 1952   Reprinted 1953, 1954, 1955, 1957, 1958, 1960
Fifth Edition, 1962   Reprinted 1963, 1965, 1967, 1969
Sixth Edition, 1971   Reprinted 1972, 1975, 1976
Seventh Edition, 1977   Reprinted 1979
Eighth Edition, 1980   Reprinted 1983
Ninth Edition, 1984   Reprinted 1987
Tenth Edition, 1988   Reprinted 1990
Eleventh Edition, 1992

Library of Congress Cataloging-in-Publication Data
Sheldon, Huntington.
     Boyd's introduction to the study of disease.—11th ed. /
Huntington Sheldon.
         p.   cm.
     Includes bibliographical references and index.
     ISBN 0-8121-1561-9
     1. Pathology.   I. Boyd, William, 1885–1979.   II. Title.
III. Title: Introduction to the study of disease.
     [DNLM: 1. Pathology.   QZ 4 S544b]
RB111.S445   1993
616—dc20
DNLM/DLC
for Library of Congress   92-49679
                                                                               CIP

Reprints of chapters may be purchased from Lea & Febiger in quantities of 100 or more. Contact Sally Grande in the Sales Department.

PRINTED IN THE UNITED STATES OF AMERICA

Print number: 5   4   3   2   1

PREFACE

This edition of the Introduction to the Study of Disease extends the range and scope of the text only slightly but presents a substantial amount of material in the form of appendices in order to make the book more readable and to condense some of the material for the reader who is already familiar with normal physiology and essential biology.

Dr. Serge Jothy has joined me in revising the text and has contributed substantially to the chapters on Inflammation, the Immune System, Neoplasia and Inherited Disease in Section I, and the Upper and Lower Digestive Tracts, the Kidney, Female Reproductive System and Blood in Section 2. Dr. Paula Traktman has revised the section on Viruses once again.

There are entirely new sections on the cytoskeleton, HIV virus and AIDS, on aging, on helicobacter and gastric ulcer, on changes in infectious disease patterns, on oncogenes and cancer, on cytokines, and on eosinophilia-myalgia syndrome.

New data on changing patterns in breast and gastric cancer, as well as epidemiological shifts in heart attacks, strokes, streptococcal disease, measles, and other common diseases are noted. Each chapter has been revised and updated but some classical illustrations are retained because of their instructional and historical value.

Irma Niemi once again typed the manuscript, collated the text and illustrations, and painstakingly assembled the many parts with unfailing good humor, skill and patience. For all her efforts we are greatly indebted.

Montreal   Huntington Sheldon, M.D.

CONTENTS

1

General Principles

1

THE LIVING BODY

The guiding principle of science is economy of explanation.—A.N. WHITEHEAD

If we are to study disease, we need to be able to distinguish what is disease from what is normal. This requires some understanding of the normal workings of the human body and the range of acceptable variation. Much of our knowledge of normal function and structure has come from comparisons between normal and abnormal. In this introduction, we outline contemporary views of how the human body is structured, from molecule to the whole person, and how the many parts function, sometimes independently, but always in relation to the whole individual. This chapter reviews anatomy and physiology at the cellular level, and outlines the mechanisms on which the living body depends for its normal function, such as circulation and digestion, and in which various disorders of function (disease) may occur, leading ultimately to failure of the whole (death).

The human body is composed of an extraordinarily large number of minute elements known as **cells,** which form definite structures or **tissues;** these again are grouped into **organs.** Certain cells with definite properties form muscle tissue, and others with quite different properties form nervous tissue; these and other tissues are combined to form organs such as the heart or brain. By definition, a tissue consists of cells of the same kind, and an organ is composed of tissues of different kinds. For example, muscle as a tissue is composed of muscle cells only, but the muscular organ, the heart, includes arteries, veins, nerves and connective tissue. To visualize the elements of cells and tissues we must use optical techniques such as the light or electron microscope, for most cells are too small to be seen with the unaided eye. The study of tissues is called **histology** (Greek *histos*, tissue, and *logos*, the study of). The word tissue itself comes from the French term *tissu*, which means weave or texture. There are four general basic types of tissue: epithelial, connective, muscular, and nervous.

Epithelial tissue (Fig. 1–1) serves to protect, absorb, and/or secrete. It is anatomically effective for these cells to be arranged in sheets to cover the surface; this is called an epithelium. One modification of most epithelial layers is the down-growth of groups of cells into the underlying connective tissue to form secretory structures known as glands. Thus, epithelia can act as protective coverings for external surfaces (skin), absorptive linings for internal surfaces such as the intestine, or secretory structures such as salivary or sweat glands.

Connective tissue (Fig. 1–2) holds together, connects and supports other tissues and cells. In addition to the connective tissue cells themselves, it is composed of a large amount of intercellular substance, which varies from one kind of connective tissue to another. Most of the intercellular substance is secreted by the connective tissue cells, whether they are cartilage cells, fibroblasts, or bone cells (osteoblasts). Depending on the type of connective tissue, the formed elements in the intercellular spaces will vary in appearance, so that we have collagen fibrils in the dermis, elastic fibers in tendons, and calcified collagen in bone (Fig. 1–3).

Muscular tissue consists of cells whose chief characteristic is their ability to contract. Different types of muscle, such as in the heart, in the gut, and in the locomotor system, are composed of cells with varied amounts and different types of fibrils. The different types of muscle also function in various ways: automatically in the heart, voluntarily in the skeleton, and rhythmically in the gut.

Nervous tissue is highly specialized for the function of permitting quick reactions both automatically, such as a reflex, and voluntarily, as when we wish to lift a spoon to our mouths.

Thus there are general functions for each of these classes of tissue: epithelial cells cover, protect, secrete,

keratin

stratified
squamous
epithelium

collagen

dermis with
skin appendages
(sweat glands
hair follicles.)

A

Villi

Brunner's
glands

Crypts of
Lieberkühn

Muscularis

B

Fig. 1–1   *A,* Photomicrograph of a section of skin shows the protective outer lining of stratified, squamous, keratinized epithelium, which lies over the dermis, the latter being composed principally of connective tissue. This epithelium serves as a natural defense to infectious organisms and prevents the body from drying by evaporation. *B,* Photomicrograph shows a section through the absorptive layer of the duodenum, where the epithelium is thrown up in many small folds and finger-like projections. This epithelium is specifically designed to increase the surface area. Microvilli at the surface of each cell serve the additional purpose of retaining extracellular enzymes to aid in absorption. (Courtesy of Dr. H. Mizoguchi.)

absorb, and may be differentiated to perform special functions. Skin, gut, liver, and milk-secreting glands are all epithelial derivatives.

Connective tissue constitutes ligaments, tendons, joints, and bones, and holds organs in place. Adipose tissue is a particular type of connective tissue.

Muscular tissue does the work in the heart, moves food along in the digestive system, and allows us to run, jump and move about.

Nervous tissue is the responsive element that permits us to perceive the world about us, and to reflect on our being.

THE HEALTHY CELL

The word "cell" originally meant a small chamber, and it is still used in that sense in relation to a jail or a monastery. But it is a chamber holding a living inmate, actually the smallest unit of living matter. Some animals, such as the ameba and the malaria parasite, consist of a single cell and are called unicellular organisms or protozoa. Although these elementary animals consist of only one cell, they breathe, digest, excrete, and move. One might recall that each of us started from the union of two cells. It has been known for some time that a fully developed higher animal can develop from a single cell that has been artificially provoked to undertake division and replication, a process called parthenogenesis. This development can even take place in an environment different from the natural one; ova can be transplanted in mammals, and development can even occur in a test tube, as the popular press is happy to report. During the normal development of a mammal, for a short while, all cells of the embryo appear remarkably similar to one another. Despite 90 years of study of embryonic development, we are still not sure why some cells differentiate into muscle, others into skin and still others into nerve or connective tissue cells.

A finished muscle cell, a finished nerve cell, and a finished liver cell are as far apart in visible structure as in what they do. Some cells pour out cement that binds them together, as in cartilage and bone. Some become as clear as glass, as in the cornea of the eye. Some develop into a system transmitting electrical signals. Each of the 70,000 billion cells in every human body specializes into something helpful to the whole. The differentiation of cells for different functions leaves us breathless—those functions we recognize in our own bodies, as well as the incredible senses of "dumb animals," such as the vision of the eagle, the olfactory sense of the dog, the radar-like sense of the bat, and the sense of touch of the mollusc. This is the wonder of life and its specializations.

The human body was likened by Rudolf Virchow (1821 to 1902) to a "cell state" with a social organization and specialization of labor. This carries with it the hazard that one group of specialized cells becomes dependent on another group of specialists, and a strike on the part of a small group may paralyze or reduce to chaos the entire community. Thus, the normal, effective contractility of the heart depends on a small bundle of conducting fibers that synchronize the different chambers. If this is impaired, the heart may stop, and every function of the whole body ceases due to lack of functional circulation of oxygen. Death results. The ameba, consisting of only one cell, has no such hazard to fear. Specialization exacts a price, in cells as well as in society.

There is a striking contrast between the durability of our body and the transitory character of its elements. Man is composed of a soft matter that can disintegrate in a few hours, and yet he lasts longer than if made of steel. Moreover, he accommodates himself marvelously to the changing conditions of his environment. The body seems to mold itself on events. Instead of wearing out like a machine, it changes. In general terms, this characteristic of *adaptation* is one of the most important features of life at any level, whether it be of a cell, tissue, or organism. We shall say more about adaptability in both health and disease.

Just as the atom is one unit of physics, so **cells are fundamental units of every living body,** whether it be animal or vegetable. In the last analysis, it is they that eat the food, drink the water, and breathe the air, all of which are necessary for the life of the body. The marvellous arrangements of structure (anatomy) and of function (physiology) are simply a complex mechanism to bring to cells food, water, and air, which are beyond their normal reach, as well as to perpetuate the species to which the organism belongs.

Every cell, whether animal or plant, consists of three principal constituents: **cell membrane, nucleus,** and **cytoplasm.** The nucleus contains: (1) **chromosomes,** which are the carriers of genes (transmitters of hereditary characteristics), and (2) the **nucleolus,** which directs the cytoplasm and seems in turn to be the target of hormones. The cytoplasm contains a variety of structural constituents known as **organelles,** or little organs. The cell is indeed a miniature universe (Fig. 1–4).

In the last 50 years enormous advances have been made in our knowledge of the structure of the cell in health and in disease. We owe these advances, in the main, to two techniques: (1) The electron microscope, which gives us a magnification of 100,000 (in place of one of 1,000) and reveals a new wealth of structure.

Fig. 1–2   *A*, Electron micrograph shows many cells in cartilage surrounded by their matrix. The perichondrium, or outer layer of the cartilage, is at the top of the field. Cartilage is an avascular tissue. All the constituents of this tissue enter by diffusion from the periphery. *B*, High-power electron micrograph shows collagen fibrils, which are identified by their characteristic repeated cross-striations. The other structures shown are portions of thin fibroblasts, limited by the bilaminar cell-surface membrane.

There are electron microscopes which make it possible for us actually to see the atom. (2) The development of new methods of cytochemistry, which demonstrate the sites of enzymes, not only in the intact cell, but also in organelles such as mitochondria. These are obtained by disrupting the cell and then separated by means of the ultracentrifuge.

Cell Membrane. The membrane or envelope of the cell is not evident with the light microscope, but it is well demonstrated by the electron microscope and by indirect evidence. Too little attention has been paid to this membrane in the past, but it is now known to be a structure no less remarkable than the contents that it encloses. It is an all-important structure, for it regu-

lates the internal environment of the cell, determining what goes in and what comes out. Thus it separates the high concentrations of potassium inside the cell from the high concentrations of sodium outside the cell, and it can push out processes to engulf harmful bacteria, which the cell then destroys: the process of phagocytosis. Water and all food particles must pass inward through the membrane freely, whereas metabolites must pass out. Virus particles are adsorbed to the surface of the cell before penetrating to the interior. It is to the surface structure that many dyes and effective drugs become attached, and antigens are bound to the surface of the cell.

The contemporary view of the plasma membrane is

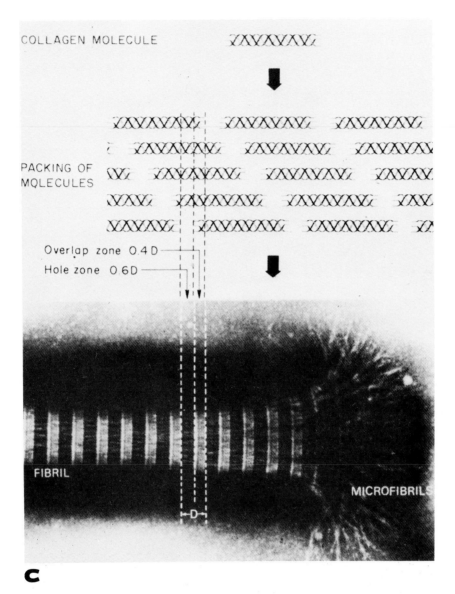

COLLAGEN MOLECULE

PACKING OF MOLECULES

Overlap zone 0.4 D

Hole zone 0.6 D

FIBRIL

MICROFIBRILS

C

Fig. 1–2   (*Continued*) *C*, High-power electron micrograph of soluble collagen shows the protofibrils and their arrangement as seen with negative staining. (From Prockop, D.J., et al.: The biosynthesis of collagen and its disorders. N. Engl. J. Med., 301:13, 1979.)

that it is composed of lipid molecules arranged with their hydrophobic regions outward in the manner of a stockade. Interspersed among the palisades of lipids are protein molecules which extend across the lipid bilayer, often as single alpha helices. Some protein molecules do not span the lipid bilayer but attach to one of the other surfaces. Some of these proteins act as pores or channels allowing small molecules access to the cell's interior. Other proteins are fixation points which attach to other cells or to intracellular molecules such as filaments. Again, some membrane proteins carry sugar or carbohydrate residues on their surfaces as oligo or polysaccharides. Many of these carbohydrates are proteoglycans, long polysaccharide chains linked to a protein core which forms a part of the extracellular matrix, such as the basement membrane of epithelial cells or the matrix of cartilage. These surface components play major roles in transport, adhesion, cell recognition and in growth and development, as well as in immune regulation (Fig. 1–5).

Nucleus. The nucleus may be regarded as the brain of the cell. When the nucleus dies, death of the cell will soon follow. There is a curious exception to this rule, for the erythrocyte (red blood cell) of man loses its nucleus when it enters the blood stream from the bone marrow, yet its life span is about 120 days. Perhaps its passive role of carrying oxygen from the lungs to the tissues makes the presence of the nucleus su-

Origin and Relationship of Mesenchymal Cells

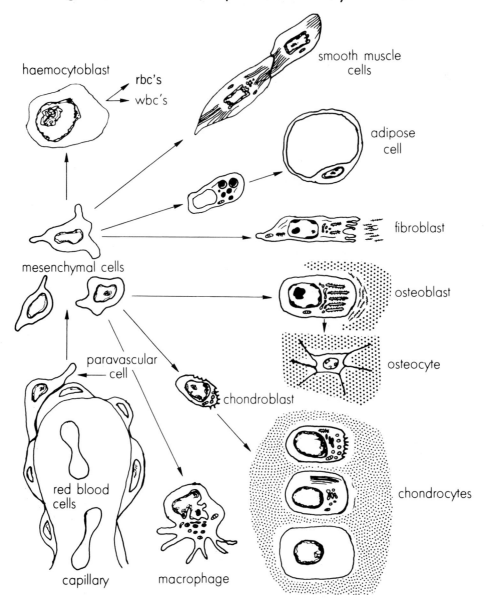

Fig. 1–3 Origin and relationship of mesenchymal cells. The primitive mesenchymal cell shown at left center of the field may differentiate into a hemocytoblast or into smooth muscle cells, adipose cells, fibrocytes, osteocytes or blasts, chondrocytes, and/or macrophages. The presumed predecessors of these cells are paravascular cells as shown in the bottom left of the field. (From Sheldon, H., and Jaeger, V.: The mesenchymal cell. In *The Musculoskeletal System. Embryology, Biochemistry, and Physiology.* Edited by R.L. Cruess. New York, Churchill Livingstone, Inc., 1982.)

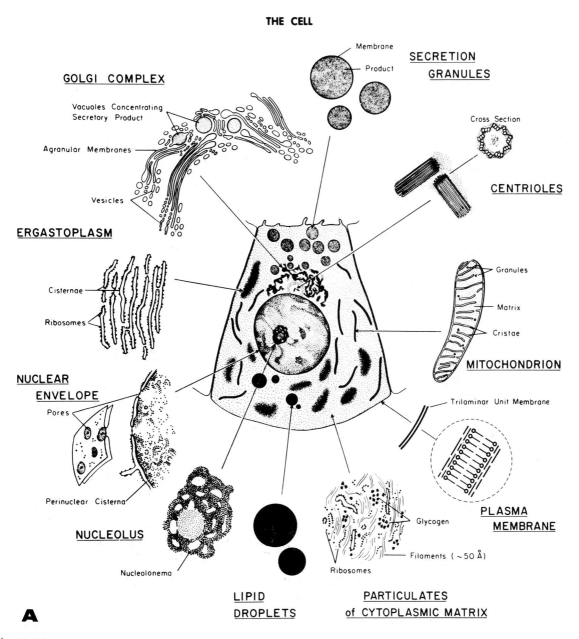

THE CELL

GOLGI COMPLEX

Vacuoles Concentrating Secretory Product

Agranular Membranes

Vesicles

Membrane

Product

SECRETION GRANULES

Cross Section

CENTRIOLES

ERGASTOPLASM

Cisternae

Ribosomes

Granules

Matrix

Cristae

MITOCHONDRION

NUCLEAR ENVELOPE

Pores

Perinuclear Cisterna

Trilaminar Unit Membrane

PLASMA MEMBRANE

NUCLEOLUS

Nucleolonema

Glycogen

Filaments (~50 Å)

Ribosomes

A

LIPID DROPLETS

PARTICULATES of CYTOPLASMIC MATRIX

Fig. 1–4   *A*, Schematic representation of a secretory cell. Arranged around the cell are the various components that have been identified with the electron microscope. The significance of these components is discussed briefly in the text. (From Bloom, W., and Fawcett, D.W.: *A Textbook of Histology*, 10th Ed. Philadelphia, W. B. Saunders Co., 1975.)

B

Fig. 1–4   *B,* Electron micrograph shows a liver cell in which the various components can be identified.

perfluous, although in some mammals such as the camel, and in cold-blooded animals (frog), the nucleus is present in the erythrocyte. The nuclear material is sequestered from other cell components (cytoplasm) by the nuclear membrane. Forty years ago, electron microscopy of this interface between the two major compartments of the cell (nucleoplasm and cytoplasm) demonstrated curious and regular structures, which have been carefully studied and shown to be a kind of pore. So each nucleus is surrounded by a system of membranes, but there are pores in the membrane that permit the exchange of material and information between the nucleus and cytoplasm. This route is important because we know that many hormones must reach the nucleus of a cell to be effective. The control of cytoplasmic protein synthesis depends on information reaching the cytoplasm from the nucleus. Perhaps in the future we will discover ways to control the ebb and flow of information through the nuclear pores.

Within the nucleus resides the DNA (deoxyribonucleic acid), the program for all cell activities. The DNA is complexed with other basic proteins in a diffuse structure known as chromatin. (These proteins are important for the structure of the total complex and probably serve a control function as well.) When the cell is resting (i.e., not dividing), the chromatin is dispersed throughout the nucleus and is barely visible.

However, when the cell prepares for mitosis (cell division), the chromatin becomes condensed into long, thin structures known as chromosomes that can easily be seen with a light microscope. Each plant and animal cell has a species-specific number of chromosomes: man has 23 pairs (46 in all). Each pair consists of two nonidentical copies of chromosomes, one derived from each parent.

A gene is a segment of a chromatin strand; there may be 50,000 to 100,000 genes strung along one chromosome. **The gene, not the chromosome, is the unit of heredity.** A structural gene is now defined operationally as a **functional unit of inheritance, situated on a chromosome and responsible for the synthesis of a specific polypeptide or protein.** This synthesis results in the production of two general classes of proteins, namely those concerned with the framework of cells (structural proteins), and those concerned with intermediary metabolism, or the rate of protein synthesis (regulatory proteins). Enzymes can be considered as a subset of regulatory proteins. Genes, therefore, contain instructions for the design of both building blocks (structural proteins) and builders (regulatory proteins) of the living machine, as well as information about how that machine is to function. It is hardly too much to say that a man's biochemistry is as individual as his fingerprints, and that both are determined by his genes.

A general concept was enunciated more than 55 years ago in the dictum ''one gene—one enzyme;'' it was subsequently amplified to ''DNA makes RNA which makes protein.'' These ideas can be better understood by the following propositions. (1) All biochemical processes in all living organisms are under the control of genes. (2) Each biochemical reaction can be resolved into different steps, governed by the availability of substrate and enzyme. (3) Each step of any reaction is under the control of a different gene. (4) Mutations of single genes affect single steps of a reaction. (5) Mutations may affect either the structure of the product of a reaction, or the amount of the product of the reaction.

Sickle cell anemia results from a single gene mutation that produces a structurally abnormal hemoglobin molecule. Other single gene mutations may result in an inborn error of metabolism, which sometimes is manifest as disease.

Abnormalities can occur in chromosomes as well as in single genes. Often a chromosomal disorder results in the loss of thousands of genes and is lethal for the new embryo, which fails to develop completely and dies during the first few weeks after conception.

The ribosomes are structural units that allow for organized and efficient protein synthesis. The mRNA

Kupffer cell

Hepatic sinusoid

Space of Disse

Lipoprotein

Agranular reticulum

Golgi complex

Bile canaliculus

Lysosome

Granular reticulum

Lysosomes

Golgi complex

Microbody

Mitochondrion

Golgi complex

C

Fig. 1–4   C, Drawing interprets the electron micrograph. Labeled are various structures that have been discovered during the last 30 years. Not all of these structures can be identified in any single micrograph. For example, in Figure 1–4 *B* no microbodies or lysosomes can be seen. (Drawing by Sylvia Colard Keene.)

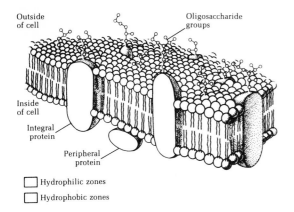

Outside
of cell

Oligosaccharide
groups

Inside
of cell

Integral
protein

Peripheral
protein

☐ Hydrophilic zones
☐ Hydrophobic zones

Fig. 1–5 The Singer-Nicolson fluid-mosaic model of membrane structure. (From Lehninger, A.L.: *Principles of Biochemistry*. New York, Worth Publishers, Inc., 1982.)

to be translated lines up in a groove on the ribosomes and is moved along it as each successive triplet is read and each successive amino acid is added to the growing protein chain. Many initiation, elongation, and termination factors are involved. In essence, however, the tRNA functions as an intermediary, an adaptor, between the nucleic acid code, and the amino acid specified. The ribosome functions as a conveyor belt. It should be mentioned that the reading of the triplets occurs in a specified phase and in a given direction (polarity). One can see how a variety of mutations or errors in DNA would change the resultant protein. A change of base might cause a new triplet or specify a new amino acid, or perhaps even the stop signal. A loss or addition of a base would put the remainder of the sequence out of phase. Errors during RNA transcription would have a similar effect on protein synthesis, but these errors would not be inherited by the next generation of cells.

Proteins, once synthesized, go to work doing the business of the cell. They may be structural components, may work as catalyzing enzymes, or may be signal proteins such as hormones that direct a range of alterations in cellular behavior.

Cytoplasm. If the nucleus is the brain of the cell, concerned with such major problems as genetic constitution and cellular reproduction, it is the cytoplasm that does most of the everyday work. Just as the cells are specialized to do different kinds of work, such as the contraction of muscle, the secretion of digestive juices, the production of hormones, and the sending out of nervous impulses, it is natural that the shape and appearance of cytoplasm should vary correspondingly. An examination of the nucleus may indicate whether the cell is living or dead, but the appearance of the cytoplasm may tell the scientist looking

down the microscope whether the cell has been sick and unable to work.

Every cell's cytoplasm contains a number of subcompartments known as *organelles*. These have been studied in detail by the modern methods already referred to: cell fractionation, high-speed centrifugation, and photography with the electron microscope. For expediency, we shall limit our discussion to 5 major cytoplasmic constituents—mitochondria, endoplasmic reticulum, lysosomes, microtubules, and intermediate filaments.

Mitochondria are thread-like bodies (Greek *mitos*, thread, and *chondrus*, granule) when viewed with the light microscope, but as seen with the electron microscope, they are rod-shaped or may look like a cucumber. Although they are barely discernible with conventional light microscopy, they are present in enormous numbers (2,500 per cell in the liver of the rat). They are surrounded with a paired membrane, so that each can be regarded as a separate chemical laboratory or membranous compartment; folds of the inner membrane project inward as shelves termed cristae (Fig. 1–6). It is on these shelves that the respiratory enzymes are arranged in an orderly way; these enzymes are responsible for the use of oxygen. Mitochondria are regarded as the main power plants of the cell. It is of interest that organisms that do not depend on oxygen may or may not have mitochondria, depending on whether they are functioning anaerobically (without oxygen). In fact, yeast may be grown aerobically and will contain mitochondria, but the same yeast grown in the absence of oxygen will lose its mitochondria. Mitochondria also contain small amounts of DNA and some RNA. Isolated mitochondria respond to hormones such as thyroxine, but we now believe that they do not synthesize their specialized respiratory enzymes themselves, despite the presence of DNA and ribosomes, but rather that such enzymes as cytochrome oxidase are assembled in the mitochondria after synthesis by the endoplasmic reticulum.

The presence of these membrane-bound cytoplasmic organelles (mitochondria) with even a little nucleic acid has suggested to some authors that mitochondria represent the symbiotic existence of prokaryotic (bacteria-like) forms, which at some remote time in evolution formed a useful alliance with nucleated cells. Whatever their origin, they are present in most living human cells and they exist in large numbers in those cells that require a large amount of energy to do their work. In fact, one may increase both the size and number of mitochondria in skeletal muscle by aerobic training. Conversely, with disuse, these mitochondria decrease in number and in size. Such

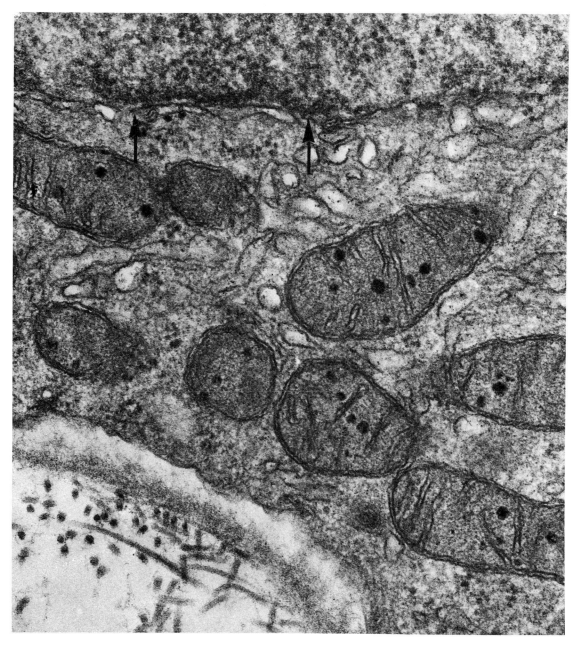

Fig. 1-6 Electron micrograph shows a small portion of a cell containing many mitochondria and bounded by a basement membrane. At the top of the field is the nucleus, and at the arrow is a nuclear pore. The mitochondria are surrounded by two parallel dense lines which constitute membranes enclosing the mitochondrial space from the cytoplasm. The mitochondria has a denser matrix than the surrounding cytoplasm and is divided into compartments by cristae. Within the mitochondria are dense aggregates that appear in this picture as black dots. Outside the border of the cell is a basement membrane. This area is seen at the bottom of the field. Extending into it are delicate fibrils of connective tissue.

observations underscore the adaptability of living cells at all levels of organization.

The term *endoplasmic reticulum* has been given to the principal membranous component of the cytoplasm, a series of vesicles and intercommunicating canals, whose primary function is to separate the cell into different compartments, much as walls may delimit the kitchen from the bedroom or bathroom, where different functions are accomplished.

Endoplasmic reticulum is a collective term for cytoplasmic membranes; we recognize both the granular reticulum (that with RNA particles attached) and the agranular reticulum. The granular reticulum is a special group of cytoplasmic membranes, which appear in greatest abundance in cells that secrete protein for export, such as plasma cells (antibodies), pancreas cells (digestive enzymes), osteoblasts (collagen), and liver cells (albumin, fibrinogen). (The granular reticulum also exists in neurons and is called the Nissl substance.) The granules of the rough endoplasmic reticulum are attached polyribosomes, which synthesize specific proteins that are directly transferred across the membrane into the cavity called a cisterna. Here the newly synthesized proteins are sequestered from the other cytoplasmic compartment and are transported by a system of channels and vacuoles through the Golgi complex (a system of smooth membranes located near the nucleus) to the exterior of the cell, where they fulfil their appropriate destiny.

All cells contain ribosomes. However, as we have described, only some cells have their ribosomes directly attached to membranes, presumably for the express purpose of directing the synthesis of protein into a particular compartment. In most cells, ribosomes lie about in the cytoplasm until they are called to synthesize proteins. During this time they can be visualized as helical clusters or pearl-necklace arrangements along a messenger RNA molecule (Fig. 1–7). Their protein product is for cellular consumption as in the erythrocyte (hemoglobin) or the muscle cell (actin or myosin).

There is another part of the endoplasmic reticulum, those membranes without ribosomes, the so-called *agranular reticulum*. This system of smooth membranes is seen most obviously in tissues that synthesize steroid hormones and lipids, that are concerned with salt and water transportation, or that are involved in detoxification, as in liver cells. In each case, the type of the membranes, their arrangement, and their basic chemical structure may be different. In general, however, it is safe to say that whereas the granular reticulum is concerned with the synthesis of protein, usually designed for secretion, the agranular reticulum functions in a different way. The Golgi complex can be considered a special example of the agranular reticulum (Fig. 1–8).

The pathway for intracellular synthesis, secretion, and transport has been elucidated during the last 45 years, principally by Palade and his group. A scheme illustrating this pathway is shown in Figure 1–9. This pathway depends on energy derived from mitochondria and on direction derived from the genome (total gene complement) to achieve its goal. It also depends on the necessary substrates, such as amino acids, essential fatty acids, carbohydrates, and vitamins or coenzymes. A single perturbation in this elaborate network will destroy the normal sequence. The substitution of a single amino-acid analog for an essential

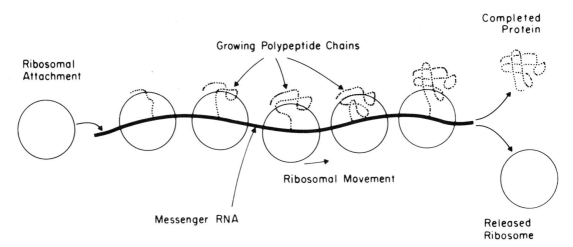

Fig. 1–7   This drawing shows a ribosome schematically attached to messenger RNA, and the nascent protein developing from the ribosome appears as a coiled set of small dots.

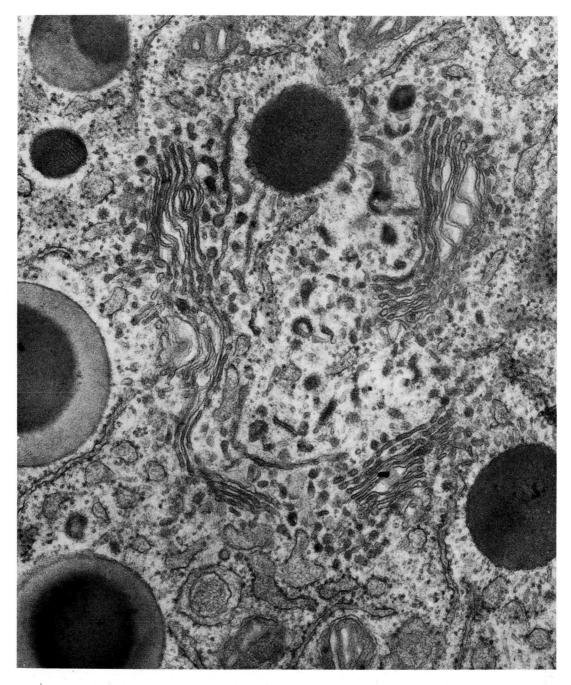

Fig. 1—8   Electron micrograph shows a horseshoe-shaped Golgi complex, where smooth membranes are arranged in parallel. The Golgi complex has been regarded as a packaging and shipping area for the segregation of materials that will be secreted by cells. The large dense granules contain enzymes in an inactive form.

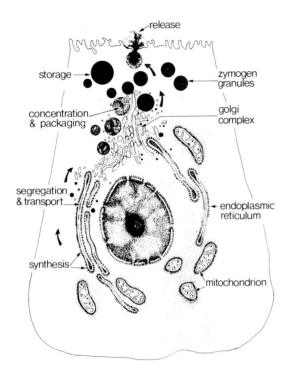

release
storage
zymogen granules
concentration & packaging
golgi complex
segregation & transport
endoplasmic reticulum
synthesis
mitochondrion

Fig. 1–9 This drawing illustrates the pathways of protein synthesis in the pancreatic acinar cell, and demonstrates the relationship between the different anatomic units and their function. (From Bloom, W., and Fawcett, D.W.: *A Textbook of Histology*, 10th Ed. Philadelphia, W. B. Saunders Co., 1975.)

amino acid will grossly distort the normal subcellular pattern as shown in the accompanying diagrams (Fig. 1–10).

Lysosomes. Membrane-bound bodies containing powerful digestive enzymes, lysosomes can be regarded as part of the digestive system of the cell, just as the mitochondria represent the power plants. One view suggests they may be called the stomach of the cell.

Different types of cells have different numbers of lysosomes, which contain different populations of enzymes. The macrophage, a wandering scavenger, contains a rich and powerful store of lysosomes, as do polymorphonuclear leukocytes, for example.

Lysosomes are conventionally united with vacuoles that contain ingested particles. The original vacuole is called a phagosome; without the presence of appropriate digestive enzymes its role is limited to the suspension of the particle. When digestive enzymes from the lysosome join the vacuole and fusion of the membranes takes place, the phagosome then becomes a digestive vacuole. Most particulate matter that has been ingested into a phagosome must be broken down before it can be assimilated into particles small enough to cross the membrane of the cell and thereby to enter into the cytoplasm proper.

Microtubules. Another cytoplasmic organelle, microtubules were only recognized relatively recently as a part of most cells. These long, straight, thin structures appear most frequently in cells with asymmetrical shapes such as neurons (axons) or spermatozoa, and have been identified as the element responsible for movement in cilia and flagella. All cells during division have masses of microtubules, for they compose the mitotic apparatus. Microtubules may serve as a cellular skeletal apparatus, or they may perform a more dynamic role by providing a mechanism for motility. It seems likely that in the case of cilia, flagella, and the mitotic apparatus, **actin** (half of the energy-producing protein, actinomyosin) is associated with the microtubules and provides the driving force for the sliding motion currently thought to be the mechanism by which this movement occurs.

Just as there may be abnormalities in mitochondria or in the endoplasmic reticulum, so there may be abnormalities in the microtubules of cells. One example discovered recently is an abnormal structure of cilia, which are responsible for clearing our airways of foreign particles, for propelling ova along the fallopian tubes, and for the motility of sperm.

Immotile but living spermatozoa were found in the semen of four men who were sterile. The sperm tail appeared as in rigor, that is, straight, stiff, and with no motility. Electron microscopy showed the spermatozoa to be relatively normal except that so-called dynein arms were not present (Fig. 1–11). Dynein arms are structures that form temporary cross bridges between adjacent ciliary filaments in normal cilia, flagella, and sperm tails, and are believed to be responsible for generating the movements of cilia or sperm tails.

Three of the four subjects had experienced, since childhood, chronic sinusitis and bronchitis, and frequent bouts of pneumonia, common cold, and ear infection.

Study of the tracheobronchial clearance in the three subjects revealed that there was no measurable mucociliary transport. Ordinary tracheobronchial clearance was nearly or totally absent when no coughing occurred, but a reasonably good substitute for this clearance could be obtained by permitting the subjects to cough. Cilia from the respiratory tract also lacked the dynein arms.

Three of the subjects had *situs inversus totalis* (their organs were placed in the reverse position in their bodies).

From these findings, two tentative conclusions are drawn. The cells of the four men cannot synthesize normal dynein arms, or if such dynein arms are formed, they cannot attach to the ciliary filaments; this causes immotility of spermatozoa and cilia. Visceral asymmetry is determined through the movements of cilia of some embryonic epithelial tissues.

The foregoing, then, illustrates how new observations on such a tiny structure as the cilia of a cell shed light on the reasons for infection, infertility, and even the mechanisms of development.

	NUCLEUS	NUCLEOLUS	ERGASTOPLASM	GOLGI	MITOCHONDRIA	ZYMOGEN
STOCK DIET						
2 HRS.						
18 HRS.						
2 DAYS						
5-8 DAYS						
10 DAYS						

Fig. 1–10 This diagram shows the effect on the nucleus, nucleolus, rough endoplasmic reticulum, mitochondria, and cell products (zymogen granules) of the administration of ethionine, an amino acid analog of methionine, to guinea pigs. Over a period of days, the pancreas cells are unable to synthesize normal products. The cytoplasm and the nucleus reflect this inability. (From Herman, L., and Fitzgerald, P.: The degenerative changes in pancreatic acinar cells caused by DL-ethionine. J. Cell Biol., 12:277, 1962.)

Fig. 1–11   *A*, This very high magnification of a sperm tail shows the normal microtubule structure and arms. The arms are better seen in the drawing, *B. C*, Section from a patient with immotile spermatozoa. The arms of the microtubules are not present. (From Afzelius, B.A.: A human syndrome caused by immotile cilia. Science, 193:317, 1976.)

Cytoplasmic Filaments. Another element of all cells which has received increasing attention over the last two decades is the complex network of cytoplasmic filaments which collectively can be considered to compose the cytoskeleton. In some cells these filaments are the predominant elements (muscle cells), and in others they are scarcely present at all (red blood cells). There are many views of how these asymmetrical, elongate cytoplasmic elements should be classified, but there is agreement that there are three general classes: large filaments such as myosin, small filaments composed of the protein actin, and a collection of filaments of intermediate dimensions which are presently divided into at least four groups (Table 1–1). Let us consider actin filaments first.

Actin filaments. Because of the ubiquitous need for contraction in all phases of cell activity it is not surprising that actin has been identified in almost every type

of cell. Actin is involved in very basic cellular activities such as mitosis, cytokinesis, cytoplasmic streaming, phagocytosis, and all types of movement both within the cell and of the cell as a whole. Three different actins have been identified—alpha, beta, and gamma actins—all of which have similar chemistry and function. Beta-actin, which is found primarily in cytoplasmic microfilaments, and gamma-actin, characteristic of smooth muscle cells, both activate magnesium ATPase activity of muscle meromyosin (meromyosin is the major protein part of the rodlike backbone of the myosin molecule; there are two types, heavy, labeled H, and light, labeled L), but they do so less well than alpha-actin, which is the actin of striated muscle. Beta and gamma actins make up 5 to 10 percent of the protein in nonmuscle cells.

All actins are made from monomeric units of the globular G-actin. G-actin spontaneously polymerizes

Table 1–1.   Principal Types of Intermediate Filament Proteins

TYPE OF INTERMEDIATE FILAMENT	COMPONENT POLYPEPTIDE (MASS IN DALTONS)	CELLULAR LOCATION
Type I	Acidic keratins (40,000–70,000) Neutral and basic keratins (40,000–70,000)	Epithelial cells and epidermal derivatives such as hair and nails
Type II	Vimentin (53,000) Desmin (52,000) Glial fibrillary acidic protein (45,000)	Many cells of mesenchymal origin, often expressed by cells in culture Muscle cells Glial cells (astrocytes and some Schwann cells)
Type III	Neurofilament proteins (about 130,000*; 100,000*; and 60,000)	Neurons
Type IV	Nuclear lamins A, B, and C (65,000–75,000)	Nuclear lamina of all cells

* Because these proteins migrate abnormally slowly on SDS gels, they were initially thought to be larger.

(From Alberts, B., et al.: *Molecular Biology of the Cell*, 2nd ed. New York, Garland Publishing, Inc., 1989.)

to form filamentous F-actin, a double stranded helix. The filaments so formed then localize in different parts of the cell depending on phase of cell cycle or current cell activity. For example, in cultured cells, bundles of fibers run parallel to the cell's axis and are known as stress fibers. During fibroblast spreading in tissue culture the microfilaments elongate in the direction of cell movement, only to disappear with the onset of mitosis. Other actin filaments then appear later in mitosis as part of the mitotic apparatus; finally, during cytokinesis, a ring of actin appears in the cleavage furrow.

Thus two differences between actin filaments of nonmuscle cells and those of skeletal muscle are apparent: individual filaments of the former are not arranged in such a well defined, interlocking manner and their supramolecular aggregates are relatively short-lived, coming and going with the needs of the cell. Similarities to actin filaments of striated muscle include requirements for Mg^{2+}-ATP and micromolar concentrations of free calcium ion. Control mechanisms of the actomyosin system of striated muscle have been quite well delineated. Postulated mechanisms for the regulation of nonmuscle actomyosin-like systems include actin or myosin linked regulation via some binding protein, protein modification (e.g., by phosphorylation), and interaction of actin with membranes.

We may leave a consideration of myosin filaments to the chapter on muscle, and turn to a consideration of intermediate filaments.

Intermediate filaments. While actin, tubulin (the subunits of thin contractile filaments), and microtubules are globular proteins, intermediate filaments are made of fibrous proteins which are elongate, asymmetric molecules which overlap to form long structures with great tensile properties.

The common property of forming a discrete fibrous system in cells and a diameter of about 100 Å when viewed in the electron microscope, have caused all these filaments to be lumped together until chemical analyses have shown that they could be divided on the basis of their amino acid sequence.

Type I filaments are those **keratins** with a molecular weight between 40,000 and 70,000 (whether they are acidic, basic or neutral) which are found predominantly in epithelial cells and epidermal derivatives such as hair and nails.

Type II filaments include three groups: a) desmin, b) vimentin, and c) glial fibrillary acid proteins.

Desmin, from the Greek *desmos*, means link. These filaments are found in smooth, skeletal, and cardiac muscle at all stages of development, but are most obvious in adult smooth muscle. Here they link sarcoplasmic electron dense bodies, believed to be analogous to striated muscle Z lines, with electron dense plaques bound to the cell membrane. In skeletal muscle desmin filaments link Z discs laterally to each other, to the plasma membrane, and to other cytoplasmic membrane organelles. They may also play a role in the development of the T tubule—sarcoplasmic reticulum system, since they have affinity for both Z disc and membrane.

Vimentin filaments are found in both mesenchymal and nonmesenchymal cells. In cultured fibroblasts these wavy filaments are found in increased concentrations around the nucleus. They appear to end on both the nuclear membrane and the adhesion plaques of cytoskeletons after detergent extraction of the cells. Their consistent association with the cell nucleus may indicate a role in maintaining it in a definite place or supporting it mechanically. Some association with normal fibroblast cell adhesion and spreading is suggested by the fact that these intermediate filaments transiently form perinuclear caps during these cell activities. Formation of these filament caps can be reproduced by treating cells with colcemid. Under these conditions the cells are found to contain equimolar amounts of two polypeptides: vimentin, MW 52,000–55,000, and desmin, equivalent to that of smooth muscle, MW 50,000–54,000. Therefore, two chemically different intermediate filaments can coexist in the small cell, although it is possible that the vimentin and desmin are copolymerized into one filament. Other functions proposed for the vimentin filaments are the intracellular transport of organelles and as an aid to cell locomotion.

Type III filaments are **neurofilament** proteins which are a major cytoskeletal element on nerve axons and dendrites.

Type IV filaments are nuclear **lamins** which may extend from the nuclear envelope to the cell periphery. They presumably play a role in tethering the nucleus.

The function of intermediate filaments is not essential to the survival of animal cells. The general thesis is that they form a network to maintain cell shape and to permit cell function to take place by tethering cells to each other, as well as resisting tension exerted by changes from within (osmotic forces) or from without

the cell. The presence of these many different types of filaments are regarded as a mechanism to permit a three dimensional framework which allows various mechanical changes to take place. It is quite clear, moreover, that these filaments relate to other cytoplasmic components such as the plasma membrane, microtubules, the endoplasmic reticulum and the nuclear envelope, as we have shown.

EXTRACELLULAR MATERIAL

The immediate environment of the cell is also of interest, for the ebb and flow of energy does not stop at the entrance to the cell. Just as one can reconstruct much of the life within a house by examination of the contents of the trash bin, so one should be aware of the materials that lie immediately adjacent to the cell. Epithelial cells sit on a basement membrane, and most of them are polarized with an outer surface and a basal surface. Along both sides they are usually attached to one another by junctions, across which they may

Fig. 1–12   This drawing illustrates the biosynthesis of collagen in the rough endoplasmic reticulum (ER) showing the vectorial transfer of a new protein into the compartment of the rough endoplasmic reticulum. (From Prockop, D.J., et al.: The biosynthesis of collagen and its disorders. N. Engl. J. Med., 301:13, 1979.)

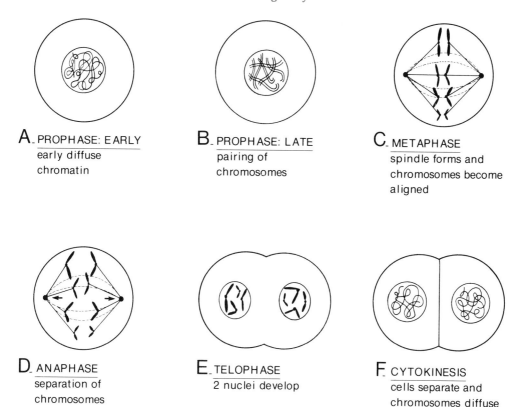

A. PROPHASE: EARLY
early diffuse
chromatin

B. PROPHASE: LATE
pairing of
chromosomes

C. METAPHASE
spindle forms and
chromosomes become
aligned

D. ANAPHASE
separation of
chromosomes

E. TELOPHASE
2 nuclei develop

F. CYTOKINESIS
cells separate and
chromosomes diffuse

Fig. 1–13 These drawings illustrate different phases in mitosis.

communicate. Their secretory products are released at their apex either onto a free surface or into a duct.

Another class of cells, the connective tissue cell, is extremely important in repairing damage to tissue and in maintaining the integrity of the interstitial space. Its principal products are collagen and complex sugars (glycosaminoglycans), and we shall have more to say about this material in the chapter on the musculoskeletal system (Fig. 1–12).

Many kinds of enzymes are normally extruded by inflammatory cells, interstitial cells, and wandering cells into the extracellular or interstitial spaces.

Mitosis. Reference has already been made to the varying life span of cells. Some are short-lived, whereas others enjoy a long life. In either case, when they die they are replaced by new cells. (An important and sad exception to this rule are the cells of the brain and spinal cord; once these are destroyed, as in cerebral hemorrhage or poliomyelitis, they cannot be replaced, although in some instances their function can be learned by other cells.) In unicellular organisms, new cells are created by the division of the pre-existing cell. In all the higher forms, new cells arise through mitosis or **mitotic division** (Fig. 1–13). A nucleus in the process of mitosis is referred to as a mitotic figure.

Mitotic figures are seldom seen in normal tissue because relatively few cells are dying and being replaced, but, as might be expected, they are common in the growing embryo. Cell division is frequent in the repair of wounds and in the replacement of excised tissue, especially in the liver. Examination of mitotic figures is of particular importance in the case of tumors, in which mitotic figures are not only numerous, but often atypical in appearance. This may enable the pathologist to decide whether he or she is examining a benign tumor or a malignant one.

THE INJURED CELL

The complex and delicate structure and function of the cell may be damaged by a variety of influences, of which chemical poisons and bacterial toxins are obvious examples. The cell becomes injured, so that it does not function perfectly. This injury is reflected in the microscopic appearance of the cytoplasm and later of the nucleus. These morphologic changes can be regarded as the fingerprints of disease; when the damage is slight, the prints can be erased. Although morphologic changes are of importance to the pathologist, they are of little interest to the reader of this book, and they will only be mentioned so that the reader will recognize the names when they are discussed. It is important to recognize that a cell may be sick without showing any morphologic change. We are now coming to think of disease in terms of molecular alterations, not merely in terms of the cell. The work of the cell depends chiefly on the integrity and availability of enzymes. An altered enzyme may escape detection by the physician. A person who dies in the convulsions of tetanus (lockjaw) has a morphologically normal nervous system, although we know that it is profoundly, indeed fatally, abnormal.

Perhaps we should state here an important concept, which is that although changes in function and structure are intimately related, and although we conventionally think that the functional change depends on change in morphology (heart failure can be shown to be due to a diseased valve), it is more likely that the earliest indications of disordered function show no disordered structure even with sophisticated modern methods.

We can also introduce the idea that, up to a point, injury to any organ, tissue, or cell may be entirely **reversible,** so that when ischemia (loss of blood supply) occurs, provided blood flow and oxygenation are restored within a few minutes, the tissue and cells will not die. However, when injury is severe (burns) and enzymes of a cell are denatured, **irreversible injury** is done, which results in an entirely different situation. We shall now consider some of the irreversible changes.

Necrosis, as the name implies (Greek *nekros,* corpse), is the local death of cells. The cellular changes characteristic of necrosis are changes that the cell undergoes after it has died while still remaining in the body, and are due to the action of enzymes contained within those cells (in lysosomes). These enzymes turn their energies on the framework of the cell itself, a process known as **autolysis.** Death of the cell may be due to (1) chemical poisons, (2) bacterial toxins, (3) physical agents such as irradiation, and (4) most commonly, loss of blood supply due to closure of an artery by thrombosis. This last phenomenon is known as an **infarct;** cellular death in this instance is caused by the sudden cutting off of the supply of oxygen to the cell, that is to say, **anoxia.** Over a period of many hours or a few days the nucleus breaks up and disappears, and the cytoplasm becomes indistinct and fades away, with eventual **liquefaction necrosis.** In the case of some bacterial infections such as tuberculosis, the structural outlines of the affected part are wiped out. This process is known as **caseation necrosis** because the gross appearance of the material is cheesy, or caseous. In an infarct, on the other hand, the general outline of microscopic structure can still be recognized, such as the tubules and glomeruli in the kidney, and the muscle fibers in the heart. The difference between the necrosis of an infarct and caseation is the difference between the site of ancient Pompeii, in which the outline of the streets can still be recognized, and the site of the destruction of Hiroshima. Different types of necrosis are outlined in Table 1–2.

Somatic death is death of the body as a whole. It occurs when respiration and the heart's action cease, although individual cells and even tissues may continue to live for short periods. Soon characteristic changes begin to make their appearance in the dead body. The most striking of these are: (1) loss of response to stimuli; (2) cessation of the circulation, which can be seen with an ophthalmoscope in the small blood vessels of the retina; (3) gradual approach to the temperature of the environment (algor mortis); (4) muscular rigidity due to chemical changes in the muscle (rigor mortis), the stiffness beginning in 4 hours or more and passing off in about 3 days; (5) a reddish discoloration of the dependent parts of the body (livor mortis) due to the sinking of the blood from gravity combined with a breaking down (hemolysis) of the red blood cells; (6) postmortem clotting of the blood. The doctor or the detective in the story book can tell to within a few minutes how long the

Table 1–2.   Types of Necrosis

TYPE	CAUSE	APPEARANCE	DISEASE
Coagulative	Ischemic cell death followed by denaturation of proteins	Basic outline of cells preserved for a period of time Loss of nuclei Increased eosinophilia of tissue	Infarcts in most tissue except brain
Liquefactive	Digestion of cells by intracellular and leukocytic enzymes	"Pus"	Brain infarcts Focal bacterial lesions (abscess)
Caseous	Tubercle bacillus inciting granulomatous inflammation with destruction of tissue	White, cheesy, "putty"	Tuberculosis
Fat	Abnormal release of pancreatic enzymes	Chalky, white flecks	Acute pancreatic necrosis

body has been dead, but so many factors, such as fever, high external temperature, and violent exercise at the time of death may influence the speed of the postmortem changes, that anything approaching accuracy is out of the question. A note of these changes, however, may be useful in making a rough estimate of the time of death for medicolegal purposes.

We may conclude our necessarily brief study of that remarkable structure, the living cell, with the vivid words of Osgood in an address to the American Society of Medical Technologists: "In summary, can you imagine a mobile, self-reproducing factory, which selects its own raw materials, manufactures not one but many products, rebuilds and repairs itself constantly, provides its own power supply, has automatic local and remote controls, transports its fuels, products and waste products with great efficiency, which may be versatile or specialized, but is integrated by efficient communication systems with the needs of the community, and always provides reserves for emergencies? Such a factory is the cell."

We have considered the cell, together with the body fluids and metabolism, which make the life of the cell possible and give it meaning as the basic unit in the living body. Let us now turn our attention to a brief discussion of the systems that bring nutrients and oxygen to the cell, prepare the food for absorption, excrete waste products, make intercommunication between the cells and organs possible, and, finally, meet the supreme challenge of reproduction. All of these will be discussed in greater detail when we study the diseases of these systems in Part 2 of this book.

BODY FLUIDS

In addition to considering the cells of the body we must recognize the importance of their environment, the interstitial spaces and the fluids which surround them. After all, the nutrients on which they depend must diffuse across a few microns of interstitial space before they can be used, and the waste products of cellular metabolism must be carried away from the cells, which would otherwise drown in their own by-products.

Body fluids are of three kinds: tissue fluid, blood, and lymph. (1) **Tissue fluid,** or interstitial fluid, surrounds and bathes the cells; it is placid, a lake, not a stream. (2) **Blood** is contained in the blood vessels, and nowhere comes in direct contact with the tissues except in the spleen. It is carried to an organ in arteries. These break up into a vast network of capillaries, through whose infinitely thin walls the fluid of the blood (plasma) is able to pass, mixing with the tissue fluid and carrying into it nutrients and oxygen that the waiting cells absorb. On the return voyage, such

metabolic by-products as lactic acid and CO_2 are carried in the capillaries to the venules and veins back to the heart. Since tissue fluid continually increases in amount, it is obvious that there must be some means of escape. This is provided by (3) **lymph,** which, like the blood, is contained in a set of vessels, the lymphatics. The tissue fluid laden with waste products from the living cells passes through the thin walls of the lymphatics and is carried away as lymph. This is a round-about way of getting back into the veins, for all the lymphatics eventually form one or two main ducts, which open into the large veins in the neck. The advantage of this method is that the lymph has to pass through a series of filters, known as **lymph nodes,** in which bacteria and other injurious agents that may have gained access to the tissue fluid are strained out and are usually destroyed. A significant proportion of the tissue fluid passes directly back through the walls of the vessels into the blood stream.

It is possible to estimate the rate of passage of water from the vessels into the tissue spaces by injecting some traceable substance, such as a radioactive isotope, into a vein and noting the rapidity with which it disappears from the blood. The rate of exchange shown by this method is incredibly fast, for **more than 70% of the water of the blood is exchanged with extravascular water every minute.** The walls of the smaller capillaries appear to be veritable sieves with regard to water.

The principal mechanism by which this exchange is achieved was elucidated by the great English physiologist Starling, who hypothesized that small molecules and water, under the influence of the hydrostatic pressure at the arteriolar end of the capillary, leave this delicate vessel, but large molecules such as the protein, albumin, and fibrinogen cannot. At the venular end of the capillary the small molecules and water are attracted by the high osmotic value of the intracapillary protein, and so water returns across the capillary cell to the circulation from the interstitial space. The pressure relationships in the circulatory systems are illustrated in the accompanying diagrams (Fig. 1–14).

It is important to recognize that if there are alterations in the pressure relationships, or in the quantity of serum protein, or in the nature of the capillary cells, there may be a disequilibrium that leads to **edema,** which is discussed in the following section. The different mechanisms that lead to an increased interstitial fluid accumulation can now be explained.

Water and Salt. The most important single constituent of the body is water, for water is essential to everything that lives. Hunger can be endured for days or weeks, but thirst is unendurable; the cells of the whole body cry out for water, not merely the parched mouth. Life started in the water in the dim and distant

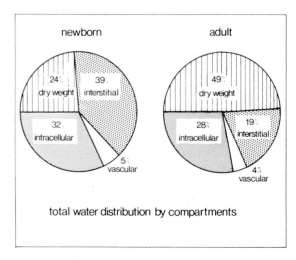

Fig. 1–14   *A,* Diagram illustrates the pressures of the pulmonary and systemic circulations. (From West, J.B.: *Respiratory Physiology.* Baltimore, Williams & Wilkins, 1974.); *B,* This drawing illustrates the equilibrium for exchange at the level of the capillary. The arteriole is shown at the left and protein is represented by stars within the capillary lumen. The large arrows show the net transfer of water and small molecules out at the arteriolar end, and the transfer of water in at the venular end. The osmostic value of the serum proteins exceeds that of the intracapillary pressure at the venular end, thereby attracting fluids back in and maintaining the circulation's integrity.

past, for the sea is the original home of all life on the globe; even vertebrate life first appeared as a marine form. We still live in a watery environment, not, as we fondly imagine, in the air. For the surface of the body in contact with the air is either dead (the horny layers of the skin) or is separated from the air by a layer of water (eyes, nose, and mouth). After all, we are completely immersed in water during the first 9 months of life before birth. The baby consists mostly of water, whereas the old man or woman shrivels up like a wilted plant (Fig. 1–15). In the salt content of the blood plasma and in the film of salt water through which we look on the outside world we carry the memory of the remote, ancient ocean in which we originated. Still more do we carry this modified salt water in the interstitial fluid, which constitutes what the great French physiologist Claude Bernard, more than 100 years ago, called the internal environment.

The water of the body, together with the salts or electrolytes (substances decomposed in solution by electricity) that are dissolved in it, is contained in two major compartments: (1) intracellular, and (2) extracellular. The **intracellular fluid** makes up nearly 30%

of the body weight, the bulk of it being contained in muscle. The **extracellular fluid** is mainly represented by the interstitial fluid, with a much smaller amount in the blood plasma. It is the fluid in the interstitial

Fig. 1–15   This diagram shows the relative distribution of water by compartments in both the newborn and the adult human being.

space that constitutes the real internal environment, and the freest communication exists through the cell membrane between the water in the compartment and the water inside the cells. The cell membranes, while freely permeable to water molecules, are selectively permeable to dissolved substances such as serum albumin. When solutes are unevenly distributed across these membranes, they cannot equilibrate their own concentrations by redistributing across the membrane. However, water easily moves across to effectively dilute the more concentrated side and concentrate the more dilute side. This movement of water across a semipermeable membrane in response to concentration difference across the membrane is termed **osmosis.** Osmolality represents the osmotic concentration of a solute. Thus, for each cell in the body the same conditions prevail as for the single-celled creatures fixed on the bed of a flowing stream that brings to them their food and oxygen and carries away their waste products. The cells are bathed in salty fluids; without that fluid they cannot live. They are indeed islands in the interstitial sea. In many diseases, such as cholera, this fluid is drained away from the body, the tissues become dehydrated, and they will die unless the water is replaced.

It is the delicate balance of electrolytes and water that serves to maintain the constancy of the internal environment, the importance of which Bernard was the first to emphasize. For the preservation of this constancy the mechanism of **homeostasis** has been evolved. Important instruments in the homeostatic orchestra are the kidney, which modulates the salt and water music; the lung, which also modifies the pH of the body; the pituitary and adrenal, which dictate obligato passages for salt and water; and the liver, which provides a bass by means of albumin synthesis. When the autoregulatory system breaks down we see the clinical picture that we call disease, a breakdown which, if sufficiently profound and prolonged, results in death due to acidosis, hyperkalemia (high serum potassium), or other fatal disorders.

The subject of the internal environment has become more important in the present day than in bygone years, not only to the physician, but also to other members of the health team, partly because of the strong likelihood of its being changed when the patient—especially the surgically treated patient—is placed in a hospital bed and fluids begin to flow into his veins, and partly because the physician, and still more the surgeon and the pediatrician, can do so much to correct disturbances of this environment, and to safeguard health and life itself in the process.

We have seen that an adequate and constant supply of tissue fluid is necessary for the health of the body cells. If this supply is insufficient, or if the fluid is withdrawn too quickly, a condition of **dehydration** develops, which can be recognized by the sunken appearance of the face and by the wrinkled condition of the skin. This may develop quickly, as after a night of hard drinking, or in acute diseases associated with severe vomiting or profuse diarrhea. Dehydration and loss of salt may be the result of excessive sweating, as is seen in the tropics or the desert and in men working under conditions of great heat. When the heat of Arabia comes out like a drawn sword and strikes you speechless, you realize that water comes before everything. In such cases it is important to drink amounts of fluid to which salt has been added. On the other hand, tissue fluid may accumulate in excessive amounts, so that the part becomes waterlogged, a condition known as **edema.** This can be recognized by the fact that when a finger is pressed into the swollen part, a temporary pit is formed, owing to the fluid's being forced away into the surrounding tissues. Edema may be caused in many ways. (1) In **inflammation,** the walls of the capillaries become unduly permeable and too much fluid passes from the blood into the tissue spaces. (2) In heart and kidney disease, edema is an important symptom; it may be caused by **fluid retention, albumin loss,** or by increased **hydrostatic pressure** in the veins and in the capillaries. (3) **Pressure on the lymphatics** by a tumor will also be accompanied by edema.

Derangements of the body fluids are discussed further in Chapter 4.

A review of the normal physiologic processes (see Appendix p. 27) may provide readers with a common framework to support the ideas and descriptions presented in the remainder of the text.

In this chapter we have reviewed the structure and function of the living body at different levels of organization; they range from man to molecule. This range can be encompassed also in the concepts of disease. We recognize diseases of the whole individual (perhaps best expressed in psychiatric disorders such as the psychoses or in a systemic disease like diabetes mellitus), diseases of a given organ (such as an infarct of the brain or heart), diseases of cells (perhaps best represented by cancer of different cell types), and finally, diseases at the molecular level (where there is frequently an inborn error that results in the accumulation of glycogen or in the synthesis of an abnormal hemoglobin).

Sickle cell hemoglobinemia (hemoglobin S) is a prototype of **molecular disease.** The particular effect of the presence of abnormal hemoglobin S is exerted at each of the levels, molecular, cellular, tissue, organ, and host. When the abnormal, genetically determined sickle cell hemoglobin is subject to a lowered oxygen tension in the circulation, hemoglobin molecules form protein rods within the erythrocyte. This is seen, for example, in the drop of blood taken from the fingertip after 3 or 4 minutes of occluding venous circulation by a rubber band in a child with sickle cell homozygous disease. The erythrocytes, instead of being biconcave discs, assume a pointed, star shape (Fig. 1–16). These cells now cannot flow normally through the capillary bed and often are stopped in the microcirculation. Frequently, these capillary thromboses, which is what they are called, precipitate more anoxia in the neighboring tissue. The neighboring capillaries and veins share the lowered oxygen tension, multiplying the anoxic effects to wider areas.

The result of this anoxia is often thrombosis and occlusion of larger, more important blood vessels that supply critical areas of the brain or kidney. The effect causes ischemia and tissue necrosis, otherwise known as an infarct. The result of the infarct is the loss of function of the particular area. Whereas necrosis in small areas, such as the bowel, spleen, or bone marrow may not cause anything more severe than pain, thrombosis and necrosis of the central nervous system, for example, usually result in a deficit of motor or intellectual function. This condition will often affect critical areas and cause death.

Thus one can consider the pathogenesis of disease at each level, ranging from the integrated action of the central nervous system to the structural integrity of the single molecule of hemoglobin in an erythrocyte.

Fig. 1–16 This pair of photographs shows the appearance of the normal erythrocyte above and of sickle-form cells from a case of homozygous sickle cell hemoglobinopathy below. (From Herrick, J.B.: Peculiar elongated and sickle-shaped red corpuscles in a case of severe anemia. Arch. Intern. Med., 6:517, 1910.)

SYNOPSIS

The hierarchy of organization of living things is: whole organisms, organ systems, tissues, cells, organelles, macromolecular aggregates, and molecular structures. Cells are the units of life.

Subcellular structures—plasma membrane, mitochondria, rough and smooth reticulum, lysosomes, microtubules, nucleus—may each be abnormal, just as there may be lesions in the brain, or lung, or other organ systems.

Structural and functional relationships are inextricably connected, and morphologic changes can be looked on as fingerprints of disease. However, serious disorders of function may occur without any visible change from normal structure.

Injuries may be reversible or irreversible, and types of injury can be classified even if poorly understood at all levels.

The structure and function of the circulatory, respiratory, digestive, excretory, nervous, and reproductive systems are reviewed briefly in the Appendix.

Terms

Cells	*Lysosome*	*tRNA*
Tissues	*Anoxia*	*mRNA*
Organs	*Chromosome*	*Transcription*
Lesions	*Homeostasis*	*Translation*
Necrosis	*Collagen*	*Replication*
Infarct	*Ribosomes*	

FURTHER READING

Afzelius, B., and Mossberg, B.: Immotile cilia. Thorax, 35:401, 1980.

Alberts, B., et al: *Molecular Biology of the Cell*, 2nd Ed. New York, Garland Publishing, Inc., 1989.

Bernat, J.L., Culver, C.M., and Gert, B.: On the definition and criterion of death. Ann. Intern. Med., 94:389, 1981.

Bistrian, B.R., et al.: Prevalence of malnutrition in general medical patients. J.A.M.A., 235:1567, 1976.

Bloom, W., and Fawcett, D.W.: *A Textbook of Histology*, 10th Ed. Philadelphia, W.B. Saunders Co., 1975.

Carlier, M.-F.: Actin: Protein structure and filament dynamics. J. Biol. Chem., 266:1, 1991.

Dustin, P.: *Microtubules*. Berlin, Springer-Verlag, 1978.

Eaton, J.W., and Hebbel, R.P.: Pathogenesis of sickle cell disease. In *Pathobiology Annual*. Vol. II. New York, Raven Press, 1981, p. 31.

Fawcett, D.W.: What makes cilia and sperm tails beat? (Editorial) N. Engl. J. Med., 297:46, 1977.

Gelehrter, T.D.: Enzyme induction. N. Engl. J. Med., 294:522, 1976.

Glimcher, M., and Nimni, M.: Collagen cross-linking and biomineralization. Connective Tissue Res., 27:73, 1992.

Guyton, A.C.: *Textbook of Medical Physiology*. Philadelphia, W.B. Saunders Co., 1981.

Hanover, J.A.: The nuclear pore—at the crossroads. FASEB Journal, 6:2288, 1992.

Hardingham, T.C., and Fosang, A.J.: Proteoglycans—many forms and many functions. FASEB Journal, 6:861, 1992.

Hasilik, A.: The early and late processing of lysosomal enzymes—proteolysis and compartmentation. Experientia, 48:130, 1992.

Hayflick, L.: The biology of human aging. Plastic and Reconstructive Surg., 67:536, 1981.

Judson, H.F.: *The Eighth Day of Creation*. New York, Simon & Schuster, 1979.

Lehman, W.: Calponin and the composition of smooth muscle thin filaments. J. Muscle Research and Cell Motility, 12:221, 1991.

Mannella, C.A., and Tedeschi, H.: The emerging picture of mitochondrial membrane channels. J. Bioenergetics and Biomembranes, 24:3, 1992.

Mellman, I., and Simms, K.: The Golgi complex—in vitro veritas. Cell, 68:829, 1992.

Moros, D.A.: The philosophy of medicine: clinical science and its ethics. Perspect. Biol. Med., 31:134, 1987.

Needleman, P., and Greenwald, J.E.: Atriopeptin: a cardiac hormone intimately involved in fluid, electrolyte, and blood-pressure homeostasis. N. Engl. J. Med., 314:828, 1986.

Palade, G.E.: Intracellular aspects of the process of protein synthesis. Science, 189:347, 1975.

Porter, K.R., and Bonneville, M.A.: *An Introduction to the Fine Structure of Cells and Tissues*, 4th Ed. Philadelphia, Lea & Febiger, 1973.

Rhodin J.A.: *Histology: A Text and Atlas*. New York, Oxford University Press, 1975.

Rothman, J.E.: The Golgi apparatus: two organelles in tandem. Science, 213:1212, 1981.

Singer, S.J.: Current concepts of molecular organization in cell membranes. Biochem. Soc. Trans., 9:203, 1981.

Spiro, H.M.: When doctors get sick. Perspect. Biol. Med., 31:117, 1987.

Thomas, L.: *The Lives of a Cell*. New York, Viking Press, 1974.

Unger, E., et al: The microtubule system and the reduplication of microtubule organizing centers in Dictyostelium Discoideum. Acta Histochemica, 92:19, 1992.

Watson, J.D.: *Double Helix: Being a Personal Account of the Discovery of the Structure of DNA*. New York, Atheneum, 1968.

Watson, J.D.: *Molecular Biology of the Gene*, 3rd Ed. Menlo Park, Calif., Benjamin-Cummings, 1976.

Wurtman, R.J., Baum, M.J., and Potts, J.T., Jr.: The medical and biological effects of light. Ann. N.Y. Acad. Sci., 453:408, 1985.

Zackroff, R.V., et al.: Intermediate filaments. In *Cytoskeletal Elements and Plasma Membrane Organization*. Edited by G. Poste and G.L. Nicolson. New York, Elsevier/North Holland Biomedical Press, 1981.

APPENDIX

Background Material for Normal Physiology

Metabolism

The sum total of the chemical reactions that proceed in that remarkable laboratory, the living cell, is called metabolism. There are many cellular laboratories that do different kinds of work, and each individual laboratory can do various kinds of work. Intermediary metabolism is the chemical transformation of foodstuffs in the body so that they can be used. The essence of metabolism is change (Greek *metabole*, change), and the change may be a breaking down (catabolism), or a building up (anabolism). The three main constituents of food are proteins, carbohydrates, and fats. All contain carbon, hydrogen, and oxygen, but proteins are also distinguished by their content of nitrogen, which has to be built into the cells to make up for the loss that occurs in the wear and tear of activity. Proteins are made up of a large number of small units differing from one another; these units are the **amino acids.** Speaking generally, proteins are used for body building, whereas carbohydrates and fats are used for the production of energy. Carbohydrates and fats have been compared with gasoline and oil in an automobile, but it is protein that replaces worn parts. We usually picture the protein of meat being built up into body protein, and so on with the other food stuffs. It is now known that the derivatives of the ingested protein, carbohydrate, and fat of the diet pass into a common metabolic pool, in which one basic foodstuff can be converted into another according to need before being built into the tissues. The essential purpose of this disintegration is to provide energy, some of which is used to perform mechanical work, some to support metabolic processes, the remainder appearing as heat. All living systems require an external source of energy for growth and activity. Plants obtain their energy directly from the sun by virtue of the photosynthesis effected by their chlorophyll. By means of photosynthesis, plants build simple substances (carbon dioxide of the air and water) into more complex ones (starch, sugar, cellulose). In all other organisms energy originally comes from the sun by way of the plants. Thus it is that animals and plants must depend on each other. When we regard a plate of beefsteak with a liberal helping of vegetables, we are really looking at a plateful of energy. Pyruvic acid is a key substance in intermediary metabolism, as it represents a stage reached by all the foodstuffs, not only carbohydrate, but also protein and fat. The various complex steps by which pyruvic acid is broken down with the liberation of energy is known as the Krebs cycle. (For his work Krebs received the Nobel prize.) The energy is trapped or bound as "energy-rich phosphate bonds," more particularly adenosine triphosphate, for convenience known as ATP. This trapped energy can suddenly be released like the combustion of gunpowder when the call comes. What brings about these dramatic changes?

Enzymes. The profound importance of the biologic catalysts known as enzymes in every phase of metabolism has now come to be fully recognized. A catalyst is a substance that can enormously speed up a reaction without itself becoming altered or forming a part of the product of that reaction, so that it can be used over and over again an almost infinite number of times. Enzymes bring about reactions that, without them, would require great heat and strong chemicals. Enzymes are protein molecules, and over 600 of them have been isolated. They are remarkably specific for all kinds of proteins, carbohydrates, and fats—specialists in the true sense of the word. Indeed the specificity is so precise that it may be likened to the fit of a key for a lock, as if to make sure that the right chemicals undergo the right reactions at the right time. The substance on which a specific enzyme acts is known as the substrate. Many enzymes are inactive unless united with a nonprotein organic molecule, known as a coenzyme, which is therefore as important as the enzyme itself. Many vitamins are coenzymes.

Enzymes may pass out of the cell and take part in the digestion of food, as is the case in the enzymes of the saliva, the gastric juice, and the secretion of the pancreas, which is poured into the intestine. Or they may act inside the cell. It is customary to name enzymes by adding the suffix "-ase" to the name of the substrate, as in maltase and lipase. Some, however, retain their original names in popular usage, such as pepsin in gastric juice and trypsin in pancreatic juice. The cellular enzymes may spill over into the blood when produced in excess, and their detection in the blood stream may be of great diagnostic value. Thus the presence of acid phosphatase may confirm a suspicion of cancer of the prostate, and the same is true of creatine phosphokinase in the case of myocardial infarction caused by coronary artery occlusion.

Enzymes belong to two great groups as regards their action on the substrate; they may be (1) hydrolytic or (2) oxidizing. The hydrolytic enzymes are those concerned more particularly with the digestion of food, and are therefore found in the mouth, the stomach, and the intestine. Hydrolysis involves the decomposition of a substance owing to the incorporation of water, followed by a splitting into simpler compounds with smaller molecules that are able to pass through the intestinal mucosa into the blood stream. Thus protein is split into amino acids (acids containing one or more amino or NH_2 groups), and the hydrolytic enzymes then recombine the products of digestion to build up complex tissue, proteins, carbohydrates, and fats.

The oxidizing enzymes are concerned more particularly with the metabolism of carbohydrates and intracellular production of energy. All the activities of the cell require energy, and this energy is derived from the oxidation of carbohydrates and, to a lesser degree, of fats and proteins. As a result of the oxidation of carbohydrate, carbon is converted to carbon dioxide (CO_2) and the hydrogen to water (H_2O), while energy is released. The body may be compared to a gasoline engine, which also burns carbon and hydrogen. In an engine, heat represents a source of energy, but in the body it is a waste product representing energy the cells have failed to use and expressed as calories.

It becomes evident that respiration is not only a matter of breathing air into and out of the lungs; it includes the cellular uses of oxygen in the metabolism of the cell (cellular respiration). The oxidative enzymes of the Krebs cycle have been pictured as arranged in an orderly manner on the shelves of the cristae of the mitochondria, the ultimate purpose of the mechanism being the synthesis of adenosine triphosphate (ATP). With this picture in mind, we can visualize how a poisonous compound such as carbon tetrachloride may play havoc with the physiology (functioning) of the liver cells by penetrating them, attacking the mitochondria, paralyzing their enzymes, and thus disrupting the Krebs cycle and the production of ATP. The cyanides and hydrocyanic acid (prussic acid) are deadly poisons because they damage the respiratory enzymes that normally transfer oxygen from the hemoglobin of the red blood cells to the cells of the tissue. Thus all the tissues immediately suffer from lack of oxygen (anoxia), although the blood cells remain oxygenated and therefore bright red. However, this is not the only cause of anoxia. Anything that interferes with O_2 delivery to the tissue will result in the condition of anoxia. Hence, obstruction of the airways carrying O_2 to the lungs may lead to anoxia because less O_2 is reaching the red cells passing through the pulmonary circulation. Similarly, a reduction in the number of the O_2 carriers will decrease the amount of O_2 carried to the tissue and poisoning of respiratory chain enzymes interferes with the release of O_2 to tissues. The important point to note is that disruption in the passage of O_2 from the air to the tissue at any level will lead to anoxia. It may be noted in passing that cancer cells appear to have fewer mitochondria than normal, perhaps because these cells are more concerned with reproduction (mitotic division) than with functional activity.

Circulation

The **circulatory system** is the mechanism by which fresh material is sent to the tissue fluid and waste material is removed from it. The fresh material is of two kinds, food and oxygen. The food is contained in the blood from the intestine, the oxygen in the blood from the lungs. Because the blood has to circulate from the intestine and lungs to the tissue fluid and back again, a pump is required. This pump is the **heart,** which is simply a hollow muscle. Contraction of the body muscles helps to force the lymph through the lymphatics, and when this is interfered with as the result of disease, massage may take its place. The blood from the tissues contains waste products, in the form of solid material in solution, and gas (carbon dioxide), also in solution. The solid material in solution is excreted, mainly by the kidneys, but also by the skin. If the kidneys go on strike, the skin may be stimulated to do at least part of the work through increased perspiration. The carbon dioxide in the blood is given off in the lungs and expired. At the same time oxygen is breathed in and taken up by the blood, as a result of which the color of the blood becomes a much brighter red. The system of blood vessels with the blood they contain (vascular system) is comparable to a system of roads and railways by means of which intercommunication between different parts of the cell state is maintained.

The tissues contain abundant reserves of water, salts, proteins, carbohydrates, and fat. These reserves can be used when the need arises. Unfortunately, oxygen is not stored anywhere; it must be unceasingly supplied to the body by the lungs, for the blood contains only a 3-minute supply at any given moment. This is why the absence of oxygen, or anoxia, can only be tolerated for the shortest time, and is rapidly fatal to a tissue such as heart muscle or to the nervous system.

An organ is like a pond completely filled with aquatic plants and fed by a small brook. The water in the pond is nearly stagnant and is polluted by waste products of the plants. The degree of stagnation and pollution depends on the volume and rapidity of the stream. This is the reason why the health of every organ suffers in the condition of prolonged heart disease known as congestive heart failure.

Blood from the body is carried to the heart by veins and

is then sent by the pulmonary artery to the lungs to be oxygenated. The blood from the lungs is also carried to the heart by another set of veins, the pulmonary veins. It is evident that if these two kinds of blood were allowed to mix in the heart, the whole object of the circulation would be defeated. The cavity of the heart is therefore divided by a longitudinal septum or partition into two sides, right and left. The right side receives the deoxygenated blood from the body and sends it to the lungs. The left side receives the oxygenated blood from the lungs and sends it throughout the body in the arteries. Like any other pump, the heart is provided with valves, so that the blood will always move in one direction. If these are diseased, the blood may leak back through the valves, with great disturbance to the circulation. The names and arrangement of the valves and of the various chambers of the heart will be considered in connection with diseases of that organ.

Respiration

The **respiratory system** is designed to bring air, or rather oxygen, from the outside to the cells in the innermost recesses of the body. The air is inhaled through the trachea or windpipe into the lungs, where it is brought into intimate contact with a vast network of capillaries through the thin walls of which the oxygen is able to pass. It is seized by the hemoglobin of the red blood corpuscles and is carried throughout the body. When the capillaries of the tissues are reached, the oxygen leaves the red blood cells, passes through the capillary walls, enters the tissue fluid, and is taken up by the cells. The energy of cells is obtained from the oxidation of food, particularly carbohydrates. At the same time the tissues give off one of their waste products in the form of a gas, carbon dioxide. The carbon dioxide passes into the venous blood, the plasma carrying three times as much as the red cells, carried back to the lungs, discharged into the air spaces of those organs, and exhaled into the outside air (Chapter 15). Tissue or cellular respiration is therefore the real meaning and reason for the rising and falling of the chest that we commonly call respiration.

Digestion

The **digestive system** is concerned with preparing the food that is to be carried by the blood to the tissue fluid for the nourishment of the cells. The tissue fluid must receive its food in the simplest form for conversion into the building stones of the body and the fuel that drives the engine. A beefsteak would be out of place in the tissue spaces; the cells would not know what to do with it. The work of preparing the food so that it may be used by the tissues is performed by the alimentary canal and by certain digestive glands, which are derived from the alimentary canal and pour their digestive juices into it. The alimentary canal consists of the **mouth,** where the food is broken by the teeth and acted on by the saliva; the esophagus or gullet, which is a mere passageway; the **stomach,** where the food is retained for some hours and is acted on by the gastric juice; the **small intestine,** where it is further digested and liquefied and from which it is absorbed; and the **large intestine,** which conducts the indigestible part of the food to the exterior. The food is converted into a soluble absorbable form by digestive juices, which are produced by collections of cells that form glands. The glands line the interior of the stomach and intestine and are also collected to form a most

important digestive organ, the **pancreas,** which pours its digestive juice into the very beginning of the intestine. Bile from the liver also enters the bowel at the same point and assists in the digestion of fats.

The **liver** plays a much more important role in the use of foodstuffs than the mere production of bile, which in many respects is simply a waste product. The three main constituents of food are proteins, carbohydrates, and fats. We have already seen that all three contain carbon, hydrogen, and oxygen, and that protein in addition possesses nitrogen.

The complex **proteins** of the food are broken down in the intestine into their simplest elements, the amino acids or building stones of the body, still characterized by the possession of nitrogen. The amino acids and carbohydrates are absorbed into capillaries in the wall of the small intestine and carried to the liver by the portal vein. In the liver the portal vein breaks up into fine capillaries, which come into intimate contact with the liver cells, each of which is a little chemical factory filled with hard working enzymes. Some of the amino acids pass on to the heart and are distributed to the tissues, where they serve the important function of body building. The rest of the amino acids lose their nitrogen in the liver, where it is converted into urea, a waste product that reaches the kidneys by the blood stream and is excreted in the urine as nonprotein nitrogen. The valuable non-nitrogenous portion (carbon and hydrogen) of these amino acids reaches the tissue cells, where it is used in the production of energy. This process of breaking down the protein of food into its constituents (catabolism) and of rebuilding these into the tissues of the body (anabolism) is graphically portrayed by Best and Taylor (*The Living Body*) in the following passage: "The utilization of protein in the construction of body tissue may be compared to the building of a number of houses of different types from materials derived from the wrecking of other structures. Each brick and stone in the old buildings must be separated and then sorted and carted to the new sites. Some of this building material will be more suitable for one type of house, some more suitable for other types. Other materials again will not be utilizable at all, and will therefore be discarded as refuse. The new buildings, though constructed from materials taken from the old, will be quite different in structure and in general plan."

The **carbohydrates** of the food are converted in the intestine into glucose or other sugars. From the intestine, glucose is absorbed into the capillaries and carried by the portal vein to the liver, where most of it is changed into a storage form known as glycogen and retained temporarily in the liver cells. Glucose is one of the important fuels of the body, necessary for muscular action and heat production. When fuel consumption is rapid, the carbohydrate depot, the liver, is called on to convert some of its glycogen into readily available glucose and to give it back to the blood for transportation to the muscles.

Some of the **fats** are carried to the liver by the portal vein; here they are converted into a form more readily available for use. The rest of the fat is absorbed into lymphatic vessels known as lacteals, and is carried by the thoracic duct to the great veins of the neck, where it enters the general circulation and is stored in the fat depots of the body.

It will be seen that the journey of the blood stream from the intestine to the tissues is somewhat in the nature of a cafeteria, various additions to the tray being made on the way. Denatured amino acids, now freed from their nitrogen and therefore no longer deserving of their name, are added by the liver; glycogen is converted into glucose when the storehouse in the liver is called on by the tissues; oxygen is added as the blood passes through the lungs; and fat is poured into the veins at the root of the neck.

Excretion

The **excretory system** is concerned with the removal of waste products from the body. This is brought about by the cooperation of a number of organs, i.e., the intestine, kidneys, skin, and lungs. The **intestine** offers the simplest example of an excretory organ. Food contains elements that are indigestible and cannot be used. These are passed on into the lower part of the bowel, the large intestine, from which they are discharged periodically as feces or stools. The **kidney** is a complex structure, the details of which will be considered in a later chapter, but the essential arrangement is not unlike that of the lung, except that fluid instead of gas leaves the blood. The arteries to the kidneys break up into fine capillaries, through the walls of which pass fluid from the blood together with waste substances in solution. The fluid or urine passes into tubules that open into a duct, the ureter; this duct carries the urine to the bladder, from which it is periodically discharged. The excretory function of the **lungs** has already been indicated. Here the waste product is carbon dioxide, which passes through the capillary walls into the air spaces or alveoli of the lungs and is breathed out through the trachea. The **skin** is an excretory organ by virtue of its sweat glands, which remove waste substances from the blood and pour them out on the surface in the fluid form of sweat. If the kidneys are not working properly, the sweating function of the skin can be stimulated by heat, and thereby relieve the kidneys of part of their load. The skin is a remarkable structure. Despite its thinness, it effectively protects the delicate internal structures and fluids against the unceasing variations of external conditions. It is moist, supple, elastic, and durable. Its durability is due to its being composed of several layers of cells that continually multiply. These cells die while remaining united to one another like slates on a roof, slates that are continually blown away by the wind and continually replaced by new ones. All the openings in the skin except the nostrils are closed by elastic and contractile rings known as sphincters. Thus it is the almost perfectly fortified frontier of a closed world.

Communication

From what has already been said, it is evident that the various highly specialized parts of the body are brought to work together for the common good. The runner breathes faster because his muscles need more oxygen; glycogen is converted into glucose when more sugar is needed for energy; the rectum, the terminal portion of the large intestine, contracts (or should contract) so as to empty itself when it becomes full of feces; the eye is closed when threatened by a flying object; the foot is raised when its owner wishes to walk. What are the integrating influences that make the organs members of one another? They are of two kinds. One is telephonic or telegraphic in type, urgent in character, demanding instantaneous response; the messengers are **nervous impulses,** electrical in nature, and they are transmitted by the nervous system. The other may be compared to a specific delivery service, slower but more detailed in character; the messengers are the **hormones,** chemical instead of electrical in nature, produced by the endocrine or ductless glands, and carried by the blood stream.

Nervous System. This system is singularly like a gigantic telephone organization, with a central exchange, an infinite number of wires, and receivers at the ends of these wires. The exchange is the brain and spinal cord, known collectively as the **central nervous system,** whereas the wires are represented by the nerves that form the **peripheral nervous system.** Some parts of the system act like automatic telephones without any conscious control; purely automatic messages are concerned in such functions as the beating of the heart, the constriction or dilation of the blood vessels, the swallowing of food, the movement of food along the intestine, the process of childbirth. The automatic messages are carried for the most part by a special set of nerves known as **autonomic** (sympathetic and parasympathetic), which form the involuntary nervous system, although reflex action also plays some part in automatic responses.

The greater part of the nervous system is operated on the principle of a nonautomatic telephone exchange. On the surface of the body as well as in its interior there are myriads of receivers that, when stimulated, transmit sensations of various kinds to the spinal cord and thence to the brain, or directly to the brain. These receivers are known as receptors, some of which are specialized for the reception of sensations of sight, sound, taste, etc. (the special senses), whereas others respond to stimulation by giving rise to sensations of touch, pain, heat, and cold. These varied sensations are carried to the central nervous system by afferent or sensory nerves, where they are sorted out and analyzed by the nerve cells of the brain. The sensory nerves form part of the voluntary nervous system, the other part of which is constituted by efferent or motor nerves. These nerves carry electrical messages from the nerve cells of the brain to the muscles, in response to which muscular contraction occurs. The actual stimulus that acts on the muscle fibers is apparently chemical in nature, for chemical substances of various kinds are liberated at the nerve endings when the nerves are stimulated. The structure of the nervous system is described in greater detail in Chapter 24.

Endocrine Glands. The other means by which intercommunication between organs is established is through the agency of the chemical messengers, the **hormones.** These are produced by the **endocrine** or ductless glands. Ordinary glands such as the salivary glands and pancreas pour out their secretions into the mouth or intestine through ducts. The endocrine glands have no ducts, and so discharge their secretions directly into the blood vessels with which they are in contact. These glands are among the most important structures in the body, for they control metabolism and regulate personality. In addition, they influence growth and reproduction. The effect that the ductless glands exert on the mind is equally striking, and the difference between endocrine health and disease may mean the difference between the finest mental power and imbecility. The principal endocrine glands are the pituitary at the base of the brain, the thyroid and parathyroids in the neck, the adrenals, the islets of Langerhans in the pancreas, and the gonads.

It would be absurd to attempt even to outline the complex functions of the endocrine organs in this place, but it may be noted that not only do they regulate the behavior of many of the tissues (e.g., the parathyroids determine the amount of calcium salts in the bones), but they also influence one another so as to act in harmony. They are like the instruments of a string quartet noted for its perfect ensemble, and the leader of the glandular orchestra is the pituitary, the master gland of the body. The pituitary produces hormones that influence the activity of the thyroid, the adrenals, and the ovaries, as well as other organs and glands.

The endocrines are stimulated to activity not only by hormones from other endocrine glands, but also by nervous stimuli. One simple example of this remarkable interrelationship must suffice. When a person is intensely activated by great rage or great fear, he is impelled to immediate muscular activity for purposes of either attack or flight. The muscles are called on to contract to the utmost of their ability, and therefore require a maximum supply of carbohydrate fuel in the shape of glucose. This is lying stored in the liver in the form of glycogen. A nervous stimulus passes from the brain along the nerves to the adrenal glands and causes them to pour out their hormone, adrenalin (epinephrine). This is carried by the blood to the liver, where it causes the conversion of inert glycogen into active glucose. The glucose is carried by the blood to the muscles, supplying them with the fuel necessary for intense and immediate activity.

Reproduction

The most complex of the mechanisms of the body is reproduction, but it is essentially simple in its elements. In the lowest forms of life, as in such a unicellular organism as the ameba, reproduction is asexual. A line of division is formed along the middle of the cell, and the cellular constituents, first the nucleus and then the cytoplasm, divide into two, one set passing to one half of the cell, the other set to the other half. Finally, the line of division becomes complete and two new individuals are formed. This is called reproduction by fission. As both cells go on living, indeed need never die, they seem to enjoy the fountain of youth and can be regarded as immortal.

In all the higher forms of life, reproduction is sexual in type and is brought about by the union of two cells especially set aside for the purpose. They are known as the male and female **gametes** or germ cells, as distinguished from the body or **somatic cells.** The sex cells are produced by the male and female sex glands or gonads, the **testicle** with its tubules lined by germinal epithelium in the male, the **ovary** in the female. The male sex cells are the **spermatozoa** or sperm, the female sex cells are the **ova.** The sperm is a highly specialized cell with an oval flattened head and a long tail-like process, which, by violent lashing movements, propels the cell with great speed. In the human female, an ovum is liberated every month from the ovary and passes along a duct, the **fallopian tube,** to reach the **uterus** or womb, from which it is soon discharged in a flow of blood known as menstruation (Latin *mensis*, month). If impregnation is to occur, the male elements, the spermatozoa, ejected by the **penis** into the **vagina,** must pass through the uterus and enter the fallopian tube. (We are apt to think that fertilization of the ovum depends on sexual intercourse, but this is not necessarily so. For instance, the female salmon lays her eggs in a quiet pool, after which the male salmon comes along and fertilizes the eggs with his sperm.) It is breath taking to learn that as many as 300,000,000 spermatozoa start the race for parenthood in mammals, but only a few hundred thousand get as far as the mouth of the cervix, probably because of dilution in the vagina and its acidic environment. A further obstacle awaits them, for many of the survivors enter the wrong tube, as only one tube contains the ovum. When the leading spermatozoon in the race encounters the ovum in the tube, its head, carrying the paternal chromosomes and genes, penetrates the tough envelope of the ovum by means of an enzyme, hyaluronidase, its lashing tail is left behind because it is no longer needed, and impregnation has occurred. The sperm's remarkable journey has taken about 12 hours. A change at once occurs in the ovum's envelope, which renders it impermeable to any subsequent sperm that might wish to enter. When the male nucleus merges with that of the female, **fertilization** has taken place, and the result is **conception** and the creation of a new life. It is hard to believe but the fertilized ovum, which is to produce all the mysteries of the human body in the course of a few months, is only the size of a grain of sand. The fertilized ovum continues on its way down the tube and enters the uterus. This time, however, it is not discharged, so that menstruation does not occur for the duration of the pregnancy. In the uterus it develops into an embryo, the original single fertilized cell at once beginning to divide and multiply, the resulting cells not separating from one another but becoming differentiated and arranged to form the infinitely varied tissues and organs, until in the fullness of time, 9 months in the case of the human being, a child is born.

There is one fundamental fallacy in the above account that the discerning reader will not fail to detect. We have seen previously that when a somatic cell divides, the chromosomes split longitudinally, one-half passing to each of the new cells, which therefore possess the correct number. How is it that the fertilized ovum, which is a combination of two cells, male and female, does not come to have twice the number of chromosomes that it ought to? The reason is that the germ cells, while still in their respective gonads, have undergone a process of **maturation** in anticipation of the impending fertilization. This is effected by a reduction division or meiosis. In the mitosis of somatic cells, each chromosome splits longitudinally and each pair separates into 2, so that each daughter cell contains the original number of 46. Since these consist of 23 pairs, somatic cells are said to have a **diploid** (Greek *diplos*, double) number of chromosomes. In the maturing germ cell there is no splitting of chromosomes, so that when division occurs each daughter cell contains only 23 chromosomes, which are said to be **haploid** (Greek, *haplos*, single) in number. **The new germ cells, both male and female, contain only half the number of chromosomes and genes.** Fusion of the two gametes after fertilization results in a restoration of the chromosomes to their original number, but now one-half are maternal and one-half paternal in origin.

Determination of Sex

The wish is sometimes expressed that something could be done to determine or to influence the sex of the unborn baby. This is particularly true in the case of farm animals. It also used to be true in the days when a king needed a male heir. It is felt that modern science, which can work other wonders, should be able to perform this miracle. The truth is that the sex of the newly created embryo has been determined at the moment of conception, and that nothing more can be done about it. To understand this we must take a second look at the chromosomes. These are divided into 44 **autosomes,** which are the ordinary chromosomes, and 2 **sex chromosomes,** which determine the future sex. In the immature female sex cell both sex chromosomes, known as

X chromosomes, are alike and equal in size so that when the cell matures and undergoes reduction division, each daughter cell has one X chromosome, which can be regarded as the hallmark of femaleness. In the immature male sex cell, on the other hand, one of the sex chromosomes is similar to the X chromosome of the female, but the other, known as the **Y chromosome,** is much smaller, and may be regarded as indicating maleness. It is evident that after reduction division of the male gamete, half of the sperm cells will receive an X chromosome and the other half a Y chromosome. If, now, the ovum containing one X chromosome should be fertilized by a sperm containing an X chromosome, a female (XX) will be produced, but if the sperm contains a Y chromosome, the result will be an XY individual, in other words, a male. The result, as far as we know, is pure chance and incapable of control.

Sex Chromatin. Unfortunately, the matter is not always as simple as has just been suggested. When the gonads develop, the testicular or ovarian hormones that they produce profoundly influence what are called secondary sex characteristics, by which one is accustomed to distinguish a boy from a girl. Occasionally, owing to some defect in the genes, this development is not normal, and we are confronted with the tragic problem of **intersex,** when the child shares both male and female characteristics. In such cases a test for sex chromatin is of the greatest value. Thanks to the work of Murray Barr and his associates in 1949 at the University of Western Ontario, we now know that the cells of the body carry the fingerprints of their genetic sex, which

may not correspond with the apparent somatic sex of the person. Barr has shown that a small mass of chromatin, the **sex chromatin,** lies against the nuclear membrane in about 85% of the cells of normal females, but in less than 10% of the cells of normal males. This chromatin mass, now known as the Barr body, is easy to see if you know what you are looking for, but no one before Barr realized its significance. The female cells are said to be **chromatin-positive** and the male cells **chromatin-negative.** The most convenient source of cells is a smear made from the mucus membrane of the mouth. It would appear, as suggested by Mary Lyon, that in the somatic cells of the female one of the two chromosomes (one inherited from each parent) is genetically inactivated, becomes tightly coiled, and forms the sex chromatin or Barr body. There is at present no explanation for the occurrence of sex chromatin in a small proportion of male cells, unless it is related to the XY sex chromosome complex. With regard to the relation of sex to disease, nearly all the serious organic ailments are more common in the male, with the notable exception of disease of the gallbladder and to a lesser degree, mitral stenosis. There appears to be an inherent weakness in the male, a sex-linked inferiority, so that by comparison with the female he is a weakling at all periods of life from conception to death. In the investigation of sterility, if the sex chromatin test reveals a discrepancy between apparent sex and chromosomal sex, the chances of fertility are practically nil. The question of sex reversal and other sex anomalies is discussed in Chapter 12, Inherited Disease.

2

HISTORICAL OUTLINE

The philosophies of one age have become the absurdities of the next.—Sir William Osler

According to ancient myth there was once a Golden Age when man lived completely free of illness, which lasted until the curious Pandora opened the box of evils and allowed disease to escape.

Whether it was the Golden Age or the Garden of Eden, there is no chance to return; disease always has been a part of all forms of life and always will be. Fossils show us that infections, arthritis, cancer, dental caries, and many other diseases have plagued men and dinosaurs since earliest time.

How man deals with disease has changed over the years, and theories about the nature of disease are as old as mankind. Theories have always been a part of a much larger system of explanations regarding the nature of life, man's purpose on earth, and his position in the universe. In this chapter we will concern ourselves with two views of the world: the natural and supernatural. A supernatural view of the world holds that the earth and everything in it is governed by gods, or other supernatural forces. These are the source of all fortunes and misfortunes, including disease. A natural view contends that what we see around us is the sum total of reality: there are no gods in control. According to the ancient Greeks, ill health was brought on by an imbalance of body fluids; now we think of viruses, chemicals and genetic defects as causes of disease. Throughout much of recorded history, man has believed that both supernatural and natural forces play a role in causing disease, although one usually dominated the other. When religion was predominant, medicine was practiced by priests or monks. Today, practitioners have a scientific rather than religious knowledge base. But in spite of a revolution in knowledge, the fundamental act of healing in which the healer listens, examines, interprets the signs and symptoms, prescribes a treatment and assigns a prognosis has remained unchanged. From the beginning the success of this healing act has depended considerably upon the patient's trust in his healer and on their sharing ideas about what makes people sick and what heals them.

The first medical practitioners may have been much like medicine men of primitive societies today. Since disease was brought by spirits, the medicine man's function was to drive the spirits away. This was accomplished using spells, incantations, and amulets to ward off the evil eye. Trephining, which consisted of opening the skull with a sharp tool to let out the evil spirit, was also used. (Skulls from archaeologic sites show growth of bone around the edges of the wound indicating that the operation was sometimes followed by survival!)

Plants and herbs were used extensively, both for their magical powers and for their clinical effects. Physiotherapy and psychosocial measures also played important roles in healing.

As civilization advanced, religion acquired a hierarchy of practitioners, and medicine became a subspecialty of religion, with its own priests, temples and gods, but with a growing body of knowledge based on experience, which was to form the basis of a natural rather than supernatural medicine. The ancient Egyptians, whose civilization thrived for some 5 millennia, became very astute observers of disease. They recorded a number of case histories on papyrus, outlining symptoms in great detail, methods of examination, diagnostic signs to look for, indications for treatment, and prognosis. Prognosis was extremely important for social reasons: the physician had to protect himself against the Egyptian equivalent of a malpractice suit if he attempted to cure a patient who then died.

The Egyptians are best remembered for their emphasis on life after death, and their embalming of bodies to preserve them until the time when the soul returned to its earthly owner. Modern study of mummies shows that the Egyptians suffered from many diseases familiar to us: poliomyelitis, tuberculosis, arteriosclerosis, pneumonia, kidney stones, and appendicitis.

In spite of their extensive experience in opening the body to embalm it, the Egyptians acquired little knowledge of anatomy. As we will see at other times in history, dissection of the body is not sufficient to provide knowledge of its structure and function. Theory must come first, and it is then used to interpret what is seen. If sickness and death are thought to result from the action of gods there is no need to search the body for "natural" causes of death. However, the Egyptians did have a theory of physiology; it was thought that all body fluids including blood, tears, sperm, urine, feces, and air came from the heart!

Other ancient civilizations were equally advanced although in different directions. The Incas of Peru placed considerable emphasis on public health; they built bathing houses, sewage systems and conducted annual house cleaning ceremonies. (They were also plagued by such modern afflictions as alcoholism and drug addiction.) They became adept surgeons and used ant heads as clamps in suturing, a technique also used in ancient India.

ANCIENT GREECE

The ancient Greeks were the first to regard disease as essentially a natural rather than a supernatural process. As a result the magic and ritual of religious medicine was discarded in favor of observation, experimentation and natural therapies which stressed diet above all else. This giant step in Western thought was hardly taken overnight; it grew slowly out of the ever-changing social context of ancient Greece, over some 1,000 years.

Religious medicine predominated initially. The early Greeks worshipped a pantheon of gods many of whom, including Apollo, contributed to the cause and cure of illness. In the 5th century B.C., Apollo was replaced by Aesculapius whose staff and holy snake remain symbols of the medical profession to this day. A sick man who wished to be cured by Aesculapius had to first follow a series of rituals and then sleep in the Temple of Aesculapius at the foot of his statue. During the night the god was supposed to appear in the sick man's dreams and prescribe treatment.

Gradually the Greeks developed a more natural understanding of the world. This turning away from religion was facilitated by the extreme political division of ancient Greece. Fragmentation of political power prevented the development of a strong priestly bureaucracy, and in the absence of a powerful priesthood, criticism and critical thought prospered. (A similar process was later to aid the scientific renaissance in 16th century Europe; schism in the church, begun by the Protestant Reformation, reduced the power of the clergy over Protestant monarchs and cultures, creating a more permissive environment for the development of nonreligious views of the world.)

Greek philosophers saw the world around them as composed of 4 basic elements: air, earth, fire and water. Later the 4 elements were identified with 4 humors of the body: blood, phlegm, yellow bile and black bile (Table 2–1). This was translated into medical practice as follows: When the 4 elements were balanced man was healthy. Excess of one over the others tipped the balance and resulted in disease. Each of the elements and each humor had two essential qualities: heat and wetness. Thus a disease caused by an excess of black bile which was dry and cold would be treated by hot and wet remedies.

Hippocrates stands out as the shining light of Greek medicine (Fig. 2–1). He is thought to have lived from about 460–375 B.C. He led the most flourishing medical school of his time and spread his teachings throughout the ancient world. A collection of 50 to 70 books called the *Corpus Hippocraticum* have been attributed to him, although modern analysis makes it clear that they could only have been written by several different authors from different periods and schools. Most likely, Hippocrates' name was affixed to those works because he was regarded as the greatest physician of the entire era. Even the famous Hippocratic Oath is now known to have been written by the Pythagoreans.

The information contained in the *Corpus Hippocraticum* is remarkably modern. Great emphasis was placed on observation, including inspection, palpation and smell. Also important were clean hands and nails, and boiled water for operations.

The end of the creative period of Greek thought is marked by two great masters, Aristotle (384–322 A.D.) the philosopher and pioneer in biology, and Galen (130–201 A.D.) the physician. Between them these two dominated science and philosophy until the 17th century.

Claudius Galen of Pergamon was born in Asia Minor but rose to fame in Rome. He was a superb

Table 2–1.   The Four Humors

ELEMENT	CHARACTERISTIC	BODY FLUID	SOURCE
Fire	hot, dry	yellow bile	liver
Earth	dry, cold	black bile	spleen
Water	cold, wet	phlegm	brain
Air	hot, wet	blood	heart

Fig. 2–1 Hippocrates. "Life is short, and the Art long; the occasion
fleeting; experience fallacious, and judgment difficult. The physician
must not only be prepared to do what is right himself, but also to make
the patient, the attendants and the externals cooperate." Thus runs the
first aphorism of Hippocrates on whom history has bestowed the title
of "Father of Medicine." His countrymen believed he was descended
from Aesculapius, the God of Healing, and most of the stories we
possess concerning his life are legends and not historical facts. He was
born about 460 BC on the island of Cos and had as contemporaries
some of the greatest men of all time: Pericles the statesman; the poets
Aeschylus, Sophocles, Euripides, Aristophanes, and Pindar; the philosophers Socrates and Plato; the historians Herodotus, Xenophon, and
Thucydides; and that unrivalled sculptor Phidias. Hippocrates died in
Thessaly, circa 375 BC. (From Major, R.H.: *Classic Descriptions of
Disease*. Springfield, Ill., Charles C Thomas.)

anatomist, physiologist and experimenter. He cut
nerves and observed the resulting loss of function,
tied arteries and thereby demonstrated that they contained blood. But Galen's knowledge of anatomy was
learned entirely from dissections on animals, and unfortunately, he assumed that human design was no
different. Galen subscribed to the 4 humors theory
of disease, but he was much more invasive than his
predecessors, using multiple drugs, bleeding, and
rectal evacuation frequently in treatment.

After the fall of Graeco-Roman civilization, Galen's
theories acquired the status of absolute truth. Experimentation and science disappeared from Western Europe and what education there was became focused
on doctrines upheld by the ever more powerful Catholic Church. The medieval era was not one for ques-
tioning authority and this included the authority of
Galen.

THE MIDDLE AGES

The medieval era extends roughly from the fall of
the Roman empire to the Italian Renaissance of the
15th century. It was a time of intense preoccupation
with death, destruction and the shortness of life. The
social and political conditions that nurtured intellectual freedom ceased to exist, but over the first millennium, considerable progress was made in many less
academic areas, especially agriculture, transportation
and clothing.

The flame of Greek and Roman learning was kept
alight by the Arabs and was not discovered by Euro-
peans until the Crusades opened communications
with the East. In the meantime, the supernatural
world view returned to the forefront. With the rise
of Christianity, pagan gods were replaced by saints.
Christianity regarded disease as punishment for sins,
or the work of the devil, and considered prayer as the
only form of therapy. Nevertheless, care of the sick
was a Christian duty and monks and nuns became an
important source of medical care.

Medical practice for most of the population was a
mixture of superstition and folklore. Certain trees,
herbs and minerals were deemed to have curative
powers. The mistletoe played a prominent role in Ger-
manic and Celtic medicine; it protected against poisons and made women fertile. Most of the lay healers
of the times were women; care of the sick was regarded as a natural extension of motherhood.

The dawn of the second millennium brought an intellectual revival and the birth of the university. The
first famous medical school of the Middle Ages was
established at about this time at Salerno. This was a
lay school of medical practitioners and teachers, many
of whom were women. The most famous treatise from
Salerno is a long medical poem entitled *Regimen Sani-
tatis Salernitum* which placed great emphasis on diet
and methods of maintaining health. The physicians
at Salerno had discovered Galen, studied anatomy by
animal dissection, practiced surgery, uroscopy and
bloodletting. The return of Galenic theory brought
naturalism back to medicine and the humoral theory
of disease again became popular.

Disease was again thought to result from an excess
of one humor in the body. Diagnosis thus depended
upon detection of this excess in body fluids such as
blood or urine. Color, odor, density and foam were
all important. Bloodletting, the practice of cutting the
patient and allowing him to bleed, was supposed to
relieve the body of excess morbid material, and to
redirect the disease from one organ to another. The
timing of treatment was heavily dependent upon as-
trology.

Diseases of the Middle Ages are dominated by leprosy and bubonic plague. Leprosy was probably a cover-all term for a number of different skin diseases, one of which was leprosy as we know it today. This highly disfiguring disease causes blindness and sensory deficits which lead to ulceration and eventual amputation of fingers and toes. The Bible pronounced lepers "unclean" and so they became outcasts and outlaws, assigned to live in special "leprosaria" on the edge of town and forced to carry a bell to warn people of their presence. The disease established itself in Europe in the 6th century AD and was endemic until 1400; by 1600 it had practically disappeared. The reasons for its decline are not clear, but the black plague of 1348 effectively wiped out most leprosaria. Tuberculosis, then on the rise, may have been partly responsible; the tubercle bacillus and leprosy bacteria have many biological similarities, and exposure to one seems to produce immunity to both. Thus TB, which is considerably more contagious, may have outdone leprosy in the competition for hosts.

The Black Death, or bubonic plague, is primarily a disease of rats spread by fleas (see Chapter 7). It was carried to Europe by the armies of the Mongol Empire, the most devastating epidemic arriving in 1348 and decimating 1/4 to 1/3 of the European population. The disease has 3 forms, two of which progress from infection to death within hours. Like leprosy, plague gradually ceased to be a major threat over the following years. This may have been due to changes in the rat population or changes in housing construction that made it harder for rats to live in close association with humans.

At the time of the Black Death naturalism was not only evident in the humoral theory of disease physiology but also in ideas about the cause and transmission of disease. The supernatural remained prominent and no doubt plague was frequently seen as an expression of the anger of God. However, plague was thought to have an earthly origin that man might control: the source was presumed to be foul smells which spread through the air. The Greeks called this disease-bringing air *miasma* (which means pollution). The association of contagious disease with unpleasant scents was reinforced throughout the Middle Ages and led to a number of public health measures. The streets were cleaned and the keeping of pigs and emptying of cesspools were forbidden. Fires were lit in the streets to cleanse the air.

Toward the end of the medieval era Galen's authority began to waiver. As early as the 13th century a physician to the French King made the bold statement that God did not exhaust his creative power in making Galen; but such criticism was rare. In the 14th century the study of anatomy showed signs of becoming more observational. Human dissection was increasingly practiced, but doctors supervised dissection while reading from Galen and saw only what Galen had described. With the experience of such calamities as the Black Death, medieval man was beset by the brutality and brevity of life and convinced that the Greeks had discovered all there was to know.

THE 16TH CENTURY: SCIENTIFIC REVIVAL

Although Galen continued to be challenged sporadically, the intellectual and social climate of the time was unable to tolerate change. A number of events were important in creating a more tolerant milieu. First and foremost, the Reformation of the early 1500s, a rebellion against the Catholic popes which established Protestantism, divided the church into national groups which seriously weakened its power. This breaking of the old hard and fast rules and disruption of authority encouraged more freedom of thought.

Secondly, the Renaissance sanctioned curiosity which led to discoveries that could not be accounted for by the Greek works. Columbus discovered America and with it a new people and new diseases. Syphilis, apparently a gift from the New World to the Old, swept across Europe like a plague in the early 16th century, yet nowhere in Greek and Roman texts was this or other American phenomena described. People began to think that modern knowledge had surpassed that of the ancients and wondered what else there was in the world that the Greeks had missed. The stage was set for innovation.

It was **Vesalius** (1514–1556), a young Belgian, who officially noticed that the organs of the human body did not always correspond to Galen's descriptions. According to Galen the human body contained a five-lobed liver, a double bile duct, and horned uterus. Vesalius saw differently and chose to believe his own eyes rather than the revered authority. He published his version of anatomy in *On the Fabric of the Human Body*. This work met initially with fierce opposition. His own teacher denounced him as a madman and in order to save his beloved tradition for posterity, dreamed up the ingenious theory that the human body had changed since Galen's time.

An alternative to the Greek theory of infection was advanced in 1546 by **Girolamo Fracastoro,** the most scientific student of epidemic disease of his time. He distinguished three types of disease transmission: spread by contact, spread by clothing or other articles, and distant spread without any form of contact (as in plague) (Fig. 2–2). He hypothesized that distant spread was accomplished by passage of minute bod-

Fig. 2–2 Bizarre protective clothing worn by Roman doctors during the 1656 outbreak of plague. With the wand they indicated their orders and avoided actual contact with the patient. The "bird bill" held filtering cloths. The stick was also used to feel the patient's pulse. (From Hastings, P.: *Medicine: An International History.* London, Ernest Benn, 1974.)

ies capable of self-replication. This became the germ theory of disease.

In the 15th and 16th centuries, the medical profession was evolving along three lines, into the apothecary, the surgeon and the physician. There were no professional general practitioners. The apothecary, originally a grocer who specialized in herbs and spices, was in charge of the "drug store." He stored and mixed drugs and applied them. He essentially carried out the treatment prescribed by the doctor. Gradually his work came to involve more and more medical practice, especially amongst the poor.

Surgery had its beginnings in the barbershop of the Middle Ages. The barber-surgeons were becoming doctors of external medicine, treating such external or visible disorders as wounds, fractures, ulcers, skin disease, and tumors. Perhaps the most famous barber-surgeon was **Ambroise Paré** (1510–1590) who, like Vesalius, forsook tradition in favor of his own observation and experience. He revolutionized the treatment of wounds.

Physicians had become highly learned so that few but the rich and powerful could afford their services. In England they were particularly scarce and general medical care of the population was left to the barber-surgeons and apothecaries. As is the case today, these "specialists" in medicine tended to collect in urban centers. The health care needs of the rural population were met by local wise women who relied largely on psychology, diet, herbs, minerals and magic.

The major threats to health in this period were dysentery, typhoid, measles and small pox. These are diseases whose transmission is considerably facilitated by close contact in unsanitary places. As the population was gradually migrating from village to town, more people were exposed to these conditions.

Sanitary practices, or the lack of them, provided fertile breeding grounds for bacteria. The sewage system of English towns consisted of open gutters running down the center of each street. Those rich enough to own cesspools pumped the contents into the street when the cesspool was full. Others simply threw all refuse into the street. The stench, which one may well imagine, was still thought to be a cause of disease.

Diet did not improve with urban migration. There were few methods of storing meat or fish and no way to keep milk without churning it into butter. Most diets were vitamin deficient, especially in the winter time. The general overall ill health of the population is reflected in the mortality rate of infants and young children. Of 1,000 newborn infants 200–500 died within a year and many of those remaining did not live to see the age of 10. One famous 16th century physician maintained that he could cure anyone provided that the patient was not younger than 7 or older than 70.

THE 17TH CENTURY: SCIENTIFIC REVOLUTION

Between 1600 and 1700 a fundamental change occurred in Western thought. The scientific boon of the 17th century led the educated European from the medieval world in which man was the center and the purpose of the universe, to the modern world which puts man on a small insignificant planet somewhere in the vast cosmos. Religion was gradually replaced by belief in science and reason. In the process man became a machine; his body, which was made of matter, became divorced from his soul. This dichotomy favored development of physiologic principles based on mechanics.

William Harvey (1578–1657) (Fig. 2–3) introduced this scientific approach and mechanistic philosophy to the study of the human body. Using mathematical, experimental and anatomic evidence he hypothesized that blood moved in a circle with the heart acting as a pump to keep the circulation in motion. Public acceptance of this concept was hampered by a missing link, namely, how the blood traveled from arteries to veins. The question was shortly solved by **Marcello Malpighi**, who used the newly discovered microscope to examine various tissues and saw tiny capillar-

Fig. 2–3 The English physician William Harvey demonstrates to King Charles I and the young Prince his theory on the circulation of the blood. (From Hastings, P.: *Medicine: An International History.* London, Ernest Benn, 1974.)

ies joining the smallest arteries to the smallest veins. Actual medical care changed little. William Harvey was known to prescribe mixtures of senna, rhubarb, agaric and other herbs, to be taken on each full moon. The use of tobacco had become a favorite habit and was thought to ward off plague. When the bubonic plague raged through London in 1665, smoking became a required activity even in some schools. One graduate of Eton College later recalled that "he was never whipped so much in his life as he was one morning for not smoking."

THE 18TH CENTURY

In Europe at this time, there was little of the stirring of spirit and uprush of new ideas that had characterized the 17th century. This was a period of consolidation, an age of criticism rather than of discovery in medicine, of philosophers and philosophizing, culminating in the French Revolution. But it witnessed the birth of pathology in the limited sense of morbid anatomy. **Giovanni Battista Morgagni** of Padua, at the age of 79 in 1761, published a book entitled *The Seats and Causes of Disease*, which at once rendered obsolete all others dealing with the diseased body. Before Morgagni, disease was considered as a general thing. Doctors speculated as to the nature of the process, built up a hypothesis no matter how fantastic, and gave it a name. Strangely enough, they did not inquire as to the seat of the disease. It was Morgagni who was the first to correlate the symptoms of the patient during life with the changes in the organs found at autopsy. He showed that it was not true that dead men tell no tales. Dead men have for centuries been telling doctors the story of how they got sick and why they died. For the first time we could think of liver disease, kidney disease, and heart disease, and have a mental picture of the clinical condition in relation to the lesions in the organs responsible for that condition. Morgagni made few real discoveries, nor did he revolutionize pathology as did Virchow in the next century; his great service to pathology was his emphasis on detail and thoroughness.

The direction taken by medical thought at this time was away from a holistic (or single-cause) explanation of disease and toward an explanation of disease that related the pain in the chest and subsequent death to a particular organ or group of cells, such as the heart, which might show a large pale soft area (infarct). This ascription of particular symptoms and signs to anatomic changes in particular organs has formed the cornerstone of rational medicine for the past 200 years. It is only recently being questioned, as newer under-standings of the interdependence of special systems (cardiovascular, respiratory, nervous) push the pendulum of thought back toward a more holistic or humoral way of looking at disease.

One of the most important discoveries of the 18th century, which had a rapid effect on the health of the population, was **Edward Jenner's** invention of small-pox vaccination. Inoculation of smallpox, whereby a small amount of pus from a smallpox pustule was introduced into a slight wound in the skin, was a widespread folk practice in some countries. The usual result was a mild case of smallpox with lasting immunity, although occasionally the inoculum did produce raging smallpox and death. Inoculation became widely used in England and the North American colonies in the early 18th century. Vaccination, however, involving the inoculum from cowpox (*vacca*, Latin for cow) avoided the occasional lethal complications of inoculation. Vaccination has eradicated smallpox (Fig. 2–4), which was the most prevalent, fatal and disfiguring disease of the 18th century in Britain. Some idea of the ravages of the disease may be gained from the old saying "mothers counted their children only after they had had the smallpox."

Typhus and diarrheal diseases were common in the 1700s; and the death rate from tuberculosis was rising. These diseases are largely the result of overcrowded cities. Industrialization was beginning and migration to the new factory towns was more common than ever. Life in the towns was far from healthy. Cold weather, bad harvests, food scarcity, and heavy drinking exacted a great toll. When mothers went to work, opiates were given to infants to quiet them.

Although conditions in the early industrial towns of England were appalling, most of the population lived in rural areas and fared considerably better. The 18th century witnessed the start of the population explosion which has continued to the present day. The cause was due to a fall in the death rate, particularly the infant mortality rate. In 1782 in Philadelphia (which had not yet witnessed the impact of the Industrial Revolution), 50% of all deaths occurred in children under the age of 10. By 1807 this statistic had fallen to 39%. (Those who survived the first 10 years lived on average to the age of 55.) The same phenomenon occurred in Europe and China. The causes of this expansion are many and complex. One theory is that infectious diseases were becoming less virulent due to biological evolution (a parasite that allows its host to live will survive better in the long run than one which kills the host). Another hypothesis concerns biologic evolution in the human immune system—it is conceivable that the high rate of infection killed off those individuals of each generation with poorer con-

Fig. 2–4 Edward Jenner vaccinating his own son against smallpox. His discovery was the greatest development in preventive medicine of the eighteenth century. (From Hastings, P.: *Medicine: An International History*. London, Ernest Benn, 1974.)

stitutions leaving behind those genetically better equipped to fight infection.

McKeown has proposed that improvements in agriculture led to better nutrition, healthier mothers and healthier babies. Agricultural productivity was considerably enhanced by improved farm machinery, fertilizers, and better storage methods. Increased amounts of feed for cattle improved the supply of protein. No doubt many other factors were also involved.

THE 19TH CENTURY

The 19th century saw a transformation in man's relationship to infection (Fig. 2–5). By 1900, some of the major means of controlling contagion had been put to use: vaccination, sewage systems, clean water supplies.

Tuberculosis was the most widespread and lethal disease of the century (Fig. 2–6). Also known as phthisis (from the Greek, meaning to waste away), consumption, or galloping consumption when it was particularly rapid, this disease was feared in the 19th century in much the same way that cancer is feared today. It was a disease of overcrowded cities, poor nutrition and squalor. Long rows of houses had been erected in the towns, without toilets, water systems or adequate ventilation; all manner of refuse and filth was thrown into the street.

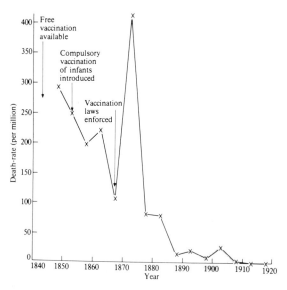

Fig. 2–5 The trend in mortality from smallpox since cause of death was first registered: England and Wales. In 1796 one-fifth of all deaths in London were ascribed to smallpox. Vaccination was first used in 1798. Today smallpox has not been seen for six years. (From McKeown, T.: *The Role of Medicine: Dream, Mirage or Nemesis?* Princeton, N.J., Princeton University Press, 1979.)

Fig. 2–6 Respiratory tuberculosis: mean annual death rates (standardized to 1901 population): England and Wales. Mortality from tuberculosis was already falling at the time when it was first recorded. A large part of the decline occurred before the introduction of effective treatment. However, when streptomycin was introduced, the mortality from tuberculosis fell sharply, a fact which is partly concealed here by the scale of the graph. (From McKeown, T.: *The Role of Medicine: Dream, Mirage or Nemesis?* Princeton, N.J., Princeton University Press, 1979.)

The working classes were seriously undernourished. They were thin, pale and short, with bowed legs and crooked spines. Their dietary staples were tea (which was warm) and bread (which didn't have to be cooked). Most houses were ill equipped for cooking and many wives worked long hours leaving little time or energy for preparing meals. Working mothers also created a problem for child care, which was sometimes solved by opiates or even infanticide. Children who survived the pneumonia, diarrhea and scarlet fever in addition to their awful living conditions joined their parents in the work force not long after they learned to walk.

Cholera made its appearance in Europe for the first time in the 19th century. It had been limited to Bengal for centuries but expansion of the British Empire in India provided new routes of spread and new susceptible hosts. Trading ships and military maneuvers carried the disease around the globe and it thrived in the unsanitary industrial cities.

In 1854, John Snow observed that most cholera deaths in the Soho district of London occurred in people drinking water from a single pump (Fig. 2–7). On examination, the well below the pump was found to be contaminated by a leaking cesspool. This discovery added impetus to the reform movement which had begun a few years before, initiated by the increasingly evident association between filthy living conditions and disease.

There were two contemporary theories of infection, the miasma and the germ theories, both of which were centuries old as we have seen. Miasmas were thought to be emanations from swamps, cesspools, and garbage dumps. The smell of filth and decay was the supposed cause of illness; septic poisons generated in putrefaction entered the body via the lungs, through wounds or with food. The obvious solution to the problem was to eliminate filth. Thus it was the miasma theory which drove reformers to build sewers, water mains and improve conditions in cities, prisons and hospitals. Florence Nightingale was a firm believer in the miasma theory. She completely revolutionized nursing and reduced the mortality rate in her hospitals from over 40 to 2%.

The germ theory was originally proposed in 1546 and was used to justify quarantine regulations against plague but had never become popular. Bacteria were discovered in the 17th century but it was not known that they caused disease. In the early 19th century, the two theories were put to the test: an outbreak of yellow fever occurred in Barcelona in 1822 and its spread was carefully studied. Germs were thought to require interpersonal contact for transmission, but there was clearly no contact between the various patients with yellow fever; and so the germ theory lost favor. (We now know that the disease is caused by a virus and transmitted by a mosquito.)

The relationship between bacteria and disease was established largely through the efforts of three men: Pasteur, Lister and Koch.

Louis Pasteur, a Frenchman, was a chemist, not a physician, but he became interested in the problem of why wine spoils, and he came to the conclusion that the fermentation of wine and beer was due to the action of living bacterial agents. From this he was led to the study of putrefaction, i.e., the decomposition of meat and other dead organic material. This was again found to be due to the same living agents, and the process could be prevented by heating organic fluids, such as milk, to a temperature below the boiling point, the procedure now known as **pasteurization.** At this time, the English surgeon, **Joseph Lister,** was pondering the problem of wound infection following surgical operations, which rendered the most brilliant operation worse than useless, and gave origin to the popular gibe "the operation was successful but the patient died," when he came across Pasteur's work. At this time the mortality rate from operations, now frequently performed owing to the use of anesthetics (Fig. 2–8), was appalling. At least 45% of amputations resulted in death from septicemia, infection, and gangrene. Lister had previously realized that putrefaction of dead organic material and infection of wounds were intimately related, and now he saw in one lightning flash that if putrefaction was bacterial in origin, so also was wound infection. Destruction of bacteria in infected wounds (antisepsis), and

Fig. 2–7   Deaths from cholera in the Soho district of London, September 1854. Using this map Snow demonstrated that most of the deaths in this outbreak of cholera occurred among those who consumed water from a pump in Broad Street. He insisted that an engineer examine the well below the pump and established that the water had become contaminated by seepage from a leaking cesspool. Additional evidence was provided by the case of a woman who lived at a distance but had her water brought from the Broad Street pump (because she liked the taste) and contracted cholera. (From Howe, G.M.: *Man, Environment and Disease in Britain*. New York, Harper and Row, 1972.)

later exclusion of bacteria from the field of operation (asepsis), wrought a revolution in surgery so far-reaching, so overwhelming, that surgery as we know it today is essentially the gift of Lister to humanity. His work alone made possible the surgery of the abdomen, chest, brain, and joints, as well as rendering a hundredfold safer operations on the limbs and the practice of obstetrics.

Robert Koch (Fig. 2–9), at first a German country practitioner, must share with Pasteur the title of the founder of modern bacteriology, for he introduced the methods of bacteriologic investigation, such as the use of pure cultures and special stains and reproduction of the disease by animal inoculation, which are employed at the present day. In addition he demonstrated the bacterial cause of many infections such as anthrax, cholera, and above all tuberculosis. In this decade a large number of infectious diseases (as opposed to wound infections) were shown to be due to

specific bacteria. Pasteur also introduced the idea of ultramicroscopic filterable viruses, agents of disease so small that they could not be seen with the microscope and were able to pass through the finest filter, although ordinary bacteria were held back by such a filter. It should be added that at the present day the electron microscope, with its enormously increased power of magnification, has brought even the smallest viruses into view, so that they no longer deserve the term ultramicroscopic.

The 19th century also witnessed considerable advances in the development of pathology. The focus of the study of disease had shifted from the body as a whole to the organs and tissues, and now was centered on the cell. **Rudolf Virchow** (Fig. 2–10) is the father of this modern pathology; he showed for the first time that the structural changes of disease may be found in the cells of a sick organ. (In the next century the focus of pathology was reduced further to

Fig. 2–8   The invention of etherization, a technique labeled in its own time as "The Death of Pain", was an understandably heralded event in the medical world, and the credit for its discovery was claimed by a number of physicians, a Dr. Marcy, Dr. Charles T. Jackson, and Dr. Horace Wells. In actuality, Dr. Crawford W. Long of Jefferson, Georgia, used ether in several minor operations in 1842, and Wells, a dentist in Hartford, Vermont, began using nitrous oxide in 1844. But the first convincing public demonstration of anesthesia took place October 16, 1846, when Dr. John C. Warren, Chief of Surgical Service at Massachusetts General Hospital, performed an operation with ether administered by Dr. W.T.G. Morton on Gilbert Abbott, a house painter suffering from a tumor of the jaw. (From Gerdts, W.H.: *The Art of Healing, Medicine and Science in American Art.* Birmingham Museum of Art, 1981. Reproduced by permission of Francis A. Countway Library of Medicine, Harvard University, Boston, Massachusetts.)

molecules!) Such scientific advances began to erode the time-worn ways of thinking about disease. Until the mid-19th century, diseases were classified into categories like "fevers" and "diarrhea." Diarrhea was one disease which might evolve into worse things like cholera if the balance of fluids in the body were not corrected. Gradually people began to think of diarrhea not as a single disease entity but as a symptom of many different diseases, each with its own course and treatment. This conceptual change contributed to a widespread scepticism in regard to the physician's ability to treat disease. In the mid-19th century the mainstays of therapy were still aggressive and unpleasant: bleeding, purging with enemas, and emetics to induce vomiting. By the end of the century, physicians had largely abandoned these methods in favor of diet and less drastic measures.

THE 20TH CENTURY

The history of medicine in the 20th century is dominated by revolutions in diagnostic techniques and therapeutics and by a rapid expansion in scientific knowledge. For centuries, healers had only their five senses to help them make a diagnosis. These they exploited fully: they listened to the heart, inspected the skin, palpated the pulse, smelled, and even tasted the urine. X-rays and biochemistry have changed all this by giving us new ways of investigating the structure and function of the body. We need not open the abdomen to search for a tumor, we can use ultrasound, CT scanning and fiberoptic scopes to assess what the naked eye cannot see and even what the hand may not feel. We examine the blood biochemically, looking for abnormal glucose in the diabetic pa-

PROFESSEUR KOCH

Fig. 2–9 Robert Koch, a physician and pioneer bacteriologist, was born in Hanover on December 11, 1843. He received the Nobel Prize for physiology and medicine in 1905. He introduced the method of making bacterial smears and fixing them with heat, was the first to isolate and obtain pure culture of anthrax bacillus, identified comma bacillus as the cause of Asiatic cholera, and discovered the organism responsible for Egyptian ophthalmia. He produced tuberculin and erroneously thought it to be the cure for TB, and later showed it to be of value in diagnosing the disease. He studied the rinderpest in South Africa and developed a means of vaccinating against it. He investigated the bubonic plague in India and malaria and sleeping sickness in Africa and discovered the methods of transmission. He elaborated general methods of bacteriologic research and developed a method of disinfection. He also developed a means of cultivating bacteria in liquid and solid media and laid the foundation for a rational system of bacterial culturing. He established rules for properly identifying causative agents of various diseases. Robert Koch died in Baden-Baden on March 27, 1910. (From *World Who's Who in Science, From Antiquity to Present.* Marquis Who's Who, Chicago.)

Fig. 2–10 Rudolf Virchow was born in Pomerania in 1821 and attended the gymnasium at Koslin. In 1839 he began the study of medicine at the Kaiser Wilhelm Akademie and received his degree at the University of Berlin in 1843. He became at once an assistant at the Charité Hospital and two years later became Prosector of Anatomy and Assistant in Froriep's clinic. In 1847 he became Privatdozent in Pathology and entered upon the great work of his life. From this period onward, Virchow seems to have been interested in only two things—the study of pathology and the study of economic and social problems. In 1848 Virchow was sent to investigate an epidemic of typhus in Silesia. His report contained not only a severe criticism of the hygienic regulations in that province, but also a harsh indictment of the prevalent social injustices. Virchow's report and his continued agitation for reforms caused trouble with the Prussian government, and he was dismissed from his position at Berlin. His fame as a pathologist, however, was already established, and he was immediately called to Wurzburg as Professor of Pathology and director of their newly founded pathologic institute. Virchow remained at Wurzburg seven years and while there completed the work that formed the basis of his cellular theory. In 1858 he returned to Berlin. His life there was one of unparalleled activity. He collected an amazing museum of pathology, was very active in teaching and research, and found time to enter political life, serving in the Reichstag for thirteen years. Here he was the leader of the Radical party and an active, outspoken, and persistent opponent of Bismarck. Students flocked from all over the world to attend his lectures and every year brought new honors and fresh testimonials of esteem. On his seventieth birthday he was presented with a gold medal by the Emperor, and his eightieth birthday took on the character of a national holiday, with delegates from all over the world assembling in Berlin to do him honor. Virchow died the following year, 1902. (From Major, R.H.: *Classic Descriptions of Disease.* Springfield, Ill., Charles C Thomas, 1948.)

tient, or enzymes released in a variety of pathologic states, from infarction to hepatitis. But no machine has yet replaced the physician's experience, and we must not forget that. Even today most diagnoses can be made with the five senses and a little reasoning.

The study of disease has shifted from structure to function, pathophysiology and biochemistry, and has led to the development of entirely new specialties.

Medical genetics really originated with the studies of **Gregor Mendel** in 1886 on the inheritance of color in sweet peas and the transmission of characteristics

from one generation to another. The ability to separate and study the chromosomes carrying their cargo of genes composed of DNA is recent, and has thrown a flood of light on such mysteries as sex anomalies and sex reversal as well as on the complex problems of inherited disease. Currently, bacteria can be cloned and genetically "reprogrammed" to produce insulin, interferon and a variety of other products. The list of possibilities is extremely provocative.

Immunology, the science of how our body recognizes itself, and how it produces soluble and cellular defenses, has developed rapidly in the last 35 years. This subject is covered in the chapter on immune mechanisms, and, of course, has directly affected the success of efforts to manage diseases by transplantation.

The discovery of **antibiotics** marked the start of the therapeutic revolution of the 20th century. Not since empirical discovery in the 17th century of the cinchona bark (which contains quinine) for malaria, had any gains been made in the treatment of infectious disease. In 1928, **Sir Alexander Fleming** observed by chance that the mold *Penicillium notatum* dissolved colonies of staphylococci. Penicillin, the active ingredient extracted from the mold, proved to be extremely difficult to produce in large amounts, and it was not until 1946 that it became available to civilians. In the meantime, sulfanilamide, a drug which evolved from the German dye industry, was discovered in 1932 to have antibiotic effects. Although not as effective as penicillin it was mass produced much earlier using methods already well known to industrial chemists.

How big was the impact of these drugs on the mortality from infectious disease? Anyone who has ever had to use them knows well their dramatic curative effects. But antibiotics have so far had a relatively small impact on population mortality statistics. By the time penicillin was available to the general public,

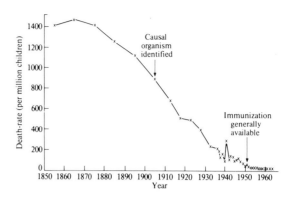

Fig. 2–12 Whooping cough: death rates of children under 15: England and Wales. Again we see the decline in mortality from a disease long before medical treatment or prophylaxis was available. (From McKeown, T.: *The Role of Medicine: Dream, Mirage or Nemesis?* Princeton, N.J., Princeton University Press, 1979.)

heart disease had replaced infection as the leading cause of death. The death rate from many infectious diseases had already fallen to low levels in the western world (Figs. 2–11 to 2–14).

Chemotherapy has become widely used in all other areas of medicine. Tranquilizers, developed in the 1950s, have replaced the straight jacket in mental illness. A combination of surgery and drugs can lengthen life in numerous cancers and even cure a few. Insulin has changed the life expectancy of the diabetic from a few years to a nearly normal life span. The pain of an arthritic hip joint may be relieved by replacing the joint with a metal prosthesis. In this way

Fig. 2–11 Diphtheria: death rates of children under 15: England and Wales. Antitoxin and immunization have obviously played a significant role in the decline in mortality from this disease. (From McKeown, T.: *The Role of Medicine: Dream, Mirage or Nemesis?* Princeton, N.J., Princeton University Press, 1979.)

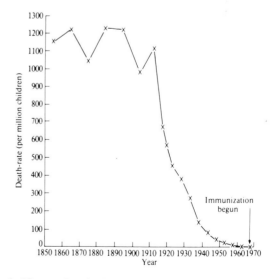

Fig. 2–13 Measles: death rates of children under 15: England and Wales. The death rate fell continuously from about 1915; treatment of secondary infections has been possible since 1935, and a vaccination has been available since 1968 (in England). (From McKeown, T.: *The Role of Medicine: Dream, Mirage or Nemesis?* Princeton, N.J., Princeton University Press, 1979.)

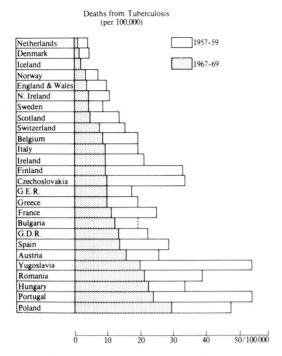

Deaths from Tuberculosis
(per 100,000)

Fig. 2–14 Tuberculosis: death rates per 100,000. The decline in mortality from tuberculosis is probably due to chemotherapy rather than BCG vaccination. The Netherlands has never had a national BCG program but they have the lowest death rates from respiratory tuberculosis as shown on the graph. (From McKeown, T.: *The Role of Medicine: Dream, Mirage or Nemesis?* Princeton, N.J., Princeton University Press, 1979.)

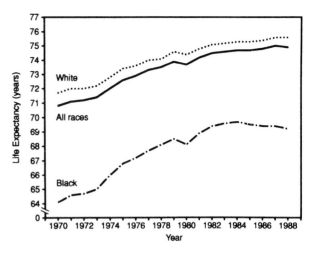

Fig. 2–15 Life expectancy in years, by year of birth and by race—United States, 1970 to 1988. (From Centers for Disease Control, Morbidity and Mortality Weekly Report, 40(29):501, 1991.)

medicine has had a significant effect on morbidity, which refers to diseases that are not lethal but may be disabling. All these gains are not without cost; iatrogenic disease (caused by doctors) remains part of our disease pattern. In addition, we have new moral questions and the financial burdens of the ultramodern hospital which are an increasing source of concern.

Over the years we have seen how our health is affected by many factors. Accidents of history have had

dramatic effects on the kinds of illnesses we suffer: the Mongols brought us plague, Columbus brought us syphilis, the British Empire spread cholera worldwide, and the conditions created by the Industrial Revolution promoted the spread of tuberculosis and typhoid. Today, disease is as much a product of lifestyle as ever. The leading causes of death in North American teenagers are accidents (usually automobile and/or alcohol related), homicide and suicide. Although cancer is our most feared killer, more years could be added to the average life expectancy by eliminating accidents than by curing cancer (Fig. 2–15, Table 2–2).

Tobacco smoking exacts an enormous cost in terms of death, disability and hospital use; it contributes to several cancers, heart disease and poor fetal health in mothers who smoke. As in the 19th century, poverty is an important source of ill health (Table 2–3). Of all

Table 2–2.   Death Rates (Age-adjusted; per 100,000 Population)

	1950	1960	1970	1980	1988*
TOTAL	841.5	760.9	714.3	585.8	535.5
Selected Causes					
Diseases of heart	307.6	286.2	253.6	202.0	166.3
Strokes	88.8	79.7	66.3	40.8	29.7
Cancer	125.4	125.8	129.9	132.8	132.7
Accidents	57.5	49.9	53.7	42.3	35.0
Homicide and legal intervention	5.4	5.2	9.1	10.8	9.0
Total for Selected Groups					
White males	963.1	917.7	893.4	745.3	664.3
White females	645.0	555.0	501.7	411.1	384.4
Black males	1,373.1	1,246.1	1,318.6	1,112.8	1,037.8
Black females	1,106.7	916.9	814.4	631.1	593.1

* Provisional data (From United States Department of Health and Human Services.)

Table 2–3. Health Indicators by Social Class, England and Wales, 1970–72

	EXPECTATION OF LIFE AT AGE 15 (MEN)	STILLBIRTHS AND INFANT DEATHS*	MORTALITY† FROM INFECTIVE AND PARASITIC DISEASES	MORTALITY† FROM CANCER
Professional occupations	57.2	20.3	61	75
Intermediate occupations (managerial)	57.0	23.6	63	80
Non-manual skilled occupations	56.0	25.8	88	91
Manual skilled occupations	55.7	29.3	86	113
Partly skilled occupations	55.1	32.4	126	116
Unskilled occupations	53.5	47.7	197	131

* Per 1,000 live and stillbirths
† Standardized mortality ratio for men aged 15–64

(From Registar General's Decennial Supplement for England and Wales, 1970–72. Occupational Mortality, Series DS no. 1 [HMSO, 1978].)

men with cancer, those in the lower classes die faster than those who are wealthy. The reasons are not entirely clear.

What effect does medicine have on this extremely complicated network of factors that produce ill health? For the individual, medicine may lengthen life, as by providing a kidney transplant or eliminating infection with antibiotics, or restoring productivity by repairing badly damaged fingers. These are the tremendous successes of modern science. But McKeown and others have pointed out that the health of the population as a whole began improving long before the modern era. It seems that on the population scale, health has always depended much more on nutrition, life style and social conditions, than on medical technology.

SYNOPSIS

The "magical" causes of disease were displaced by the beginnings of science in Greek times.

Renaissance medicine began with the study of anatomy and the understanding of the function of different organs.

The concept of disease as arising in a specific organ or system, rather than as a "humor," is based on the correlation of the patient's signs and symptoms with the findings at autopsy.

The fact that biologic agents cause disease was established only after the development of techniques for microscopy and culture of organisms.

Modern medicine begins in the twentieth century with the application of chemotherapy, radiation, genetic knowledge, biochemical technology, and modern surgical and invasive techniques to the study and management of the sick person.

Disease changes with time.

The understanding of disease depends both on the technologic development of the era and on the cultural and intellectual attitudes to the problem.

Disease results from the failure of an organism to adapt successfully to genetic variations, to invasion by biologic agents, to repair of trauma, or to complications of aging.

Disease is perceived as a change from the normal or "steady" state and is expressed by the organism's reaction pattern. Disease need not be physical or "organic."

Terms

William Harvey
Giovanni Battista Morgagni
Florence Nightingale
Rudolph Virchow

Robert Koch
Chemotherapy
Antibiotic
Dietetics

Immunology
Morbidity
Mortality

FURTHER READING

Altman, L.K.: *Who Goes First*. New York, Random House, 1987.

Bergman, N.A.: Humphrey Davy's contribution to the introduction of anaesthesia: a new perspective. Perspect. Biol. Med., 34:534, 1991.

Castiglioni, A.: *A History of Medicine*. New York, Knopf, 1947.

Fabrega, H.: Concepts of disease: logical features and social implications. Perspect. Biol. Med., 15:583, 1972.

Forrest, R.D.: Development of wound therapy from the Dark Ages to the present. J. Roy. Soc. Med., 75:268, 1982.

Major, R.H.: *Classic Descriptions of Disease*, 3rd Ed. Springfield, Charles C Thomas, 1948.

Matossian, M.K.: Fertility decline in Europe, 1875–1913—was zinc the cause? Perspect. Biol. Med., 34:604, 1991.

McNeill, W.H.: *Plagues and People*. Garden City, N.Y., Anchor Books, 1976.

Murphy, E.A.: A scientific viewpoint on normalcy. Perspect. Biol. Med.,9:333, 1965.

Osler, Sir William: *The Evolution of Modern Medicine*. New Haven, Yale University Press, 1921.

Rosenberg, C.E.: The therapeutic revolution: medicine, meaning and social change in 19th century America. Perspect. Biol. Med., 20:485, 1977. Science, Vol. 200, No. 4344, May 26, 1978. Sci. Am., Vol. 229, No. 3, September 1973.

Smith, C.E.: The Broad Street pump revisited. Intl. J. Epidemiol., 11:99, 1982.

Sontag, S.: *Illness as Metaphor*. New York, Farrar, Straus and Giroux, 1978.

3

CAUSES OF DISEASE

To talk of disease is a sort of Arabian Nights entertainment.—Sir William Osler

WHAT IS DISEASE?

Before beginning a discussion of the possible causes of disease, it may be well to ask, "What is disease?" This is a question that is easier to ask than to answer. To the patient it means discomfort, dis-ease, dis-harmony with his environment; to the physician or surgeon it may be revealed by a variety of symptoms and signs; and to the pathologist it may be represented in one or more structural changes (lesions), which may be gross, i.e., seen with the naked eye, or microscopic, only made visible with the light or the electron microscope. The study of lesions forms a part of the science of pathology. Pathology itself can be defined as that branch of medicine that deals with the nature of disease.

But to return to the question, What is disease? Perhaps the best answer we can give is that **disease is the pattern of response of a living organism to some form of injury.** In order for disease to be present there is usually some alteration in normal function. This broad definition must include disease as a response to all kinds of injury, ranging from infection with a virus to stress from crowding or depression from loss.

One way to look at disease is to ask the question, Who dies of what today? Another is to ask the question in another way, namely, what diseases are prevalent in humans on a worldwide basis, deferring the question of whether the diseases cause death or merely decrease the life expectancy or impair the well-being of the individual. These questions address **mortality** on one hand and **morbidity** on the other.

Table 3–1 shows estimates for a number of diseases on a worldwide basis postulating the possibilities of eradication. Smallpox was an example of such a disease which has been successfully eradicated because a) no reservoir of the virus existed except in humans, b) nearly all people with the disease could be identi-

fied easily because of their rash, c) a natural infection conferred lifelong immunity, and d) a safe, inexpensive, effective, stable vaccine was available.

If one turns from the list of diseases in Table 3–1 which are deemed eradicable to the broader list of diseases in Table 3–2, we see a different pattern because the numbers are estimates of the annual worldwide causes of death. It is interesting that diarrheal diseases which are infectious (and frequently contagious) exceed cancer, and that two respiratory diseases (also infectious) exceed cancer by a factor of 2. Many other diseases would also be considered preventable or eradicable by many authorities.

However, if one considers the pattern of causes of mortality by comparing causes of death in the developed countries (approximately 25% of the world population) there is a different story. Of 11 million deaths annually in Europe, North America, New Zealand, and Japan, 2.4 million deaths are due to ischemic heart disease, 2.3 million to cancer, 1.5 million to stroke, and 0.8 million to violent causes including motor vehicle accidents and suicides. Infections and parasitic diseases account for only 5% of deaths in developed countries.

One additional way of looking at disease is to examine trends of disease incidence as shown in Fig. 3–1. Here one can observe in the United States that diseases for which there are readily available vaccines are manifestly increasing at a time when one would expect a decrease.

For the incidence of morbidity one depends on reporting of diseases to central agencies such as the Centers for Disease Control in the United States and NATO internationally. For the incidence of mortality or the causes of death one must rely on death certificates. The degree of certainty in either case is always open to comment. Historically, the branch of health sciences most concerned with these matters was pa-

Table 3–1. Disease Candidates for Worldwide Eradication—International Task Force for Disease Education, 1989

DISEASE	CURRENT ANNUAL TOLL WORLDWIDE	CHIEF OBSTACLES TO ERADICATION	CONCLUSION
Guinea worm	10 million persons infected; few deaths	Lack of public and political awareness; inadequate funding	Eradicable
Poliomyelitis	250,000 cases of paralytic polio; 25,000 deaths	No insurmountable technical obstacles; increased national/international commitment needed	Eradicable
Onchocerciasis	18 million cases; 340,000 blind	High cost of vector control; no therapy to kill adult worms; restrictions in mass use of invermectin	Could eliminate associated blindness
Yaws and endemic syphilis	2.5 million cases	Political and financial inertia	Could interrupt transmission*
Rabies	52,000 deaths	No effective way to deliver vaccine to wild animal disease carriers	Could eliminate urban rabies
Measles	2 million deaths, mostly children	Lack of suitably effective vaccine for young infants; cost; public misconception of seriousness	Not now eradicable
Tuberculosis	8–10 million new cases; 2–3 million deaths	Need for improved diagnostic tests, chemotherapy, and vaccine; wider application of current therapy	Not now eradicable
Leprosy	11–12 million cases	Need for improved diagnostic tests and chemotherapy; social stigma; potential reservoir in armadillos	Not now eradicable

* Because persons may be infected for decades and the organisms cannot be distinguished from those that cause venereal syphilis, elimination of transmission—not eradication—is the goal.

(From Centers for Disease Control, Morbidity and Mortality Weekly Report, 39(13):211, 1990.)

Table 3–2. Estimated Annual Deaths Worldwide

Cardiovascular disease	12 million
Diarrheal diseases	5 million
Cancer	4.8 million
Pneumonia	4.8 million
Tuberculosis*	3 million
Chronic obstructive lung disease	2.7 million
Measles*	1.5 million
Malaria	1–2 million
Hepatitis B	1–2 million
Tetanus* (neonatal)	775,000
Whooping cough*	500,000
Maternal mortality	500,000
AIDS	200,000
Shistosomiasis (parasite)	200,000
Amebiasis (parasite)	40,000–110,000
Hookworm	50,000–60,000
Rabies	35,000
Typhoid	25,000
Yellow fever (epidemic)	25,000
African sleeping sickness	20,000
Ascariasis (parasite)	20,000

* Vaccine-preventable diseases

(Source: World Health Organization.)

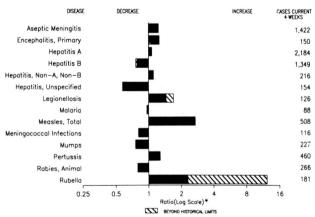

*Ratio of current 4-week total to mean of 15 4-week totals (from comparable, previous, and subsequent 4-week periods for past 5 years).

Fig. 3–1 Notifiable disease reports, comparison of 4-week totals ending October 27, 1990, with historical data—United States. (From Centers for Disease Control, Morbidity and Mortality Weekly Report, 39(43):780, 1990.

thology, and more latterly, epidemiology and public health.

Pathology was originally an investigation into structural changes revealed in the autopsy room. At first only gross changes (naked eye) and later (from 1850) microscopic findings were demonstrated. From the very beginning the aim was to explain the patient's signs and symptoms. In 1483 Leonardo da Vinci dissected an old man in Florence "to see the cause of such a quiet death". When the investigation of disease moved from the autopsy room to the bedside of the living patient, the study was called clinical pathology, or in recent years, because so much of this work is done in the laboratories, the term laboratory medicine has gained in popularity. Our knowledge of the processes and patterns of disease and the techniques for investigating them has continued to grow at an increasing rate. It is now obvious to everyone that the practice of medicine without adequate laboratory facilities denies the patient some important advantages. The diagnostic laboratory is no longer run by a single individual, but rather by a team of experts in various fields—medical, scientific, and technical. The amount of work required from clinical laboratories has led to the introduction of automation, which in turn has resulted in an enormous increase in the volume of work that can be done. But we must not forget that the object of the whole exercise is the care of the patient, a matter to which we shall return in the final chapter.

Anatomic or histologic lesions in tissue may bear an obvious relation to the symptoms, as in the case of acute appendicitis or poliomyelitis. But there may be lesions without symptoms, as in early cancer or pulmonary tuberculosis. Finally, there may be symptoms without anatomic lesions, as in the psychosomatic (Greek *psyche*, spirit and *soma*, body) diseases and the various psychoses. As we have already seen, it is possible that future research may reveal hitherto unsuspected biochemical lesions in these cases also. For disease itself is merely life under abnormal conditions. The presence of lesions distinguishes organic disease, in which there are observable gross or microscopic changes in an organ, from so-called "functional disease," in which there is some disturbance of function without any observable organic change. Although it is true that at the present time diagnosis consists largely of the naming of lesions (e.g., cancer of the lung, coronary artery thrombosis), **disease should be viewed as disordered function rather than only as altered structure.**

Since the time of Virchow (1858), it has been popular to think of disease as arising in disorders of cellular function, and it has become fashionable to talk of molecular disease (Pauling, 1952), but it seems wise now to recognize that this trend to "atomism" in the study of disease may be less than illuminating. In fact, as suggested in an earlier chapter, new knowledge about hormonal control mechanisms suggests that there is a greater interdependence of the different organ systems than has been suspected.

We may classify disease in anatomic or physiologic terms, e.g., "diseases of the heart or nervous system," or "diseases of the endocrines or circulatory system." We may also think of disease according to its causative agent, so we can talk of tuberculosis (caused by the tubercle bacterium), or talk of viral diseases. Or we can consider disease in terms of the reaction patterns to the injury, e.g., pneumoconiosis (lung damage in persons who have inhaled various kinds of dust). None of these methods of classifying disease is exclusively right or wrong, and all help to organize the ways in which we try to cope with the incomplete understanding we have.

One point, however, seems clear: patterns emerge to show us that some illnesses are confined exclusively or principally to a single anatomic compartment and that others involve many systems or the whole host, so we have come to talk also about **systemic diseases.** That is not to say that an infection is always local, as in an abscess, because we all know that infections may spread, but some diseases involve many organ systems, in fact the whole body, and exact their toll because of this. An example is diabetes mellitus, in which there may be lesions in blood vessels of the eye and kidney, as well as heart and aorta, all related in some poorly understood way to disordered metabolism of glucose.

Fortunately, there is a natural tendency to recover from disease, more especially from acute illnesses. Perhaps the best example is the spontaneous healing of a clean wound, which we all take for granted. This healing power, however, presents us with great difficulties in assessing the value of new therapeutic measures, especially new drugs. Is the happy outcome merely a natural event thanks to mother nature, or is it the result of the therapy?

One important point in the understanding of disease is knowing what happens in most cases when there is no therapeutic intervention or attempt at modifying the disease by medical or surgical or other means. This knowledge of the "natural history" of a disease is sadly lacking in many instances because, simply, it would be unethical not to offer some help to an afflicted person. However, there are always cases in which a person denies or fails to seek assistance for a pain, or a mass, or a recurrent problem, for whatever reason, until the process is far advanced.

Through such anecdotal experiences we have accumulated some knowledge of the natural history of various diseases.

It is interesting, for example, to know that there is a study of patients who acquired primary syphilis but who were not treated either with penicillin or with any other drug. After 25 years, only about one quarter of these untreated persons developed any of the legendary and debilitating signs or symptoms of tertiary syphilis that may affect the central nervous system (general paresis), dorsal columns of the spinal cord (tabes), or cardiovascular system (aortic aneurysm, aortic valvular insufficiency, or coronary artery ostial narrowing). This suggests that the natural history of the disease syphilis is more benign than previous generations, in a more prudish era, were wont to believe. But these observations, that only about one quarter of those affected by the spirochete become seriously incapacitated, still suggest that to go without treatment is a type of Russian roulette that has little appeal when one considers the unpleasant outcomes of tertiary syphilis.

It is often said that the nature of disease is changing, that we hear much more about people dying of heart failure and cancer than used to be the case. This does not mean that these diseases have become actually more common, although more people do die from them.

The outcome of disease varies between the extremes of complete recovery and death. The prediction of this outcome is called prognosis; it is a forecast of what may be expected to happen. If one knows the pattern of disease and if the patient's disease conforms to the pattern, then one can forecast or anticipate what may occur and thereby offer a prognosis. Clinical diagnosis is the art of recognizing the pattern from only pieces of the puzzle. Diagnosis is often difficult, but accurate prognosis is much more difficult and requires a complete knowledge of the various patterns that may develop from the pieces of this puzzle. It is largely the result of experience and judgment, and depends to a great extent on a complete comprehension of the natural history of the disease in question. That is what is likely to happen in the way of interaction between the injury process and the host response.

ETIOLOGY

The study of causation of a pathologic process is known as the **etiology** (Fig. 3–2). **Pathogenesis,** a term easily confused with etiology, is the process of production and development of the lesion. It might

Fig. 3–2 This fifteenth-century woodcut of the tree of life shows leaves falling into the sea and onto the land. The interpretation that the genesis of animal life comes from such sources is clearly at variance with our modern knowledge. It is important to recognize that simple association is not the same as causality.

be supposed that the relation of etiologic agent to disease, of cause to effect, was a relatively simple matter. Often the reverse is the case. Perhaps we are misled into imagining that only one cause is responsible. We say the cause of tuberculosis is the tubercle bacillus, but we know that many people may inhale these bacilli yet only one may develop the disease, and that the bacilli may lurk in the body for years and only become active as the result of an intercurrent infection, prolonged stress, or starvation. In fact, Rich derived an equation to describe the development of disease in which he proposed that the occurrence of disease is directly proportional to the number and virulence of organisms and inversely proportional to the native and acquired resistance of the host (constitutional factors).

Obviously, the pathologist who investigates the causation of a disease must consider such elements as heredity, sex, age, environment, immunity, allergy, nutrition, and previous exposure to injury. It becomes evident, then, that there is no simple answer to such questions as, what is the cause of cancer or of arterio-sclerosis?

The following classification may prove helpful in our attempts to cope with the infinitely large number of diseases to be identified now and in the future.

CLASSIFICATION OF DISEASES

Hereditary *athrogenesis*	Vascular *blood*
Congenital *anacephalic*	Metabolic *diabetes*
Traumatic *injury*	Nutritional *lead poisoning*
Physical *burn*	Psychologic
Chemical	Iatrogenic *physician induced*
Infectious *bacteria virus*	Idiopathic *unknown*
Inflammatory *AID*	Tumors

HEREDITY AND CONSTITUTION

Heredity. During the last two decades it has become increasingly clear that heritable disorders of structure and function may explain many diseases that have been poorly understood. Often the inherited abnormalities are subtle and their contribution to signs and symptoms of disease are debated. On the other hand, we have known since the time of Garrod (1909) of the relationship between the inborn error of metabolism and how it causes a failure of function. The field of medical genetics has advanced with exponential speed. It is based on several technologies: cytogenetics and the recognition of karyotypic or chromosomal abnormalities, human population studies and pedigree analysis, and modern biochemical methodologies that permit refined analytic procedures to distinguish small differences in serum, blood, urine, and cells of human beings—differences not detectable heretofore.

It is important to recognize that, whereas hereditary disease implies a genetic basis for the disease, mutations do occur in persons. It is also important to recognize that not all hereditary diseases appear or become identifiable at birth. It may well be that some heritable diseases that only appear at age 30 or 40 such as Huntington's chorea, a disease of the central nervous system that results in loss of motor control, may become detectable in the childhood period with more modern methods.

In addition, one must be aware that not all abnormalities seen in the newborn have their origin in genetic disorders. We now recognize that the fetus is unusually susceptible to a variety of influences during uterine life and not only the infectious diseases such as German measles, but the diet and drugs of the mother may directly affect the development of the fetus. Thus we distinguish between *congenital* disease (appearing at birth) and genetic disease, and between *genetic* disease that is heritable and that occurring spontaneously, due to a mutation.

Constitution. Constitution comprises those features of the mind and body that a man derives from both heredity and environment. It is the sum total of his being. There can be little doubt that nutrition is a factor of great importance, especially in the early formative years of life. Every hour the cells of the body take up elements from the food, including vitamins, and if these are deficient in quantity or quality, the constitution as a whole cannot fail to suffer. It has been said, with what truth we are unable to tell, that if all the diseases in the textbooks could be removed by the wave of a wand, doctors would still be left with 80% of their patients. Their ill health would be due not so much to any known disease as to the failure of the constitution to adapt itself to the life the patient is leading. A good constitution is not to be confused with a good physique; it is something more and something more valuable. Those who have it seem able to do whatever they wish without impairing it in any way. When it is poor, small causes may impair health or even endanger life. The athlete with the most perfect physique may be prostrated by every infection that he encounters.

Genetic Information. We now have available to us several different methods of finding information about a person's genetic makeup. There are various substances in the body whose presence, absence, or variations provide this information. Four groups of substances can be isolated and examined in the pursuit of genetic information: genes, chromosomes, red blood cell antigens, and white blood cell antigens or HLA (human leukocyte antigens). These are called **markers** because the presence, absence, or variations are visible manifestations of the genes in the same way that blue eyes or dark skin are manifestations of the genes. Looking at skin color provides information about one genetically determined category, namely race. Looking at red blood cell antigens also yields information about genetic categories, namely, blood type (A, B, AB, O).

Examination of bands on chromosomes and of the chromosomes themselves (karyotyping) provides a picture of the shape, size, and number of chromosomes as well as (recently) location of bands on chromosomes. Some human characteristics have been linked with these chromosome traits, for example, normal female sex is associated with two X chromosomes of a certain size and shape. Thus, in the case where a child's sex is not clear, the chromosomes are useful markers or indicators of the true genetic situation.

Red blood cell antigens were discovered after disastrous attempts at blood transfusion. Certain individuals were discovered to be (genetically) so different that their blood could not be exchanged. The donor and recipient must be of genetically compatible types, and the A, B, AB, O groups serve as markers or indicators of who the compatible individuals are.

More recently, unsuccessful attempts at tissue transplantation led to the discovery that the red blood cell marker system does not provide sufficient information about compatibility. White blood cells also have surface antigens that must be matched if graft rejection is to be minimized. HLA, then, serve as markers of different genetically determined groups.

HLA have been found to have other uses outside of tissue transplantation. Not only are they markers of tissue compatibility; they have also been associated with various diseases. Some groups of persons suffering from the same disease appear to have the same combination of HLA antigens. (Each HLA antigen has been designated by a specific letter and number; hence HLA B27, HLA W6.) Investigators noticed that all sufferers of ankylosing spondylitis (a form of arthritis) had HLA B27, although not all persons with HLA B27 either have or get ankylosing spondylitis. Current theory describes the presence of HLA B27 as a marker or indication that the person may be susceptible to ankylosing spondylitis, although given the right environmental conditions, he or she may never develop the disease. Thus the HLA marker system provides us with information about disease susceptibility; it allows us to distinguish between those who are most likely and those who are unlikely to contract the disease, and that is all. It provides us with no certainties, because it appears that other nongenetic factors are crucial to the development of disease.

The following story provides an example of this concept. In June 1962, the United States Navy cruiser *Little Rock* departed from Trieste, Italy. Two days later, 602 of the 1,276 crew members came down with dysentery caused by the Shigella bacteria. Two weeks afterwards, 10 of the sailors who had been infected showed symptoms of Reiter's syndrome—swollen joints and skin infections—although no cases of this developed in the uninfected sailors. (Reiter's syndrome has been known to follow a Shigella infection.) Years later, 6 of the 10 sailors were located for HLA testing and it was discovered that 5 of them had HLA B27. (The sixth had had a much milder form of the disease.) Thus it appears that some people are born with a genetic susceptibility to Reiter's syndrome, a susceptibility that can be identified by the presence of HLA B27, but these persons will probably not develop the disease unless they encounter a triggering environmental factor, the Shigella.

Many other diseases have since been linked with HLA antigens. Most of these have long been recognized as hereditary to some extent, but now there is

Table 3–3. HLA Antigens and Disease

DISEASE	HLA ANTIGEN SHOWING CHANGE IN FREQUENCY
Ankylosing spondylitis	↑ B27
Reiter's syndrome	↑ B27
Juvenile rheumatoid arthritis	↑ B27
Adult celiac disease	↑ B8, D3
Addison's disease	↑ B8, D3
Chronic active hepatitis	↑ B8, D3
Graves' disease	↑ B8, D3
Juvenile diabetes	↑ B8; ↑ B15; ↑ D3; ↑ D4
Myasthenia gravis	↑ B8, D3 (♀ <35 yrs.)
Hodgkin's disease (>5-year survival)	↑ A3; ↑ A11
Multiple sclerosis	↑ D2

(Courtesy of Dr. R.D. Guttmann)

a way to pinpoint who in a family is most susceptible and who runs no risk. Eventually, we may be able to state that all disease is hereditary, meaning that we are all born with our own set of susceptibilities, and sooner or later the right environmental conditions will trigger development of the disease (Table 3–3).

Population geneticists currently speculate that a given disease can exert a selection pressure during evolution. This speculation is based on the recent observation that the HLA type Bw53 is exceedingly rare in most parts of the world except in regions of Africa that have been endemic for malaria for thousands of years. In these regions 25% of people are Bw53 positive. Malaria is a disease with several grades of severity and what was remarkable in this report was that children with lethal forms of malaria did not belong to this Bw53 positive group. On the contrary, healthy individuals, or those affected with a mild form of malaria, were often Bw53 positive. This unfortunate group of malaria patients do not usually reach reproductive age, leaving behind the Bw53 positive group who have, therefore, a selective genetic advantage through evolution. We will discuss in Chapter 23 that a genetic form of anemia also protects against malaria. This is a challenging concept and, of course, it remains to be established whether other diseases can select for some genetic traits.

TRAUMA

Trauma or mechanical injury may damage a part to such an extent that the tissues may be killed. It may take the form of a blow, a wound, a fracture of bone, or a sprain of a joint. Mechanical injury may act as a predisposing cause of a nontraumatic disease. One of the best examples is acute osteomyelitis, an acute inflammation of bone and bone marrow caused by microorganisms, usually staphylococci, which settle in the bone, often at the site of a traumatic injury. It is the possibility that the disease may be predisposed or precipitated by trauma that makes Worker's Compensation cases so difficult to decide. Trauma may injure a bone, causing a fracture, or it may injure the soft parts, with a resulting wound or bruise.

An injury of the soft parts associated with rupture of the skin is known as a **wound.** It is obvious that there can be a great variety of wounds. The wound may be clean or infected, incised, punctured, penetrating, and so on. Trauma may injure the soft tissues even though the skin is not broken. The finer vessels, especially the capillaries, are ruptured, so that there is bleeding into the tissue spaces. The result is a **bruise** or **contusion,** which is at first red, then greenish or yellow before it fades. This is the basis of the so-called "black eye." The changes in color are caused by changes that the red blood cells undergo after the blood has been trapped in the interstitial spaces where the blood vessels have been ruptured (hematoma).

To put traumatic injury in perspective as a cause of death, one might note that among all causes of death during the years 1986–1988, accidents (including motor vehicle accidents) ranked fourth after heart disease, cancer, and stroke, accounting for 40 people per 100,000 population. It is interesting that this statistic has changed for the better during the last 20-year period, declining about 30%, and is attributed largely to the use of seat belts and a lower rate of alcohol intake. Unintentional injuries, particularly among children, have also receded, a particularly welcome finding since they are mainly preventable.

PHYSICAL AGENTS

Trauma, as described above, is the most obvious physical agent causing injury (Figs. 3–3, 3–4). Other physical agents that may prove dangerous are unusually high or low temperatures, irradiation, and increased or decreased atmospheric pressure.

Temperature. High temperature may produce local or general damage. Local damage takes the form of **burns.** The burn may be first degree (slight reddening of skin), second degree (blistering), or third degree (destruction of whole thickness of skin). The threat to life depends as much on the size of the area burned as on the severity of the burn, because of the leakage of fluid and the concomitant shock.

Heat stroke may be caused by direct exposure to the sun (sunstroke), or to a high temperature. The heat-regulating mechanism of the body seems to be paralyzed, so that the temperature shoots up to an alarming degree, collapse and unconsciousness develop, and death may result; this is particularly true for temperatures above 42°C. Heat-related deaths are another cause of mortality which has received recent

Distribution of occupational traumatic deaths, by cause—United States, 1980–1981*		Occupational traumatic death rates per 100,000 workers, by industry—United States, 1982*	
CAUSE	PERCENTAGE	INDUSTRY	RATE
Highway motor-vehicles incidents	34.1	Mining and quarrying	55
Falls	12.5	Agriculture	52
Industrial vehicles or equipment	11.4	Construction	40
Blows (other than by vehicles or equipment)	8.0	Transportation and public utilities	26
Electrocutions	6.8	Government	10
Gun shots	4.5	Services	6
Aircraft crashes	3.4	Manufacturing	6
Entrapment	3.4	Trade	5
Fires	3.4		
Plant machinery operations	3.4		
Explosions	2.3		
Gas inhalations	2.3		
Other	4.5		
Total	100.0		
*Adapted from Bureau of Labor Statistics: Occupational Injuries and Illnesses in the United States by Industry, 1981. U.S. Department of Labor Bulletin 2164, January 1983.		*Adapted from (7) Accident Facts, National Safety Council, 1983 Edition.	

Fig. 3–3 Trauma associated with occupation. (From Centers for Disease Control: Morbidity and Mortality Weekly Report, 33(16):214, 1984.)

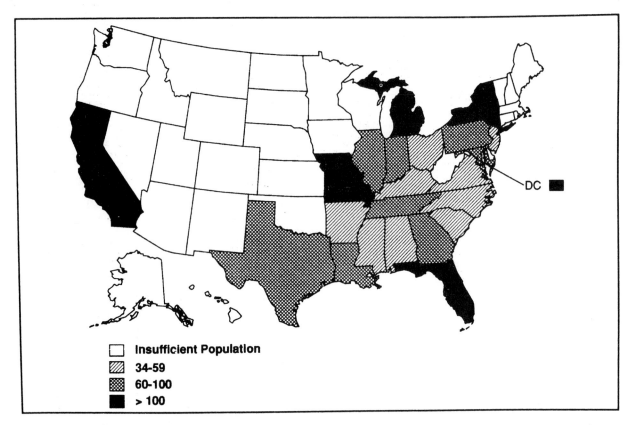

Fig. 3—4   Homicide rates per 100,000 population for black males 15–24 years of age, by state—United States, 1987. (From Centers for Disease Control: Morbidity and Mortality Weekly Report, 39(48):872, 1990.)

attention. Figure 3–5 illustrates the number of deaths which parallel the average temperature in Missouri in June to August. The majority of these have been in persons older than 65 years and most are a result of heat stroke.

Low temperature may cause **frostbite** which usually involves exposed parts such as the ears, the tip of the nose, the hands, and the feet. The fluid in the cells becomes converted into ice crystals which rupture them. The result varies, as in the case of burns, from mild blistering to necrosis and gangrene (Fig. 3–6).

Electrical Hazards. The enormous grid of power lines and the ready availability of electricity in the western world is taken for granted, but few of us recognize the hazards to life this provides until an accident occurs. Summer thunderstorms with lightening, and hospital or household hazards, are usually thought of, but the important concept is that small currents (200 micro amps) may be sufficient to cause ventricular fibrillation when the normal protection of dry skin is altered, as in incisions or wetness. We have heard of one freak occurrence where a person found it necessary to empty his bladder in a place where the stream of urine fell on a live circuit, and the current

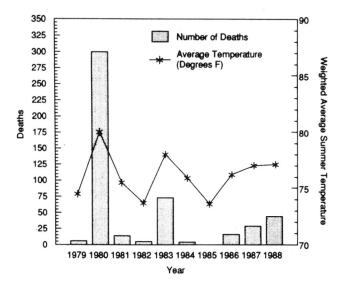

Fig. 3—5   Heat-related deaths and average summer (June-August) temperatures—Missouri, 1979–1988. (From Centers for Disease Control, Morbidity and Mortality Weekly Report, 38(25):437, 1989.)

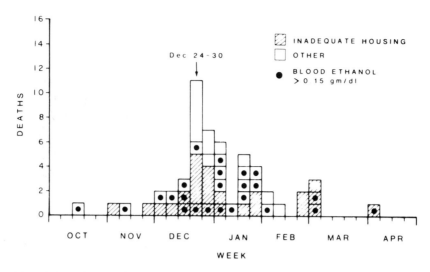

Fig. 3–6   Exposure-related hypothermia deaths and associated factors by week—Washington, D.C., October 1, 1972 to April 30, 1981. (From Centers for Disease Control: Morbidity and Mortality Weekly Report, 31(50):670, 1982.)

was conducted through the stream to the bladder, alternately closing the urethral sphincter with electricity and temporarily paralyzing the victim. Fortunately, the sparks-stream episode was shortlived, but many other instances of human exposure to electrical current have had fatal results.

Radiation Injury. Different tissues differ widely in their sensitivity to radiation. Different kinds of animals also vary in a similar and, at present, inexplicable manner. In general terms it may be said that those cells are especially radiosensitive that normally continue to multiply throughout life, owing to their own short life span. Such are the cells of the lymphatic and hematopoietic or blood-forming systems, and the germinal cells of the gonads. We could expect a lymphocyte, with its life span of a few hours, to be more sensitive to radiation than a nerve cell that never divides. (See Appendix, p. 76.)

Cancer Cells. The cells of a neoplasm, like the normal cells from which they originate, differ widely in their response to irradiation. (Irradiation is the deliberate or therapeutic use of radiation.) Rapidly dividing cells may be expected to respond well, but the radiotherapist must beware of generalizations and know the peculiarities of individual tumors. Thus, such tumors as malignant melanoma and osteogenic sarcoma may be teeming with mitoses and yet be quite radioresistant. Lymphosarcoma, composed of short-lived lymphocytes, is particularly radiosensitive, and may melt away as quickly as the proverbial snowball in hell. Unfortunately, there is a profound difference between radiosensitivity and radiocurability, for even the most radiosensitive of tumors have often a small proportion of cells that survive and

transmit the property of resistance to their progeny, so that eventually the entire mass may be radioresistant. We shall see the same thing happens in the case of antibiotics and bacteria.

Atmospheric Pressure. As in the case of temperature, the pressure of the atmosphere may be too high or too low.

Increased Pressure. People so affected are those involved in construction of underwater structures (when caissons are used), in construction of tunnels under rivers, and in deep-sea diving. Additional pressures of two or three atmospheres may be experienced, which result in additional air becoming dissolved in the blood plasma. When a person passes too rapidly from a high to a normal atmospheric pressure, the dissolved air is released as bubbles in the blood. The oxygen is absorbed, but the nitrogen may form bubbles or emboli in the small arteries to the brain with resulting damage. Pains develop in various parts of the body (the bends), and there may be temporary or even permanent paralysis. The condition in general is known as **caisson disease**.

Decreased Pressure. Effects of decreased pressure may be experienced by aviators flying at altitudes over 30,000 feet unless the plane is pressurized. The gases in the body cavities such as the intestine expand, causing marked discomfort, and gas bubbles are released in the blood and cause air embolism, with results similar to those of caisson disease.

CHEMICAL POISONS

The subject of poisoning, or toxicology, is a large and specialized one that need not detain us long. Poisonous chemicals may be introduced into the body under four different circumstances: (1) by **accident,** especially in the case of young children, (2) for **suicide,** (3) for **homicide,** (4) as an **industrial hazard.** These days, when every industry seems to use a new and different chemical, the last named has become of particular importance. Strong acids and alkalis burn and kill the skin or the mucus membrane of the mouth and stomach if taken internally. Lead poisoning (plumbism) deserves special mention, because it belongs to both the first and fourth groups. Children are apt to put painted objects in their mouths and repeatedly swallow small amounts of the lead in the paint. Lead was used in many industries—painting, glass making, lacquering, among others. Poisons such as lead, mercury, arsenic, and phosphorus interfere with the working of some cell enzymes, thus producing sickness and even death.

With more travel, more people have opportunities for exposure to exotic poisons. Marine bites as a cause of injury have recently been reviewed as a cause of illness.

INFECTIONS

Biologic agents are the cause of infections. They may be minute and exist only as nucleic acid (viruses), or gigantic and complex, as are some intestinal parasites (nematodes, cestodes). Basically, one can think of infectious diseases as a form of parasitism, in which man is the host and the parasite is more or less successful, depending on the nature of the response that it elicits in man. Disease is the product of the interaction between the agent and the host; thus we may be visited by many bacteria, without developing any signs or symptoms, but at other times the same organisms may elicit a strong response that causes destruction and loss of function in various parts of our bodies. The most successful agents are not those that cause death of the host quickly. In fact, a virulent organism will prevent itself from becoming disseminated should it destroy the host: viruses, bacteria, fungi, and parasites are more successful if they effect a symbiotic relationship.

By far the most common cause of disease is **bacteria.** Finally there are **filterable viruses,** forms of living matter so minute that they pass through the pores of filters fine enough to hold back bacteria, so tiny that they cannot be seen with the most powerful light microscope.

Bacteria can be divided into three main groups: (1) **cocci,** which are round, (2) **bacilli,** which are rod-shaped and (3) **spirilla,** or spirochetes, which are spiral like a corkscrew. They cause disease either by their presence in the tissues or by producing toxins (poisons), which either act on the surrounding structures or are carried by the blood stream to distant organs; in both instances they cause inflammation and necrosis either directly or indirectly.

It would be useless to list all the bacteria that cause disease, for it would be merely a list of names with little meaning. Some of these are considered in Chapter 7, and others in connection with the organs that they are most prone to attack.

It is the physician's role to diagnose the presence of disease in the patient and to try to determine the cause of that disease. However, as the physician usually sees only a small number of patients, he may not see a disease often enough to properly gauge its importance in terms of the whole population. The investigation of disease in large groups is called epidemiology. **Epidemiology is the observation of the occurrence of disease in populations.**

Epidemiology depends on the scientific collection of data. First, populations and diseases are investigated individually. The study of populations is called **demography** and involves determining the numbers, ages and distributions of people in various regions of the country. When these data are illustrated, a population distribution similar to Figure 3–7 is obtained.

Study of disease involves investigation of its causes and etiologies as well as its course of development or pathogenesis and its manifestations or signs or symptoms.

Finally, these data are combined and the diseases are studied in the context of populations (Fig. 3–8). **Prevalence** of a disease is defined as the number of cases of a disease in a given population. When a population is followed for a length of time, **incidence** of disease can be calculated as the number of new cases of a disease per unit of time. Prevalence and incidence are informative parameters in the description of disease but must be interpreted with caution. For example, the high prevalence of a disease in an area where the inciting organism is commonly found (Fig. 3–9) is not as significant as a similar finding in an area where the organism is relatively uncommon (Fig. 3–10). In the former case, the disease can be termed **endemic** while in the latter it is **epidemic.** *Histoplasma capsulatum* is an organism common in states in the Ohio and Mississippi River Valleys. Its distribution is illustrated in Figure 9–1. It is not surprising therefore to find a large number of cases of histoplasmosis in this area. On the other hand, it is relatively uncommon on the west coast. A similarly large number of cases arising in, say, California should arouse greater interest. This can either be traced to the introduction of the organism by a person who is infected

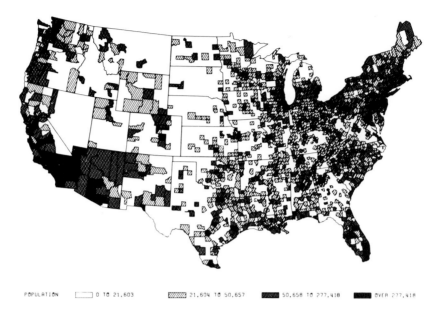

Fig. 3–7   Population distribution, by county, United States, 1980. (From Centers for Disease Control: Morbidity and Mortality Weekly Report, 30(54):18, 1982.)

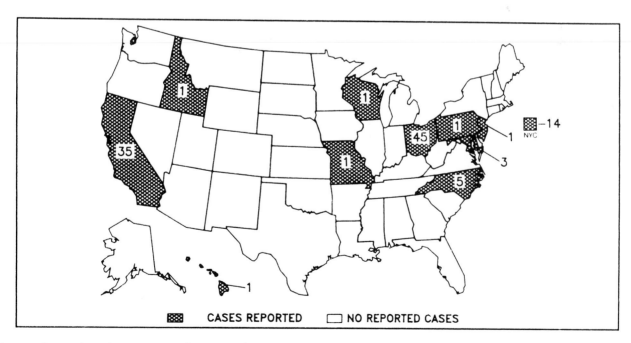

Fig. 3–8   Reported measles cases—United States, Weeks 3–6, 1989. (From Centers for Disease Control: Morbidity and Mortality Weekly Report, 38(7):116, 1989.)

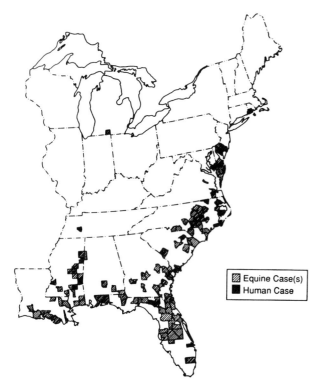

Fig. 3–9 Equine and human eastern equine encephalitis cases, by county—United States, 1989. (From Centers for Disease Control: Morbidity and Mortality Weekly Report, 39(24):414, 1990.)

but not symptomatic (carrier), (as in malaria) (Fig. 3–11), or to persons who have become infected and who have not yet become symptomatic. These individuals are usually referred to as index cases.

Epidemiology is concerned with both small and great numbers. The cause of a single, isolated case of a disease is often as hard to find as the cause of a massive outbreak. In this respect it is easy to see how epidemiology is sometimes referred to as investigative medicine. Because of the attention given not only to the organisms responsible for the disease but to the habits and characteristics of the people infected, epidemiology has uncovered such novel agents of disease as tampons in the case of toxic shock syndrome, and legionella, and has often traced epidemics to a single index case, the classic example being typhoid Mary.

Finally, epidemiology has a role in illustrating the changing trend of disease. That certain patterns of disease occurrence exist is illustrated by the seasonal rhythm of chickenpox (Fig. 3–13). On a larger scale one can see the shift in causes of mortality that has taken place in this century. In 1900 the leading cause of death was pneumonia. By 1990 that had been supplanted by cardiovascular disease. Within diseases themselves changes are remarkable. Thus certain

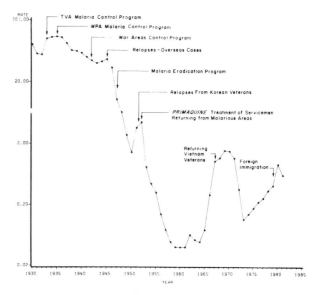

Fig. 3–10 The decrease in the number of reported cases of malaria for 1981 is attributed to a substantial decrease in cases among foreign-born civilians who had acquired malaria before entry into the United States. Seventy-three per cent of all malaria cases reported for 1981 were in foreign-born civilians, compared with 81% for 1980. Of those infections acquired in the United States, 10 were congenital infections, 2 were due to blood transfusions, and for one the source of infection could not be determined. (From Centers for Disease Control: Morbidity and Mortality Weekly Report, 30(54):53, 1982.)

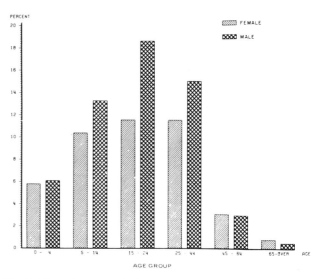

Fig. 3–11 Refugees—Indochinese refugee arrivals in the United States, by age and sex, United States, 1981. (From Centers for Disease Control: Morbidity and Mortality Weekly Report, 30(54):122, 1982.)

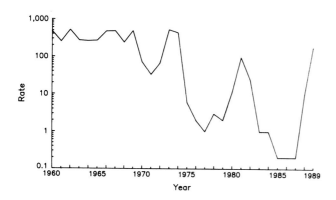

Fig. 3–12   Annual measles incidence rate per 100,000 population—Hungary, 1960-May 1989. (From Centers for Disease Control: Morbidity and Mortality Weekly Report, 38(39):665, 1989.)

types of cancer have been shown to be increasing in frequency while others have been declining. Epidemiology has suggested factors that might be responsible for this phenomenon but has not reached any conclusions. On the other hand the decreasing morbidity due to measles and rubella is easily shown by the accompanying diagrams (Figs. 3–12, 3–14, 3–15) and is readily explained by the introduction of mass vaccination programs in the past decade. However, the prevalence of a disease is not a constant, and the most recent experience with measles illustrates the difficulties of management of a serious disease when its con-

sequences are underestimated by the public and the vaccination rate falls, or there is the introduction of a susceptible (immigrant) population. Recent epidemics of measles are serious problems for this last decade of the 20th century.

Epidemiology, therefore, is a science concerned not only with the identification of disease in large groups but is also a measure of the effectiveness with which we deal with disease.

In the case of cardiovascular disease and cancer, whose etiologies are unknown, studies of populations have made possible the identification of agents or characters that are often found in association with people stricken with these diseases, and which may be suggested as contributors to the development of these pathologies. These factors, which include smoking in the case of lung cancer and a sedentary lifestyle in cardiovascular disease, are termed risk factors (Fig. 3–16). It must be noted that these are only patterns of association and cannot be considered causative agents since not all people with these factors will go on to develop the disease.

INFLAMMATION

Whereas most infections produce inflammation in the host, not all inflammation is due to infectious agents. The body responds to any injury such as

**CHICKENPOX— Reported cases per 100,000 population, by month,
United States, 1977-1981**

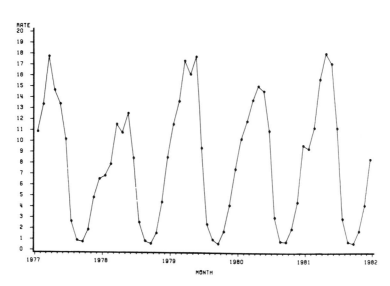

Fig. 3–13   Chickenpox continues to be the second most frequently reported infectious disease in the United States. The seasonal pattern has remained constant; peak incidence for 1981 was reached between March and May. (From Centers for Disease Control: Morbidity and Mortality Weekly Report, 30(54):30, 1982.)

*Data for 1986 are provisional.

Fig. 3–14 Measles cases, by year—United States, 1950–1986. (From Centers for Disease Control: Morbidity and Mortality Weekly Report, 36(20):301, 1987.)

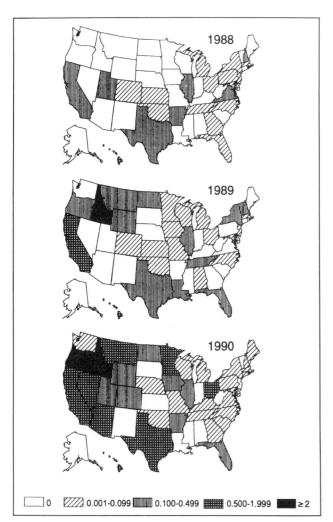

Fig. 3–15 Incidence rates per 100,000 population of reported rubella—United States, 1988–1990. (From Centers for Disease Control: Morbidity and Mortality Weekly Report, 40(6):95, 1991.)

wounding or burns with inflammation: heat, swelling, redness, pain.

Recently, another type of injury has been identified as responsible for arousing the fever, chills, and leukocytosis that herald inflammation. We now know that there are many instances in which our bodies elaborate and circulate antibodies in response to an injury or exposure to an antigen, e.g., response to poison ivy or a bee sting. This type of inflammation can cause just as serious a disability as an infection with a bacterium. In fact, we now believe that many chronic and a few acute diseases (rheumatoid arthritis, glomerulonephritis, serum sickness) are diseases in which inflammation is the only part of the disease that we really comprehend; the exact mechanism of injury and the nature of the antigenic stimulus are still unclear. Some of these diseases respond dramatically to anti-inflammatory agents such as cortisone or aspirin, but these drugs are palliative and do not cure the disease. In our classification of diseases, therefore, we should distinguish inflammation from infection. It is important to keep this in mind as we read on, because there are even instances in which the inciting agent may be some tissue or altered tissue of the body itself, leading to the concept of **autoimmune** diseases.

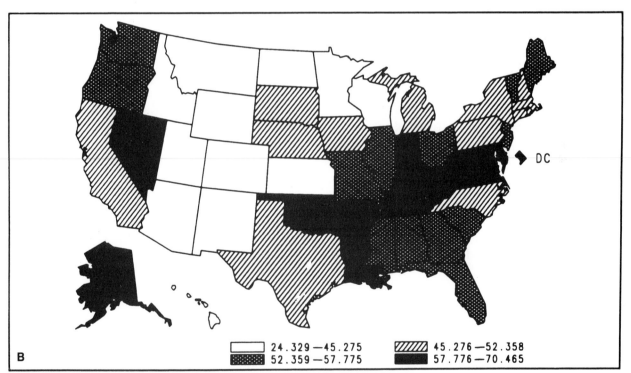

Fig. 3–16   *A*, Percentage of current smoking among adults ≥ 35 years of age, by quartile—United States, 1985. (From Centers for Disease Control: Morbidity and Mortality Weekly Report, 38(32):553, 1989.) *B*, Age-specific lung cancer mortality rates per 100,000 persons, by quartile—United States, 1986. (From Centers for Disease Control, Morbidity and Mortality Weekly Report, 38(29):504, 1989.)

VASCULAR DISEASE

Perhaps the most common disease of the civilized world is atherosclerosis or arteriosclerosis. It is not clear whether this disease of blood vessels is acquired or has a hereditary factor, but it is clear that occlusion of branches of the arterial tree causes untimely death in more than 500,000 North Americans each year. It is most convenient at present to consider it as a multifactorial disease that has an increased incidence in those who have hypertension, hypercholesterolemia, or diabetes mellitus, in those who are overweight, or in those who smoke. There is increasing evidence to support the idea that a sedentary life accelerates the process and that exercise may ameliorate or delay the onset of arteriosclerosis. We also believe now from human observations that atherosclerosis is reversible.

Loss of blood supply to a part is called **ischemia.** This is a local loss of blood supply in contrast to anemia, which is a general condition of bloodlessness affecting the entire body. The result is **anoxia** or loss of oxygen to the part. As food and oxygen are carried by the blood, it is evident that if the supply of blood is diminished by narrowing of an artery, the part of the body deprived of its blood supply will suffer and become diseased. An example of this is seen in arteriosclerosis of the vessels supplying the leg; the tissues of the foot will finally die, a condition formerly known as **gangrene.** An even more important example of ischemia is blockage of the coronary arteries to the heart muscle, either by arteriosclerosis or by thrombosis, resulting in sudden death, in arrhythmias, or in permanent damage to the heart (infarction).

METABOLIC DISEASES

Diseases of this type can be thought of as those in which disorders in the production of enzymes, hormones, or secretory products can be identified. These diseases commonly are hereditary, such as the glycogen storage diseases, and have been found for all kinds of metabolism whether it is an amino aciduria, hypertriglyceridemia, or defect in mucopolysaccharide synthesis. But some metabolic diseases are acquired later in life, perhaps due to changes in the function of an organ or organ system caused by viral infection, or by destruction by such forces as the presence of tumor in a vital organ, or by necrosis of an endocrine gland due to infarction, presence of a cyst, or inflammation.

This heading is a catch-all because it depends on your point of view whether you wish to include diabetes mellitus here or under, for example, hereditary diseases. In fact, as we gain newer knowledge, diseases may be shunted around like boxcars in a railyard in our classification. Recently there has been some evidence that diabetes mellitus occurs in young people following a viral infection. So is diabetes mellitus a metabolic, a hereditary, or an infectious disease?

This does not really damage the validity of the pigeonhole, because there are many diseases in the same category. For example, is atherosclerosis a metabolic or a vascular disease? Clearly, the use of any classification system is simply to aid you in organizing the information that comes your way. Diseases of the endocrine system can be catalogued under metabolism, along with disorders of fluids and electrolytes, such as shock and dehydration.

NUTRITIONAL DISEASES

The idea that disease may be due to something lacking, rather than to some positive hostile factor such as bacteria, injury, or poison, is a sophisticated one, but enormously important and far-reaching. It has always been recognized that starvation will affect the health of the body and will eventually result in death. But there may be an insufficient supply of some particular element in the food, such as a particular amino acid or essential lipid. Perhaps more important as a cause of disease is an inadequate supply of **minerals** and of the essential coenzymes known as **vitamins.** Even though actual disease may not be present, perfect health is impossible if there are deficiencies in the food. This is particularly true of the growing period of life.

With every year that passes, the importance of nutritional deficiencies is becoming more apparent. It is the quality rather than the quantity of the food that is essential (Fig. 3–17). During starvation, the demands of the body are so much lowered that true deficiency disease may not become apparent. However, if the food is abundant in carbohydrates, but deficient in minerals or vitamins, the health of the cells is impaired and evidence of disease becomes manifest.

The most common worldwide cause of disease attributable to nutrition may be inadequate caloric intake, as in many parts of Asia today. In North America there is a malnutrition of a different kind. Large populations eat carbohydrates exclusively; on the other hand, some eat an expensive, high-protein, high-fat diet that they do not need. Eating is a cultural and social activity, and most people do not understand or consider the rationale of eating. Although most of this section on nutritional disease will be devoted to deficiencies, it is worth mentioning that problems also arise at the other end of the spectrum, where too much food rather than too little is the problem. Obe-

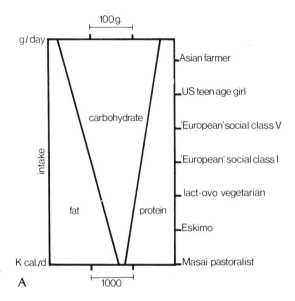

Fig. 3-17 *A,* This graph shows the relative proportions in the diet of different persons of fat, carbohydrate and protein. The Asian farmer subsists on a principally carbohydrate diet, whereas the Eskimo lives on a diet rich in fat and protein. (From Thorn, C.W., et al. (eds.): *Harrison's Principles of Internal Medicine,* 8th Ed. New York, McGraw-Hill, 1977.)

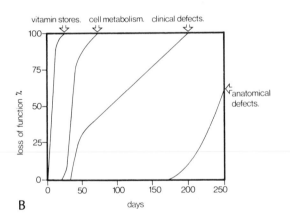

Fig. 3-17 *B,* This graph shows the time span related to the loss of function before anatomic defects occur in vitamin deficiencies. Clearly, cell metabolism and clinical defects occur first. (Adapted from Marks, J.: *The Vitamins in Health and Disease.* Boston, Little, Brown & Co., 1968.)

sity is a major health problem in many countries. For example, in Karelia, Northern Finland, there is the highest incidence of death from heart attacks in the world. This population is well nourished and also has a high incidence of hypertension. In general, obese persons run a greater risk of developing hypertension, cardiovascular disease, diabetes, and gallstones. The mortality rate is higher than for people of normal weight. Each pound of fat has been estimated to add as much as a kilometer of blood vessels that increase

the work of the heart, to say nothing of the load added weight places on the joints of the skeleton. To complicate matters further, each pound of additional adipose tissue is a living thing, not an inert brick of lard. Like all living things it requires energy, usually in the form of glucose. Thus, once you have transformed 25 or 30% of your body into adipose tissue, you have acquired a hungry population of cells which continually cry for more nourishment. Most obese people feel they have to eat because the hypoglycemia (low blood sugar) they experience is a very real part of being fat; this vicious cycle is hard to break. Excess adipose tissue uses glucose, makes you hungry, you eat more, you make more adipose tissue, you continue to feed the adipose parasite.

The most obvious method of production of nutritional deficiency is lack of certain elements in the diet. But the same result may be brought about in a number of other ways. If a patient has persistent vomiting, he cannot assimilate his food, no matter how excellent it may be. Conditions such as gastric ulcer and diabetes may necessitate the long-continued use of diets that may be deficient in particular foods. Widespread disease of the intestine, commonly associated with diarrhea, may interfere so seriously with the absorption of food that deficiency must result.

Resistance to infection appears to depend to some extent on the food supply and particularly on proteins, for it is from proteins that antibodies to bacteria are manufactured. Chronic starvation is associated with a lowered resistance to such infections as tuberculosis. A tragic demonstration of this fact was provided by the high incidence of tuberculosis and other serious infections among the peoples of Europe impoverished by a great war. Although this association between starvation and infection has frequently been noted, it has not yet been firmly established.

Earlier work on nutritional deficiency, particularly vitamin deficiency, was concerned with full-blown diseases such as scurvy, rickets, and beriberi. It is now realized that minor manifestations of deficiency are much more common, although they have been overlooked in the past. In certain localities where, for geographic reasons, there is a lack of such essential foods as milk and fresh vegetables, a large proportion of the population may exhibit symptoms and signs of deficiency disease, although they may be unconscious of the fact.

Table 3-4 is a summary of some of the principal clinical features of the vitamin deficiencies in man. The reader is also referred to the section on deficiency disease in the Appendix p. 73.)

The various vitamins are necessary for perfect health. Deficiency in any one of them may lead to

Table 3–4. Vitamin Deficiency Diseases

Vitamin A	Night blindness, xerophthalmia, keratomalacia
Thiamin (B_1)	Beriberi
Riboflavin (B_2)	Cheilosis, eye lesions
Niacin (nicotinic acid)	Pellagra (skin, alimentary canal, central nervous system)
Vitamin B_{12}	Pernicious anemia
Vitamin C	Scurvy
Vitamin D	Rickets, osteomalacia
Vitamin K	Hypoprothrombinemia, tendency to bleeding

disease. It is important, however, to remember the following facts, which are apt to be overlooked in view of the flood of articles on vitamins in the press and periodicals, not to mention the persuasive pamphlets from the pharmaceutical houses. (1) Under modern conditions, outspoken deficiency disease is uncommon except in the third world, although minor degrees of deficiency are far from rare. (2) An average mixed diet including fresh fruit and green vegetables contains an ample supply of vitamins. (3) Whereas pure vitamin deficiency can be produced in the experimental animal, in human cases an inadequate diet is likely to be lacking in more than one vitamin, so that the clinical picture will tend to be mixed. (4) More than $100,000,000 are spent annually by the United States public buying vitamins. (5) It is better and infinitely cheaper to get your vitamins from the grocery store, where they have been manufactured by nature, than from the drugstore, where they have been manufactured by man. Although this is true for healthy persons, it may not be true for those suffering from avitaminosis. When the condition is of long duration, it may be necessary to administer artificially prepared vitamins for a correspondingly long period before the needs of the tissue are fully satisfied and the normal balance of vitamins is restored. Finally, it must be borne in mind that vitamins, although essential to life, are no substitute for food. They provide no energy, calories, or body-building materials, and are merely accessory to diet.

A final note might be added to point out that although the politicians may claim all men are equal, it is clear that we are all different. Our normal complements of enzymes vary just as do our heights and weights and our intellectual capabilities. Relative deficiencies leading to disease are not only a function of supply or a function of demand, but also depend on the rates at which we use substrate or manufacture coenzymes. Charles Scriver has wisely illustrated this concept of disease in the accompanying diagram (Fig. 3–18).

DRUGS

The causes of disease are endless, and it is sad to implicate man as the agent of his own ills. But, as we have already seen, what is powerful for good may also be potent for evil. The picture of disease is changing before our very eyes, and while some diseases are passing away as the result of modern therapy, new diseases are taking their place, and many of these new diseases are due to drugs. These are usually drugs used by the general public, but they may be drugs prescribed by the doctor (Fig. 3–19). In these days when tranquilizers take the place of baby-sitters, antibiotics are regarded as the cure-all for the most minor infections, and steroid therapy is a panacea, it is small wonder that old maladies are replaced by new, manmade ones.

There has never been a period in human history when such a deluge of new drugs has been poured forth. The public press daily reports a quota of miracle drugs, which the public demands. No drug is completely safe. If the reader will consult the table of contents of Spain's *The Complications of Modern Medical Practices*, he will see the truth of this statement. A most tragic example is, of course, thalidomide given to pregnant women with results that we all know. The use of oral contraceptives involves a distinct danger of thromboembolism, stroke, and hypertension.

A Non-categorical Approach to Origin of Disease

Fig. 3–18 Necessary and sufficient "causes" of PKU and scurvy. (From Scriver, C.R.: Treatment of inborn errors of metabolism. The nature:nurture argument specified. In *Advances in the Treatment of Inborn Errors of Metabolism*. Edited by M.D'A. Crawford, D.A. Gibbs, and R.W.E. Watts. New York, John Wiley & Sons, 1982.)

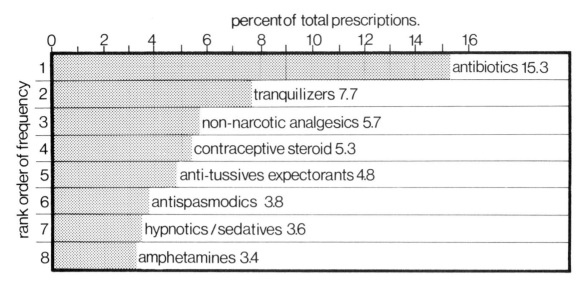

Fig. 3–19   This set of bar graphs shows the percentage of total prescriptions ordered in the 1970s for North America. (From Stolley, P.D., et al.: Drug prescribing and use in an American community. Ann. Intern. Med., 76:537, 1972.)

PSYCHOGENIC DISEASE

Clearly, it is possible to identify situations in which, by their reaction pattern or attitude, subconscious or otherwise, people become incapacitated and are unable to enjoy a normal life. In other words, they become ill. The death of a loved one may lead to depression, which in turn takes away the appetite not only for life, but for simple sustenance. This self-imposed starvation resulting from depression can have real consequences.

IATROGENIC DISEASE

We alluded previously to diseases caused by the medical profession (Greek *iatros*, doctor), and we shall come back to the subject frequently. This cause ranks as one of the most important in western medicine today.

IDIOPATHIC DISEASE

This heading for disease simply covers our ignorance; it refers to those diseases of unknown cause. We recognize many patterns of disease for which we can relate the anatomic lesions and physiologic dysfunctions to a causative agent. Thus we speak of tuberculosis of the lung as a disease caused by the tubercle bacillus (infectious etiology). Some disease processes are so poorly understood that we can only accept at present that we do not know their etiology, although we may collect cases in which the same pattern repeats itself in many people. Cancer is of unknown etiology, as are ulcerative colitis and rheuma-

toid arthritis, although in each instance we have theories as to the possible causes of these processes. Thus we may classify the processes, if we wish, under the heading Idiopathic.

TUMORS

One cause of disease is the presence of abnormal growth. Normally in the adult, cell replication constitutes an adaptive response; for example, replacement of old or damaged cells. However, in some instances a group of cells will proliferate as if out of control, without regard for the health or survival of the body. This process is called neoplasia and results in a tumor (Fig. 3–20).

Tumors interfere with body function in several ways. First, they occupy space, and in doing so they may obstruct essential pathways or compress essential structures, and thereby destroy normal tissue. Second, some tumors have been found to secrete substances that act like hormones and thereby interfere with endocrine function. They can be benign or malignant, but the extent of damage to the body depends on additional important factors, such as location. A benign tumor in the pituitary will have far-reaching consequences through uncontrolled hormone production, whereas a malignant tumor in the abdominal cavity can grow to the size of a basketball without killing the patient.

MAKING THE DIAGNOSIS

Although every patient who visits a physician does so with good reason, every physician is faced first

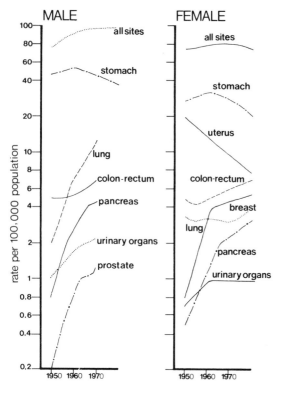

Fig. 3—20   This set of graphs shows the frequency of different types of cancer in men and women in North America in 1950, 1960, and 1970. Note the decline in cancer of the stomach in men and women; the decline in carcinoma of the uterus in women, which includes carcinoma of the cervix in this graph; and the extraordinary rise in carcinoma of the lung for both sexes. Naturally, some of these changes are due to better methods of detection. (From Hirayama, T.: Changing patterns of cancer in Japan with special reference to the decrease in stomach cancer mortality. In *Origins of Human Cancer, Book A*. Edited by H. H. Hiatt, et al. New York, Cold Spring Harbor Laboratory, 1977.)

with the question, "What is the cause of this patient's discomfort or disease?" To make a diagnosis of a particular disease is often not easy, and the increasingly sophisticated techniques available today are expensive and sometimes time consuming as well. They are also subject to error, if not of a technical sort, then of interpretation. This section outlines both traditional and newer methods used to determine the pattern that we recognize as disease.

Clinical Methods. By this term we mean the deductive and inductive reasoning that relates the presence of certain symptoms or signs in a patient to the patterns of disease we have learned about in other patients. Clearly, there are situations in which the difficulties in medicine are complicated by the appearance of a new disease (e.g., Legionnaires Disease, Lassa fever) or by new manifestations of a known disease to such an extent that it cannot be identified, but these are rare. **Symptoms** include the complaints of the pa-

tient, either voluntary or elicited by careful cross-examination. It is often possible to make a correct diagnosis from the symptoms alone. Thus the agonizing pain in the chest in coronary thrombosis, or the digestive distress and pain relieved by taking food, so characteristic of ulcer of the stomach, may tell the doctor in clear and unmistakable language the disease from which the patient is suffering. In the majority of diseases, there is a close relationship between the symptoms of the patient and the lesions that the pathologist may be able to demonstrate. Thus if the air spaces of the lung are filled with inflammatory material in pneumonia, it is only natural that the patient should be severely short of breath. This close relationship of lesions to symptoms is one of the chief reasons why a knowledge of pathology is of value to the doctor. Unfortunately, the number of symptoms of which a patient can complain is unlimited, and pain, shortness of breath, fever, and loss of strength can be caused by many different diseases. On this account the doctor has to turn to physical signs for further help.

Physical signs are elicited by physical examination of the patient. By listening to the heart a murmur may be heard, palpation of the kidney may show it to be enlarged, and pressure over the appendix may elicit tenderness even though the patient has not complained of pain. These signs are of the greatest help in diagnosis.

Simple visual inspection of the patient may tell the doctor or the nurse all that needs to be known. The patient with pneumonia can be recognized by reason of the rapid respiration, cough, and flushed feverish appearance. In chronic heart failure there is shortness of breath (dyspnea), swelling of the legs, and the bluish tinge of cyanosis. In an acute heart attack, such as that of coronary thrombosis, the face is clammy and ashen in color, the expression that of deep anxiety, and there is a strange immobility, as if the patient feared to move a muscle. In nephritis, the face and eyelids are swollen and the skin presents a typical pallor. Acute intestinal obstruction can be suspected from the sunken appearance of the eyes due to extreme loss of fluid (dehydration), the leaden skin, and the board-like rigidity of the abdomen. The wasted and emaciated appearance (cachexia) of the cancer patient is only too readily recognized. Among the most characteristic of clinical pictures are those of certain diseases of the endocrine glands, as illustrated by the pigmentation of the skin in Addison's disease associated with destruction of the cortex of the adrenals, and the striking contrasts presented by Graves' disease due to hyperactivity of the thyroid and by myxedema due to hypoactivity of the same gland.

What may be called the "scopes" can be included in a discussion of physical signs. The scopes in use today range from short metal specula used for rectal or vaginal examinations to the long, flexible, fiberoptic scope that can visualize the ampulla of Vater, nearly 100 cm from the mouth of the patient. The laryngoscope reveals the interior of the larynx, the bronchoscope the interior of the bronchial tree, the gastroscope the interior of the stomach, the sigmoidoscope the interior of the colon (sigmoid), the cystoscope the interior of the bladder, and so on. In the case of the ophthalmoscope, a beam of light is directed into the eye, the interior of which is illuminated and can be studied.

Laboratory Methods. These comprise tests that cannot be done at the bedside, but require the use of laboratory apparatus such as the microscope and the test tube with all its complicated extensions. It must be emphasized that laboratory tests, with which must be included x-ray examination, do not provide the doctor with a ready-made diagnosis; they merely give him additional information, which, taken in conjunction with the clinical evidence (history of the illness, symptoms, and signs), enables him to arrive at a correct diagnosis—we hope.

These tests constitute what has now become the specialty of **clinical pathology,** and comprise the examination of fluids (including blood) and cells taken from the patient during life.

Laboratory tests are numerous and complex. Indeed entire books are devoted to them. Only a few of the more important will be mentioned here. In what follows we have kept to the barest outline, intended as a preview of some more detailed accounts in the second part of this book.

Urinalysis is the most common of all laboratory tests. Examination of the urine serves not only to give indirect evidence of kidney function, but may also reveal disease of the bladder and urethra. Other diseases not connected with the urinary tract may be detected by urinalysis, e.g., the presence of sugar in the urine in diabetes. As a matter of fact, the urine represents the main route by which abnormal substances are eliminated from the blood. It is obvious how many of these substances, such as minerals and hormones, may be revealed by skillful urinalysis.

Examination of stomach contents and **feces** gives valuable information as to the presence of disease in the stomach and intestine.

A **blood count** shows the number and condition of both the red blood cells and the leukocytes. The red cells are diminished in number or are altered in size or shape in various forms of anemia. The number of the leukocytes is increased in acute infections (appendicitis, pneumonia) and in the blood disease leukemia.

Blood chemistry is of ever-increasing importance. Thus the blood sugar is increased in diabetes, the urea nitrogen is increased in renal failure, the phosphorus may be abnormal in rickets, and various enzymes may be increased in amount, whereas others not normally present may make their appearance.

The **cerebrospinal fluid** shows changes in many diseases of the nervous system. Thus the diagnosis of acute meningitis is made by finding large numbers of leukocytes in this fluid, together with the bacteria causing the infection. The fluid, which is obtained by means of lumbar puncture, is a mirror in which is reflected disease of the brain and spinal cord.

Bacteriologic examination is of the greatest importance in the diagnosis of many of the infectious diseases such as diphtheria, pneumonia, and tuberculosis. A blood culture may show the presence of streptococci or other organisms in the circulating blood.

Serology consists of the examination of the blood serum for substances that indicate the presence of bacterial infection. It must be understood that these are not tests for the bacteria, but for substances such as antibodies produced by the body in response to the infection.

Tissue diagnosis is the microscopic examination of pieces of tissue. When such a piece is removed during life for the purpose of diagnosis, the procedure is called a **biopsy,** in contrast to the examination of tissues at autopsy. It is usually done to determine whether a tumor is malignant.

The **electrocardiogram** is an electrical record of the contractions of the heart. All contracting muscles produce an electric current, and such a current is produced by the contractions of the auricles and ventricles. The current is made to write a permanent tracing (electrocardiogram), which is of one pattern when the heart muscle is healthy, but of a different pattern when the muscle is diseased. These "fingerprints" of the heart's action are of great value to the heart specialist.

Radiography. The radiologist provides invaluable assistance to the clinician in search of a diagnosis. X-rays have the power of passing through solid objects and affecting a photographic film on the other side of that object, but their use is limited by the fact that they can only show differences in density. An opaque object, such as a bullet, will stand out clearly; large solid organs can be seen on the film, but the outlines of hollow structures, such as the stomach, intestine, gallbladder, and bronchi, are indistinguishable. It is these outlines, however, that are most likely to be altered in disease.

New chemical and mechanical diagnostic techniques (see Appendix, p. 78.) have become so much a part of modern diagnosis that we forget that there was a time when they did not exist. Even today, in other parts of the world, accurate diagnoses are made without these machines, depending only on human knowledge, skill, and senses. Richard Selzer, in his book *Mortal Lessons*, describes the diagnostic techniques of the personal physician to the Dalai Lama, Yeshi Dhonden, who once visited the United States. His methods are virtually incomprehensible to us, yet they are successful, as can be seen in the following passage:

He bows in greeting while his young interpreter makes the introduction. Yeshi Dhonden, we are told, will examine a patient selected by a member of the staff. The diagnosis is as unknown to Yeshi Dhonden as it is to us. The examination of the patient will take place in our presence, after which we will reconvene in the conference room where Yeshi Dhonden will discuss the case. We are further informed that for the past two hours Yeshi Dhonden has purified himself by bathing, fasting, and prayer. I, having breakfasted well, performed only the most desultory of ablutions, and given no thought at all to my soul, glance furtively at my fellows. Suddenly, we seem a soiled, uncouth lot.

The patient had been awakened early and told that she was to be examined by a foreign doctor, and has been asked to produce a fresh specimen of urine, so when we enter her room, the woman shows no surprise. . . . Yeshi Dhonden steps to the bedside while the rest stand apart, watching. For a long time he gazes at the woman, favoring no part of her body with his eyes, but seeming to fix his glance at a place just above her supine form. I, too, study her. No physical sign nor obvious symptom gives a clue to the nature of her disease.

At last he takes her hand, raising it in both of his own. Now he bends over the bed in a kind of crouching stance, his head drawn down into the collar of his robe. His eyes are closed as he feels for her pulse. In a moment he has found the spot, and for the next half hour he remains thus, suspended above the patient like some exotic golden bird with folded wings, holding the pulse of the woman beneath his fingers, cradling her hand in his. . . . It is palpation of the pulse raised to the state of ritual. . . .

At last Yeshi Dhonden straightens, gently places the woman's hand upon the bed, and steps back. The interpreter produces a small wooden bowl and two sticks. Yeshi Dhonden pours a portion of the urine specimen into the bowl and proceeds to whip the liquid with the two sticks. This he does for several minutes until a foam is raised. Then, bowing above the bowl, he inhales the odor three times. He sets down the bowl and turns to leave.

We are seated once more in the conference room. Yeshi Dhonden speaks now for the first time, in soft Tibetan sounds that I have never heard before. He has barely begun when the young interpreter begins to translate, the two voices continuing in tandem—a bilingual fugue, the one chasing the other. It is like the chanting of monks. He speaks of winds coursing through the body of the woman,

Table 3–5. Age-adjusted Death Rates* for 1987 and Percent Changes in Age-adjusted Death Rates for the 15 Leading Causes of Death from 1986 to 1987 and 1979 to 1987—United States

RANK†	CAUSE OF DEATH (ICD-9)	AGE-ADJUSTED DEATH RATE FOR 1987	% CHANGE 1986 TO 1987	% CHANGE 1979 TO 1987
1	Diseases of the heart (390–398, 402, 404–429)	169.6	−3.1	−15.0
2	Malignant neoplasms, including neoplasms of lymphatic and hematopoietic tissues (140–208)	132.9	−0.2	1.6
3	Cerebrovascular disease (430–438)	30.3	−2.3	−27.2
4	Accidents and adverse effects§ (E800–E949)	34.6	−1.7	−19.3
	Motor vehicle accidents (E810–E825)	19.5	0.5	−15.9
	All other accidents and adverse effects (E800–E807, E826–E949)	15.2	−3.2	−22.4
5	Chronic obstructive pulmonary disease and allied conditions (490–496)	18.7	−0.5	28.1
6	Pneumonia and influenza (480–487)	13.1	−3.0	17.0
7	Diabetes mellitus (250)	9.8	2.1	—
8	Suicide (E950–E959)	11.7	−1.7	—
9	Chronic liver disease and cirrhosis (571)	9.1	−1.1	−24.2
10	Atherosclerosis (440)	3.6	−2.7	−36.8
11	Nephritis, nephrotic syndrome, and nephrosis (580–589)	4.8	−2.0	11.6
12	Homicide and legal intervention (E960–E978)	8.6	−4.4	−15.7
13	Septicemia (038)	4.5	4.7	95.7
14	Certain conditions originating in the perinatal period¶ (760–779)	—	−2.2	−28.9
15	Human immunodeficiency virus infection (new code: 042–044)	5.5	—	—
	All causes	**535.5**	**−1.1**	**−7.2**

* Per 100,000 population, age-adjusted to 1940 U.S. population.
† Based on number of deaths.
§ When a death occurs under "accidental" circumstances, the preferred term within the public health community is "unintentional injury."
¶ Based on infant mortality rates.

(From Centers for Disease Control, Morbidity and Mortality Weekly Report, 39(12):194, 1990.)

currents that break against barriers, eddying. These vortices are in her blood, he says. The last spendings of an imperfect heart. Between the chambers of her heart, long, long before she was born, a wind had come and blown open a deep gate that must never be opened. Through it charge the full waters of her river, as the mountain stream cascades in the springtime, battering, knocking loose the land, and flooding her breath. Thus he speaks, and is silent.

"May we now have the diagnosis?" a professor asks.

The host of these rounds, the man who knows, answers.

"Congenital heart disease", he says. "Interventricular septal defect, with resultant heart failure."

A gateway in the heart, I think. That must not be opened.

Table 3–6. Ratio of Age-Adjusted Death Rates* for the 15 Leading Causes of Death, by Sex and Race—United States, 1987

RANK†	CAUSE OF DEATH (ICD-9)	MALE TO FEMALE	BLACK TO WHITE§
1	Diseases of the heart (390–398, 402, 404–429)	1.9	1.4
2	Malignant neoplasms, including neoplasms of lymphatic and hematopoietic tissues (140–208)	1.5	1.3
3	Cerebrovascular disease (430–438)	1.2	1.8
4	Accidents and adverse effects¶	2.7	1.2
	Motor vehicle accidents (E810–E825)	2.6	0.9
	All other accidents and adverse effects (E800–E807, E826–E949)	3.0	1.7
5	Chronic obstructive pulmonary disease and allied conditions (490–496)	2.0	0.8
6	Pneumonia and influenza (480–487)	1.8	1.5
7	Diabetes mellitus (250)	1.1	2.3
8	Suicide (E950–E959)	3.9	0.5
9	Chronic liver disease and cirrhosis (571)	2.3	1.8
10	Atherosclerosis (440)	1.3	1.1
11	Nephritis, nephrotic syndrome, and nephrosis (580–589)	1.5	2.8
12	Homicide and legal intervention (E960–E978)	3.2	6.0
13	Septicemia (038)	1.4	2.7
14	Certain conditions originating in the perinatal period** (760–779)	1.3	2.6
15	Human immunodeficiency virus infection (new code: 042–044)	9.1	3.2
	All causes	1.7	1.5

* Per 100,000 population, age-adjusted to 1940 U.S. population.
† Based on number of deaths.
§ Both groups include Hispanics.
¶ When a death occurs under "accidental" circumstances, the preferred term within the public health community for the cause of death is "unintentional injury."
** Based on infant mortality rates.

(From Centers for Disease Control, Morbidity and Mortality Weekly Report, 39(12):195, 1990.)

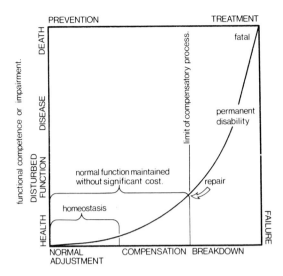

Fig. 3–21 This graph shows the range of adaptation from health through to death.

Through it charge the full waters that flood her breath. So! Here then is the doctor listening to the sounds of the body to which the rest of us are deaf.

To conclude our discussion of disease, it may be useful to regard disease as the failure of the organism to adapt to whatever changes are wrought in its external and internal existence. This can be illustrated in the form of a graph, as shown in Figure 3–21. The natural result of failure of adaptation is death.

DEATH

We have been discussing various causes of disease and how to circumvent them. There remains the fact that for every living being there is an end to life, whatever the cause. That end we call death. The age-adjusted death rates from the U.S. statistics are shown in Tables 3–5 and 3–6.

If we consider the termination of life of each of our cells, we die a thousand million deaths, but in most parts of the world it is the cessation of the heartbeat that has been used as the criterion of death. As everyone knows today, the heartbeat may often be restored by prompt medical attempts to convert the fibrillation or to restore the rhythm. From the biologic point of view, death is a process, not just a particular moment, and we are all partaking of that process unwittingly all the time.

It would seem simple to say that when the heart has ceased to beat, the lungs to breathe, or the brain to think that a man is dead, but we know there is a wide variation in the ability of different tissues to survive the loss of their essential circulation. Muscle cells, particularly smooth muscle, may be reanimated after days of anoxia. Liver and kidney cells can repopulate large areas that have been destroyed, and these organs can be restored to normal function after hours of anoxia. However, the neurons of the brain are incapable of regeneration and rarely survive more than 15 minutes without normal oxygen and glucose.

It is not strange to redirect our definition of death from the heart and respiratory functions to the essential features of a particular person, his personality, attitudes, emotions, and intellect, which compose his character. These are all manifestations of his cerebral functions and depend on the integrity of these selfsame susceptible neurons.

Today, the most accepted definitions of death consider that when the normal signs of responsiveness are absent, and when the brainstem and spinal reflexes are also gone, death has occurred. Electrical activity of the central nervous system as shown by electroencephalography demonstrates only flat waves. This observation should be repeated at least once in 24 hours. When these findings have been confirmed by a second physician the patient can be considered biologically and medically dead.

At this point, the question of continuing supportive medical measures becomes a consideration. Much debate surrounds the suitability of such active intervention, or on the other hand, the decision to withdraw such support, once started. These decisions differ in every case and are beyond the scope of this chapter.

The knowledge that dialysis for renal failure and transplantation of kidneys have altered the prognosis of thousands of patients that would have been hopeless nearly four decades ago underscores the important question of who is to give and who is to receive in these circumstances. Hundreds of successful renal transplantations and scores of cardiac transplantations, as well as many successful liver transplantations, all testify to the importance of these efforts. One outcome of this has been to cause us to define death in a new and more complex way.

As a cautionary note, it is important to remember that the attribution of one cause of death or another in any particular case is still open to discussion since our systems vary widely from place to place, as shown in Figure 3–22.

We might conclude this section on the causes of disease with the thought that when all natural frailties are considered, it seems strange that a harp with so many strings should stay in tune so long.

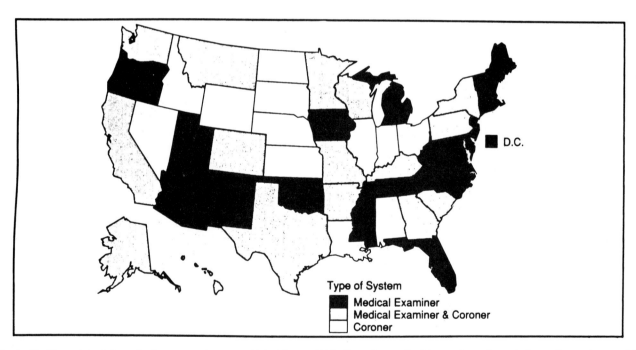

Fig. 3–22 Type of death investigation system, by state—United States, 1987. (From Centers for Disease Control, Morbidity and Mortality Weekly Report, 38(1):3, 1989.)

SYNOPSIS

Disease is the pattern of response of a living organism to some form of injury.

The pattern of disease is determined as much by the reaction of the host as it is by the nature of the injury.

The morphologic manifestations of disease (lesions) are no more or less important than the disorders of function. The symptoms of disease (subjective) are as significant as the signs (objective).

Our ideas of the causes of disease are changing and reflect the scientific knowledge of biology of the time and our cultural paradigms.

Classification of disease is an arbitrary but useful way to systematize our knowledge. It does not matter what the basis of the taxonomy is, so long as it is used in a rational way.

Techniques for establishing a specific diagnosis include history taking, physical examination, routine laboratory examinations, special laboratory examinations, radiologic methods, and invasive techniques such as biopsy.

The principle of causality in our understanding of disease may be misleading. The association between two phenomena does not imply a causal relation.

Terms

Lesion	*Infarction*	*Prevalence*
Prognosis	*Iatrogenic*	*Morbidity*
Etiology	*Idiopathic*	*Mortality*
Pathogenesis	*Dyspnea*	*Attack rate*
Inflammation	*Cachexia*	*Epidemic*
Ischemia	*Death*	*Endemic*
Anoxia	*Incidence*	

MAGNETIC RESONANCE IMAGING (MRI).

The most modern diagnostic method is the application of nuclear magnetic resonance analysis to the intact patient. Impetus to the development of this imaging technique came from results which suggested that normal and malignant tissue have different relaxation times. The principle behind MRI is to use magnetic field gradients to obtain spatial (3 dimensional) information. While conventional radiology using x rays depends on the differential absorption of energy by tissues in the path of the beam and provides information on only the mass of the interposed tissue, nuclear magnetic resonance technology uses two or three magnetic fields which translate the energy of the living tissue into signals of different frequencies. These signals are then reconstructed by computer in the same way as CT scans or PET scans to provide anatomical coordinates for study.

Advantages of MRI are that it is noninvasive, does not use x rays, and has the potential of demonstrating physiological and chemical information in the living patient. Disadvantages are only the present inexperience with the extremely expensive apparatus and its complexity. For some time, like early CT scanning, its use will be limited to large centers and small numbers of patients until its promise is developed.

FURTHER READING

Auerback, P.S.: Marine envenomations. N. Engl. J. Med., 325:486, 1991.

Barsley, A.J.: The paradox of health. N. Engl. J. Med., 318:414, 1988.

Black, P. McL.: Brain death. N. Engl. J. Med., 299:393, 1978.

Burkitt, D.P.: Relationship as a clue to causation. Lancet, 2:1237, 1970.

Burnet, F.M.: A modern basis for pathology. Lancet, 1:1383, 1968.

Copeland, D.D.: Concepts of disease and diagnosis. Perspect. Biol. Med., 20:528, 1977.

Doll, J.R.R.: The pattern of disease in the post-infection era: national trends. Proc. R. Soc. Lond. (Biol.), 205:47, 1980.

Dubos, R.J.: Infection into disease. Perspect. Biol. Med., 1:425, 1957.

Feinstein, A.R.: Boolean algebra and clinical toxonomy. N. Engl. J. Med., 269:929, 1963.

Ferrucci, J.T., Jr.: Body ultrasonography. N. Engl. J. Med., 300:538, 1979.

Gardner, I.D.: The effect of aging on susceptibility to infection. Rev. Infect. Dis., 2:801, 1980.

Geller, S.A.: Autopsy. Sci. Am., 248:124, 1983.

Giulian, G.G., et al.: Elevated fetal hemoglobin levels in sudden infant death syndrome. N. Engl. J. Med., 316:1122, 1987.

Glasser, J.H.: The quality and utility of death certificate data. Am. J. Public Health, 71;231, 1981.

Goldenberg, D.M., et al.: Use of radiolabeled antibodies to carcinoembryonic antigen for the detection and localization of diverse cancers by external photoscanning. N. Engl. J. Med., 293:1384, 1978.

Hochberg, M.E.: Non-linear transmission rates and the dynamics of infectious disease. J. Theor. Biol., 153:301, 1991.

Howard, J.C.: Disease and evolution. Nature, 352:565, 1991.

Kaslow, R.A., and Shaw, S.: The role of histocompatibility antigens (HLA) in infection. Epidemiol. Rev., 3:90, 1981.

Kilbourne, E.M., et al.: Risk factors for heatstroke. J.A.M.A., 247:3332, 1982.

Kohn, R.R.: Cause of death in very old people. J.A.M.A., 247:2793, 1982.

Lasagna, L.: The diseases drugs cause. Perspect. Biol. Med., 7:457, 1963.

Mann, G.V.: The influence of obesity on health. N. Engl. J. Med., 291:178, 1974.

Mathers, C.: Who dies of what (these days)? Med. J. Australia, 154:227, 1991.

Maupin, G.O., Fish, D., Zultowsky, J., et al.: Landscape ecology of Lyme disease in a residential area of Westchester County, New York. Am. J. Epidemiol., 133:1105, 1991.

Melamed, Y., Shupak, A., and Bitterman, H.: Medical problems associated with underwater diving. N. Engl. J. Med., 326:30, 1992.

Moss, N.H., and Mayer, J.: Food and nutrition in health and disease. Ann. N.Y. Acad. Sci., 300, 1977.

Nathanson, N.: Epidemiology. In: *Virology*, 2nd Ed. Edited by B.N. Fields, D.M. Knipe, et al. New York, Raven Press, Ltd., 1990.

Osborn, J.E.: The AIDS epidemic multidisciplinary trouble. N. Engl. J. Med., 314:779, 1986.

Pace, N.: Weightlessness: a matter of gravity. N. Engl. J. Med., 297:32, 1977.

Paffenbarger, R.S., et al.: Physical activity, all cause mortality, and longevity of college alumni. N. Engl. J. Med., 314:605, 1986.

Petersen, P.: A perspective of infection and infectious disease. Perspect. Biol. Med., 23:255, 1980.

Rawlings, J.S., and Weir, M.R.: Race-specific and rank-specific infant mortality in a U.S. military population. Am. J. Dis. Child., 146:313, 1992.

Roueché, B.: *Eleven Blue Men and Other Tales of Medical Detection.* Boston, Little, Brown & Co., 1954.

Scriver, C.R.: Treatment of inborn errors of metabolism. The nature:nurture argument specified. In *Advances in the Treatment of Inborn Errors of Metabolism.* Edited by M.D'A. Crawford, D.A. Gibbs, and R.W.E. Watts. Proceedings of the Second Clinical Research Center Symposium, September, 1981. New York, John Wiley & Sons, 1982, pp. 289–303.

Scriver, C.R.: Window panes of eternity. Health, disease, and inherited risk. Yale J. Biol. Med., 55:487, 1982.

Selzer, R.: *Mortal Lessons, Notes in the Art of Surgery.* New York, Simon & Schuster, 1976.

Shute, N.: *On the Beach.* New York, Morrow, 1957.

Sullivan, L.W.: Healthy people 2000. N. Engl. J. Med., 323:1065, 1990.

Upton, A.C.: Low-dose radiation. Postgrad. Med., 70:34, 1981.

Wagner, Jr., H.N.: Highlights of Nuclear Medicine. I.J.N.M., 5:1, 1990.

West, J.B.: Human physiology at extreme altitudes on Mount Everest. Science, 223:784, 1984.

Withers, R.T., et al.: Some aspects of metabolism following a 35 km road run. Eur. J. Appl. Physiol., 63:436, 1991.

Zylke, J.W.: Declining childhood immunization rates becoming a cause for concern. J.A.M.A., 266:1321, 1991.

APPENDIX

Deficiency Disease in General Including Vitamin Deficiencies

Mineral Deficiency. Among the important minerals that may be deficient in the food are calcium, iron, and iodine. **Calcium** is necessary both for the formation and the continued health of bone. If it is deficient in the diet during early childhood, there is danger that rickets may develop; bones that are deficient in calcium are soft and easily bent, so that bowlegs and other deformities occur. In adult life calcium deficiency may lead to softening of the bone or osteomalacia. **Iron** is absolutely necessary for the synthesis of hemoglobin, and when it is deficient in the diet, anemia inevitably develops. Normal adults have 2 to 6 g of iron, of which 80% is in the hemoglobin of the erythrocytes, and 20% is in stores in the liver, spleen, or in cellular enzymes (cytochrome), or myoglobin. Normally, adults lose about 1 mg per day in the urine, stool, or sweat, and this is matched by absorption from the small bowel from dietary sources. Menstruation increases this loss to 30 mg for each period, and in pregnancy, 500 mg of iron goes to the fetus. With extra exercise (marathon training) there is an increased loss, just as there is with hemolysis (breakdown of red blood cells) whatever the cause. As will be seen when diseases of the blood are studied, anemias are now divided into iron-deficiency anemias and other forms of anemia. It is of interest to note that the most important member of the latter group, pernicious anemia, is also a deficiency disease. **Iodine** is essential to the proper functioning of the thyroid gland, and when it is deficient, one form of goiter develops. Although minerals are essential for the health of the body, the actual amounts needed are minute. For instance, the amount of iodine needed to prevent the development of goiter is only 10 to 20 mg a year. Iodine is added to salt in the western world to prevent iodine deficiency.

Potassium deficiency has come to assume a position of special importance. The deficiency of the mineral is due to loss from the body, not to an insufficient supply in the food. At least 98% of the potassium of the body is located in the intracellular fluid, mainly in the muscle cells, in contrast with sodium which is mainly in the extracellular fluid. Potassium deficiency (hypokalemia) may develop from a variety of causes, of which the most important are: (1) stress, usually the result of surgical trauma; the cells of the postoperative patient leaking potassium into the extracellular fluid and thence at once into the urine, and the leak being activated by aldosterone liberated as part of the reaction of the adrenal cortex to stress; (2) vomiting and diarrhea, when severe and prolonged; (3) deficiency caused by therapy, especially the continued intravenous administration of salt and glucose solutions, or the use of modern antihypertensive drugs that may lower the serum potassium level to a dangerous degree. The muscles suffer most, with lack of tone, weakness, and finally, paralysis. Abdominal distention so common in the postoperative patient is caused by lack of tone of the muscular wall of the intestine due to potassium depletion caused by stress. Cardiac dilatation and myocardial failure with marked changes in the electrocardiogram are among the most serious of its effects.

Other minerals or trace elements that are important in man include zinc (Zn^+), which plays a role in the healing of surgical incisions and any injury; magnesium (Mg^{++}), which is essential for protein synthesis; phosphorus (PO_4^{++}), which is fundamental to energy production and to the normal development of bone; and, naturally, sodium and chloride.

Vitamin Deficiency. An adequate supply of protein, carbohydrate, fat, and mineral salts is not sufficient for the needs of the living body. Certain "accessory food factors" are also necessary for life. These are called vitamins. They are formed or synthesized by plants, not by animals. Man's supply therefore comes directly from plants, or from animals (including fish) that have eaten the plants and have stored the vitamins—unless these happen to be bought at the corner drugstore. They need only be present in minute amounts, but their absence (avitaminosis) leads to profound pathologic changes. Some deficiency diseases, such as rickets and scurvy, have been known for centuries. Although it was not recognized that they were due to a simple deficiency in diet, empiric methods of treatment were successfully employed. The old explorers recognized the value of fresh fruit in the prevention of scurvy, and cod liver oil has been used in the treatment of rickets for more than 100 years.

The original list of 4 vitamins (A, B, C, D) has been greatly extended, and the end is not in sight. Moreover, vitamin B, a complex, has been separated into a number of distinct chemicals. With such complexity, the alphabetic system of names has broken down, and the chemical names have come into general use. Vitamins are organic catalysts of exogenous origin, which are intimately related to the enzyme systems. They play the part of coenzymes in the chemical mechanism of the cell by which foodstuffs are metabolized. In many respects they resemble hormones, the chief distinction being that hormones are endogenous in origin, whereas vitamins are exogenous, the body being unable to synthesize them.

It is customary to divide the vitamins into 2 groups, the fat-soluble and the water-soluble. The **fat-soluble vitamins** are A, D, E, and K, and the **water-soluble** ones are B and C.

Avitaminosis or vitamin deficiency may be due to 2 different conditions. (1) The supply of the food factor may be inadequate. This is known as primary deficiency, and is exogenous in origin. This is no longer of great importance in developed countries, except among food faddists and other health cranks, but it is widely prevalent in the underdeveloped countries, particularly in Africa and in the Orient. (2) The supply is adequate, but for various reasons it cannot be used properly. This is secondary conditioned deficiency. Conditioning factors may be: (1) **reduced intake,** as may occur in prolonged vomiting, esophageal obstruction, and loss of appetite; (2) **malabsorption,** such as occurs in chronic inflammation of the pancreas and small intestine; (3) **excessive demand,** seen especially in infancy and puberty, but also during pregnancy and lactation; (4) **reduced**

storage facilities, the best example being cirrhosis of the liver in the chronic alcoholic. Before proceeding to a consideration of the various vitamin deficiencies, it should be pointed out that man seldom shows the picture of pure vitamin deficiency seen in the experimental animal, and that the administration of a single vitamin in a chemically pure state may not serve to correct the condition. We now know enough, however, to prevent the 5 major vitamin-deficiency diseases, namely **beriberi** (vitamin B complex—thiamin), **pellagra** (vitamin B complex—niacin), **scurvy** (vitamin C), **rickets** (vitamin D), and **keratomalacia** (vitamin A).

Vitamin A. This fat-soluble vitamin is found in butter, cream, egg yolk, and fish liver oils, as well as in yellow and green vegetables such as carrots, spinach, peas, and beans. The plants do not really contain vitamin A, but a yellow pigment called **carotene** that is converted by the liver into the vitamin. The vitamin A content of milk and butter depends on the carotene content of the plants the animal eats. Even the vitamin in fish liver oil comes from marine plants (plankton). Minute invertebrates feed on the plants; they are devoured later by small fish; these in turn serve as food to large fish in whose livers the vitamin is stored.

Lack of vitamin A in the diet leads to change in the epithelium lining the mucus membranes in the respiratory and digestive tracts as well as in certain glands such as the lachrymal and salivary. These mucus surfaces are especially susceptible to infection. In children, in whom the deficiency is most likely to develop, drying of the cornea, known as xerophthalmia (Greek *xeros*, dry) may occur owing to lack of secretion of the lachrymal glands. Bronchopneumonia in children may be caused by the changes in the mucus membrane of the bronchial tree. A peculiar symptom is night blindness, or inability to see in a dim light. This is due to deficiency in the visual purple of the retina, a substance necessary for vision in poor light.

Under ordinary conditions of life, vitamin A deficiency is seldom seen in Europe and North America, although it is common in India, China, and other countries where the diet is often of low quality. When war brings restriction in diet, however, night blindness and xerophthalmia may become common, the former being particularly dangerous during blackouts. Governments have recognized this to such an extent that they have added vitamin A to bread when necessary.

Vitamin B Complex. One of the earliest discoveries regarding vitamins was that beriberi, a disease of the Orient, was due to eating "polished rice," i.e., rice from which the outer covering and the germ had been removed in the milling process. The vitamin responsible was called vitamin B. It is now known that what was thought to be a single vitamin is really a complex, from which a number of components have been separated. The 3 best known of these are thiamin, niacin, and riboflavin. This group of vitamins is one of the most widely distributed, being present in all natural foodstuffs. The various members of the group are water-soluble, so that they are readily absorbed, but they pay a penalty, because much is lost in the process of refining and of converting natural into artificial foods, as in the case of white bread and polished rice. Fortunately, most of the B complex vitamins used by the body are produced by the bacteria in the intestine.

Thiamin (formerly vitamin B_1) is the antiberiberi factor. The principal features of beriberi are peripheral neuritis (marked by weakness of the limbs), widespread edema, and myocardial weakness. When rice is polished, the skin and the germ, which contain the vitamin, are removed, so that in rice-eating countries such as China, beriberi is a common disease. Thiamin is now added to enriched white wheat flour, to restore what is lost from the whole wheat in milling.

Riboflavin (formerly vitamin B₂) is also desirable for the enrichment of bread, but the supply is still inadequate. Mild symptoms of its absence (ariboflavinosis) are not uncommon among the undernourished and among those women who subsist on absurdly inadequate diets with the object of improving their figures. Severe manifestations are seen principally in the southern United States and in Newfoundland. There may be fissured lesions at the corners of the mouth (cheilosis) and erosions around the eyes and the sides of the nose. The tongue may acquire a characteristic magenta color. The most serious disturbances are those involving the eye. In persons whose occupation exposes them to bright light, including workers with the microscope, there may be eyestrain and redness of the conjunctiva and the lower lids. In advanced cases there is invasion of the cornea by capillaries. In the past, these ocular symptoms were never attributed to the real cause, namely, vitamin deficiency. The principal source of riboflavin is milk.

Niacin (formerly nicotinic acid) is the pellagra-preventing vitamin. **Pellagra** is a disease common in Italy and the southern United States, but it is not confined to these regions. It is characterized by reddening and scaling of the skin on the exposed parts of the body, as well as by gastrointestinal, nervous, and mental disorders. The tongue may become smooth and fiery red. Although a deficiency disease, it is also in some way connected with eating diseased maize.

Vitamin B₁₂ is a growth factor in the maturation of red blood cells in the bone marrow. It is derived from the food, but it is absorbed from the intestine only in the presence of an "intrinsic factor" secreted by the stomach. Absence of this factor leads to the development of pernicious anemia, in which the progenitors of the red blood cells in the marrow do not develop into adult erythrocytes, but enter the blood stream as abnormally large red cells (macrocytes), which have a shortened life span, even though the bowel is full of vitamin. Vitamin B₁₂ deficiency is therefore an excellent example of a conditioned deficiency, depending on absence of the gastric intrinsic factor.

Vitamin C (Ascorbic Acid). This is the antiscorbutic vitamin, which prevents scurvy. It is particularly abundant in tomato, orange, lemon, and grapefruit. It is destroyed by heat and drying, so that preserved foods and fruits are lacking it. In vitamin C deficiency, the level of ascorbic acid is low in the urine and very low in the blood. By estimation of this level, deficiency of the vitamin can be readily detected. Linus Pauling, Nobel Prize winner, believes that taking large doses of vitamin C in the form of powdered ascorbic acid leads to increased vigor, increased protection against infections, and increased rate of healing of wounds.

When ascorbic acid is lacking, the cement substance, which holds together the endothelial cells lining the capillaries, becomes deficient. The vessels thus develop leaks through which bleeding occurs into the tissues. The health of the ground substance of the connective tissue in general also suffers.

Scurvy is the manifestation of vitamin C deficiency. It used to be a common disease among sailors, soldiers, arctic explorers, and others deprived of fresh fruit and vegetables. The old Elizabethan seaman, Captain Hawkins, called it "the plague of the sea and the spoil of mariners," adding that "the sea is natural for fishes and the land for men." That was all changed by Captain Cook's discovery that limes and lime juice would prevent the disease, and now even that is not necessary, for the vitamin can be put up as tablets of ascorbic acid.

Hemorrhage occurs owing to lack of cement substance in the capillaries. The gums are soft, spongy, bleed readily, and are heavily invaded by bacteria, while the teeth fall out, so that the condition of the mouth becomes foul and distressing. The skin presents numerous small hemorrhages (petechiae). There is hemorrhage into the joints and the internal organs. Owing to the deficient ground substance of connective tissue, there is delayed healing of wounds. After healing they tend to break down under strain. If the scorbutic condition is not relieved, it may end fatally, and in the past it frequently did so.

Vitamin D. Much of the romance of the vitamins centers around this member of the group. Several factors are concerned in the action of this vitamin, and the unraveling of these might easily have taken half a century, but the whole problem was cleared up in little more than half a dozen years by workers in many widely separated countries.

Vitamin D is the antirachitic vitamin; it prevents rickets. It does this by controlling calcium metabolism. It is a fat-soluble vitamin, and so, as might be expected, it is found in milk, butter, egg yolk, and other fats, but by far the most abundant supply is in cod liver oil.

One of the remarkable discoveries was that the vitamin is formed by the action of ultraviolet light on certain waxy compounds known as sterols, particularly ergosterol, found in yeast, and cholesterol, present in the skin. When the skin is exposed to abundant sunlight, a sufficient amount of the vitamin is formed from the cholesterol. In dark and gloomy climates, however, and in the slums of cities, there is not enough light to form the vitamin. It is prepared commercially by irradiating yeast, which is rich in ergosterol, by the mercury vapor lamp, and is then called viosterol. The vitamin has been synthesized in the laboratory; it is a yellow, crystalline substance, which has been named calciferol, because of its influence on calcification.

Without a sufficient supply of vitamin D, the proper calcification of bone in the child cannot take place, and rickets is the result. It is also required for the formation of normal teeth in the growing child. Marked deficiency of the vitamin is rare in adults, but when present it may produce osteomalacia. This disease is more likely to be seen in countries such as India and China, where the diet is deficient. It is most common in women, who are not often exposed to sunlight in those countries.

Rickets is a disease of young children. The bones are not properly formed, owing to insufficient deposition of both calcium and phosphorus. The bones are therefore soft and bend easily, so that deformities (e.g., bowlegs) result. (These deformities are described in more detail in connection with disease of bones.) The disease occurs usually in bottle-fed babies, and in young children brought up in the slums of smokey cities in northern latitudes. It is unknown in the tropics. As we have seen, it may be due to one of two factors, or often to a combination of the two: (1) insufficient vitamin D in the diet; (2) insufficient sunlight (ultraviolet), which could produce the vitamin by activating the cholesterol in the skin. There are also rare causes of rickets that may be inherited. Treatment of rickets is more successful if the correct cause is established.

There have also been tragic instances in which excessive amounts of vitamin D have been administered on the basis of "where a little is good, a lot is better". Excess vitamin D can lead to calcification in the brain and other organs.

Vitamin E. This vitamin is necessary for normal reproduction, and so it has been called the antisterility vitamin. The chief sources are the germ of various cereals and green vegetable foods. Wheat germ oil contains a large amount of the vitamin. Knowledge of its actions is limited to animals. Deficiency in female rats causes the embryo to die early, and in males spermatozoa are not produced because of degenerative changes in the testes. This has not been established for human beings.

Vitamin K. The story of vitamin K is as remarkable as that of vitamin D. In 1930 a Danish observer, Dam, noticed that chicks fed on a deficient diet developed hemorrhage, and that this was prevented when they were given alfalfa. There was evidently some factor in the alfalfa that was necessary for the coagulation of the blood and without which hemorrhage would occur. Soon this factor was extracted and crystallized. It was called Koagulations vitamin, German for the "vitamin that promotes coagulation;" this became shortened to vitamin K.

The **prothrombin** of the blood must be at a normal level if the coagulation of blood, which is necessary to stop hemorrhage, is to occur normally. It was soon found that animals deficient in vitamin K were also deficient in prothrombin, and so it became apparent that vitamin K is necessary for the formation of prothrombin. The mere presence of a sufficient amount of vitamin K in the food is not enough; it has to be absorbed before it can be used for the manufacture of prothrombin.

The next discovery was that the vitamin is not absorbed unless bile is present in the intestine. It had long been known that operations on jaundiced patients were apt to be followed by hemorrhage, often fatal, at the site of operation. In jaundice, the bile is unable to reach the intestine. Now it was clear that the reason for the bleeding tendency in jaundice was lack of vitamin K, that lack being due to failure in absorption, which in turn was due to absence of bile in the bowel. The prothrombin in the blood was found to be low in cases of jaundice, as was to be expected.

This was a discovery of great practical importance, because now it is possible to raise the prothrombin in the blood of jaundiced patients before operation. This is done by administering bile salts, combined with vitamin K. The vitamin is absorbed, the prothrombin rises to normal, and the operation can be performed without the danger of hemorrhage.

Another condition in which the prothrombin is low is hemorrhagic disease of the newborn. Shortly after birth the baby may show a tendency to bleed, and if there has been any birth injury to the head, there may be fatal intracranial hemorrhage. This is due to vitamin K deficiency in the baby, and can readily be prevented by administering the vitamin to the mother before delivery.

Radiation Injury

There never has been a time when the question of radiation hazards was of graver concern than it is at present.

These hazards are of three kinds, which in their order of importance may be termed diagnostic, therapeutic, and fallout hazards. **Diagnostic radiation,** when used with judgment (Fig. A3–1A), presents so small a hazard to health that it is completely outweighed by the potential for good. If overdone and repeated too frequently, it may be a source of danger. **Therapeutic radiation** obviously involves greater hazard, because the radiotherapist's goal is to disable or kill cancer or other undesirable cells, and in the process the normal tissue may easily be injured. In some cases the injury may be much more serious and devastating than that inflicted by the surgeon's knife. The effect of radiation depends on (1) size of dose and (2) sensitivity of tissue, to which must be added the area involved in the radiation. The dosage is expressed as roentgens or r, in honor of Roentgen, who first observed the rays or radiations from the vacuum cathode tube. **Fallout radiation,** which gives rise to total body radiation (Fig. A3–1B), may be the result of atomic or hydrogen bomb bursts in war, of atomic weapon tests, or of accidental leakage from atomic energy installations. A dose of 400 r over the total body surface is believed to be enough to kill half of a given human population.

Skin. The skin is most frequently involved, because all therapeutic external radiations must pass through the skin. **Acute radiodermatitis** is really a burn of the skin, but one that takes many days or a week or two to develop. It is equally slow in healing, and scarring may go on for many months, causing marked deformity. **Chronic radiodermatitis** is likely to be the result of frequent small doses. It was a common lesion on the hands of radiologists before the danger was realized and efficient screening was practiced. The epidermis is thinned and devitalized, so that minor injury may result in localized areas of necrosis that often take months to heal. The surrounding capillaries are dilated, so that the skin is red. Finally, carcinoma may develop, often after an interval of many years since the last exposure to radiation.

Lymphoid and Hematopoietic Tissues. These are the most sensitive to radiation. Damage to these tissues is most likely to be seen in total body radiation. As the life span of the lymphocyte is only a few hours, extensive injury to lymphoid tissue is immediately followed by a marked drop in the number of lymphocytes in the circulating blood. The hematopoietic cells of the bone marrow are even more sensitive than the lymphocytes. There is a striking drop in the number of circulating granular leukocytes and blood platelets, the maximum effect being seen about the end of the first week of total body radiation. By that time the bone marrow is almost acellular. If the patient survives, he is sure to suffer from recurring infections due to the lack of leukocytes as well as failure in antibody formation owing to the loss of lymphocytes, and from frequent hemorrhages due to the lack of platelets. Long-continued exposure to small doses of ionizing radiation may cause neoplasia rather than destruction of the marrow cells, which results in leukemia, an occupational hazard of radiologists before this danger was recognized. Leukemia is also liable to develop in patients receiving long-continued heavy radiation for the disabling disease of the spine, ankylosing spondylitis.

Gastrointestinal Tract. The epithelium of the stomach and intestine is continually being renewed, so that it is highly radiosensitive, but the deep location of these structures serves to protect them against external radiation of moderate intensity. When radium is implanted for the treat-

Fig. A3–1 *A,* The normal background of man-made radiation, such as x-rays, luminous watch dials, and television screens is shown in column 6 at *A,* internal emitters such as potassium 42, calcium 45, and radon at *B,* gamma rays from radium thorium and granite at *C,* and cosmic rays at sea level at *D.* The estimated total global fallout from atomic testing through the year 1961 is shown in column 7, and the annual dose suggested by the International Commission on Radiological Protection as the maximum permissible dose for the general population from all sources is shown in column 8. Compare this with the doses that would be received in the vicinity of atomic explosion shown in columns 1 and 2. The estimated level of exposure that doubles the mutation rate in mammalian germ cells is shown in column 5*B.* This diagram shows the effect of radiation at different distances from the center of an atomic blast. (*A* and *B* from Ervin, F.F., et al.: Human and ecologic effects in Massachusetts of an assumed thermonuclear attack on the United States. N. Engl. J. Med., 266:1127, 1962.)

ment of carcinoma of the cervix, the mucosa of the rectum and colon may be seriously injured, with changes comparable to the lesions of radiodermatitis. In about 2% of presumably oversensitive persons inflammatory lesions with ulceration may develop in the anterior wall of the rectum from 6 months to several years after completion of the treatment. These ulcers are painful and the partitions between the rectum, bladder, and vagina may break down with distressing results. Even if the lesions heal, there may be extensive scarring with stricture (narrowing) of the rectum.

Germ Cells. The germinal cells of the ovary and testis are highly radiosensitive, so that these organs have to be shielded with particular care in persons liable to be exposed to radiation, especially workers with radioactive material. The testicles are naturally more exposed than the deeply situated ovaries. If the cells are killed, sterility is the result. If, on the other hand, one of the chromosomes or even one of its genes is damaged, the result may be a mutation, which becomes hereditary, transmitted to future generations. This is the basis of the genetic hazard of fallout radiation resulting from the atomic bomb explosions or tests.

Acute Radiation Syndrome. This syndrome, caused by whole body radiation due to atomic fallout from the air, must be distinguished from **radiation sickness,** the result of intensive local radiotherapy, which is characterized by loss of appetite and nausea, but rarely by vomiting. The essential lesion of total body radiation is cell depletion. This applies particularly to the intestine, the bone marrow, and the testis, but with a marked difference in the latent period. After a single small total body exposure, maximum damage to the small bowel occurs within a few days, to the granulocytes of the marrow in 3 to 5 weeks, while the sperm cells reach their minimum number in about a year. In the low dose range (100 r) death is due to depression of the bone marrow; in the middle-dose range (500 r) it is due to damage to the gastrointestinal tract; in the high-dose range (2,000 r) it is the result of failure of the central nervous system. There is a wide variation in individual susceptibility both in the experimental animal and in man. There were many thousands of survivors of the Hiroshima and Nagasaki blasts who resumed their previous occupations with full vigor. Of these we hear little.

The **clinical picture** is as follows. Within two hours of exposure there is a sudden onset of anorexia (loss of appetite), nausea, fatigue, malaise, and drowsiness. By the third day the patient feels well. Some three weeks later he begins to suffer from chills, fever, malaise, and shortness of breath. These are followed in a day or so by (1) diarrhea and other evidence of ulceration of the bowel, (2) hemorrhages into the skin and from the mucus membranes due to destruction of the megakaryocytes in the bone marrow which make the blood platelets, (3) severe infections in the mouth and elsewhere due to the disappearance of the polymorphonuclear leukocytes and of the lymphocytes which make antibodies, and finally (4) severe anemia due to destruction of the blood-forming cells of the marrow.

A moving account of the development of the acute radiation syndrome in an entire community representing the last survivors of a world war fought with atomic weapons will be found in Nevil Shute's novel, *On the Beach*.

In addition to the foregoing account of radiation effects, three other types of hazard deserve mention. First, those exposed to an event such as the Chernobyl or Goiana disaster run the risk of developing cataracts, leukemia, and possibly a variety of neoplasms. Second, there is a danger that

radioactive isotope strontium-90, formed during an explosion, will be incorporated into vegetation, and eventually into milk, and then into the bones of mammals such as man. Finally, we must not forget that we are all constantly exposed to other forms of radiation such as microwaves from television sets and microwave towers. Prolonged exposure to microwaves produces headaches, a general feeling of malaise, a reduced white blood cell count, and possibly more change in our physiology and cellular function than we have detected to date.

Diagnostic Imaging—Radiology, Ultrasound, and Nuclear Medicine

X-rays are high-energy, electromagnetic waves with the ability to penetrate solid objects. The penetrance, and thus the transmission, is related to the energy of the wave and thickness, density, and relative atomic number of the object being exposed. These are collectively referred to as the attenuation characteristics. X-rays are conventionally generated by a tube external to the portion of the anatomy being radiographed (Fig. A3–2). The waves then pass into the object, where they may be absorbed, scattered, or transmitted. Those that are transmitted are routinely recorded on radiographic film, a photographic emulsion in which the degree of blackening is proportional to the degree of trans-

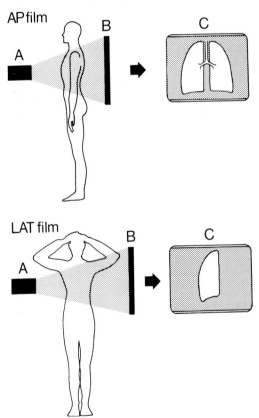

Conventional Radiology:

AP film

LAT film

Fig. A3–2 This diagram shows the source, or x-ray tube, at *A*, and the film on which the image is recorded at *B*, and the image of a developed, conventional x-ray at *C*.

mission. For many newer techniques, such as CT scanning (Fig. A3–3), the transmitted waves stimulate detectors similar to a Geiger counter. The output signals may be integrated and a visual image transmitted to a screen. Thus not all radiographic techniques use film in the conventional sense. Four major densities are described in radiology—air, fat, water, and metal. Air is the least dense and exhibits the greatest transmission. Fat is denser and transmits less; water is next, followed by metal, which is the densest and transmits least. This is why the normal air-filled lung appears black, and normal calcium-containing bone appears white.

Most of the body tissues, however, have approximately the density of water. Different organs may be identified from others by the air within them (bowel), or by the fat around them (kidney). It is difficult at times to separate one organ from another. Therefore, radiologists administer different contrast agents to outline particular organs in a selective fashion. Barium, a heavy metal, is a positive contrast agent denser than the tissues it outlines. A liquid suspension of barium is predominantly used for revealing the anatomy of the gastrointestinal tract. Iodine, also a heavy element, is used in a wider variety of examinations. Iodinated agents administered either orally or intravenously may outline the biliary tree (cholangiography, oral cholecystography), thereby enabling the radiologist to determine function as well as structure. Iodine may also be administered intravenously to demonstrate the kidneys, ureters, and bladder (intravenous urography). Some insight into the function of the organs is also provided because of the rate at which the contrast agent is taken up and excreted. Iodinated agents may also be administered directly, by catheter into blood vessels (angiography) (Fig. A3–4), into the urinary bladder and/or ureters (retrograde urography), into the pancreas (endoscopic retrograde pancreatography), into the lungs (bronchography), or by direct needle puncture into the liver (percutaneous transhepatic cholangiography), into the spinal canal (myelography), and by other techniques into other organs. These studies demonstrate structure but not function. Air (a negative contrast agent) has been used, for example, to outline the ventricular system of the brain (pneumoencephalography), which is used less and less because of the efficacy of the CT scanner.

Many of these examinations are performed under fluoroscopy. The fluoroscope is basically a screen that emits an image on stimulation by x-rays. Fluoroscopy allows the radiologist to visualize what is happening directly as it happens, rather than "after-the-fact" static images. The radiologist may record what he or she sees by cineradiologic film or on videotape, and is able to evaluate the moment-to-moment activity of a particular organ, such as the beating heart, the contracting bowel, or the moving diaphragm. Fluoroscopy may be used in conjunction with other procedures. For example, needle biopsies have been performed under fluoroscopic guidance, drugs may be delivered to specific parts of the body, catheters may be specifically

Computerized Tomography:

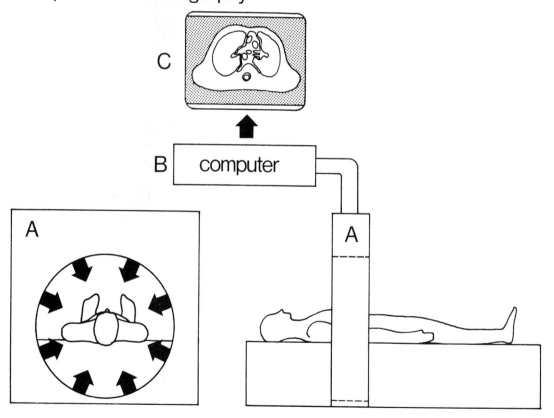

Fig. A3–3 This diagram illustrates at A the position of a patient inside the net of x-ray tubes, which are represented by black arrows. The images are interpreted by the computer and are reconstructed in cross-section representation as shown at C. Several images of CT scanning are shown in the chapter on the Central Nervous System.

Fig. A3–4   This x-ray shows the presence of iodinated, radiopaque material in the arterial tree of a patient, outlining the hepatic, renal and splenic arteries as well as the aorta. This is called an arteriogram and the technique is called angiography.

placed under fluoroscopic control, and calculi have been removed from the biliary tree with the aid of fluoroscopy.

Another technique of great importance is laminography, or tomography, which focuses on a particular section of the body by blurring out structures in front of and behind the plane of interest. This too can be used with contrast agents.

The development of **computerized tomography** (CT) has allowed the radiologist to visualize structures in a transverse plane. This device is sensitive to the attenuation characteristics of various structures. It employs computer technology to reconstruct transverse images on the basis of information fed into the computer by a series of detectors that are stimulated by x-rays transmitted in the transverse section.

Ultrasound, like CT scanning, enables one to see body section cuts in planes other than longitudinal. Ultrasound employs high-frequency sound waves rather than x-rays. The image depends primarily on the reflection of these waves, not their transmission. Waves are reflected at the interface of 2 objects of different acoustic density. A uniform cystic structure reflects waves at its front and back walls, but the uniform fluid in between is "echolucent" (Fig. A3–5). However, a solid, nonuniform structure has many internal interfaces, and is therefore "echogenic." The sound waves are generated, and the reflected waves detected, by the same device, a piezoelectric transducer. Only waves reflected from surfaces perpendicular to the angle of the beam are received by the transducer. The return signal from the transducer is fed into the electronic circuitry of the ultrasound machine, and an image is produced. The recorded image may be static (B mode), it may detail motion on a strip recording (M mode), as in echocardiography, or it may demonstrate active motion on a "real time" scanning device, as in fluoroscopy. Ultrasound, like fluoroscopy, has also been used to guide needle biopsies, for the puncture of cysts, for the placement of needles for amniocentesis, and as a guide to the obstetrician.

Ultrasound:

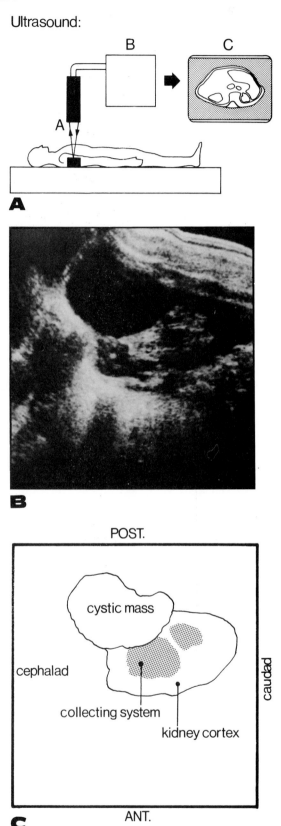

Fig. A3–5   A, This drawing shows the patient in relationship to the ultrasound emitter (B) and transducer (A), and shows the image that is created (C). B, This film shows an ultrasound image of the kidney. An interpretive drawing of the cystic mass is shown on the right.

Nuclear medicine as a diagnostic tool employs radionuclides, that is, elements that emit gamma rays and/or other charged particles. The best-known examination in nuclear medicine is the thyroid scan, which involves the uptake of radioactive iodine by gland tissue (Fig. A3–6). Gamma rays, like x-rays, are electromagnetic waves with similar properties. However, unlike x-rays, which are generated in the electron orbits of an atom, gamma rays originate in the nucleus of an atom by a radioactive decay of the nucleus. In addition, rather than being generated by an external source and recording an image by transmission, gamma rays are emitted from within organs in which radionuclides have accumulated. Emission, like transmission, is affected by wave energy and by the attenuation characteristics of the organs involved. These emitted rays do not expose films directly, as do x-rays, but rather stimulate light-emitting crystals or other types of radiation detectors in devices known as scanners or gamma cameras. The output of these detectors is then fed through electronic amplification circuitry and an image is produced.

Radionuclides may be administered orally or intravenously, and their accumulation within an organ depends on the carrier to which they are attached and on the function of the organ involved. Therefore, function takes precedence over anatomic detail. The nuclides most commonly used are Tc99m and I131, although I123, I125, Ga67, thallium, and others are available. Carriers include such compounds as methylene diphosphonate, a calcium-seeking agent that localizes in areas of active calcium hydroxyapatite turnover (bone); sulfur colloid, which is taken up by the reticuloendothelial system of the liver, spleen, and bone marrow; hepatoiminodiacetic acid, which is taken up and excreted by liver cells; hippuran, which undergoes active secretion by the renal tubules (Fig. A3–7); and albumin macro-aggregates, which embolize the microvasculature of the lung. Gallium is actively taken up by white blood cells and therefore accumulates in areas of inflammation.

Moreover, there is a therapeutic side to nuclear medicine. Radioactive iodine, an emitter of *beta* particles as well as of gamma rays, given in appropriate doses, is used to treat hyperthyroidism and either local or metastatic thyroid carcinoma.

Newer techniques involve the labeling of radionuclides to antibodies of tumor-marker antigens such as carcinoembryonic antigen (CEA), or other specific endogenous proteins, for example parathyroid hormone, so that those proteins may be quantitated or identified; the use of computers to study the active function of the heart; and the use of

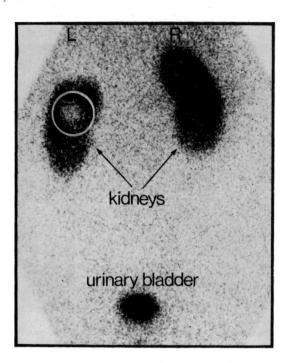

Fig. A3–7   This scan shows the presence of a normal kidney on the right, and the absence of uniform scanning on the left. Such an area could be due to a cyst or to the presence of a tumor or an abscess, for example.

radioactive blood-soluble gases to measure regional blood flow. Newer short-lived lower-dose nuclides are also being developed.

Although some of these techniques have supplanted others, these examinations are generally used in a complementary fashion. However, with benefits provided by new investigational techniques come risks. The CT scan of the thorax, for example, is noninvasive and shows the anatomy in great detail, but the dose of radiation is higher than with the equally noninvasive routine chest x-ray. Ultrasound avoids the use of damaging ionizing radiation; however, the long-term effects of high-frequency sound waves are not known. Contrast agents such as iodine are invaluable in defining anatomy, but they run the risk of allergic reactions. Ionizing radiation in general has deleterious effects on actively growing cells. However, when in the hands of persons skilled in its proper use and aware of its dangers, its long-term benefits far outweigh its risks.

A new method using gamma cameras and computer analysis called PET scanning for *Positron Emission Tomography* has made possible the visualization and localization of small amounts of isotopes in organs of the body. For example, when visual cells in the brain are working, reading a signal, their metabolism increases and they consume more oxygen and glucose than when the eyes are closed. If, in an experimental situation, radioactively labeled glucose is injected into the arteries of the brain, and the eye is opened to a strong, visual image, a gamma computer can show the increased concentration of the isotope in the part of the brain that is working to read the image. This scintillation imaging holds real promise, not only to understand normal function, but possibly also to localize tumors when they are small enough that they can be easily removed, before they invade and destroy tissue and the host.

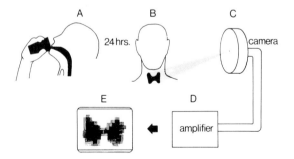

Fig. A3–6   This drawing shows the administration of a radioactive substance at *A*, the delay of 24 hours and the concentration of this radioactive iodine in the thyroid at *B*, and the scintillation counter at *C*, which records the uptake of the emissions and projects them, *D*. The result is the computer-aided image at *E*.

4

DISTURBANCES OF BLOOD FLOW AND DERANGEMENTS OF BODY FLUIDS

All problems are divided into two classes: soluble questions, which are trivial, and important questions, which are insoluble.—G. SANTAYANA

NORMAL FLUID EXCHANGE

Before we consider abnormal or pathologic changes in blood and body fluid, let us review the forces in the circulatory system that provide nourishment to all our tissues and that keep the "vital juices flowing." The central pump, the heart, provides energy with each contraction (systole) sufficient to move the plasma and blood cells around the arterial, capillary, and venous circuit, so that no cell is without oxygen or glucose or chokes in its own waste for more than a few seconds during the 70 or more years of a normal human life. How does this miniature irrigation system achieve this goal? The English physiologist Starling was perplexed by this problem. Although he understood that the pressure of 150 mm of mercury (mm Hg) in the aorta was sufficient at the time of each ventricular contraction to provide a reservoir of energy to pump blood through the circulation, he could not see how fluid from the small capillaries, if it moved into the interstitial space, moved back into the capillary bed. If the circulation was to continue to function, there had to be some mechanism to return fluids from the tissue spaces to the vascular compartment, to keep the blood volume constant. The lymphatic circulation certainly did not accumulate all this material. Starling proposed that one of the forces at work in the microcirculation was the hydrostatic pressure at the arteriolar end of the capillary bed, the net effect of which was to move water, salts, and small organic molecules across the capillary wall to the neighboring cells, to which they provided nourishment. At the same time, at the venous end of the capillary, small molecules, salts, and water had to return to the vascular lumen. This could happen if there were an equal and opposite force to the hydrostatic

pressure to attract the small molecules back into the circulation, and Starling proposed that the osmotic pressure of the plasma proteins was just such a force. This is shown in Fig. 4–1. Large molecules such as albumin, fibrinogen, and prothrombin cannot normally move across the capillary wall.

This microcirculation, then, provides for a constant exchange between the vascular and interstitial compartments, bringing oxygen, glucose, calcium, sodium, and fatty and amino acids to the cell, while at the same time returning lactate, carbon dioxide, urea, and other conventional waste products to the general circulation.

Simple perturbations in this scheme can be imagined. If there are inadequate numbers of protein molecules (hypoalbuminemia), free water will not return to the vascular compartment (Fig. 4–2). If the hydrostatic pressure is raised at the venular end, water will not return to the capillary (Fig. 4–3). If the capillary walls become indiscriminately permeable, the whole system fails because there is no maintenance of the vascular volume (shock) (Fig. 4–4). We shall consider these changes under appropriate headings.

EDEMA

An abnormal collection of fluid in tissue spaces (extravascular compartment) is called **edema.** This may be local, for example when the lymphatic or venous drainage in a person's leg has been partially blocked. Edema may also be generalized in all the dependent portions of the body, as when venous pressure is raised because of congestive heart failure. It may also occur in the pulmonary circulation. This last situation

NORMAL

Fig. 4–1   *A*, This diagram illustrates the gradient of pressures from the arteriolar to the venular end in the capillary bed. Joining the arteriole and venule is the capillary, the arrows indicating the relative forces moving fluids into the interstitial space and into the lymph. (After Landis, E.M., and Pappenheimer, J.R.: Exchange of substances through the capillary walls. In *Handbook of Physiology*. Section 2: Circulation, Vol. II. Edited by Hamilton and Dow. Washington, D.C., American Physiological Society, 1963.)

NORMAL

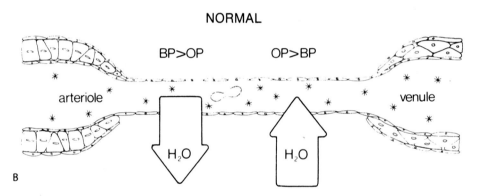

Fig. 4–1   *B*, This diagram demonstrates the cellular nature of the arteriolar capillary and venular bed and illustrates diagrammatically the red blood cells and proteins (shown as stars).

EDEMA

Fig. 4–2   The protein most responsible for the osmotic pressure gradient is albumin (symbolized by the stars within the capillary lumen). If the body loses albumin (e.g., by excretion through a diseased kidney), or if it has a problem in production (e.g., a diseased liver), hypoalbuminemia will result. Here, the level of albumin in the blood is too low to produce a sufficient osmotic pressure gradient across the capillary wall, and flow cannot return as normal. This is symbolized by the smaller, unequal arrow on the right side of the diagram and the notation that the blood pressure (BP) is equal to the osmotic pressure (OP) (unlike the normal situation shown in Figure 4–1B), resulting in edema.

HEART FAILURE

Fig. 4–3 This diagram illustrates what happens to the equilibrium at the capillary bed when the venous pressure is raised. Here, the hydrostatic pressure is raised either because of an obstruction (e.g., tumor), or because of congestive heart failure. Raised hydrostatic pressure at the venous end interferes with the normal gradient and fluid cannot return to the capillary. Excess fluid in the interstitial space is called edema.

is perhaps the most common emergency in an acute myocardial infarct in which the left ventricle fails and the venous pressure rises, leading to pulmonary edema and extreme shortness of breath. When edema fluid accumulates in the interstitial tissues of the leg or the hand, one may displace the fluid by pressure in the same way that one might leave a fingerprint on an over-ripe melon. However, when there is edema in the lung, one cannot see or feel the interstitial fluid externally; nevertheless, it is often possible to hear, with the stethoscope, moisture in the alveoli that sounds like tissue paper rustling or, in extreme cases, like bubbles with each breath. These are called rales and are a clinical sign of pulmonary edema of which anxiety and breathlessness are symptoms. Pulmonary edema constitutes a medical emergency, whether the cause is high altitude, sickness, or acute heart failure (Fig. 4–5).

There are three general causes of edema. The first of these, and perhaps the easiest to understand, is the **general or systemic loss of selective permeability of the capillary wall.** This may occur in anoxia, shock, or severe allergic response. This permeability permits all contents of the capillary (large and small molecules) to escape into the interstitial space, and it effectually brings about a major loss of blood volume, thereby precipitating a state of shock because of the lack of tissue perfusion. The loss of the selective permeability, which normally retains plasma proteins within the capillary bed, occurs locally in inflammation and is responsible for the local production of increased tissue fluid. When this fluid accumulates in a compartment, such as the pericardial sac or pleural space, it is often referred to as an **effusion** (Fig. 4–6). Collections of fluid can be readily aspirated and examined for their specific characteristics, which merely suggest the mechanism that has caused their accumulation. If the fluid accumulates in the peritoneal cavity, it is referred to as **ascites.**

Thus it is that one may well find in the same patient both the presence of pulmonary edema and a pleural effusion. This brings us to a second major general

SHOCK

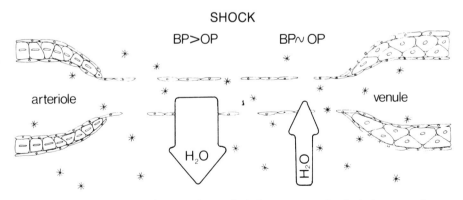

Fig. 4–4 Owing to inflammation, the capillary may become abnormally leaky. Protein (and cells) leak out into the tissue, which causes local edema (as in the swelling of an infected finger). Because of this change in permeability, the normal gradients for exchange cannot be maintained and there is a net loss of fluid to the interstitial space that results in edema. These diagrams (Figs. 4–2 to 4–4) thus illustrate three mechanisms that result in edema: hypoalbuminemia, increased hydrostatic pressure, and increased capillary permeability.

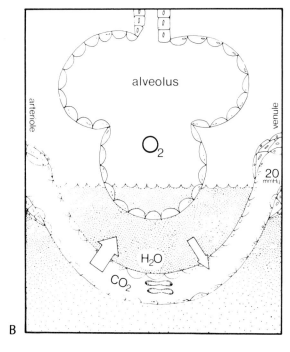

PULMONARY EDEMA

Fig. 4–5 This figure illustrates the normal and edematous lung. In *A*, venous pressure is normal, as is fluid exchange between capillary and tissue space. In *B*, venous pressure is raised, as in left heart failure. This increased pressure interferes with fluid exchange; water and small molecules pass out of the capillary under normal arteriolar pressure, but are then prevented from returning by the high venous pressure. Thus fluid accumulates in the interstitial space and interferes with gas exchange, because the distance between capillary and alveolus is increased. Eventually, fluid passes into the alveolus, where it may be perceived as bubbling rales on auscultation of the chest.

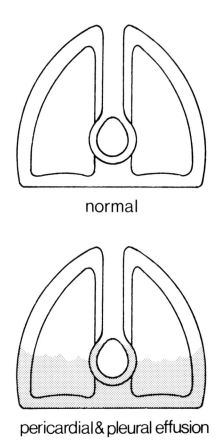

Fig. 4–6 This drawing shows the presence of a pleural effusion in schematic diagram. It also shows a pericardial effusion caused either by increased hydrostatic pressure or by disequilibrium of the normal distribution of fluid between the circulation and the tissue spaces. The normal relationships show the heart in the center of the drawing lying within its sac (pericardium) and the lungs on either side, lying in the pleural spaces.

cause of the displacement of vascular equilibrium that leads to edema. **Any increase in pressure at the venous end of the capillary bed, or increase in venous pressure anywhere,** whether it is right heart failure or a small benign pelvic tumor pressing on an ovarian vein, **decreases the ease with which interstitial fluid returns to the capillary at the venular end.** The fluid that has passed out of the normal capillary (small molecules and water) remains in the interstitial space. Eventually it may find its way back to the circulation. Such a fluid without any protein (or only small amounts) is called a **transudate** to distinguish it from the protein-rich fluid (greater than 3 g per 100 ml) that is generally referred to as an **exudate.** Thus the pleural effusion (and the edema fluid in the lung) in congestive heart failure are typically clear and have a low specific gravity, whereas the effusion seen with pneumonia (an inflammation) may have a higher specific gravity, may even form fibrin threads because of the protein (fibrinogen) present, and may show the presence of white blood cells. All of these characteristics testify to the loss of selective permeability that is characteristic of an exudate. If the fluid in the pleural space contains enough white blood cells to be considered as pus, we speak of a purulent exudate, and if there is a great amount of fibrin, we talk about fibrinopurulent exudate, but we are getting ahead of ourselves and beginning to talk aspects of inflammation.

The third general cause of increased interstitial or tissue space fluid (edema) is any **decrease in the osmotic pressure of plasma proteins.** As we have said, the principal serum protein responsible for osmotic pressure is serum albumin, synthesized in the liver. The pool of serum albumin so essential to maintaining the vascular equilibrium can be reduced in several ways. It may simply be lost by the body more rapidly than it is made, as happens with the kidney disease, glomerulonephritis. This renal loss is referred to as proteinuria, or more specifically as albuminuria, and is detected routinely on urinalysis. We shall discuss this further in the chapter on kidney disease.

A second reason for the fall of serum albumin (hypoalbuminemia) is the failure of the liver to synthesize adequate amounts of albumin. One reason may be simply starvation, in which the ingredients (amino acids) for albumin synthesis (protein) are not available in the diet. With the prolonged loss of albumin, one of the tissue compartments, the peritoneal cavity, may accumulate vast amounts of watery fluid (ascites) to produce a bloated belly, as seen in the prison camps of World War II and in the starving populations of poor countries. Another cause of hypoalbuminemia is the failure of liver cells to function, because they themselves have been poisoned or injured, as in toxic or viral (hepatitis) injury to the liver. Here again, the dramatic accumulations of edema fluid in the peritoneal cavity (transudate) may reach 10 or more liters.

Sometimes there are local accumulations of fluid following surgical explorations or operations. Occasionally, this happens to the arm or the side from which a breast tumor has been removed. This form of edema may be attributed to interference with another circulation, namely that of the lymphatics. If the lymphatic drainage system is blocked, fluid accumulates. We can distinguish between lymphedema and edema caused by venous obstruction, but in the end, because the lymphatics drain through the thoracic duct into the venous system, one might consider the disorder to follow the same general principle as its cause, namely, interference with the hydrostatic forces normally at play.

HEMORRHAGE

When a vessel ruptures, blood escapes naturally into the surrounding tissue or onto a free surface. The hemorrhage may be large and form a swelling known as a **hematoma.** Or the hemorrhages may be as small as a pin's head and are then called **petechiae.** The significance of bleeding depends on the size and the site of the hemorrhage. If it occurs into a muscle, it does little damage, but if it takes place in the brain or on a free surface such as the interior of the stomach, where it cannot be arrested, it may cause death. Rupture of an artery or vein may be produced in several ways: (1) The most common cause is **trauma,** a wound or bruise (Fig. 4–7). (2) An ulcer or a cancer in the neighborhood of a large vessel may finally perforate the wall and give rise to profuse hemorrhage; this may happen in the esophagus or the stomach (Fig. 4–8), or in a tuberculous cavity in the lung. (3) The wall of the vessel may be weakened by a condition such as **atherosclerosis,** and finally give way under the pressure of the blood; this is what often happens in cerebral hemorrhage (Fig. 4–9). Sometimes this is preceded by a localized bulging of the vessel wall, known as an **aneurysm.**

The remarkable thing about hemorrhage is not that it should occur, but that it should ever stop. If a hole is made in a pipe through which water is passing, the water will flow out until the pipe is empty. It is true that if we fill the pipe with a glue-like material too thick to pass through a small hole, none will escape, but such a material would never be able to flow through the small arteries and the minute capillaries. The wonder in the case of hemorrhage is how a fluid thin enough to pass through the finest channels

Fig. 4–7   This large black mass is an extradural hemorrhage that occurred following traumatic injury to the head. The skull fracture led to arterial bleeding, and the hematoma has compressed the underlying brain substance, as can be seen immediately beneath the extradural hematoma. (McGill University, Department of Pathology Museum.)

Fig. 4–8   The circular structure in the center of the photograph is an ulcer in the first portion of the duodenum. At the base of this ulcer can be seen a small dark dot, which is an eroded artery. This peptic duodenal ulcer eroded into a blood vessel and caused a massive hemorrhage into the gastrointestinal tract. (McGill University, Department of Pathology Museum.)

ceases after a short time to flow through a comparatively large opening in the vessel wall.

The arrest of hemorrhage is brought about by the **coagulation** or clotting of the blood. As long as the blood is inside the vessel, it does not clot, but when it escapes into the surrounding tissue or onto the surface of the skin, it begins at once to coagulate. Soon the clot is able to plug the hole in the vessel, unless that hole is much too large. The clotting of blood is due to the interaction of substances in the plasma such as **fibrinogen** and **thrombin.**

Thrombin is formed by the interaction of prothrom-

Fig. 4–9   This cross section of brain shows an intracerebral hemorrhage (dark area) which has occurred in the thalamus of the brain and has shifted structures across the midline. This hemorrhage occurred in a patient who had hypertension and was attributed to rupture of an arteriosclerotic blood vessel. (McGill University, Department of Pathology Museum.)

bin and calcium. Prothrombin is a substance of great importance; when a person suffers from vitamin K deficiency, his prothrombin level is low and the blood loses the ability to clot. Heparin (antithrombin) prevents this mechanism from making the blood clot in the vessels of a normal person; it acts by preventing prothrombin and calcium from uniting to form thrombin. Heparin is present in minute quantities in the blood. It was first obtained from the liver, hence its name (Greek *hepar*, liver), but it is also present in large amounts in the lung and intestine. When blood is shed, blood platelets are activated and liberate thromboplastin, which neutralizes heparin, and when it is eliminated, the whole complex machinery of clotting is set in motion. A clot is formed of interlacing threads of **fibrin.** These threads seal over the opening in the vessel in much the same way as the threads of a spider's web might do. The plug is greatly reinforced by the blood platelets, particles that float in the plasma and aggregate to form a sticky mass that effectually seals up the hole in the vessel wall. In time this emergency plug is converted into fibrous or scar tissue, just as an inflammatory exudate becomes changed into scar tissue, and the opening is closed permanently. The coagulation mechanism is more complex than is outlined here, and the reader is referred to Chapter 23, entitled "Blood and Lymph Nodes."

Occasionally, although fortunately rarely, the mechanism for the temporary arrest of hemorrhage is defective, so that the blood continues to flow out of the vessel. This condition is most marked in the hereditary disease called **hemophilia,** sufferers from which are known as "bleeders" who may die of hemorrhage from a trivial wound, cut, or tooth extraction. Their essential defect is a lack of a globulin fraction of the plasma known as the antihemophilic factor (AHF). When this factor is added to hemophilic blood, it causes coagulation to occur, and when it is injected into the patient, clotting time is reduced. Prothrombin seems not to be used properly in the hemophiliac. Hemophilia is a good example of sex-linked heredity; only the males of a family exhibit the disease, and only the females transmit it (Fig. 4–10). Most readers are familiar with the story of the Czar of Russia's only son, so well told in *Nicholas and Alexandra* by R. Massie.

THROMBOSIS

Speaking teleologically, clotting of the blood should occur when the blood escapes from the vessel, but not when it is flowing through the lumen of the vessel. Should this occur, it is called thrombosis; the clot within the vessel is known as a thrombus. It consists

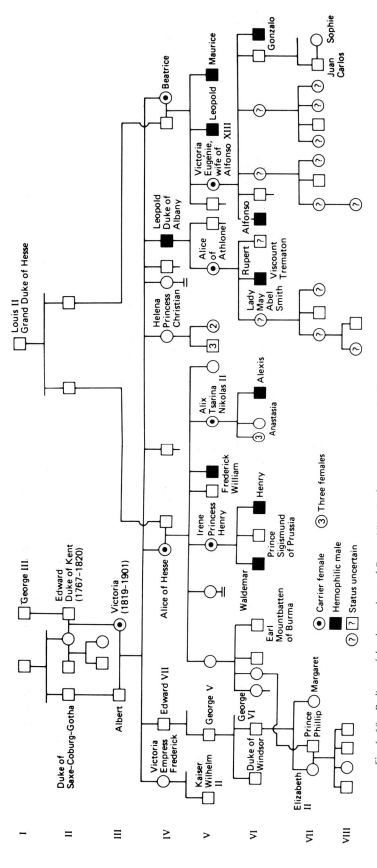

Fig. 4–10 Pedigree of the descendants of Queen Victoria showing carriers and afflicted males possessing the X-linked gene conferring the disease hemophilia. (McKusick, V.: *Human Genetics*, 2nd Ed. Englewood Cliffs, N.J., Prentice Hall, 1969.)

mainly of platelets that adhere to the vessel wall, fibrin, and red blood cells trapped in the mesh, which gradually form a mass that may finally close the lumen of the vessel and stop the flow of blood through it. A thrombus may be defined as a mass formed from constituents of the blood on the inner surface of the heart or a blood vessel. The difference between a clot formed postmortem or in a test tube, and one that forms in the flowing stream of an artery, vein, or chamber of the heart, is that in a tube or after death the heaviest elements, the red blood cells, gravitate to the bottom and the lighter fibrin forms a jelly-like clear layer on top, whereas during life thrombosis occurs in layers. First, a layer of platelets attaches to the injured vessel, then some fibrin forms and snares some red blood cells. The process then repeats itself. These layers were described and are referred to as the lines of Zahn, after their discoverer. It has been said with some truth that throughout his entire existence man is almost constantly hemorrhaging or thrombosing.

The causes of thrombosis are threefold, as Virchow stated over 100 years ago (Virchow's triad). They are: (1) **slowing of the blood stream,** (2) **changes in the vessel wall,** and (3) **changes in the blood itself**. As the first of these factors is more common in veins than in arteries, it is natural that thrombosis usually should occur in veins. The normal vessel has an exquisitely smooth lining known as the endothelium. When this is destroyed by injury or inflammation, platelets adhere to the rough spot and gradually build up a thrombus from the blood as it flows past. The slower the flow, the more likely are the platelets to fall out of the stream and to adhere to the vessel wall, so that thrombosis is associated with varicose (dilated and tortuous) veins (Fig. 4–11) and a slowed circulation. Thrombosis frequently follows abdominal operations, particularly on the pelvic organs. Closely related to this is the thrombosis that may occur in the puerperium, the period following childbirth. This phenomenon is due to the unusual dilatation and stasis in the pelvic veins caused by the growing uterus. When the child has been delivered, the veins cannot involute so rapidly and remain a site for stasis, thrombosis, and potential embolization.

Stasis is the name given to slowing of the circulation. It occurs most frequently in inactive or immobilized persons. In addition to inactivity, any impairment of cardiovascular function (heart failure) may also lead to slowing of the blood stream.

Changes in the vessel wall can occur acutely or with chronic disease. After any surgical intervention, there may have been local pressure from a retractor or an anoxic injury due to transient ischemia that would

Fig. 4–11   Varicose veins. Although these are dramatic and aesthetically unpleasing, they are infrequently a cause of thrombophlebitis and pulmonary embolism. The deep femoral veins are the most likely source of pulmonary emboli. (The Evans Collection, Osler Library, McGill University.)

affect the venous or arterial endothelium. This local acute injury sets the scene for thrombosis. On a long-term basis, there may be loss of the endothelium with the progression of atherosclerosis in the arterial tree. This loss also predisposes a patient to thrombus formation, particularly in the abdominal aorta, and occasionally in smaller vessels such as the coronary arteries or the circle of Willis at the base of the brain.

Changes in the blood itself can occur with lesions that result in deoxygenation, such as intracardiac shunts due to congenital heart disease. The body makes up for the deoxygenation by a compensatory increase in red blood cell numbers (polycythemia). When the blood cell number increases, the circulating blood itself (plasma and cells) becomes more viscous. This viscosity often precipitates thrombus formation. Thus cerebral thromboses are a complication of congenital, cyanotic heart disease. There are changes in the clotting and fibrinolytic mechanisms that may alter the blood's predisposition either to remain liquid and free-flowing or to form thrombi in the arterial or venous system.

While the principal sites of thrombosis are the veins and the heart, thrombosis may also occur in arteries, particularly in the coronary arteries, the cerebral arteries, and the arteries to the leg in elderly persons. In all of these cases there may be preliminary narrowing of the lumen by arteriosclerosis. The veins of the leg are frequently affected because of the tendency for postoperative and puerperal thrombosis to involve these veins. Thrombosis of the veins of the leg is also common in chronic heart failure, owing to the sluggish circulation, particularly when a patient is confined to bed for some time. A number of cases of thrombosis in the legs followed by fatal pulmonary embolism occurred during World War II in London air raid shelters in elderly persons who sat all night in deck chairs, the wooden supports of which pressed continuously on their thighs. The leg is swollen owing to interference with the return of blood, and the thrombosed vein may be felt as a hard tender cord. In the heart, a common site of thrombus formation is an inflamed valve, on which the platelets are deposited as the blood flows past, until they form a large thrombus that, in this situation, is known as a vegetation. Even more common is thrombus formation in one of the atria, particularly in the part called the atrial appendage, a kind of cul-de-sac in which the blood is apt to stagnate.

Thrombosis may be a serious complication of surgical operations, particularly in operations on large blood vessels such as arteries. This can now be anticipated by the use of heparin, which prevents the platelets from sticking together and to the vessel wall, so that a thrombus is not formed. Heparin has also been used to prevent thrombosis in the veins of the leg after an operation. The action of the substance dicumarol resembles that of heparin in prolonging the coagulation time, but it has the advantage over heparin of a much more prolonged action, and it can be taken by mouth instead of by injection.

The subsequent fate of a thrombus varies: (1) The thrombus may become converted into fibrous tissue with permanent closure of the vessel. (2) It may contract or become canalized so that blood can flow through the lumen once again (Fig. 4–12). (3) Finally, parts or all of the thrombus may become detached from the vessel wall and enter the blood stream as a floating body known as an **embolus,** a catastrophic occurrence, as we shall see in the next section. This detachment of the thrombus is particularly likely to occur when there is sepsis at the site of thrombosis as the infection predisposes the thrombus to break down and become loosened (Fig. 4–13). Another factor may be rough handling of the part. It is evident that a thrombosed leg has to be treated with the greatest care, and that anything in the nature of massage must be avoided.

Fig. 4–12 An arterial thrombus showing canalization. Photomicrograph. (Bell, E.T.: *Textbook of Pathology*, 8th Ed. Philadelphia, Lea & Febiger, 1956.)

Fibrinolysis. Blood clots are not necessarily permanent structures, and nature tries to remove an obstructing thrombus by means of fibrinolytic enzymes in the blood. One enzyme, called plasmin or fibrinolysin, is a globulin. It exists in the form of a precursor, plasminogen, and it digests the fibrin of the thrombosis. Unfortunately, nature is often far from successful in its efforts, although it must be admitted that myocardial infarction associated with thrombotic occlusion of the coronary arteries is accompanied by the production of fibrinolysin. In view of the serious damage that a thrombus can do in obstructing such arteries as the coronaries and cerebrals, not to mention the veins, great efforts have been made to find some substance that would dissolve the thrombus. Today several fibrinolytic enzymes are available for direct in-

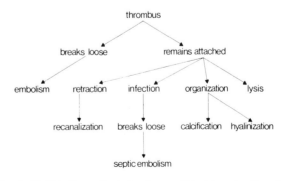

Fig. 4–13 This figure illustrates the possible fates of a thrombus. (Adapted from Walter, J.B.: *An Introduction to the Principles of Disease.* Philadelphia, W. B. Saunders Co., 1977.)

travascular use or by injection. Early results indicate that they may be very useful in some clinical situations.

EMBOLISM

An embolism may be a thrombus that has become detached and has entered the blood stream. As it is most commonly a vein that is the site of the thrombus, and as the veins become larger as the heart is approached, it follows that the embolus will meet with no obstruction in its voyage to the heart. But no sooner has it passed through the right side of the heart and entered the pulmonary artery that carries the blood to the lungs than the chances of arrest of the thrombus increase with every millimeter the embolus

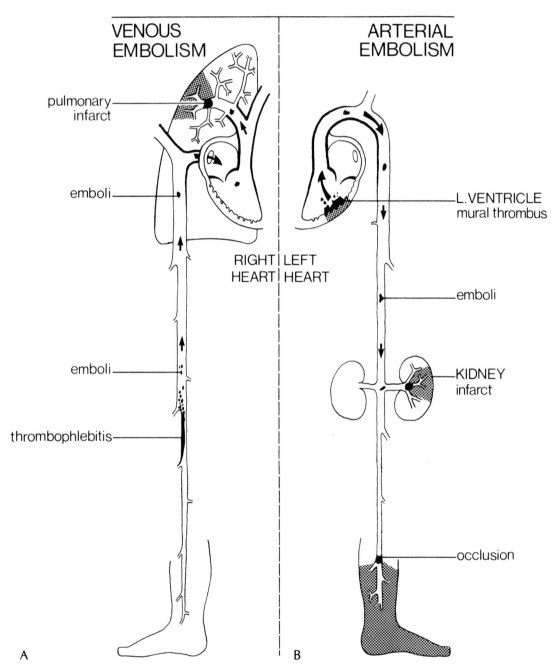

Fig. 4–14   This set of diagrams illustrates the complications and eventual fates of embolism. In *A*, a venous embolism arises in thrombophlebitis in a leg vein. It may pass through the inferior vena cava into the right heart and out to the pulmonary artery, causing pulmonary infarcts. Arterial embolism, shown in *B*, arises on a mural thrombus in the left ventricle, possibly arresting in a branch of the cerebral blood vessels, causing kidney infarcts, or occluding peripheral vessels.

travels, for the arteries become narrower the farther they pass from the heart. Finally, the embolus will lodge in one of the arteries of the lung. The vessel blocked depends entirely on the size of the embolus. Indeed, the main pulmonary artery may be blocked if the embolus is sufficiently large.

Embolism refers to occlusion of some part of the cardiovascular system by impaction of a foreign mass transported to the site through the blood stream.

An embolus may originate in the heart instead of in a vein, usually on the left side of the heart (Fig. 4–14). The original thrombus may have been a vegetation on a valve (Fig. 4–15), as has already been described, or it may be formed in one of the chambers of the heart, usually the left atrium. In either case, the destination of the embolus is now different, for it enters the aorta, the great vessel that leaves the left side of the heart, and passes not to the lungs but to the brain, kidneys, and other organs.

There are other types of emboli besides those that originate as a thrombus. The most important of these are fat emboli, air emboli, septic emboli, and tumor emboli. **Fat embolism** occurs as the result of crushing injuries to bones, which allow the fat in the bone marrow to enter the veins in that substance in the form of globules. Fat embolism may be the cause of death in such injuries as car accidents, in which the blood loss, shock, and mechanical injuries can be managed, but the pulmonary and cerebral emboli cannot.

Air embolism is due to the entrance of air into the veins either during a surgical operation or because of the injection of air into the uterus during an attempt to produce an abortion. An air embolus is a bubble too large to dissolve that may eventually occlude a small vessel. The oxygen in the bubble is useless to the cells in the area because they can only use dissolved oxygen.

Septic emboli occur in bacterial endocarditis and when bacterial colonies either are growing in veins or gain access to the circulation.

Tumor emboli are groups of cancer cells that have invaded a vein, become detached, and are then carried to the lungs or other organs. It is by this means that cancer is disseminated throughout the body with the formation of secondary growths known as **metastases.**

Effects of Embolism. When an embolus lodges in an artery, it blocks the lumen and cuts off the blood supply to the organ or part supplied by that artery. The effect depends on the size of the embolus and on the circulatory arrangements of the part. It is obvious that if an embolus is large enough to block the main artery to an organ or a limb, the effect will be as disastrous as the cutting off of the main water supply to a city. In the case of a smaller embolus, the question of the vascular connections is all-important. In most parts of the body there is what is called a **collateral circulation,** a communication between two sets of arteries. The blood to the hand is carried by two main arteries, one on each side of the wrist, and between the branches of these there pass numerous small communicating vessels (Fig. 4–16). Should one of the main arteries be blocked by an embolus or be ligatured, the communications from the remaining artery become greatly dilated, so that sufficient blood can still reach the area supplied by the blocked vessel. Under these circumstances, an embolus does little or no harm. The availability of collateral circulation determines the outcome of occlusion in the systemic circulation.

There is another consideration, namely, that organs such as the lung and liver have a double blood supply. Each segment of the lung is perfused by blood from

Fig. 4–15   This figure shows the aortic valve with the two coronary artery ostia arising above the valve cusps. Just below the free margin of the valve cusps is an irregular fibrinous material which is gray and shaggy. This is an area of endocarditis from which platelet and bacterial emboli were liberated into the arterial blood stream. These may lodge in the brain, kidneys, spleen, or terminal branches of the arterial tree. Occasionally they may even find their way into those coronary arteries. (McGill University, Department of Pathology Museum.)

Fig. 4–16   This drawing shows the advantage of a collateral circulation. The ulnar artery can be occluded and still the fingers may be supplied by the radial artery.

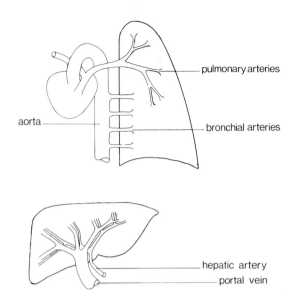

Fig. 4–17 These diagrams show the dual circulation to the lung and the liver. The lung receives venous blood from the right heart through the pulmonary arteries (one circulation). This blood is oxygenated in the lung, returns to the left heart, and is pumped out into the aorta. The bronchial arteries supply the lung with oxygenated blood from the aorta (the other circulation). The liver similarly receives both venous and arterial blood. The portal vein carries deoxygenated blood from the spleen, stomach, intestine, and other parts of the digestive system. The hepatic artery carries arterial blood from the aorta. One important advantage of a double circulation is a reduced susceptibility to infarcts. Both circulations must be impaired in order for the tissue to become ischemic.

Fig. 4–18 This photograph shows the thoracic and abdominal aorta, the renal arteries, and the kidneys, as viewed from the posterior aspect. At the arrow is the right renal artery which is occluded. The right kidney shows a large area of recent infarction (the pale area with the dark border). This has been caused by occlusion of the renal artery by embolic material from a mural thrombus. (McGill University, Department of Pathology Museum.)

both the pulmonary artery (pulmonary circulation) and the bronchial artery (systemic circulation) (Fig. 4–17). This dual supply provides a safety factor, for if there is a small embolus to a small branch of the pulmonary artery, that part of the lung does not die, since it is also supplied by its respective bronchial artery. However, if there is a degree of heart failure present, the auxiliary circulation may be inadequate, and the embolism may cause an infarct despite the dual circulation.

Infarction. It is a different matter, however, if the main artery to a limb, such as the femoral artery in the thigh, is blocked. Here there can be no efficient collateral circulation and the tissues are completely deprived of their blood supply and die. A similar state of affairs exists in a number of organs such as the brain, heart, kidney, and spleen. Each organ is supplied by arterial blood and drained by a system of veins. If the arterial supply is occluded by a thrombus or embolus, by mechanical means (traumatic injury), or even by surgical intervention (ligature or clamp), the organ thus deprived of blood may undergo ischemic coagulative necrosis, provided the interruption lasts for a significant time. This is called ischemic

(or anoxic) infarction, and is demonstrated in the kidney (Fig. 4–18) and the spleen (Fig. 4–19), where the infarcts appear as pale areas. The arterial blood does not reach parts of the organs and the cells become mummified following prolonged anoxemia (Fig. 4–20B).

Another cause of infarction is occlusion of the venous system (Fig. 4–20A). This may occur by simple thrombosis or by a thrombus initiated by compression from outside a vein (as in many cases of cancer). In

Fig. 4–19 This section of the spleen shows 2 large infarcts, one in the center of the picture, and one in the right hand corner. The infarcts are pale areas caused by arterial occlusions. (McGill University, Department of Pathology Museum.)

A

B

Fig. 4–21   This photograph shows small bowel (white) which is normal, and infarcted bowel (dark) caused by thrombosis of the mesenteric vein. (McGill University, Department of Pathology Museum.)

Fig. 4–20   *A* and *B*, These diagrams illustrate 2 mechanisms that cause infarcts. In *A*, occlusion of the outflow (venous) from an organ or a part of the circulation results in infarction because once the venous-capillary pressure equals arterial levels, no further oxygenated blood can perfuse the organ. This leads to anoxic death in an organ that is paradoxically suffused with erythrocytes. These infarcts look red (hemorrhagic) because the capillary walls are stuffed with red blood cells, but they also become permeable because of the anoxemia, and leak blood into the tissue space. *B* illustrates a more common situation, in which arterial occlusion (embolism, thrombosis) blocks perfusion of the organ, leaving it bloodless and therefore anoxemic. These infarcts are pale or white. The capillaries, if they are subsequently perfused, will leak (reflow phenomenon).

cases of venous occlusion, arterial blood enters the organ and perfuses the tissue, but cannot leave because the vein is obstructed, much as a beaver dam may raise the water level in the forest and drown the trees. So, in the case of venous thrombosis, blood rich in oxygen reaches the tissue, but cannot leave, and anoxemia occurs in this stagnant area. Then the capillaries become permeable and congestion passes to hemorrhage. This lesion is an infarct, but its appearance is different; the tissue is suffused with blood and the infarct appears as a hemorrhagic area. A good example of this is thrombosis of a mesenteric vein (Fig. 4–21). Here the bowel becomes darkly hemorrhagic due to segmental occlusion of the venous return. This kind of ischemic necrosis used to be referred to as gangrene.

It is evident that infarction is the result of a sudden cutting off of the blood supply to part of an organ with an insufficient collateral circulation. **An infarct may be produced by thrombosis as well as by embolism.** Thus an infarct of cardiac muscle is nearly always caused by thrombosis of one of the coronary arteries;

an infarct of the brain may be caused by either thrombosis or embolism of the cerebral arteries. The most frequent and important sites of infarction are the heart, lung, brain, spleen, kidney, and intestine.

Before leaving the subject we might recapitulate the importance of pulmonary embolism and infarction. The effect on the patient depends principally on the size of the embolus and collateral circulation and its competence. If the embolus is small, it will not be arrested until it reaches a correspondingly small arterial branch, and the area of the infarct produced will be equally small. The patient will experience a sharp pain in the chest, and may cough up a little blood during the next few days, after which recovery will be complete (Fig. 4–22).

Of course, if there is a competent bronchial (systemic) circulation, there need not be any infarct. The course of events is tragically different when the embolus is large enough to block the main pulmonary artery or one of its principal branches. After an uneventful, postoperative convalescence, suddenly, almost out of a clear sky, there is a strange restlessness, rapidly ensuing shock, air hunger, and collapse, and death usually in 2 to 15 minutes. The exact explanation for sudden death is not easy. We have suggested that the cause is the shock of the abrupt pulmonary ischemia. But when the surgeon ties off the main pulmonary artery before removing a lung for cancer, he does not expect the patient to die. Perhaps a more probable explanation is the release of **serotonin** from the blood platelets at the site of embolism. Serotonin, a vasoconstricting substance obtained from clotted blood as long ago as 1884, is stored in the platelets, readily released, and stimulates smooth muscle, including that of the bronchi. The full tragedy of this accident is evident in those cases in which the embo-

Fig. 4–22 This photograph of the external surface of the lung shows two large, dark areas in the center of the field. These areas are infarcts of the lung caused by recent pulmonary emboli. (McGill University, Department of Pathology Museum.)

lism occurs about a week after an abdominal operation or after childbirth, when the patient is convalescing splendidly, but after sitting up in bed suddenly feels faint, drops back on the pillow panting for breath, and is dead in the course of a few minutes. Often, however, embolism is a complication of medical rather than surgical cases, and it is particularly likely to complicate heart failure.

In all these cases the patient is confined to bed, and the condition (failing heart, childbirth, abdominal operation, immobility) tends to interfere with the flow of blood from the veins of the leg to the heart. It is in these veins that thrombosis occurs; the thrombus becomes dislodged by some sudden movement, and pulmonary embolism is the result. Precautions can be taken to prevent the stagnation of circulation that leads to thrombosis. Voluntary movements of the legs, frequent changes of position, and elevation of the foot of the bed all contribute to this end. In order to counteract the tendency to thrombosis, which is

associated with prolonged rest in bed after pelvic operations and childbirth, it has become the fashion to make the patient get up, if only for a short time, at a much earlier date than in the past.

ISCHEMIA—ITS CAUSES AND EFFECTS

Ischemia is the condition in which the blood supply to a part is diminished or stopped. It is a local rather than a general bloodlessness. As blood is carried to the part by an artery, it is evident that ischemia will be caused by anything that narrows or closes the lumen of an artery, provided the collateral circulation is not sufficiently adequate to compensate fully for the primary loss of blood supply.

The closure of the artery may be sudden or slow, and the effect varies accordingly. We have already studied the effect of sudden closure of an artery, whether by the formation of a thrombus or by the lodgment of an embolus. If the collateral circulation is inadequate, the result will be an infarct. Slow closure is due to the disease of arteries known as arteriosclerosis or atherosclerosis, commonly called hardening of the arteries (Fig. 4–23). The exact cause of this condition is not known, a matter that is discussed in Chapter 14, but it is a common condition in advancing years, just as is graying of the hair. The blood vessels begin to feel the effect of the sharp tooth of time. The subject of atherosclerosis is currently of much interest, partly because autopsies on United States soldiers as young as age 19 who were killed in Vietnam showed atherosclerosis of their coronary arteries. This evidence suggests that the American way of life was creating lesions in apparently healthy young persons. On the other hand, there are many octogenarians who die of other causes and who appear to have little atherosclerosis at autopsy. The saying that "a man is as old as his arteries" is profoundly true. The essential change is a nodular thickening of the intima or inner coat of the artery, as a result of which the lumen slowly becomes narrowed, until finally a mere chink may be left through which the blood can only trickle with difficulty. The smooth endothelium lining the vessel becomes lost in time where atherosclerosis exists, so that the inner surface is now roughened. Since platelets tend to stick to the rough surfaces, a thrombus may form, which suddenly completes the closure of the already narrowed vessel. This is what happens in **coronary artery thrombosis,** one of the most common causes of sudden death in persons over 50 years of age. The coronary arteries are the vessels that supply blood to the heart muscle, the most essential muscle in the body, and if that supply is suddenly cut off, the heart will stop beating.

The effect of ischemia is gradual death of the specialized cells of the part, i.e., nerve cells in the brain, heart muscle cells, and so on, and their replacement by scar tissue, so that the organ loses the power to do its proper work. In the brain there is failure of recent memory and of the power of accurate thinking, and there may be actual softening of the part of the brain affected owing to infarction.

Closure of the arteries in the leg and, rarely, in the arm may lead to death of the parts farthest from the heart, the toes or fingers. Here another change becomes evident, for bacteria invade the dead tissue through the skin and cause decomposition and putrefaction of the ischemic tissue. The necrotic part undergoes a series of color changes, becoming first green and finally black. The necrosis spreads slowly up the limb as the narrowing of the arteries becomes more extreme and widespread. Diabetes often leads to the occurrence of marked atheroma in the arteries of the leg, so that necrosis is a common complication in diabetic patients.

When a patient shows evidence of marked interference of the circulation in the leg, special care is necessary to prevent any injury, however trivial, that may start the process in the devitalized tissues, a process that may eventually require amputation of the affected foot. Additional care must be taken in cutting the nails, lest the toe be injured. Bandages must not be too tight, and the limb must be kept warm to encourage any circulation that may still remain in the collateral vessels. However, too much heat in the form of an electric foot warmer or a hot-water bottle is a particular source of danger.

ARTERIAL HYPERTENSION

Blood pressure in health is the result of a number of forces, the chief ones being the contractions of the heart and the peripheral resistance provided by the arterioles. In spite of rapid fluctuations in both the peripheral resistance and the cardiac output from minute to minute, depending on whether you sit or stand, are tranquil or excited, are drinking tea or eating cake, the systemic blood pressure remains remarkably constant in a normal person.

Hypertension or high blood pressure is defined by the life insurance companies as any elevation of the systolic pressure above 140 mm Hg and of the diastolic pressure above 90 mm Hg. This may be true statistically, but it does not follow that these figures can be applied to every person and thus label him as hypertensive. Pressure determinations, to carry any significance, should be made on three separate occasions with the patient in a relaxed and basal state.

Fig. 4–23   This photograph of the abdominal aorta and iliac vessels shows a markedly deformed vessel with thrombosis of the wall with thrombi superimposed on the markedly atherosclerotic vessel. Compare the appearance of this aorta with that in Figure 4–18, where only below the renal arteries is there any evidence of arteriosclerosis. (McGill University, Department of Pathology Museum.)

For some reason not understood at present, arteriosclerosis is not a general process affecting all the arteries in the body, but a selective process that picks out an artery here and there. The three principal sufferers are the heart, kidneys, and brain, to which may be added the arteries of the leg. Not all of these are attacked in the same person, so that one person may have symptoms pointing to injury to the heart, another to the kidneys, and a third to the brain. Strokes and transient ischemic attacks are usually due to thrombosis and not to hemorrhage, as used to be believed. It is probable that a hereditary or inherited weakness plays a part in the selection, for several members of one family may die of coronary thrombosis at about the same age.

This is particularly important because a diagnosis of hypertension carries with it an obligation to consider some form of treatment since serious hypertension implies a shortened life expectancy. A rise in the diastolic pressure is much more important than a similar rise in the systolic pressure. **Hypertension** is at present divided into two forms, **primary** or essential, of which the cause is unknown, and which constitutes about 90% of all cases of hypertension, and **secondary,** in which there is some associated lesion, such as chronic nephritis or tumor of the adrenal cortex, that is proven to be responsible for the elevated blood pressure.

Essential Hypertension

This is the term commonly used for the primary variety, that is where there is no demonstrable cause for the elevated blood pressure. It is divided in turn into so-called benign and malignant forms. The **benign form** is characterized by a gradual onset and a long-continued course, often of many years. The **malignant form,** fortunately much less common, is frequently of abrupt onset and runs a course measured in months rather than years, so that it justifies its name. It often ends with renal failure (uremia) or cerebral hemorrhage.

Etiology. The very names primary and essential indicate our ignorance of the etiology of the condition, but that does not prevent us from speculating on the causes. There is considerable evidence, both experimental and human, to suggest that the kidney and the adrenal cortex exert a regulating effect on the blood pressure (Fig. 4–24). Over 100 years ago Richard Bright pointed out the association between **chronic nephritis** and hypertrophy of the left ventricle. When the arteries to both kidneys in the dog or one kidney in the rat are gradually constricted by a clamp (Goldblatt phenomenon), the resulting **renal ischemia** causes hypertension. The same thing happens in man when the main renal artery to one kidney is narrowed by disease. The **adrenal cortex** exerts its influence on blood pressure by regulating salt and water content (therefore the blood volume). One of the most striking features of Addison's disease, which is the destruction of both adrenals, is low blood pressure. **It is clear that both the kidney and the adrenal are associated in the control of blood pressure in health.**

A newly characterized family of chemicals, called prostaglandins, has an opposite effect, namely an ability to lower blood pressure in some circumstances. These chemicals are also synthesized partly in the kidney and have been implicated, although largely in a speculative way, in disorders of blood pressure.

Any evidence for a disorder of prostaglandin secretion (inadequate amounts) or renin secretion (inappropriate amounts) or disorders in receptors is not available presently to explain the observation that a significant population have elevated diastolic and systolic blood pressures, often appearing in middle age. Some suggestions about the possible causes of essential hypertension include the observation that the number of functioning glomeruli decrease with age, starting generally at about 40. We do know that salt in the diet has a marked hypertensive effect and that anything which tends to conserve sodium or decrease its excretion may contribute to hypertension.

New experimental data on genetically transformed rats and on rats with hereditary hypertension suggest that the gene for renin, or a gene located close to the renin gene, plays a role in determining blood pressure in animals, although we have been unable to identify renin abnormalities as the cause of essential hypertension in man. It is clear, however, that blockade by drugs of the renin system is currently one of the best ways to treat hypertension of unknown origin.

Secondary Hypertension

Raised blood pressure may be associated with renal disease, endocrine tumors, and constriction of the arteries. **Renal lesions** may take the form of (1) **glomerulonephritis,** which causes diffuse glomerular ischemia, (2) **chronic pyelonephritis,** and (3) **stenosis of the main renal artery** on one or both sides by atheroma. **Endocrine tumors** may be (1) **pheochromocytoma of the adrenal medulla,** which produces vasoconstricting hormone, or (2) **adenoma of the adrenal cortex,** which produces excess salt-retaining hormone with resulting **aldosteronism.** Constriction of the arteries may take the form of **coarctation of the aorta,** in which the hypertension is restricted to the upper part of the body and the upper limbs. This last is a cause of hypertension in childhood, and one readily cured by operation. The **arteriolar narrowing of age** is associated with hypertension, but which is cause and which effect is difficult to know.

DERANGEMENTS OF BODY FLUIDS

Millions of years ago, the first land animal crawled out of the sea where, with relatively little effort, he maintained an equilibrium. To float and move about in the sea is much easier than standing upright and running, or even crawling on all fours or your belly. The preservation of an internal aqueous environment on land requires work, too; to conserve water and to excrete wastes requires energy from cells of the kid-

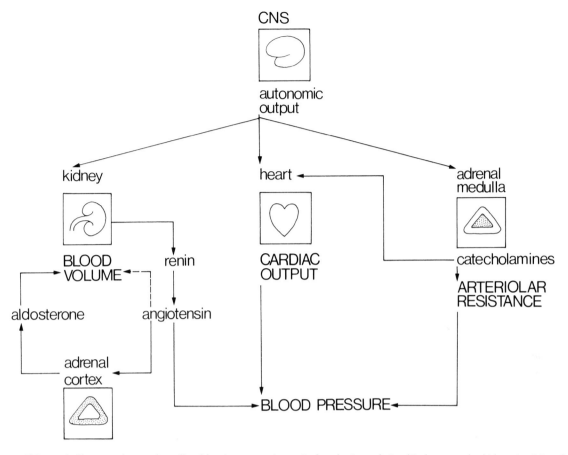

Fig. 4–24 This graph illustrates factors that affect blood pressure. In particular, the interrelationship between the kidney (renin) and the adrenal cortex (aldosterone) shown in the lower left corner has been of great diagnostic and therapeutic interest.

ney, lung, and skin. For each of us there is a brief but visible recapitulation of evolution in the months before our birth.

For a tadpole, who diffuses away ammonia into the pond water, to adapt successfully to terrestrial life, gills must be exchanged for lungs, a tail for feet, and osmotically important material (albumin) must be synthesized for the functioning of the circulation. New enzymes capable of excreting nitrogen in a relatively innocuous form (urea) are evoked during metamorphosis from the liver. In disease, some of the principal disorders of human beings are those of overly diminished body fluids, whether they circulate, are in the interstitial compartment, or are intracellular. Intoxication or depletion of the substances that are present in these various compartments is the source of many ills. This section will treat some of these disorders, such as water and electrolyte balance, acid-base balance, dehydration, and shock.

Water Balance

The importance of water has already been discussed in Chapter 1. Water comprises about 50% of the weight of the body, is present in the vessels (in the form of plasma), in the interstitial space, and in the cells. These may be regarded as three compartments, among which a continual exchange of fluid is taking place. Water lost from one compartment can be supplied from another compartment. Thus plasma that is lost may be replaced by fluid from the interstitial compartment. There is 12 times as much water in the cells as in the blood, and 4 times as much in the interstitial space (Table 4–1). Water balance is the remarkably constant balance between the fluid in the vessels and the fluid in the tissues, both cellular and interstitial. It is in the cells themselves that the correct content of water is so important. The balance will be influenced by both the intake and the output of water. Water balance, for the most part, is regulated by water loss, which averages about 2,500 ml a day in the adult, and proportionately more in children, whose surface area is large in relation to their weight. The loss takes place by four routes: (1) from the intestine, (2) from the lungs in expired air, (3) from the skin, and (4) from the kidneys. The kidneys are mainly responsible for removing excess fluid in health, although the large

Table 4–1. Body Water Distribution in an "Average" Normal Young man

SOURCE	ml/kg OF BODY WEIGHT	% OF TOTAL BODY WATER
Plasma	45	7.5
Interstitial lymph	120	20.0
Dense connective tissue and cartilage	45	7.5
Inaccessible bone water	45	7.5
Transcellular	15	2.5
Total extracellular	270	45.0
Total body water (H$_2$O)	600	100.0
Total intracellular	330	55.0

(From Perez-Tamayo, R.: *Mechanisms of Disease*, Philadelphia, W. B. Saunders Co., 1961.)

amount that may be lost in severe and continued diarrhea or in the profuse sweating brought about by natural or artificial heat is obvious. The renal glomeruli filter water and sodium chloride, but these are reabsorbed by the renal tubules in quantities necessary to maintain the correct balance. The entire mechanism, called **homeostasis,** maintains the constancy of the internal environment.

It is this mechanism that serves to maintain the constancy of the acid-base balance, the osmotic pressure, the concentration of the different solutes or of ions, the blood sugar no matter how much glucose is consumed, the body temperature despite changes in the outside temperature, and the blood volume even after severe hemorrhage or copious intravenous fluid infusion. It is on the internal environment that the multiplicity of laboratory tests are now performed to determine the state of health of a person. For further reading on fluid balance see the Appendix p. 104.

Dehydration

Under normal conditions more water is taken in than is needed, and the excess excreted in the urine by the kidneys. If the **intake is insufficient,** the output due to evaporation from the skin and the lungs and the excretion in urine and feces results in a negative water balance and a state of **dehydration.** The same result is produced by **excessive loss** of water through the skin, lungs, kidneys, or gastrointestinal tract. A patient suffering from Asiatic cholera may become completely dehydrated in the space of 24 hours. Death occurs when the loss reaches 15% of the body weight. As this percentage is reached twice as quickly in an infant as in an adult, it is evident that the water in the tissues will be exhausted at twice the rate of those of an adult, and that the infant will die in half the time. **Dehydration is therefore a much more acute problem in infants and young children than in adults.**

From what has been said, it is obvious that fluid balance depends not only on water but also on salt. If both water and salt are lost, as in vomiting and diarrhea, or even in profuse and continued sweating, such as occurs in the tropics or in persons working at blast furnaces, salt must be replenished as well as water. One of the hormones of the adrenal cortex, aldosterone, controls the excretion of sodium chloride by the kidneys. If this hormone is insufficient, excessive salt is lost in the urine, the salt content of the plasma falls, water is not retained in the tissues, and dehydration results. This is seen to a marked degree in Addison's disease, which is due to destruction of the adrenal cortex.

Decrease of body water from whatever cause is naturally first seen in the intravascular compartment, with a reduction in blood volume, carrying with it the possibility of shock. The regulating mechanism at once comes into play, withdrawing fluid from the interstitial compartment, and finally the intracellular fluid. This is significant, for cellular dehydration creates thirst that may become so intense as to be unendurable, and it interferes with cellular enzymes to a degree that may be fatal.

Disturbance in the water (and salt) balance may occur in a number of diseases, some of which will be discussed in this book. Examples are shock, acute intestinal obstruction, renal failure, and Addison's disease.

Shock

Shock may be defined as the **condition arising from a reduction in tissue perfusion.** When prolonged, it not only leads to interference with cellular function, but also may lead to death. The person in shock experiences many physiologic derangements, extremely disturbing and anxiety-producing. A few summers ago, while tending honeybees, I had become sensitized to bee venom and was sufficiently stung to develop an acute anaphylactic reaction (see Chapter 6), which is usually accompanied by shock. The sweating, tachycardia, weakness, dizziness, and transient cerebral ischemia when my blood pressure fell to 80/40 was an awesome experience.

Without knowing the state of the circulation, the systolic or diastolic pressures, or the central venous pressures, it takes only one experience to recognize the outward signs of shock in a person. He or she looks pale and apprehensive, and beads of perspiration stand out on the skin. The patient in shock may either lie still or be restless. His responses to questions are abbreviated, as he conserves whatever energy remains. The skin, hands, and feet are blue and cool to the touch in the most common types of shock, and the pulse rate is increased over normal.

Shock is not a disease: it is a physiologic state that changes rapidly as the underlying cause and homeostatic reactions to it progress. It is important to emphasize here that although we may be able to recognize different types of shock, and in doing so to treat them differently, we do not completely understand the process. For example, in the past 35 years, we have gone from treating shock with vasopressor agents to increase the peripheral resistance, to using vasodilators to decrease the peripheral resistance and therefore the work of the heart in one particular type of shock (Fig. 4–25).

For the purposes of this chapter, we can discuss four general causes of shock.

(1) Shock caused by a **loss of blood volume** (e.g., hemorrhage). This is called hypovolemic shock and is the type most commonly associated with traumatic injuries and obvious blood loss, or blood loss into some portion of a body cavity.

(2) Shock caused by **failure of the heart** to pump blood through the circulation (e.g., myocardial infarct). This is probably the most common cause of shock in the North American population, and we refer to it as cardiogenic shock.

(3) Shock caused by **vasodilatation**, in which the arteriolar bed and capillary branches fail to maintain their normal diameter or become leaky and allow blood to pool in the tissues of the body. This may occur in anaphylactic (severe allergic) shock, in which

the various mechanisms result in a decreased venous return to the heart, or can be caused by specific interference with vasomotor nerves or by substantial tissue injury. In a few instances, a person who has received what appears to be superficial trauma may die with shock, and the cause may never become apparent anatomically. This type of shock is referred to as neurogenic or vasomotor shock.

(4) Shock that occurs in patients with severe infections, particularly those caused by gram-negative bacteria such as *E. coli*, is known as **septic shock.** The mechanisms that have been used to explain the cause of this shock include the production of a toxin by the organism, and also the overwhelming insult to the body by the presence of millions of bacteria.

The importance of these different general causes is that, if one mistakenly treats the shock caused by myocardial infarct with transfusion because the shock is thought to be caused by some hidden hemorrhage, the patient will not fare as well as if the correct diagnosis of the cause of the shock had been made. Treatment that increases cardiac output is in vain when the patient has an overwhelming bacterial sepsis. We shall now discuss some of the mechanisms whereby shock causes injury to the patient that may be reversed, or that may become irreversible and result in death.

First let us consider the final common path that makes shock such a life-threatening condition. Without regard for the initiating event (myocardial infarct, hemorrhage, anaphylaxis) the result of the reduction in tissue perfusion at the cellular level is the interference with the normal aerobic metabolism of all tissues. This cellular hypoxia is reversible for some time, as we have discussed in Chapter 1. However, an inevitable result is the increased production of lactate as the tissues attempt to survive without adequate oxygen and shift into anaerobic metabolic pathways. The increasing leakiness of all cells and the production of lactate progressively move the pH of the blood away from the normal of 7.4 toward a more and more acidotic range. Metabolic acidosis itself compounds the injury to cells, and at some stage an irreversible phase is entered whereby the cells can no longer produce energy by any mechanism. For example, dogs that are bled and then retransfused within two hours have a 10% mortality rate, whereas those that are not retransfused until four hours later have only a 10% survival rate.

It is not difficult to understand that if there is a transient, sudden loss of blood pressure, the body in its wisdom perceives that something is wrong and takes immediate steps to restore the circulatory pressures to normal. Sometimes we experience this when

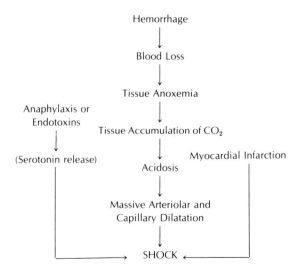

Fig. 4–25   This diagram shows the steps in the development of shock and illustrates the interrelationship of a variety of causes at the tissue level.

we get up from a chair and feel dizzy, or "black out," which is due to the failure to keep the circulation to the brain at a normal pressure because there has been a pooling of blood in the lower limbs. When faced with a blackout, the heart may immediately beat more rapidly (increased cardiac output restores the cerebral circulation). Almost as quickly, there is a narrowing of the arterioles in the systemic circulatory bed, which increases peripheral resistance. A concomitant increase in the pressure at the venous end of the microcirculation increases venous return of blood, which in turn allows the heart to fill more effectively, and thereby increases cardiac output. Some of these effects are mediated by reflex arcs; the baroreceptors in the carotid arteries inform the brain that the blood pressure is too low, and as a result the brain sends signals to the vagus nerve, which regulates the heart rate. Similar effects are mediated by chemical messengers or hormones; shock signals the adrenal medulla to release epinephrine and norepinephrine, which have a direct effect on the heart and the arteriolar bed.

Some responses to shock, such as the shift in major circulatory pathways, shunting blood from the gastrointestinal tract or peripheral musculature to the brain and heart, may take longer, and it is much longer still before major readjustments in the distribution of fluids between the vascular bed and the interstitial or cellular spaces become evident. A fall in hematocrit (see Chapter 23) that indicates major blood loss may not be evident for an hour or more, just as the readjustment to a minor loss of blood, as when one donates a pint for the Red Cross, may be delayed and not revealed in the hematocrit for several hours. When the kidneys are not perfused, whether because of a low cardiac output or because of pooling elsewhere, urine will not be made normally. This decrease in the amount of urine produced may not become apparent for several hours. Shock therefore is a complex, physiologic phenomenon.

Newer methods of diagnosing shock and of distinguishing between possible etiologies of shock have made the management of it simpler in some ways and more complex in others. We have talked about increased heart rate (pulse) and have indicated that it reflects a compensatory effort to increase the cardiac output. Blood pressure, shown in the accompanying diagram (Fig. 4–26), is many things; we conventionally speak of the pressure taken in the brachial artery as blood pressure, but changes in the venous pressure and in pressures in the pulmonary circulation are also important reflections of the state of the circulation and of its principal pump, the heart.

Having established the nature of the peripheral arterial pressure, and determined that it is low, for the

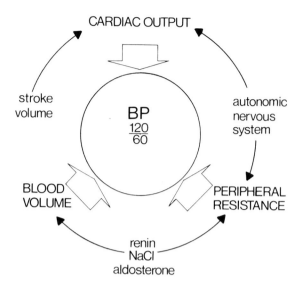

Fig. 4–26   This figure shows the major factors that affect the blood pressure.

surgical patient, where the diagnosis is an issue and the prognosis of the patient is grave, it is relevant to obtain additional pressure measurements by the use of direct catheterizations. The **central venous pressure** (pressure in the superior vena cava) normally is 5 to 10 cm of water or less than 2 mm Hg. Any change in this pressure must be explained. If the heart is failing, the central venous pressure will be raised. This is a direct reflection of failure of the right heart, which is one step removed from the left ventricle. If there is volume overload, the increased central venous pressure can be caused by excess intravenous therapy. Changes in the central venous pressure occur during therapeutic intervention with drugs and transfusions. Such changes serve to confirm the appropriateness of the diagnosis and therapy. However, these assessments reflect only indirectly the functions of the left heart, as we have stated, because the pulmonary circulation and right heart pressure are being read indirectly.

A more modern attempt to assess directly the function of the left ventricle is to insert a catheter into a branch of the pulmonary artery. This catheter, with a balloon at the tip, is inflated when it is in a branch of the pulmonary artery, and the measurements derived are called the pulmonary wedge pressure. This catheter is now much closer to the left ventricle and atrial pressures and is named after its inventors, Drs. Swan and Ganz. The pressures thus recorded reflect the left atrial pressure just as the central venous pressure reflects the right atrial pressure. Naturally, these invasive procedures have potential and real hazards: the catheter can introduce infections, precipitate thrombus formation and emboli, and may obstruct the blood vessels in which it is placed. Catheters may also cause reflex cardiac arrest or arrhythmia. Therefore they are used only when the data is important for the management of the patient's shock.

A final way to determine the extent, prognosis, and severity of shock is to measure blood gases. The PO_2, PCO_2, and blood pH all directly reflect the capacity of the circulation to maintain life. A progressive decrease in the PO_2 indicates that somewhere there is inadequate oxygenation, which may be due to respiratory disease at the outset, but which may also reflect inadequate perfusion of the lung. A progressive rise in the PCO_2 again may be caused by inadequate ventilatory mechanisms. However, it may also be due to an inappropriate circulation through the lungs. A fall in the blood pH may be the result of the accumulation of retained acid products as in chronic renal failure, but such a fall in pH may rapidly occur when anaerobic metabolic events cause many tissues of the body to accumulate lactate. Thus changes in the PO_2, PCO_2, and arterial pH and a rise in blood lactate are all indicators of the shock syndrome.

We have come to recognize both the anatomic and the physiologic effects of reversible shock, in that specific organs such as the lung and kidney may have impaired function for days and weeks in the patient who has survived the acute and critical episode. Therefore we talk about shock lung and shock kidney. Fortunate, indeed, is the patient who eventually recovers, because he has teetered on the edge of the precipice over which so many acutely ill patients have fallen.

SYNOPSIS

Edema may be caused by increased capillary permeability, decreased plasma proteins, or increased hydrostatic pressure in veins or lymphatics.

Thrombosis may be caused by stasis of the circulation, by injury to the endothelial lining of the vessel, or by changes in the character of the blood itself.

Emboli may arise anywhere in the circulation (heart, veins, arteries) and usually travel to where the vessel size limits their progress. Emboli may result in infarction or sudden death (pulmonary emboli), or may be asymptomatic.

Thrombosis and embolism may both cause and result from infarction.

Shock, a significant reduction in tissue perfusion, may be caused by blood loss, heart failure, or loss of peripheral resistance.

Terms

Edema	*Hematoma*	*Infarction*
Hemorrhage	*Petechiae*	*Hypertension*
Ascites	*Aneurysm*	*Metabolic acidosis/alkalosis*
Effusion	*Fibrinolysis*	*Respiratory acidosis/alkalosis*
Transudate	*Thrombosis*	*Shock*
Exudate	*Embolus*	

FURTHER READING

Brace, R.A., and Christian, J.L.: Transcapillary Starling pressures in the fetus, newborn, adult, and pregnant adult. Am. J. Physiol., 240:H843, 1981.

Clowes, G.H.A., Jr., and O'Donnell, T.F., Jr.: Heat stroke. N. Engl. J. Med., 291:564, 1974.

Dalen, J.E., and Alpert, J.S.: Natural history of pulmonary embolus. Prog. Cardiovas. Dis., 27:259, 1975.

Diamond, J.M.: Osmotic water flow in leaky epithelia. J. Membrane Biol., 51:195, 1979.

Gamble, J.L.: *Chemical Anatomy, Physiology and Pathology of Extracellular Fluid,* 6th ed. Cambridge, Harvard University Press, 1954.

Glouse, L.H., and Comp, P.C.: The regulation of hemostasis: the protein C system. N. Engl. J. Med., 314:1298, 1986.

Goldstein, J.L., and Brown, M.S.: The LDL receptor locus and the genetics of familial hypercholesterolemia. Annu. Rev. Genet., 13:259, 1979.

Kashtan, J., Conti, S., and Blaisdell, F.W.: Heparin therapy for deep venous thrombosis. Am. J. Surg., 140:836, 1980.

LeQuesne, L.P.: Relation between deep vein thrombosis and pulmonary embolism in surgical patients. N. Engl. J. Med., 291:1292, 1974.

Light, R.W., et al.: Pleural effusions: the diagnostic separation of transudates and exudates. Ann. Intern. Med., 77:507, 1972.

Loeb, J.N.: The hyperosmolar state. N. Engl. J. Med., 290:1184, 1974.

Man, S.O., and Carroll, H.J.: The anion gap. N. Engl. J. Med., 297:814, 1977.

Massie, R.: *Nicholas and Alexandra.* New York, Atheneum, 1967.

Moore, F.D., et al.: *The Body Cell Mass and Its Supporting Environment.* Philadelphia, W.B. Saunders Co., 1963.

Morris, B.J.: The renin gene in hypertension. Today's Life Science, 2:36, 1990.

Parving, H.H., et al.: Mechanisms of edema formation in myx-edema. N. Engl. J. Med., 301:460, 1979.

Raine, A.E.G., et al.: Atrial natriuretic peptide and atrial pressure in patients with congestive heart failure. N. Engl. J. Med., 315:533, 1987.

Relman, A.S.: Lactic acidosis and a possible new treatment. N. Engl. J. Med., 298:564, 1978.

Thompsom, J.E.: Acute peripheral arterial occlusion. N. Engl. J. Med., 290:950, 1974.

Tremper, K.K.: Oncotic pressure and wedge pressure. N. Engl. J. Med., 297:616, 1977.

APPENDIX

Further Reading Regarding Fluids, Electrolytes and Regulation of Acid-Base Balance

Electrolyte Balance

Some substances in body fluids are present in the form of salts, such as sodium chloride or calcium phosphate, which are **electrolytes;** that is when placed in water, they become dissociated into electrically charged particles called **ions.** This dissociation was first observed 150 years ago when an electric current was passed through a solution of inorganic compounds with the result that some elements passed to the negative pole and the adjacent fluid became alkaline, whereas others went to the positive pole and the fluid became acidic. Ion is derived from the Greek word meaning to pass or go. The ions may be positively charged **cations,** so-called because they collect at the negative or cathode pole, the more important being sodium (Na^+), potassium (K^+), and calcium (Ca^{++}). The negatively charged ions are **anions,** which pass to the positive pole or anode, the chief being chlorine (Cl^-), carbonates, and phosphates. Substances are not electrolytes unless they become dissociated into charged particles. All the sodium and potassium and much of the calcium of the body are ionized. Cations include all the metals and hydrogen. Anions include the nonmetals, the acid radicals, and the hydroxyl (OH^-) ion. The ions of the electrolytes with their positive and negative charges and their consequent chemical combining power determine the constancy of the acid-base balance.

Electrolytes exert an important effect on the amount of water in the various compartments because of the osmotic pressure that they produce. (Osmosis is the passage of a fluid through a semipermeable membrane to that side that has the higher concentration of molecules.) A semipermeable membrane offers no obstacle to the passage of electrolytes, but does not permit the passage of large molecules, e.g., those of proteins such as albumin, prothrombin, fibrinogen, and globulins. The salt content in the cellular compartment is different from that in the interstitial and vascular compartments.

The normal figures for the principal electrolytes in the plasma, which vary within narrow limits, are given below, together with round or average figures, which are easier to remember:

Sodium	135 to 155 mEq/L (150)
Chloride	97 to 105 mEq/L (100)
Potassium	3.6 to 5.0 mEq/L (4)
Bicarbonate	25 to 32 mEq/L (30)

The equivalent weight of an electrolyte is the weight in grams that combines with or displaces 1 gram of hydrogen. Because the concentrations of electrolytes in body fluids are so low, we express them as milliequivalents per liter (mEq/L). This is in place of milligrams per 100 ml, as has been used in the past, and which must still be used for nonelectrolytes that cannot be dissociated into ions. The use of milliequivalents facilitates the expressions of the total amounts of cations and anions in body fluids. Thus plasma contains about 155 mEq/L of cations and an equal number of anions.

The electrolytes present may determine the amount of body fluid. Their relative proportions determine the reaction of that fluid and influence the action of nerve on muscle. The total electrolyte concentration is essentially the same in all 3 phases of body fluid, but the relative amounts of the different electrolytes vary widely. In the extracellular fluid (plasma and interstitial fluid), the important ions are **sodium, chloride,** and **bicarbonate,** of which sodium is the principal basic ion (cation), and chloride and bicarbonate are the chief acidic ions (anions). In the intracellular fluid, **potassium** is the chief cation and **organic phosphate** the corresponding anion.

Acid-Base Balance

In addition to changes in the volume of the fluids in the various compartments, we must consider changes in the ionic equilibrium that affect the reaction of the acid-base balance of the fluid. The **concentration of hydrogen ions** in the body fluids indicates their reaction, and this is expressed as the **negative** logarithm of this concentration. In practice this is abbreviated as pH. Thus 10^{-7} becomes pH 7.0, which is the hydrogen ion concentration of pure water, representing electroneutrality, and is taken as the reference point for expressing the ionic concentration of other solutions. The pH of normal serum is 7.4, and the normal limits of variation are narrow, between 7.35 and 7.45. An increased concentration of hydrogen ions, or a shift of pH toward 7, indicates acidosis, whereas a decreased concentration toward 7.5 signifies alkalosis.

It is of extreme importance that the H^+ ion concentration be maintained within normal limits because of the effect of pH on the conformation of proteins. If the pH shifts appreciably, proteins such as enzymes cannot function. The **regulation of the acid-base balance** depends on 3 principal factors: (1) buffer systems; (2) excretion of acid or alkali by the kidneys; (3) excretion of carbon dioxide by the lungs.

Buffer Systems. Body fluids contain substances known as buffers, which "soak up" excess acid or alkali and thus minimize changes in hydrogen ion concentration. They convert strong acids and bases into weaker ones, so that the narrow limits of hydrogen ion concentration are not transgressed. Hydrochloric acid is a "strong" acid because in solution it is highly ionized, and as a result nearly all its hydrogen is present in the ionized form, whereas carbonic acid is a "weak" acid, because only a small number of dissociated ions are in solution. The chief buffers of the blood are carbonic acid (H_2CO_3), its bicarbonate salt ($NaHCO_3$), and hemoglobin, which is weakly acidic. **Sodium bicarbonate buffers strong acids, whereas carbonic acid buffers strong bases such as sodium hydroxide, converting it into sodium bicarbonate and water,** with only a few OH ions. Both plasma proteins and hemoglobin are buffer systems. Hemoglobin is the buffer of carbonic acid derived from carbon dioxide and changed into carbonate in the red cells as part of the mechanism of respiration.

Respiratory Control of pH. The respiratory center in the brain is extremely sensitive to changes in the H^+ concentration of the plasma. The amount of sodium bicarbonate present in the extracellular fluid available for the neutralization of acids stronger than carbonic acid is known as the **alkali reserve.** It is a measure of the degree of disturbance of the acid-base balance. The plasma bicarbonate is expressed as the **carbon dioxide combining power. The simplest measurement for the demonstration of acidosis or alkalosis is the estimation of this combining power,** which is done by gas analysis. The quantity of carbon dioxide normally present as bicarbonate is 55 to 75 volumes per cent. In moderate acidosis the carbon dioxide combining power is less than 40 volumes; in alkalosis it is above 80 volumes. As bicarbonate

is continually being formed by tissue metabolism and as carbonic acid is readily eliminated as carbon dioxide, it is easy to appreciate the paramount importance of respiration in conjunction with bicarbonate in maintaining the acid-base balance.

Renal Control. Although carbonic acid is regulated by respiration, all the other electrolyte components of the plasma structure are under the control of the kidneys. There is a constant production of acid products such as sulfuric and phosphoric acids from protein metabolism, lactic acid from muscle activity and ketone acids, in high-fat diet when the carbohydrates are low. These acids must be eliminated without a loss of base, so that the alkali reserve will not be depleted. Urea is formed from the blood by the cells of the renal tubules; ammonia is formed in turn from the urea; and the ammonia thus formed combines with the acid phosphate and sulfate radicals to be excreted in the urine.

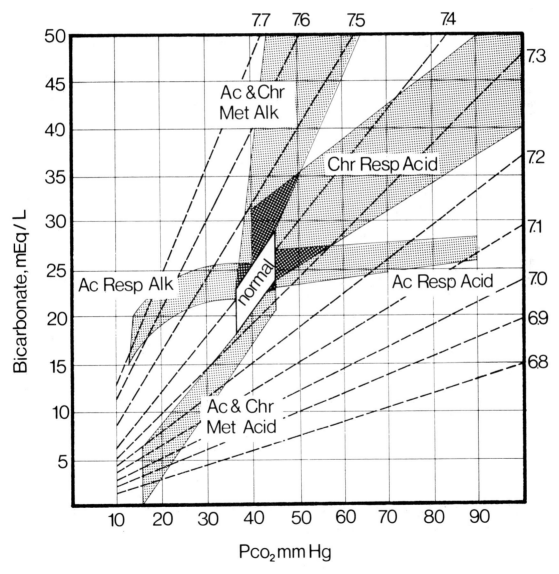

Fig. A4—1   This nomogram illustrates the range of normal pH, bicarbonate, and PCO_2, and demonstrates the mean $\pm$ 2 standard deviations for the compensatory response of patients. (From Arbus, G.S.: An *in vivo* acid-base nomogram for clinical use. Can. Med. Assoc. J., 109:291, 1973.)

Another renal device for conserving fixed base is the ability of the kidney to separate sodium from fixed acid salts in the tubules and return it to the blood, where it combines with bicarbonate while the acid radical is excreted in the urine in the form of free acid.

Acidosis. We have already seen that the alkali reserve of the blood is represented by bicarbonate. Any change in this reserve is reflected in the plasma carbon dioxide level. The buffer system $\dfrac{H_2CO_3}{NaHCO_3}$ has a normal ratio of 1/20. Four things may happen to upset this ratio. Acid may be increased if the numerator, carbonic acid, is increased, or if the denominator, sodium bicarbonate, is decreased; the reverse is true of alkali. A primary alkali deficit with resulting acidosis is the most important disturbance of the acid-base balance. The mechanism for the change may be metabolic or respiratory.

Metabolic Acidosis. This condition develops whenever the available alkali is diminished. Such a state of affairs may arrive in one of three ways: (1) An **excess of acid ions** may develop as the result of disease that uses up the bicarbonate. This may occur in diabetic acidosis or in the ketosis of starvation. (2) An **inadequate excretion of acids** due to renal failure. This is retention acidosis. (3) **Loss of sodium bicarbonate,** as in chronic diarrhea, the secretions of the bowel being alkaline. The ratio of carbonic acid to carbonate may fall from a normal of 1/20 to 1/10, with a fall in pH to as low as 7.1.

Respiratory Acidosis. When there is interference with the exchange of gases in the pulmonary alveoli, an insuffi-cient amount of carbon dioxide is blown off. The retention of carbon dioxide leads to an increased carbonic acid concentration in the blood and acidosis. The carbonic acid-bicarbonate ratio may be only 1/15. The exchange of gases may be depressed by advanced chronic pulmonary disease such as fibrosis or emphysema, or by impairment of the respiratory muscles.

Alkalosis. It is only natural that alkalosis is not nearly so common as acidosis, nor does it have the same clinical significance. Again it may be metabolic or respiratory in character.

Metabolic Alkalosis. Here there is a primary bicarbonate excess. Occasionally this is due to an increased intake of alkalis, as in overdone sodium bicarbonate therapy for duodenal ulcer. Much more important is the loss of fixed acids, as in the depletion of free hydrochloric acid in the vomiting of duodenal ulcer. When chloride is lost, its place is taken by bicarbonate.

Respiratory Alkalosis. This is the result of a primary carbon dioxide deficit. The usual cause is the deep and rapid breathing that may accompany hysteria or fear. It may also result from the anoxia of heart disease or of high altitudes. The increased ventilation blows off such large volumes of carbon dioxide that the concentration of carbonic acid in the blood falls in relation to the bicarbonate, so that a relative alkalosis results. If the pH is above 7.6, the spasmodic attacks known as **tetany** may occur, owing to increased neuromuscular irritability. These relations are all demonstrated in Figure A4–1.

5

INFLAMMATION AND REPAIR

Research is to see what everybody else has seen and think what nobody has thought—A. SZENT-GYORGY

INFLAMMATION

The reaction of living tissue to injury is called inflammation. It is a tapestry, woven of cells and their products, enzymes, soluble factors, of blood vessels and their contents; its texture and appearance change with time. It is best viewed as a process that starts with an injury and that ends with what we call healing. Yet the boundaries between injury and inflammation, and between inflammation and healing, are indistinct. The process depends on a number of factors, including general features of the host, such as nutrition and age, and specific local and tissue factors, such as the blood supply and the presence of foreign bodies or bacteria in the injured area. The type of injury itself, whether a burn, an ischemic injury, or a surgical wound, and its size often determine the nature of the actions that are collectively called inflammation. Inflammation has many different aspects; it can be recognized by the presence of redness, swelling, pain, heat, and a loss of function. These aspects of inflammation were recognized more than 2,000 years ago and were known in the ancient world by the Latin terms *rubor, tumor, dolor, calor,* and *functio laesa,* which respectively mean redness, swelling, pain, fever, and loss of function.

An important concept is that inflammation is a defense reaction whose purpose is to protect the host. Having said that, it is important to recognize that this defense reaction also has some disadvantages. The ways in which we have come to understand inflammation have been from observations in man after injury and in disease states, and from studies on experimentally induced inflammation, as in the capillary network of rats, mice, frogs and rabbits.

Inflammation, whatever its cause, is called by the suffix *itis* (as in appendicitis or cholecystitis, which mean, respectively, inflammation of the appendix and of the gallbladder). Inflammation is important in that its symptoms and signs such as pain, swelling, and fever, lead the person to inquire about its cause. Moreover, the cause of inflammation is not decided simply by describing its existence. The causes of inflammation in any organ may include obstruction, infection, injury and a compromised vascular supply, as well as physical and chemical injury (Fig. 5–1). Biologic agents such as bacteria are often the inciting agent, but frostbite or sunburn may also initiate such inflammatory responses as heat and pain. Attempts to understand the general and specific reactions to injury in living tissue have been made more difficult by the imperceptible transition from acute reaction, through more vigorous and obvious responses to the melting away of the angry signs and the restoration of the tissue to normal, or healing. The lines between injury, inflammation, and healing are arbitrary at best, and should be considered only as a way of explaining what little we know of this complex process.

Before considering inflammation in more detail, it is useful to outline a classification of inflammation so that our descriptions and interpretations may be kept in perspective. Inflammation may occur in any tissue or in any organ, as we have already said, but there may be differences in the changes that take place in different tissues.

First, there are acute, limited areas of redness and painful swelling, which may disappear in a few days. Because of its short duration, and because of the histology of the tissue and cellular responses, we call this response **acute inflammation.** Examples are insect bites, small abrasions or cuts, mild burns, or other injuries that are generally considered to be minor. Sometimes acute inflammation can be quite extensive and involve viscera such as in a lung abscess caused by accidentally aspirated food. In all cases, the site of acute inflammation is remarkable for the presence of numerous polymorphonuclear leukocytes.

Occasionally, acute inflammation does not resolve.

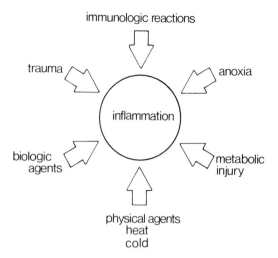

Fig. 5–1 This diagram illustrates some of the multiple causes of inflammation. Naturally, in many instances, more than one factor may be responsible for the inflammatory response.

In this case, one outcome of the host's reaction to minor injuries may be the continued evolution of the inflammatory response, so that it lasts for many days or weeks, and may spread to involve adjacent or distant tissues. The response may persist because of continued or repeated insults, and it may be considered **chronic** because of the length of its duration. It also may be considered chronic if one examines the tissue microscopically and finds a pattern of tissue and cell response that differs from the acute response. Whereas acute inflammations characteristically show large numbers of polymorphonuclear leukocytes, chronic inflammations consist of lymphocytes, monocytes, and plasma cells, collectively called mononuclear cells (Fig. 5–2).

There is a third type of inflammation that can be separated from the typical acute and chronic types; this is designated **granulomatous** inflammation. Granulomatous inflammation is a subset of chronic inflammation and is distinguished from simple chronic inflammatory responses by the broader range of cell types found in tissues. Typically, the site of granulomatous inflammation contains macrophages enlarging to a point where they resemble epithelial cells, hence the name of epithelioid cells which is given to them. In addition, they often fuse to form multinucleated giant cells. Lymphocytes are found at sites of granulomatous inflammation.

Having attempted to distinguish these three types of inflammation, let us consider a typical injury and discuss the sequence of responses in a normal adult human being.

Injury by bacteria is one of the most common causes of inflammation. Everyone has had a boil or an ab-

scess. The bacterium (a staphylococcus for example), a usual contaminant of the skin, gains access to the host when the primary line of defense (the epithelium or the skin) has been breached by a splinter, a cut, or a wound. The bacterium is now able to cause local injury by the production of toxins and enzymes that may have a lethal effect on the cells of the host in the immediate vicinity of the bacterium. Cells of the host release, in their dying stages, proteins, enzymes, and peptides, many of which have general and specific designations, and have been shown to affect directly the neighboring tissues' components, such as the capillaries, venules, and arterioles. Bacteria that are able to multiply rapidly may increase the circle of injury and may recruit more of the host's tissue into the zone of destruction.

Capillaries in the tissue that surrounds the injured area become permeable to large and small molecules and to white blood cells that would normally stay within the circulation. These changes in the microcirculation, which can be seen with the light microscope, are responsible for the increasing redness of the inflamed area. The permeability of the capillaries allows

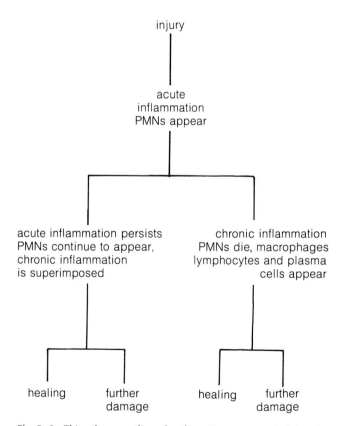

Fig. 5–2 This scheme outlines the alternative responses to injury in terms of acute inflammation on the left, and of chronic inflammation on the right.

Table 5–1.   Bodily Changes in First Phase of Metabolic Response to Injury

CIRCULATORY	METABOLIC	BLOOD
Tachycardia	Hepatic glycogenolysis	Increase in platelets and fibrinogen
Increase in cardiac output	Hyperglycemia	Decrease in prothrombin time
Generalized vasoconstriction	Increase in O_2 consumption	Accelerated coagulation
Splenic contraction	Decrease in adrenal cholesterol and vitamin C	Leukocytosis
Hypertension	Increase in urinary corticoids	Accelerated sedimentation rate and rouleaux formation
		Hypoferremia
		Fibrinolysis
		Eosinopenia

(From Perez-Tamayo, R.: *Mechanisms of Disease*, Philadelphia, W. B. Saunders Co., 1961.)

fluid to accumulate in the injured area and causes the swelling that is so typical of all inflamed tissues.

Responses at different levels of organization are shown in Table 5–1. This sequence may also be outlined thus: The liberation of low-molecular-weight substances (vasoactive peptides, histamine, lymphokines) from injured tissue stimulates local nerve endings. The process causes pain and elicits a brief phase of vasoconstriction and blanching in the injured area. This axon reflex was described more than 60 years ago. Following the transient vasoconstriction, the blood vessels become dilated and blood flow slows in the injured area.

Stasis within the microcirculation has many results. Red blood cells clump together and the channels widen as more and more erythrocytes move sluggishly through this inflamed area. One reason for the apparent increase in the number of red blood cells is that the capillaries are no longer normally intact, but rather lose both high- and low-molecular-weight substances into the interstitial tissue. This permeability sets in motion the disequilibrium of Starling's forces, so that fluid is no longer returned at the venous end of the capillary circulation (Fig. 5–3). Naturally, this disequilibrium contributes to the turnover of the inflamed tissue.

Injury to the endothelial walls of the microcirculation renders the surface of the capillary cell sticky, which enables white blood cells that normally flow past to attach themselves to the wall. In an inflamed area, whole segments of capillaries may soon be covered by white blood cells much as barnacles attach themselves to old pilings. This phenomenon is called pavementing and is regarded as an early stage in the sequence of the cellular phase of inflammation. These white blood cells also respond to the presence in neighboring tissue of foreign bacteria or antibody-antigen complexes.

The direct migration of the inflammatory cells toward an injured area is called **chemotaxis** (Fig. 5–4). This phenomenon has great value as a second line of defense in infections. Polymorphonuclear leukocytes are active, motile cells containing large amounts of enzymes capable of degrading biologic materials, as well as of isolating them, and of removing the noxious effects of these materials from the host. We now know that there are congenital disorders of the polymorphonuclear leukocytes themselves, of their structure, of their complement of enzymes, and of their motility, and that many agents can interfere with their normal response to such chemotactic agents as the presence of complement and antigen/antibody macromolecular complexes. Nearly 100 years ago, Dr. Almoth Wright, in London, used early knowledge of phagocytosis in his attempts to treat infectious disease; he is caricatured by George Bernard Shaw in *The Doctor's Dilemma*, as Sir Colenso Rigeon, whose battle cry is "Stimulate the phagocyte" as the panacea for all illness.

Accumulating evidence suggests that the importance of the polymorphonuclear leukocyte as a line of defense cannot be underestimated. There are many ways in which a loss of this phagocytic capability renders the host susceptible to acute and chronic illness. When the white blood cell count falls below 2000 per cubic milliliter, patients are often put in protective isolation, and when the count falls further (below 600), leukocyte transfusions are given.

We might now consider the normal protective barriers before we reconsider their role in inflammation and in healing.

The intact, functioning, mammalian host has a remarkable series of defense mechanisms against injury. They can be considered under several different headings, and, for simplicity's sake, we shall divide them into three categories. First, the external, epithelial, and mucosal barriers (skin, respiratory tract, bowel), which protect the *milieu intérieur* (Fig. 5–5). The second level of defense consists of the cellular and humoral apparatus, granulocytes, round cells, the microcirculation, and the "immune system," subject of a chapter of its own. The third category, which

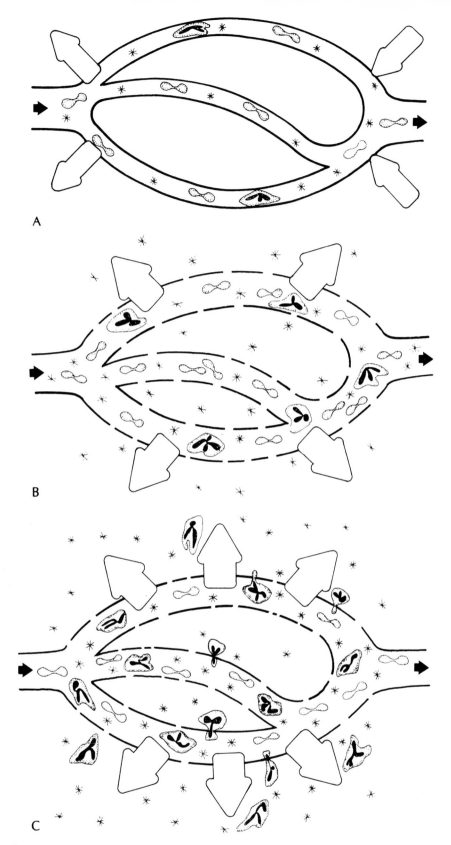

Fig. 5–3   *A,* This diagram illustrates the normal equilibrium in the microcirculation. The small black arrows show the direction of flow from the arteriole through the capillary to the venule, and the large white arrows show the passage of small molecules and water out at the arteriolar end and into the microcirculation at the venular end. The asterisks represent protein molecules. Red and white blood cells are also shown. *B,* This represents a transudate. The large white arrows show the escape of small molecules at both ends of the capillary bed. The presence of small amounts of protein is represented by asterisks, outside the microcirculation. *C,* This represents an exudate. There is a large amount of protein (asterisks) outside the capillary bed, as well as the presence of white blood cells.

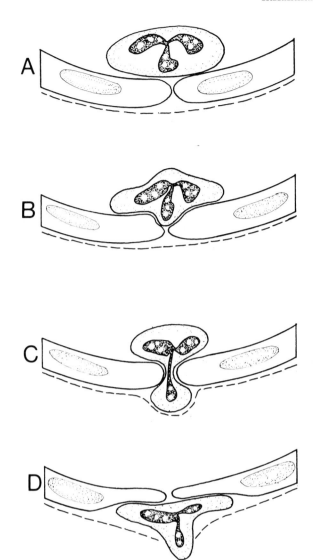

Fig. 5–4 *A, B, C,* and *D,* This diagram shows one mechanism whereby white blood cells may leave the microcirculation, crawling through or between the endothelial cells of the capillary. This process is known as diapedesis, and it occurs under the influence of chemotactic signals. (From Marchesi, V.T., and Gowans, J.L.: The migration of lymphocytes through the endothelium of venules in lymph nodes: an electron microscope study. Proc. R. Soc. Lond. Biol., 159:283, 1964.)

separate us from the external world. Whereas the skin and its specializations, at first glance, might seem as uncomplicated as a plastic poncho, serving only to keep the inner man from being washed away by the tempests of life, every square centimeter of our skin is adapted specially to keep us from drying out and to prevent the normal bacterial flora and fauna from having a free lunch. Specific, definitive adaptations are best seen in the eye, where this transparent area of skin is kept moist by tears, a fluid in which there is significant antibacterial activity (lysozyme). This enzyme has the ability to lyse bacterial colonies in dilute solutions, and maintains a sterile film of transparent cells through which we view the world.

The respiratory tract, which is normally exposed with each breath to millions of potentially injurious agents every day, has the wonderful and effective external surface, mucus, that covers the epithelial cells and that serves as a trap for bacteria and microscopic particles of dust, smog, pollen, and soot, much as a flypaper catches flies. However, unlike the flypaper, which must be changed when it is covered, the mucus blanket is continuously renewed, and, better yet, is constantly swept towards the mouth by the ciliated epithelial cells of the airways. This combination of mucus and cilia protects the underlying epithelial barrier from bacteria and the injury they cause. Cigarette smoke, alcohol, and chronic irritation from environmental toxins all interfere with the maintenance of this respiratory barrier. Viruses that infect the respiratory cells and kill the ciliated epithelium destroy the effectiveness of this barrier and permit bacterial overgrowth to occur. In fact, the danger from influenza epidemics in the past has not been from the tracheobronchitis caused by the viral infection, but rather from the superimposed bacterial pneumonias, once this defense mechanism has been destroyed.

The other extension of a mucosal barrier to infection is, of course, the oral cavity and the rest of the digestive tract. This tube is lined by millions of cells that are constantly renewed. Again, the rich mucus barrier throughout its length buffers the billions of bacteria that normally populate our intestines. Seldom do these bacteria come into direct contact with the underlying epithelial cells or penetrate further to cause disease. Peristalsis, which is a rhythmic movement of the smooth intestinal muscle, moves the ingested contents sufficiently rapidly to forestall stasis under normal conditions. Only in blind pouches, such as the appendix or colonic diverticuli, do biologic agents linger sufficiently to injure the tissue locally.

As the name implies, primary defenses displayed by skin and mucosal barriers are chronologically the first ones to help us deal with inflammatory assaults. Next are cellular and humoral responses.

we designate as systemic defense mechanisms, includes fever, leukocytosis, and general humoral or adaptive responses to injury of any kind (Fig. 5–6).

Primary Defenses

Particularly in man, the skin and mucosal barriers that protect us from injury have been well developed to provide a continuing, stable, internal environment where the essential functions of the various organs may flourish. This environment is made possible by special adaptations of the epithelial boundaries that

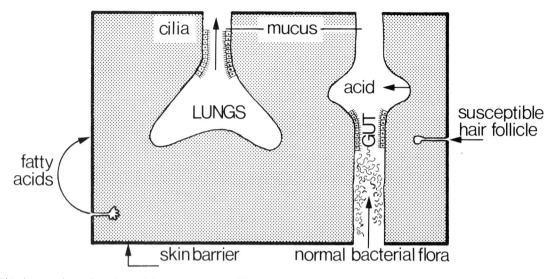

Fig. 5–5 This diagram shows the primary defense mechanisms of the body. The skin is a waterproof barrier covered with fatty acids. The respiratory tract is lined by mucus and cilia, and the gastrointestinal tract contains mucus as well. (From Roitt, I.: *Essential Immunology*. Oxford, Blackwell Scientific Publications, 1977.)

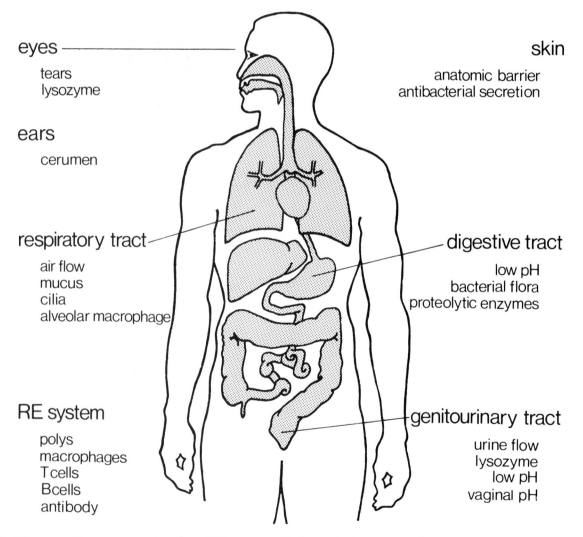

Fig. 5–6 This drawing illustrates many adaptations of different parts of the human body that act as defense barriers. The reticuloendothelial (RE) system is distributed throughout the body. The other defense mechanisms are labeled in the figure. (Adapted from Barrett, J.T.: *Basic Immunology and Its Medical Application*. St. Louis, C. V. Mosby, 1976.)

Cellular Responses to Injury

This is a good place to introduce the *dramatis personae* of the hematopoietic system, of whose many roles none is more important than providing the cells that will participate in and control the inflammatory response. Fig. 5–7 lists the cells of this system and suggests their relationship to the progenitor stem cell. Here we shall not discuss the sequence of steps in maturation of the erythroid and megakaryocyte series, which culminates in the mature red blood cell and platelet response, as this is presented in Chapter 23. Rather, we shall consider the white blood cell series, paying particular notice to those cells with granules. The mononuclear cells (lymphocytes, monocytes, plasma cells) are considered in more detail in the next chapter, but will be mentioned briefly here.

The myeloid series produces large cells with granules. The granules are modified lysosomes. These granules, which contain active enzymes that are occasionally secreted into the environment, are usually reserved for intracellular digestion. It is the staining quality of each type of granule that gives these cells their names (eosinophil, basophil, neutrophil), and the whole group is called **polymorphonuclear leukocyte**. Each granulocyte seems to be associated with particular aspects of inflammation, yet they all act as a secondary defense line.

The life span of these cells after they are mature is short (4 to 6 days), and they are constantly liberated

into the peripheral blood from the bone marrow in numbers that range around 5,000 to 6,000/mm^3. Neutropenia is the name given to a significant drop in the number of neutrophils. When the neutrophil count falls below 1,000 per mm^3, there is a serious risk from infections, and if it falls below 100 per mm^3, 70% of patients develop bacterial infections with a mortality rate that may reach 70%. It is estimated that the daily output in man of neutrophils is about 11×10^{10} cells. The proportions of these cells as compared to the total number of leukocytes normally are 60% neutrophils, 2% eosinophils, and 0.5% basophils, if one counts 100 cells on a smear (differential count). The other leukocytes in the blood are lymphocytes and monocytes.

The main function of neutrophils is phagocytosis of microorganisms. Patients with abnormal neutrophils, or absent neutrophils, suffer multiple, frequent, prolonged infections. There are examples of particular defects, such as the "lazy leukocyte syndrome," where the polymorphonuclear leukocytes are relatively immotile, failing to respond normally to chemotactic substances; however, these leukocytes have a normal complement of digestive enzymes. Other variations are polymorphonuclear leukocytes in which there are giant granules that seem to interfere with normal function. Overall, these conditions are quite rare. In all these cases, the discovery of the defect has stemmed from thorough investigations to explain the reason for persistent and recurring infections in a particular person.

The second major group of white blood cells that must be considered whenever the inflammatory response is mentioned comprises those called mononuclear cells to distinguish them from granulocytes. Mononuclear cells include lymphocytes and monocytes.

The lymphocytes are extensively discussed in the next chapter since they are the major participants of the immune reactions. We only need to mention in this section that they can be recruited at the site of inflammation by other cells. The monocyte is a mononuclear cell present in the blood but which has the remarkable property of being able to migrate outside of the vascular space into tissues where it can stay as long as it is necessary to accomplish its tasks in the inflammatory response. When monocytes are fixed in the tissue they are called by the name of histiocytes or, more commonly, macrophages. Some of them actually stay permanently in normal tissues where they are required for the proper function of the organ they inhabit.

Macrophages in the simplest sense have been recognized for 100 years as the cellular crows of our hematopoietic system; they always appear where there

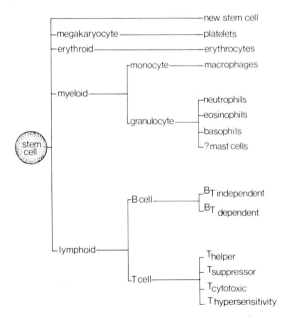

Fig. 5–7 This diagram illustrates the relationship of the lymphoid elements, the myeloid elements, and the erythroid elements in the blood, on the left, all arising from the stem cell, to the specific cells on the right. (From Roitt, I.: *Essential Immunology*. Oxford, Blackwell Scientific Publications, 1988.)

is dead or dying material to be scavenged. They are found in the lung after pneumonia has run its course, and they carry away the cellular debris to regional lymph nodes. Some macrophages are permanent residents of the lung (alveolar macrophages), and some are domiciled in the liver (Kupffer cells). Now there is evidence that they also affect the early stages of infection, particularly with organisms such as the tubercle bacillus in which humoral immunity is not effective, by both ingesting and transporting such bacteria to regional lymph nodes, where cellular immune mechanisms are alerted to the danger, and where specific reactivity is initiated (Fig. 6–3).

It has recently been discovered that macrophages secrete at least three classes of enzymes into the immediate environment where they are activated (Fig. 5–8). Some of these enzymes are active on the extracellular materials such as collagenase, elastase, and plasminogen activators. Other enzymes are principally concerned with the intracellular digestion, such as acid-activated lysosomal enzymes (phosphatase, sulfatase, and assorted nucleases). The former group of enzymes seem to be secreted in such large amounts that they may even be found in the interstitial space, perhaps when the cells have broken down.

One might wonder about the possible disastrous consequences of having so many enzymes released freely in the immediate surrounding of the inflammatory reactions. Fortunately the organism has an ingenious antagonistic way of dealing with it. Indeed, monocytes and macrophages contain and release antiproteases that neutralize the proteases shed by inflammatory cells. On this theme there is an inherited condition called alpha$_1$-antitrypsin deficiency in which patients do not produce enough of this antiprotease. As a result of this deficiency, the patient's lung parenchyma is progressively destroyed following pulmonary inflammatory lesions. This results in emphysema and is discussed in Chapter 15.

When polymorphonuclear leukocytes and macrophages perform phagocytosis they also release reactive oxygen metabolites such as hydrogen peroxide. This produces free radicals which have a dramatic damaging effect on membrane lipids and DNA, resulting in cell death.

Finally, a family of substances that macrophages may secrete comprise materials that affect the activities of cells in the immediate vicinity of the macrophage, much as in times of danger a fire alarm may be rung. These materials may inhibit cell growth, or

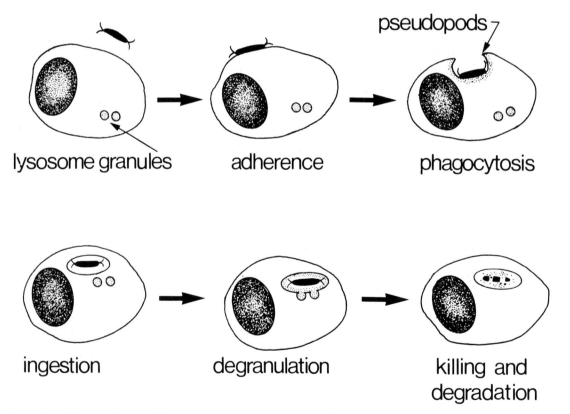

Fig. 5–8 This scheme illustrates the role of lysosomes in phagocytosis and intracellular digestion. The bacterium at the top of the drawing is ingested in a vacuole that is subsequently joined by the lysosomes, which contain enzymes that aid in the killing and degradation of the bacteria. (From Pelczar, M. Jr., et al.: *Microbiology*, 4th Ed. New York, McGraw-Hill, 1977.)

they may fall into the category of lymphocyte-stimulating substances. They are called interleukins and are discussed along with other cytokines in the following section on humoral responses to injury. The complex interactions between macrophages and lymphocytes will be considered in more detail in the chapter on immune mechanisms.

Each white blood cell can only attempt to isolate, ingest, and immobilize such threats as bacteria. Leukocytes in large numbers, in a contained space, can radically change the nature of the microenvironment. Their active metabolism consumes oxygen, glucose, and reduces the local pH, as they ingest the bacterial invaders. The liberation of large quantities of enzymes, including many nonspecific nucleases as well as hydrolytic and proteolytic enzymes that are often activated at low pH, limits the growth of microorganisms. If these organisms have not already been killed by intracellular digestion, they may be unable to withstand the hothouse climate that the short-lived polymorphonuclear leukocyte has created. This "soup," with degraded tissue cells, inflammatory cells, micro-

organisms, enzymes and inflammatory mediators, is called pus, and the cavity in which it collects is named an abscess.

In some instances, the bacteria are hardier and survive both ingestion and the enzymatic attack of the specialized leukocyte lysosomes. Bacteria such as the waxy-coated tubercle bacillus and some other spore-forming bacteria are notoriously resistant to ingestion. In fact, they can survive for many months in macrophages, outliving several generations of polymorphonuclear leukocytes.

A particular type of adaptive response to foreign material is the evolution of a population of cells that wall off the foreign material, whether it is silk suture, silica dust, or an indigestible biologic agent such as foreign vegetable matter, or, for that matter, bacteria such as we have just mentioned. These collections of chronic inflammatory cells appear as a halo about the object and may include cells with several nuclei (giant cells) (Fig. 5–9). Such a cellular reaction, typical for chronic inflammations, is called a **granuloma.** The characteristic morphologic lesion always suggests

A

B

Fig. 5–9 *A*, This diagram shows the relationship of the monocyte-macrophage in the formation of a granuloma. The epithelioid cells are derivatives of monocytes. In *B*, one sees a microphotograph of this type of giant cell.

persistent irritation. Sometimes the inciting agent is a biological pathogen, such as a tuberculosis bacillus, a spirochete, or a fungus. Special stains may reveal the organism within the boundaries of the granuloma. In other instances, no particular agent can be identified, and in another small group of cases, the pathologic process can be attributed to some types of hypersensitivity.

Humoral Responses to Injury

It has been known for more than 60 years that after an injury of any kind, there is a sequence of changes in the local vascular bed that have been described as a triple response: a red line that changes to a spreading flush, which is replaced by a pale wheal. The raised area then becomes pale and subsides after a period of up to an hour. Lewis described this change and the accompanying pain. We shall first turn to the mediators of these responses that result in an abnormal increase in permeability of the local blood vessels.

Current views separate the substances that have been identified in inflammation; the principal ones are now described.

Histamine. This substance is a naturally occurring, labile, highly active derivative of the amino acid histidine that probably is liberated from mast cells in all tissues. Mast cells are found mostly along the course of capillaries in all tissues. Histamine causes capillary dilatation and may either constrict or dilate arterioles and venules. Its effects on smooth muscle depend on the tissue and the animal species. The circumstantial evidence that supports histamine's importance in inflammation is the suppression of this effect by the administration of histamine antagonists.

5-Hydroxytryptamine (serotonin). Widespread in tissues of the body, this substance is a powerful permeability factor and may also play other roles in the body, possibly as a transmitter substance both in the diffuse endocrine system and in the central nervous system.

Kallikreins. This family of enzymes is involved in chemical reactions producing bradykinin, a powerful molecule capable of increasing vascular permeability for a few seconds at an early stage of acute inflammation. This process is linked to the activation of the coagulation system. The bradykinin and other kinins thus generated cause vasodilatation, increase capillary permeability, provoke pain, stimulate smooth muscle, and are increased at sites of acute inflammation.

Prostaglandins and leukotrienes. This large family of arachidonic acid derivatives affects the normal economy of the body in various ways. There is abundant evidence that the injection of prostaglandins may mimic the early phases of inflammation and that they affect the microcirculation. We will review briefly prostaglandins and discuss the functions of three of them: thromboxane, prostacyclin, and leukotrienes. It is important to note here that we are not concerned with details of the chemistry of these substances, which can be pursued elsewhere.

Prostaglandin is the generic term for a family of polyunsaturated fatty acids which were first identified in the 1930s. One early observation was that human semen has the ability to stimulate smooth muscle. This was observed by gynecologists who were studying the earliest phase of insemination. They noted that when semen came in contact with the cervix there was contraction of the uterus. Van Euler then identified the active substance as derivative of arachidonic acid originating in the seminal vesicles. In fact, arachidonic acid is found in the membranes of most cells of the body. It occurs as a fatty acid component of membrane phospholipids. You recall from the section on cell death that a common feature of most forms of cell injury, whether they are triggered by ischemia or inflammation, is the activation of phospholipases that will release the fatty acid components from the membrane phospholipids. The fate of arachidonic acid depends on which cell type it is released from, and on which enzyme it is activated. As illustrated in Fig. 5–10, there are two main pathways in the metabolic conversion of arachidonic acid, one governed by cyclooxygenase, the other governed by lipoxygenase. The cyclooxygenase pathway is particularly important because there are specific drugs such as aspirin, indomethacin and corticosteroids that can block it. Prostaglandins, prostacyclin and thromboxane are generated by the cyclooxygenase pathway.

It is important to recognize that the members of this large cyclooxygenase family do not necessarily all have the same effects. For instance, prostacyclin and thromboxane have two opposite effects on platelets and blood vessel tension (Fig. 5–10). These opposite effects probably represent a fine regulation by the host of the local inflammatory reaction. It remains that the predominant vascular feature or acute inflammation is vasodilatation, and this is mostly explained by the action of prostaglandin E and prostacyclin. Also it is interesting that the two major effects of thromboxane, namely platelet aggregation and vasoconstriction, are mechanisms which can be considered lifesaving or major defense mechanisms since, in the event of major physical injury, both are directed toward staunching the flow of blood.

In studies on inflammation as long ago as 1938 other substances have been recognized, such as a material

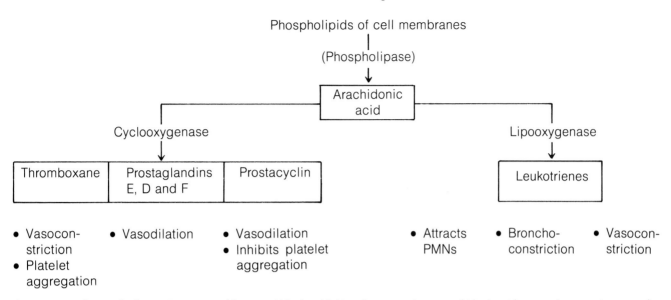

Fig. 5–10   Mediators of inflammation generated from arachidonic acid. Note that conversion or arachidonic acid occurs via two main routes, the cyclooxygenase and the lipooxygenase pathways.

which caused smooth muscle to contract following injury to the lung. This material has now been identified also as a derivative of arachidonic acid through the lipooxygenase pathway and is a member of a family of similar substances which have been designated **leukotrienes** since they are released by leukocytes.

Leukotrienes are about 1,000 times more active than histamines in causing contraction of human bronchial muscle. They are also potent vasoconstrictors and increase vascular permeability (Fig. 5–10). Their presence in acute inflammatory conditions is well demonstrated and their appearance in immunologically injured tissue is now clear. Leukotrienes have been implicated in immediate hypersensitivity reactions and in asthma.

Cytokines. Recently, important soluble mediators of inflammation have been completely purified. This has allowed the cloning of their genes and has introduced a timely clarification. Indeed, we found that various factors, described under different names, were in fact the same molecules. Modern terminology uses the term cytokine (Table 5–2). Cytokines often share some common characteristics; for instance, a given cytokine can originate from more than one type of cell and will itself often act on more than one cell target. This clearly means that the development of a timely and well regulated inflammatory response will involve not one cytokine and two types of cell, but rather a network of cytokines and the recruitment of many different cell types. Secondly, these cytokines

are mostly involved in stimulation of the growth or differentiation of cells participating in the inflammatory response. Finally, most of these cytokines have been purified and cloned so that their exact mechanism of action can be elucidated and, in addition, some of them can be used therapeutically to modify or augment an otherwise inappropriate inflammatory or immune response. This is the case, for example, of IL-2 which is used in humans to stimulate the proliferation of lymphocytes, and of GM-CSF, used to treat neutropenia. Several cytokines participate in the inflammatory response, and since most of them involve immune competent cells, they belong to the subgroup of interleukins (IL). Others, like GM-CSF, target on granulocyte and macrophage precursors stimulating them to produce more mature daughter cells.

Basophils and mast cells, and also other cells, produce a factor called platelet activating factor (PAF) which is a potent inducer of platelet aggregation and activation, causing the release of histamine.

Complement. We will see in Chapter 6 when we discuss immunological reactions, that serum component participates in the formation of the antigen/antibody complex. This third partner, called complement, is not an innocent bystander. Indeed, the binding of complement has two consequences that are relevant to the processes of inflammation. First, it exerts a strong chemotactic effect attracting polymorphonuclear leukocytes. Second, complement activation causes an increase in vascular permeability by trigger-

Table 5–2. Cytokines Participating in Inflammation

	MAIN CELLULAR SOURCES	MAIN EFFECTS
IL-1	Several cell types including: macrophages, fibroblasts, epidermal cells, lymphocytes, some brain cells	Fever; stimulation of lymphocytes; stimulation of liver to produce acute phase proteins; activation of lymphocytes; induction of mediators of inflammation, e.g., prostaglandins; mobilization of neutrophils to site of inflammation
IL-2	Helper T lymphocytes	Lymphocyte proliferation
IL-3	Helper T lymphocytes	Growth and differentiation of pluripotent hemopoietic stem cells
IL-4	Activated T lymphocytes	Stimulation of B and T lymphocytes, and hematopoietic cells, especially mast cells; promotion of granulomatous inflammation
IL-5	T lymphocytes	Stimulation of eosinophils; acts on B lymphocyte differentiation
IL-6	Several cell types including: T lymphocytes, macrophages, fibroblasts, some brain cells, some epithelial cells	Stimulation of B cells and plasma cells; stimulation of liver cells to produce acute phase proteins; acts on hematopoietic cells
IL-7	Stromal cells of spleen, bone marrow and thymus	Differentiation of immature B lymphocytes; differentiation of T cells
GM-CSF	Several cell types including: fibroblasts, macrophages, endothelial cells	Production of neutrophils, macrophages and eosinophils
Interferon gamma	Activated T lymphocytes	Expression of histocompatibility antigens on a number of mesenchymal and epithelial cells

Abbreviations IL = interleukin; GM = granulocyte-macrophage colony stimulating factor. Note that most cytokines can be produced by more than one cell type and, in turn, often have different cellular targets.

ing histamine and leukotriene release from neighboring leukocytes.

Additional aspects of the role of antibody in inflammation are discussed in the next chapter.

Fibrin. When inflammation occurs, one important molecule that normally circulates in the vascular compartment in a precursor form is able to escape into the interstitial spaces. Fibrinogen, a high-molecular-weight protein synthesized by the liver, is normally inactive and contributes to the intravascular osmotic pressure. When capillary permeability is increased, fibrinogen escapes from the lumen and is converted to fibrin by the inflammatory response. It turns into threads of fibrin that are woven into a mesh or network in the interstitial space. These threads act as a lattice on which polymorphonuclear leukocytes can gain a foothold. Lattice-building facilitates the process of phagocytosis, particularly in the lung (Fig. 5–11).

Fig. 5–11 This photomicrograph of the lung in lobar pneumonia shows abundant polymorphonuclear leukocytes, and, at the arrow, fibrin strands and leukocytes passing through the pores of Kohn between 2 alveoli.

This lattice is not immovable and some steps of the inflammatory process itself are associated with the lysis of the fibrin network.

Systemic Defense Mechanisms

Under this umbrella we consider fever, leukocytosis, pain, and some less-well-understood changes that accompany major stress.

Fever. Normal temperature includes the recognition that each of us has a daily rhythm of body temperatures. This normal rhythm peaks about 6 p.m. each day, with an increase of as much as half a degree Celsius over the basal level. This is normal temperature, far short of the bone-aching, hectic, sheet-drenching expression of the physiology of a temperature of 104°F or 42°C.

The causes of fever are legion, but the mechanisms are well described. Any substance capable of causing fever is generally called a **pyrogen.** There are bacterial pyrogens and chemical agents, such as etiocholanolone, a steroid, that also raise the body temperature. There are endogenous pyrogens derived from leukocytes of the polymorphonuclear class as well as from macrophages and monocytes. The relevant mediator in this respect is interleukin-1 which is released by the activated macrophage. In elegant studies, Bodel showed that cells, including the monocyte, macrophages, Kupffer cells, and granulocytes, when isolated, contain no pyrogen, but that after stimulation, they produce pyrogen for many hours or for several days. Pyrogens, whether they are exogenous or endogenous to the host, act on the neurons of the thermoregulatory center of the anterior hypothalamus. The signals that adjust this thermostat increase the metabolic rate, oxygen consumption, and the respiratory rate. Interleukin-1 does not work alone in producing fever and requires secondary components such as prostaglandins. The end result producing fever is the inability of the organism to dissipate the excess heat. It is desirable to bring down fever by any means, for example, baths, ice, water, and drugs such as aspirin.

Leukocytosis. An increase in the number of circulating white blood cells in the peripheral blood has been referred to earlier as an example of systemic response to injury. The presence of injury is often revealed to the physician by the increase (normal 5,000 to 7,000 white blood cells/mm^3) in numbers up to 30,000/mm^3. The spectrum of change includes a departure from the normal pattern of white blood cells to one in which even immature forms are seen on examination of the smear of the peripheral blood.

Pain. We might say a word here about pain, as it is another component of our defense system, one that is easy to understand in the light of an injury such as a burn, but is nonetheless important to put into perspective because, most frequently, pain is accompanied by inflammation, and vice versa.

In the most general sense, pain is a response to injury. The mechanism by which it is induced is currently the focus of much interest. The subject is larger than we can encompass here, but a simple consideration of pain may draw attention to its relation to inflammation and may suggest some more important aspects of pain as a part of the picture of disease.

First, pain may be caused by direct stimulation of nerve endings, which are in some instances directly designed to respond to inflammation, just as other nerve endings respond to light, odor, or temperature. The skin, an organ in its own right, contains naked nerve endings that signal pain, just as others signal pressure or temperature change. Other organs, such as the gut, do not respond in exactly the same way, and the sensation of pain is perceived in the gastrointestinal tract only when there is stretching, as in overdistension of the stomach, or when the mucosa is removed and free nerve endings are exposed, as in an ulcer. Both ischemia and anoxia, in skeletal and cardiac muscle, signal pain. Traction of an artery may give pain when an arterial puncture is performed. Veins, however, are relatively insensitive, as anyone who has given blood can testify. However, all structures of the body, except perhaps the brain itself, respond to inflammation by signalling pain. The substances credited with this perception are polypeptides and substances of low molecular weight, such as histamine, acetylcholine, 5-hydroxytryptamine, bradykinin, all included in a class known as **mediators** of inflammation. These substances may be secreted by cells that are distributed through all tissues, such as mast cells, or they may be the product of dead or dying cells, or the result of interaction between the injured tissue and serum proteins in an inflamed area. These substances may be activated by a cascade of enzymatic reactions, and they leak, during inflammation, out of the microcirculation. Whatever its origin, pain is often the earliest and one of the most important signs that an injury has occurred.

It is of interest, because of the difficulty in deciding what the true cause of the pain may be, to recognize that pain that appears to come from one place does not necessarily arise in the tissues or organs underlying the apparent location. For example, pain during a myocardial infarction may be felt to radiate down the inner aspect of the left arm. This phenomenon is called referred pain, and several explanations have been offered, none of which is entirely satisfactory. Two existing theories are: (1) pain is referred between

parts of the body that share the embryologic deriva-
tion and innervation, and (2) it is referred through
connection in the spinal cord.

There is a large variation in the perception of pain
in different persons. The awareness of pain can be
dulled by drugs (morphine). Rage and fear may suppress pain, so that one may not even be aware of an
extensive injury. Pain remains one of the commonest
and most important signs of disease, and of all the
processes in disease states, inflammation is one of the
most common.

It is possible to spend many pages characterizing
pain of different origins, its onset, duration, and factors that either alleviate or exacerbate it, and to relate
these characteristics to different types of disease or
organ systems, but that is beyond the scope of this
chapter.

Results of Inflammation

The effective inflammatory response meets the
challenge of injury with the varied panoply we have
sketched. Microcirculatory, cellular, humoral, and
systemic reactions are like an ancient Roman army
meeting the foreign enemy's spearmen and gladia-
tors. The net result is to isolate, wall off, starve out,
or annihilate the invader, if indeed it is injury due to
a biologic agent, and to prepare the way for the next
sequence of events, the repair of the damage (healing). In general terms, the inflammatory response has
modified the vascular supply to the injured area and
has alerted the host by a variety of signals to send
troops continuously to the beleaguered zone, to initiate the machinery for antibody synthesis, and to arm
the host for faster metabolic activity. The localization
of the injury by slowing the flow in and out of the
inflamed area, the presence of a scaffolding (fibrin) on
which the active cellular defenders can climb, hand
over hand, and can engage in combat with the bacterial invaders, and the general alarm reaction initiated
through the release of interleukins and adrenal, cortical and medullary hormones all take place in an effective sequence unless the host is debilitated, or unless
aspects of the response are inhibited by drugs such as
are used to treat cancer or to suppress the inflammatory response. In brief, the results are an effective con-
tainment of the injury.

Complications of Inflammation

There are other sides to the inflammatory process,
particularly when it is elicited by a bacterial or infectious agent, and we shall consider them under the
general heading of complications of inflammation.

The more common outcomes of inflammation are
shown in Figure 5–12.

Let us consider the prototype of a bacterial attack
introduced through a puncture wound of the skin,
where the original inflammatory response is not successful in containing and destroying the implanted
microorganisms. When the inflammatory sequence is
successful, there is no spread or evolution of the injury. When spread does occur, it is the result of the
penetration of the microorganism into the blood
stream. If the numbers of bacteria are sufficient and
virulent, we call this **septicemia,** and its effect is to
escalate the warfare from a small affair to a systemic
and life-threatening episode. Norman Bethune, the
Canadian missionary surgeon who was a hero of
modern China for his battlefield efforts during their
Revolution, died from septicemia following his accidental inoculation when he cut himself while operating in an infected area. With the development of antibiotic and drug sensitivity assays, the outcome of septicemia is not necessarily fatal today. One result of the
embolization of bacteria, represented by septicemia,
is the potential for seeding bacterial colonies to grow
in an infinite number of anatomic sites, in addition to
the site of entry. Widespread abscesses may form in
many organs of the body. This outcome of uncontrolled infection is due to an ineffective inflammatory
response.

The most common evolution of inflammation in response to bacterial injury is the development of an
abscess. An **abscess** may be defined as a cavity filled
with pus in a tissue. The importance of an abscess is
not that it exists, but that in order to exist it has had
to make a place for itself in a vital organ, and by so
doing has inevitably destroyed some of the tissue of
that organ. It is one thing to have an abscess under a

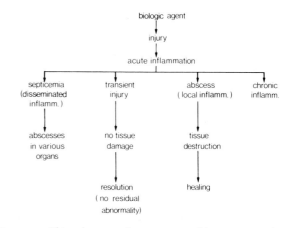

Fig. 5–12 This scheme outlines some possible outcomes of acute
inflammation.

tooth, and quite another to have an abscess in the speech center of the brain. The evolution of the abscess is the story of inflammation, but its physiologic consequence may be to destroy irretrievably some functioning tissue. The history of an abscess begins when the bacterial invaders gain a foothold in a particular tissue and the defensive reaction walls off the bacteria and builds a boundary of fibrin and cells around the margin. At the same time, a large number of phagocytes, attracted by the prey, sally into the area where tissue is dying and where bacteria are multiplying. Subsequently, the limited life span of the polymorphonuclear leukocytes reduces them and the ingested bacteria to a yellowish liquid without life, but rich in enzymatic debris. This is pus. The eventual fate of the liquid-filled cavity is to rupture, usually to the surface if the abscess is in the skin, a most common site. Abscesses deep in vital organs such as the liver may rupture through the surface of the organ into the appropriate body cavity, in that case the peritoneum, and spread the infection (peritonitis), or they may become enclosed again in some larger space, for example, between the liver and the diaphragm. In lung abscess, inflammation may frequently extend to the pleural surface and may involve the pleural space. Pus in the pleural space is commonly referred to as an empyema.

When an abscess lies deep in the tissues and eventually finds its way to rupture and drain the necrotic, purulent material, it creates a track leading from the abscess to the surface that is called a **sinus.** Should the abscess join two mucosal surfaces (bowel to bowel), or an internal organ and the skin, this connection is often referred to as a **fistula,** or abnormal communication between two compartments.

Because the rich enzymatic content and the presence of fibrin in acute inflammation are not easily resolved, the effect of inflammation on otherwise normal organs is to create a fabric of new contacts or adhesions between surfaces that had been smooth, shiny, and normally lubricated. This phenomenon allows spatial adjustments to take place as necessary within cavities such as the peritoneum. These fibrinous adhesions, as they are called, are testimony to the fire within. The adhesions may bind the surface of the lung to the chest wall, the epicardial surface of the heart to the pericardium, or the surfaces of the small or large bowel to one another. One result of this new, unplanned contact is the colonization of these fibrin links by permanent fibrous bridges, predisposing patients to obstruction in the gastrointestinal tract.

Anergy. We should note that in some cases the expected does not happen. In the very old, very young, and very sick, inflammation does not occur in a nor-

mal way. The failure to mobilize the defensive reactions has been termed anergy. In so many instances it is the presence of pain, fever, and leukocytosis that signifies the presence of injury. The diagnosis of appendicitis is easier since we have come to understand the pattern. The diagnosis of meningitis is usually made more obvious because of the inflammation that involves nerve roots. Can you imagine the diagnostic dilemma when, in a case of appendicitis, there is no pain in the right lower quadrant, no fever, or no leukocytosis, and the patient becomes progressively sicker? Or the situation where coma supervenes without the telltale sign of a stiff neck in meningitis? In these situations, the appropriate therapy is not given because the diagnosis is obscured by the absence of the usual pattern of inflammation. Thus inflammation is more than a biologic phenomenon. In the practice of medicine it often presents the clue to the correct diagnosis.

There are intermediate forms of anergy in which the patient is capable of mounting an inflammatory response, but at a lower level than required. This is found in otherwise normal persons who have become severely ill from a number of causes. Their partially compromised state can be easily detected using skin tests with antigens eliciting delayed hypersensitivity and the information has a prognostic significance.

Chronic Inflammation. Depending on the host's defense mechanisms or the virulence of the causative agent, acute inflammation can progress to a chronic process. This can also occur if the same episode of acute inflammation occurs at the same site. Sometimes, however, chronic inflammation can start as such without prior clinical manifestations of acute inflammation. In any event, the chronically inflamed site contains mononuclear cells such as lymphocytes, macrophages and plasma cells in various proportions. The patient experiences smoldering pain which fluctuates with time. If the chronic inflammation is located in a joint, such as in rheumatoid arthritis, there is also remodeling of tissue resulting in deformity and loss of motion. Chronic inflammation can persist for life, and sometimes afflicts the morale of patients who cannot accept to live with its symptoms. Curiously, in some circumstances it can also subside after many months and even years, probably as a result of a favorable repair mechanism.

Some cases of chronic inflammation are accompanied by the deposition of an amorphous substance called amyloid. Extensive deposition of this material in multiple organs corresponds to the systemic disease amyloidosis. The amyloid substance is a protein and has a natural tendency to have a pleated molecular configuration which helps in its identification by a special stain. In fact, there are several types of proteins that can become processed and deposited in this way. The important organs in which deposition occurs with significant clinical implications are: liver, kidney, heart and spleen. In addition, the brain of patients with Alzheimer's disease contains focal lesions in which amyloid is found. This has important implications to be discussed in Chapter 24.

HEALING OR REPAIR

The aim of the efforts deployed by the body in response to injury is to restore the organism to its original state, if possible, and the steps toward this goal can be arbitrarily separated. However, it is difficult to state categorically at any one moment where inflammation ends and where healing begins.

For the purpose of this chapter, it is well to remember that we are discussing generalities about biologic phenomena that are derived from many different specific examples. For instance, healing in the skin is different from healing in the cornea, which has no blood vessels. Healing in the heart is different (because it is constantly working) from healing in a skeletal muscle that has been splinted. Healing in the liver is different from healing of the femur. In these instances, healing may be different because the nature of the injuries may vary. Mechanical trauma, a one-time occasion, may initiate a series of responses that appear different, with a beginning, a middle, and an end, from the healing that takes place in the face of chronic irritation or metabolic injury, as in nutritional cirrhosis.

With these provisos, we shall consider an arbitrary division of the process from injury to restoration of normal function, and then we shall discuss specific examples of healing in different tissues.

An arbitrary list of steps, starting with injury, could be stated as follows:

1. **Injury.** This can be of many kinds, from thermal burns and surgical incisions to infections and ischemic necrosis. Important considerations are the size, extent, and degree of local hemorrhage, and the kind of tissue damage. Obviously a small puncture with a sterile needle invokes a different type of healing from a fracture of a long bone with massive hemorrhage.

2. **Inflammation.** The vascular, cellular, and systemic responses already discussed are an important preparation for restoration of normal structure and function.

3. **Debridement.** Although the removal of dead, dying, injured, or foreign material from an injury could just as easily be considered part of inflammation, it is an essential part of healing. In the presence of foreign bodies (splinters, glass, bacteria), the process of healing is aborted and inflammation persists, invariably distorting the restoration to normal. This debridement is effected most conventionally by enzymatic means. However, it is one of the achievements of medicine that the intervention of the physician, who removes the nonviable materials, actually accelerates the repair process. In older times, maggots were sometimes used to debride complicated wounds, and more recently, purified enzymes (streptokinase) have been used occasionally for that purpose.

4. **Repair.** The ingrowth of new capillaries, the migration of fibroblasts, the elaboration of collagen, ground substance, and elastic fibers, and the recovery of areas where the epithelium has been lost are all unequivocal steps in healing. When a group of epithelial cells of the skin or intestinal mucosa have been killed by whatever means, the neighboring cells perceive in some way this loss of integrity of the membranous barrier and begin to migrate over the basement membrane in efforts to resurface the lost area (Fig. 5–13). This migration can be seen within minutes of injury, and within hours there is an increase in mitosis in the adjacent cells, which begin to multiply in order to replace the lost cells. The signal for this re-epithelization is believed to be the loss of the cell-to-cell attachments typical of all epithelia. Normally, cells cease replicating when their borders are attached to other cells; this is called contact inhibition.

5. **Remodeling.** The final phase in repair is the remodeling of the newly manufactured tissue in response to the demands of normal use. Typically, a new scar on the skin of the arm or the hand is first as smooth as glass, but with use and time it develops wrinkles and calluses just like the old skin. However, it may not develop the freckles or the hairs that were once there, since the regeneration may not include all the elements of the original tissue. Nowhere is remodeling so elegantly seen as in the final healed result of a fractured long bone in a young person.

For an illustration of healing, we shall take a simple skin wound, in which the incision has sundered the epithelium and the subcutaneous tissue down to the underlying muscle (Fig. 5–14). It is the typical kitchen knife accident, treated at home with a small adhesive bandage and soon forgotten as healing takes place over the ensuing four or five days. The wound kills a few hundred thousand cells of the epidermis, splits the basement membrane, and ruptures small and large blood vessels in its path. These blood vessels bleed briskly into the defect between the severed edges; the coagulation cascade is initiated by the liberation of tissue thromboplastins from the damaged cells.

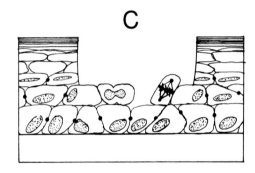

Fig. 5–13 These drawings show: *A*, the injury of the epithelium; *B*, the mitosis and migration of the germinal cells; and *C*, the continuing attempt to repair the epithelial lesion.

Next is the initiation of the inflammatory response by the kinins and the peptides liberated from the damaged tissue. Simultaneously, the epithelial cells that have lost their neighboring contact begin to move to find a similar cell. This movement causes a flow of epithelial cells toward the free or cut margin. The attenuation of the covering sheet of cells is met later by new cells arising from mitosis in the germinal epithelium of the epidermis. If the cut margins are brought together by an adhesive bandage, suture, or pressure, as in Fig. 5–15, then the migrating epithelial cells may meet their counterparts and join in a single sheet within a day or so. This renewal of epithelium and approximation of the underlying tissue is called **healing by first intention.**

In the deeper layer of the skin wound, fat cells have been ruptured, elastic fibers severed, nerves rendered, and the fabric of the interstitial tissue altered by the cataclysm of microcosmic catastrophe. Bringing together the severed edges staunches the blood flow, accelerates coagulation, and apposes the tissues. The inflammatory process is soon in progress, and there are attempts to realign the vascular network. New capillaries form from the neighboring ones. Fibroblasts differentiate from paravascular cells or are transformed from existing quiescent fibrocytes. Soon the cytoplasmic machinery prepares collagen in soluble or monomeric (unpolymerized) form to be delivered into the interstitial space, where the collagen will mature, polymerize (aggregate to form macromolecules), and form fibrils of indeterminate length but of great tensile strength. The sequence of events during healing is shown in Fig. 5–16, which illustrates the time course of the deposition of extracellular materials and its relationship to the tensile strength of the wound.

The rate at which the repair by newly formed collagen, a "magic weave" repair, takes place is of real consequence to the restoration of normal function of a tissue. Not until the restoration of the mechanical integrity of the tissue has occurred is it safe to remove the surgeon's sutures, or to apply physical stress to

Fig. 5–14 This drawing suggests the changes that take place with time in the restoration or healing of a wound. At the top (*A*), a fresh injury with red blood cells, fibrin, and platelets indicated, the fibrinogen as the single lines, the platelets as the triangles. At the bottom (*B*) an organized clot has formed.

the recent incision line. For example, the simple stress of a cough may initiate the breakdown of the gossamer-like fabric of fibrin and cells of a 2-day-old wound. The patient in whom wound dehiscence (rupture) most commonly occurs after an operation is the person with chronic lung disease who coughs constantly. Other important causes of failure of normal healing are malnutrition, vitamin deficiency, absence of essential elements such as zinc, and the presence of infection. A marginally successful blood supply or atherosclerosis also predisposes a person to inadequate healing and wound dehiscence.

A second pattern of healing is best illustrated when the injured edges are not brought together within a short time (hours), and where the edges are left separated, either exposed to the air or separated by a large clot or by necrotic tissue (Fig. 5–17). The defect created by the injury may be deep or superficial, small or extensive, but the distances to repair in cellular terms are vast. The process of repair must proceed from the base of the wound and must attempt to fill in the defect from the bottom. This pattern of healing is called healing by **second intention**, and is much

slower than healing by first intention. Because of its very nature, this slower pattern of healing often leads to a palpable or visible defect years later in the form of scar tissue. In man, the process consists of budding capillary loops growing slowly into the crusted, overlying area (scab), which is composed of serum proteins and clot. The appearance of the capillary loops, with their accompanying perivascular cells and fibroblasts, is red and friable, bleeding at the slightest provocation, and has a granular appearance. It is called granulation tissue. Scar tissue such as is formed in a defect caused by a burn or an extensive loss of epithelium may conform to the original shape and size of the damage; however, in general, scar tissue has the tendency to contract as it gets older. Marked deformities and shortening in the area may result (contractures), leading to a loss of function. The victims of the atomic bomb in Hiroshima had to undergo many plastic reconstructive procedures because of the contractures on the exposed areas of their skin. Another outcome of scar formation may be the exuberant overgrowth of the new connective tissue that results

Fig. 5–15 *A* and *B*, This figure illustrates the importance of apposition in a fresh injury, showing the approximation of the wound edges.

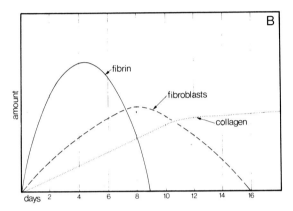

Fig. 5–16   *A,* This graph shows the sequential changes of polymorphs, lymphocytes, and monocytes in comparative numbers. *B,* This shows, at the same time, changes in the presence of fibrin, fibroblasts, and collagen.

the heart cannot regenerate new muscle, and although the remaining fibers compensate by increasing in size (hypertrophy), the necrotic area is replaced in six weeks by firm, white connective tissue that has no contractile capacity. Some organs, such as the kidney, may respond to injury by replacement with new tubular cells, so that a scar does not appear. However, in other instances where the damage is considerable or continuous, there may be scar tissue present as testimony to the previous injury. The fibrous tissue of the scar can cause compression or even occlusion of hollow organs. This is what happens in chronic salpingitis when the affected woman becomes sterile because of the occlusion of the fallopian tubes by an inappropriate repair process. The most successful of the many appearances of healing is the replacement of damaged tissue by identical but new tissue. Unfortunately, this cannot take place in many tissues of man, where the important cells have lost their power to undergo mitosis (for example, neurons in the brain, heart muscle cells), but in other organs (the liver and epithelium of the gastrointestinal tract, for example), repair can be effected by simple, natural replacement. The many factors that come to bear on the healing process are shown diagrammatically in Fig. 5–18.

Principles of Management. In the treatment of any disease, the health care personnel may adopt one or both of two methods: he or she may assist the healing powers of Nature, and/or directly attack the cause of the illness. Rest of the inflamed part is one of the most important of all therapeutic measures. Activity may act as an additional irritant, and may disperse the bacteria through the tissues and increase the area of inflammation. It tends to break down the barrier that the leukocytes try to build around the bacteria. Thus

in a protuberance above the old surface plane. This raised, healed area, seen frequently in surgical wounds, is called a keloid. After many months or years, it may subside to match the surrounding tissue elevations as remodeling takes place.

We have discussed healing in the skin and have described what happens in a system that is largely 2-dimensional. Healing occurs, of course, in many organs besides the skin. After a myocardial infarction,

Fig. 5–17   This drawing illustrates granulation tissue. The capillary buds and the presence of perivascular cells are shown in the drawing.

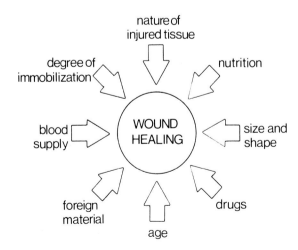

Fig. 5–18   This illustrates the many different factors that may modify wound healing.

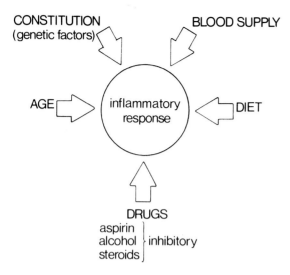

Fig. 5–19 This scheme illustrates factors that can alter the inflammatory response.

good, for it may open fresh channels for the spread of the infection. Drainage is essential in infections of enclosed spaces such as the pleural and peritoneal cavities.

Depending on the cause of the inflammatory process and whether it is accompanied by edema or not, cold or heat may be applied

A direct attack on the invading bacteria by antibiotics has come to occupy so dominant a place in the treatment of inflammation due to infection that we sometimes lose sight of the healing powers that used to be our only hope, powers that proved to be sufficient in most cases (Fig. 5–19).

Finally, we have anti-inflammatory agents which are active against acute and chronic inflammation. However, the aids to the healing process reviewed earlier far outweigh the value of individual drugs.

In conclusion, we should recognize that whereas inflammation and healing have been represented here as beneficial biologic responses, in each instance there are examples in which the deleterious effects of the process may outweigh the benefits. Chronic inflammation, as in rheumatoid arthritis, can destroy joints and permanently cripple; the formation of adhesions and scar tissue can obstruct vital pathways, as in mitral stenosis, or in the case of hydrocephalus following meningitis. We must therefore recognize these processes for what they are—responses to stimuli that depend on many factors for their outcome.

Table 5–2 lists the important soluble cytokines secreted by various cells participating directly or indirectly in the inflammatory reactions.

the inflamed finger is splinted, the inflamed arm is placed in a sling, the inflamed eye is shaded so that it cannot be used.

A second principle is drainage. The quickest way to get an abscess to heal is to open it and to drain the pus. This procedure not only allows the infecting bacteria to escape, but it also relieves the tension in the inflamed area, and thus encourages the further flow of healing substances from the blood vessel, in addition to relieving the pain. However, if pus has not yet formed and if a barrier of leukocytes has been built around the bacteria, the knife may do more harm than

SYNOPSIS

Physical, chemical, bacterial, and immunologic injuries all lead to inflammation.
Inflammation and healing are a continuum.
Humoral, vascular and cellular phases of inflammation are well coordinated.
A large number of mediators are involved in the inflammatory humoral response and some of them can be specifically blocked by therapeutic drugs.
Systemic responses to inflammation are leukocytosis and fever.
Acute, subacute, chronic, and granulomatous inflammations differ in cellular and temporal terms.
The advantages and disadvantages of inflammation are opposite sides of the same coin. Inflammation is advantageous when it is properly regulated in its duration and extent. On the contrary, an excessive or uncontrolled inflammatory response leads to further tissue injury and sequelae.
Factors that enhance healing include rest, adequate nutrition, a good blood supply, normal protein metabolism, and adequate stores of nutrients.

Terms

Phagocytosis	Lymphocyte	Cytokine
Chemotaxis	Plasma cell	Mediator
Polymorphonuclear leukocytes	Granuloma	Septicemia
Pyrogen	Giant cell	Fibroblast
Macrophage	Interleukins	Granulation tissue

FURTHER READING

Adams, D.O.: The granulomatous inflammatory response. A review. Am. J. Pathol., 84:164, 1976.

Alam, R., et al.: Monocyte chemotactic and activating factor is a potent histamine-releasing factor for basophils. J. Clin. Investig., 89:723, 1992.

Atkins,. E., and Bodel, P.: Clinical fever: its history, manifestations and pathogenesis. Fed. Proc., 38:57, 1979.

Bonta, I.L., et al.: Tumour necrosis factor in inflammation: relation to other mediators and to macrophage antitumour defence. Pharmacol. Res., 24:115, 1991.

Boucher, N.L.R.: Experimental aspects of hepatic regeneration. N. Engl. J. Med., 277:686, 1967.

Bruyen G.A.W., et al.: Mechanisms of host defense against infection with streptococcus pneumoniae. Clin. Infect. Dis., 14:251, 1992.

Colten, H.R.: Tissue-specific regulation of inflammation. J. Appl. Physiol., 72:1, 1992.

Delrosso, M.: Relationship between coagulation and inflammation. J. Immunol. Res., 3:185, 1991.

Deuel, T.F., and Kawahara, R.S.: Growth factors and wound healing: Platelet-derived growth factor as a model cytokine. Annu. Rev. Med., 42:567, 1991.

Editorial. From regeneration to scar formation: the collagen way. Lab. Investig., 64:131, 1991.

Fine, R.: Inhibition of alveolar macrophage chemotaxis by ethanol and prostaglandin E_1. Am. Rev. Respir. Dis., 117:273, 1978.

Goodwin, J.S., and Webb, D.R.: Regulation of the immune response by prostaglandins. Clin. Immunol. Immunopathol., 15:106, 1980.

Hulth, A.: Fracture healing. A concept of competing healing factors. Acta Orthop. Scand., 51:5, 1980.

Jäättelä, M.: Biologic of disease. Biologic activities and mechanisms of action of tumor necrosis factor-α/cachectin. Lab. Investig., 64:724, 1991.

Keller, H.U., Hess, M.W., and Cottier, H.: Granulocyte chemokinesis and chemotaxis. In Cellular Interactions. Edited by Dingle and Gordon. Elsevier/North Holland Biomedical Press, 1981.

Kluger, M.J.: Fever: Role of pyrogens and cryogens. Physiol. Rev., 71:93, 1991.

Knockaert, D.C., Vanneste, L.J., Vanneste, S.B., et al.: Fever of unknown origin in the 1980s. Arch. Int. Med., 152:51, 1992.

Kuehl, F.A., and Egan, R.W.: Prostaglandins, arachidonic acid and inflammation. Science, 210:978, 1980.

Majno, G.: The Healing Hand: Man and Wound in the Ancient World. Cambridge, Harvard University Press, 1974.

Marx, J.L.: Coagulation as a common thread in disease. Science, 218:145, 1982.

Medved, L., et al.: Electron microscope investigation of the early stages of fibrin assembly. Twisted protofibrils and fibers. J. Mol. Biol., 216:503, 1990.

Moldauer, L.L, et al.: Interleukin[1] tumor necrosis factor-alpha (cachetic) and the pathogenesis of cancer cachexia. Clin. Physiol., 7:263, 1987.

Movat, H.Z. (ed.): Inflammation, Immunity and Hypersensitivity. Hagerstown, Md., Harper & Row, 1972.

Newhouse, M., Shanchis, J., and Bienenstock, J.: Lung defense mechanisms. N. Engl. J. Med., 295:990, 1976.

Oster, W., and Schulz, G.: Interleukin 3: biological and clinical effects. Intl. J. Cell Cloning, 9:5, 1991.

Peplow, P.V., and Mikhailidis, D.P.: Platelet-activating factor (PAF) and its relation to prostaglandins, leukotrienes and other aspects of arachidonate metabolism. Prostaglandins, Leukot. Essent. Fatty Acids, 41:71, 1990.

Roberts, R., and Gallin, J.I.: The phagocytic cell and its disorders. Ann. Allergy, 50:330, 1983.

Samuelsson, B.: Prostaglandins, thromboxanes, and leukotrienes: formation and biological roles. Harvey Lectures 75, 1. New York, Academic Press, 1981.

Samuelsson, B., Dahlen, S.E., et al.: Leukotrienes and lipoxins. Structures, biosynthesis and biological effects. Science, 237:1171, 1987.

Serafin, W.E., and Austen, K.F.: Mediators of immediate hypersensitivity reactions. N. Engl. J. Med., 317:30, 1987.

Sharma, J.N., and Mohsin, S.S.J.: The role of chemical mediators in the pathogenesis of inflammation with emphasis on the kinin system. Exp. Pathol., 38:73, 1990.

Spitznagel, J.K.: Antibiotic proteins of human neutrophils. J. Clin. Invest., 86:1381, 1990.

Stemerman, M.B.: Vascular injury: platelets and smooth muscle cell response. Phil. Trans. R. Soc. Lond., B294:217, 1981.

Stossel, T.P.: Phagocytosis. N. Engl. J. Med., 290:717, 1974.

Unanue, E.R.: Cooperation between mononuclear phagocytes and lymphocytes in immunity. N. Engl. J. Med., 303:977, 1980.

Vane, J.R.: Prostacyclin. J. Roy. Soc. Med., 76:245, 1983.

Von Euler, U.S.: History and development of prostaglandins. Gen. Pharmac., 14:3, 1983.

6

THE IMMUNE SYSTEM AND ITS DISORDERS

The development of immunity, in the broadest sense, is a process by which the body learns from experience of past infections to deal more efficiently with subsequent ones.—MACFARLANE BURNET

Early in the course of evolution, animals learned to protect themselves against external enemies by developing armor, spines, or poison. Some enemies gained access to the interior of the body and adopted the life of a parasite. They were recognized by the wandering cells we have described in Chapter 5 (macrophages), and attempts to evict the newcomers were not always successful. An acceptance or tolerance of the newcomer was often acquired by the host after it had remained for some time. This tolerance demanded some adaptation to the foreign agent, which frequently secreted substances or was acknowledged to be different from the host by virtue of different biochemical markers on its surface. Perhaps the visitor was successfully repulsed after a lengthy battle. We now know that if the host is visited again by the same unwanted guest, the cellular and humoral mechanisms are able to recognize the intruder because of the previous visitation, and react more vigorously to reject him, we say, because of their previous **sensitization.**

Classically, immunity takes two forms: the cellular response, in which lymphocytes and their relatives are concerned with a direct confrontation, and the humoral response, characterized by antibodies that circulate in the serum after having been produced by a cell somewhere in the body following the original sensitization. However, the immunologic mechanisms are not so simple, because every cell and every host has genetically determined markers on all its cells from the time of its creation. These substances are the hallmark of our individuality. Blood group determinants A, B, and O, the Rh factors, and transplantation antigens are all examples of these inherited differences among persons.

The capacity to develop antibodies to any antigen is related both to the presence of lymphocytes in the blood and to the presence of lymphoid tissue somewhere in the body. This unique defensive system permits the host to mobilize a cytologic army (lymphocytes) against invaders, and to spread the serologic equivalent of gas warfare (antibody production). However, this complicated defensive apparatus can sometimes backfire, as when the wind blows poison gas back over the troops who launched it. The immunologic defense system can be turned on tissues of the host itself. The concept of **autoimmunity** is described later in this chapter. There are also a number of circumstances in which the immune system is either genetically deficient or becomes suppressed during life. The latter situation is epitomized by the acquired immune deficiency syndrome (AIDS), which is also discussed below.

We shall outline first the normal function of the immune system: the cells involved and the types of antibody and immunologic reactions. We shall then discuss two general disorders of this system: first, when it is deficient, and second, when it is over-reactive. Finally, we shall consider immunity as it relates to transplantation and to autoimmune disease.

CELLS OF THE IMMUNE RESPONSE

There are several populations of cells that function directly in the immune response. First is the lymphocyte, a cell capable of detecting foreign cells or material. There are two main kinds of lymphocytes: "B cells," derived from the bone marrow, and "T cells," derived from the thymus (Fig. 6–1). Essentially, B cells originate in the bone marrow and mature in peripheral organs. T cells also originate in the bone mar-

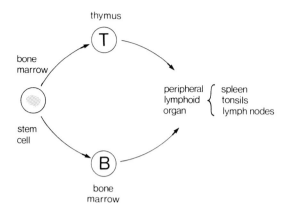

Fig. 6–1   Differentiation of lymphocytes. Cells of the immune system begin as multipotential (stem) cells in the bone marrow. They may differentiate into several types of blood cells and lymphocytes (see Fig. 5–7). The two types of lymphocytes mature in different locations as described in the text, then migrate to lymph nodes throughout the body.

row but undergo processing in the thymus, hence their name, whereby some of them are deleted. Subsequently, T cells colonize the same types of peripheral organs as the B cells, which include lymph nodes, spleen, and intestine. They are also present in the peripheral blood in which they traffic between various organs to carry on their immunologic duties.

Both the B and T lymphocytes have a sophisticated way of expressing their genes. The relevant genes code for immunoglobulins in the case of B cells, and for the T cell receptor in the case of T cells. Interestingly, these two genes have a certain degree of homology in their organization and mode of expression. In the resting stage the genes are organized in a number of physically separated exons. When the lymphocyte is stimulated some of these exons become rearranged in the DNA. When this segment of DNA is transcribed into m-RNA the rearranged genes are spliced together into mature molecules of messenger RNA. Eventually the messenger RNA is translated into surface immunoglobulin or T cell receptors, depending on whether this occurs in a B cell or a T cell. Because there are several exons in the gene and a very large number of ways to rearrange them, there is an enormous potential diversity in the number of gene products that can be produced. For instance, it has been calculated that gene rearrangements in B cells can produce a repertoire of more than 10 million different types of immunoglobulin molecules. The whole process is comparable to the task of those professionals in the perfume industry who combine a number of different primordial scents to produce a unique product.

In a given lymphoid organ, such as a lymph node or the spleen, there is a mixture of different lymphocytes each housing its specific pattern of rearranged genes. Conversely, when there is a lymphoma or a lymphocytic leukemia, only one type of gene rearrangement can be observed when the DNA of the affected lymphoid organ is examined. Based on this observation new diagnostic methods have been introduced which allow the detection of monoclonal rearrangements of genes even when there is a very small proportion of lymphomatous or leukemic cells in the organ to be tested.

Both types of lymphocytes originate from stem cells in the bone marrow; some stem cells later migrate to the thymus, where they develop into mature T cells. Finally, T cells migrate to various lymphoid tissues around the body. Several lymphoid elements affect the differentiation of B cells (Fig. 6–2).

"B cells" were originally so called because in birds these lymphocytes arise in the bursa of Fabricius, a lymphoid organ lying in the avian rump. B cells retain immunoglobulins or antibodies attached to their surface membranes. When these antibodies come into contact with an antigen (foreign macromolecule, particle or cell), the antibody on the cell surface interacts with the antigen, and B cell differentiates into a plasma cell. Plasma cells then actively produce and secrete antibodies specific for the antigen that originally stimulated the differentiation of the original B cell. Antibodies circulate in blood, and for this reason the B cell antibody response is often called the **humoral** component of the immune response.

T cells do not have soluble antibody on their surfaces; nevertheless, they react specifically with antigen, then they proliferate. The specificity of the antigen recognition is guaranteed by the T cell receptor present on the surface of the T cell. Because the types of reactions mediated by T cells can be experimentally transferred to recipient subjects by white blood cells and not by serum, the T cell system is referred to as the **cellular** component of the immune response, or "cell-mediated immunity." Among the most important functions of the T cells are protection of the host against tumors, intracellular bacteria, viruses, parasites, and the rejection of transplants. The basic mechanisms which account for most of these diverse functions are as follows. Some of the T cells are cytotoxic to incompatible transplanted cells or cells infected by a virus. Others participate in the release of various mediators at the site of hypersensitivity reaction. Another type of lymphocyte is involved in inducing or helping the stimulation of B cells and cytotoxic cells. Conversely, another subpopulation suppresses a number of events associated with immune responses

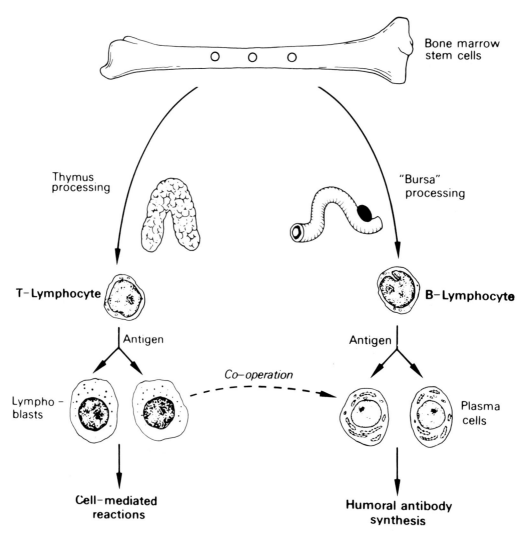

Fig. 6–2   This figure illustrates the processing of lymphocytes. Proliferation and transformation to cells of the lymphoblast and plasma cell series occur following antigenic stimulation. Cooperation between T and B cells can take the form either of help or of suppression. (From Roitt, I.: *Essential Immunology*, 3rd Ed. Oxford, Blackwell Scientific Publications, 1977.)

so that they do not develop out of control, a situation which might be harmful to the host.

How do we recognize these various subpopulations of T lymphocytes? Even though they look the same under the microscope, they carry on their surface specific proteins called CD (cluster designation) that can be recognized by corresponding monoclonal antibodies. For instance, the CD4 membrane protein is found on cells that have helper/inducer functions, whereas the CD8 protein resides on T lymphocytes with cytotoxic/suppressor functions. We have in our blood about twice as many CD4 as CD8 cells. CD4:CD8 ratio is markedly decreased in AIDS as we will discuss shortly.

A numerically minor but functionally important population of lymphocytes is called natural killer (NK) cells. They do not carry the usual markers associated with T cells and owe their name to the fact that they can kill a number of other cells, including tumor cells, cells infected by a virus, and, at least in the test tube, normal cells. Obviously they must be regulated in vivo so that they do not kill other cells indiscriminately, but they have the remarkable property of performing their function without requiring sensitization prior to killing. NK cells can be amplified in vitro by the use of a cytokine called interleukin-2 (IL-2), and in therapeutic trials that have been introduced recently they were found to have a significant reducing effect when reintroduced in some patients with two types of cancer: melanoma and renal cell carcinoma (see Chapter 11).

The second general type of cells important in the

immune response belong to the reticuloendothelial (RE) system. These cells are nonspecific "scavengers" of foreign or antigenic material; they ingest material that is recognized by the lymphocytes as being foreign. RE cells form a diverse group, but all are phagocytic. The most important cells we shall consider are the monocytes and their tissue counterparts, the macrophages (which are also called histiocytes).

Macrophages do not require prior sensitization by an antigen. They are found in a large number of normal and abnormal tissues, as well as in typical lymphoid organs such as the spleen and the lymph nodes. Macrophages are thought to derive from circulating blood monocytes that have migrated to tissues where they reside. The reader should consult Chapter 5 to study the role of the macrophage in inflammation and repair. We will address here their role in the immune reaction. The two most important immunological functions are production of interleukin-1 (IL-1), and presentation of antigens to the lymphocytes. IL-1 is a cytokine and can be produced by a large number of cells but the macrophage is the most effective cellular source. Conversely, IL-1 acts on a variety of cells but its significance in the immune response derives from the potent activation it exerts on resting T cells. The other aspect of macrophage function, antigen presentation, occurs after it has phagocytosed or pinocytosed the antigen. The antigen is processed through various biochemical alterations inside the macrophage and is then re-expressed at the surface where it is presented to the T cell. Finally, another immunologically related macrophage function is the killing of tumor cells.

On the basis of what was stated on the role of the macrophages in IL-1 production and antigen presentation to the T lymphocyte, it is easy to understand that they play both an early and a central role in the immune response. One has, however, to explain what attracts and stimulates macrophages in the first place. A great part of the mechanism of macrophage attraction is the presence on their surface of receptors for the Fc portion of immunoglobulins and for complement. Therefore, if a cellular or particulate antigen is bound to an antibody, especially in the presence of complement, then it becomes more palatable for the macrophage.

The phenomena of macrophage-lymphocyte interaction and of macrophage activation are new insights into the complex nature of the defense mechanisms that are taken for granted when they work normally (Fig. 6–3). Moreover, defects or alterations in these activities provide new explanations for the susceptibility of some persons to infections. Tables 6–1 and

Fig. 6–3   A schematic representation of macrophage and lymphocyte interaction. The macrophage finds antigenic material in the tissue and brings it to the lymph node. The antigen stimulates T and B cells to differentiate into effector T cells and plasma cells, capable of responding specifically to that antigen. It is thought that at some stage in this differentiation memory cells are formed which remain in the lymph node and await the next exposure to the same antigen.

6–2 list some mechanisms that activate and depress macrophages.

To summarize, although macrophages do not determine the specificity of the immune response, they are important in its initiation.

We also have in our lymph nodes and skin, cells with long dendrite-looking cytoplasmic extensions which, because of this morphological feature, are called dendritic cells. They resemble the usual type of macrophages by their effectiveness at antigen presentation. However, they differ from them because they perform poorly at phagocytosis.

Table 6–1.   Macrophage Activators

1. Specific fixed cellular antibodies
2. Antigen-antibody complexes and complement
3. Glass or plastic surface
4. Phagocytosed particulate material (carbon), etc.
5. Microbial products (cell wall, etc.)
6. Interferon
7. Lymphokines

Table 6–2.   Macrophage Suppressors

1. Corticosteroids
2. Antimetabolites and anti-inflammatory agents
3. Reticuloendothelial system blockade
4. Silica, Thorotrast
5. Irradiation
6. Certain viruses, fungi, protozoa
7. Specific antimacrophage serum

ANTIGENS

Before we dive deeper into the turbulent waters of the immune response, let us discuss what we are responding to immunologically. An antigen is a substance that, when introduced into the body, provokes an immune response to which an antibody reacts specifically. This antigen could be a bacterium or another biologic agent, a toxin, a protein, or almost any other kind of macromolecule. For cellular or viral antigens, the antigen which combines with antibody is not the whole cell or virus but some protein or molecule on the surface (or possibly inside).

Antigens are usually foreign to the host. Occasionally, the immune system loses part of its ability to distinguish between self and nonself, so that a tissue or a substance belonging to the host is perceived by the lymphocytes as antigen, and is subsequently attacked. The result is so-called "autoimmune" disease.

There are small, simple substances (molecular weight of less than 1,000) that do not evoke an immune response by themselves, but that can do so if complexed with larger carrier molecules. In this bound form these substances behave as antigens and react with antibodies, once the latter are formed. Such small substances are called **haptens.**

ANTIBODIES

In the simplest sense, the term antibody means exactly that: a substance that has been raised in the self as an antagonistic (protective) response to some non-self material (antigen). Antibodies have the unique ability to distinguish among almost identical antigens, much as a cylinder lock distinguishes among nearly identical keys. Antibodies were recognized in theory long before they were identified, and it was not until the era of modern physical chemistry that antibody activity was shown by electrophoresis to reside in the globulin fractions of human serum.

The term antibody currently designates a member of the family of serum proteins often referred to as **immunoglobulins.** Serum has been shown to contain at least five different immunoglobulins, which are designated by their abbreviations IgG, IgM, IgA, IgD, and IgE (Table 6–3 and Fig. 6–4). All these different classes of proteins are approximately the same size (molecular weight 160,000), except for IgM, which is much larger (molecular weight 900,000). Immunoglobulin molecules in each class are made up of two heavy chains and two light chains, but each molecule may be different by virtue of the specific nature of its amino acid sequence and 3-dimensional arrangement. Of the five types of gamma globulin, IgG represents the largest proportion (80%) in the normal serum. This antibody is directed against common infectious agents such as viruses, bacteria, and toxins. IgG is the only type of immunoglobulin capable of crossing the placental barrier and, therefore, capable of protecting the fetus during the maturation of its immune system.

IgM, the largest molecule, constitutes between 5 and 10% of the circulating antibody, and is important to the primary immune response. This large molecule

Table 6–3. Biologic Properties of Major Immunoglobulin Classes in the Human

	IgG	IgA	IgM	IgD	IgE
Major characteristics	Most abundant Ig of internal body fluids, particularly extra-vascular where it combats microorganisms and their toxins	Major Ig in seromucous secretions where it defends external body surfaces	Very effective agglutinator; produced early in immune response— effective first line defense vs. bacteremia	Present on lymphocyte surface	Raised in parasitic infections Responsible for symptoms of atopic allergy
Complication fixation					
Classical	+ +	−	+ + +	−	−
Alternative	−	+	−	−	−
Cross placenta	+	−	−	−	−
Fix to mast cells (in homologous skin) and basophils	−	−	−	−	+
Cytophilic binding to macrophages and polymorphs	+	−	−	−	−

(From Roitt, I.: *Essential Immunology,* 3rd Ed. Oxford, Blackwell Scientific Publications, 1977.)

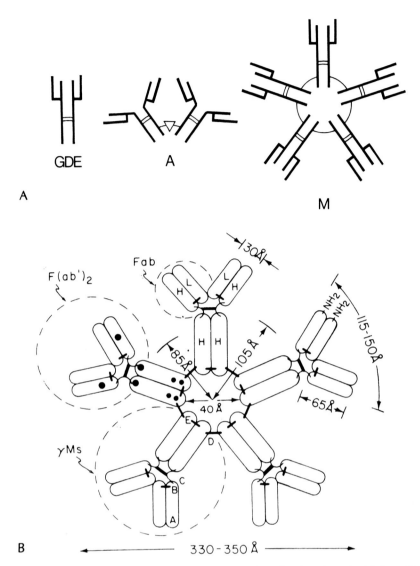

Fig. 6–4 *A*, This figure shows schematic representations of the 5 types of antibody molecules. The unit of light and heavy chains constitutes the molecules of IgG, IgD, and IgE shown at the left. IgA is shown schematically in the center, and IgM, the largest molecule, is at the right. The pieces of the molecule IgM are represented in the diagram *B*, and the dimensions are shown in the scale at the bottom.

may have as many as 10 antibody reaction sites (Fig. 6–4).

IgA globulins differ in that they are found in secretions such as tears, saliva, and mucus of the respiratory tract. Therefore, we think of them as antibodies that help to protect the mucosal barriers, which are exposed and susceptible to attack by bacteria. IgA globulins represent about 5 to 10% of the normal total antibody in the host. There are IgA molecules in the serum as well as in the secretions, and these molecules may not be identical.

IgE is concerned with acute allergic responses such as asthma, hay fever, and anaphylaxis, and aid in protection against parasites. IgD is found as a surface marker on B cells, usually in association with IgM. Its function is unclear.

Antibody Synthesis

It seems that for an antibody to appear in the serum in response to an infection such as an acute streptococcal sore throat, it is necessary for several cellular reactions to take place: processing by macrophage, recognition by B-lymphocyte, synthesis, and secretion of antibody in a significant amount which requires time, perhaps as much as 2 or 3 weeks.

None of this takes place in man during the days immediately after birth, and the predominant immu-

---

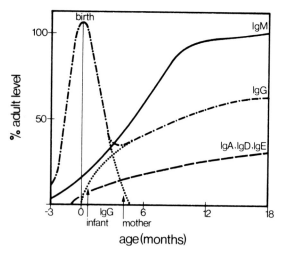

Fig. 6–5   The development of serum immunoglobulin levels in human beings. This diagram illustrates the time course of development of different immunoglobulins up to the age of 18 months. (From Roitt, I.: *Essential Immunology*, 3rd Ed. Oxford, Blackwell Scientific Publications, 1977.)

nologic protection of a newborn is the passively acquired antibody transferred from the mother while the child is in utero (IgG can cross the placenta). Immunologic competence matures slowly and IgA begins to be synthesized at about three weeks of age, IgG at six weeks. During these first weeks the lymphoid tissue of the newborn is developing.

It is of interest that the synthesis of different classes of antibodies occurs at different rates (Fig. 6–5), as well as in different amounts and at different times, depending on whether it is a primary exposure to an antigen or a secondary or anamnestic response (see

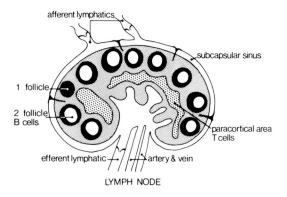

Fig. 6–6   A diagrammatic representation of a human lymph node. A primary follicle contains an aggregation of B cells that has not yet been stimulated by antigen. After antigenic challenge, these form secondary follicles containing pale-staining germinal centers of large, proliferating lymphoid cells and macrophages. T cells reside in the paracortical areas. (Adapted from Roitt, I.: *Essential Immunology*, 3rd Ed. Oxford, Blackwell Scientific Publications, 1977.)

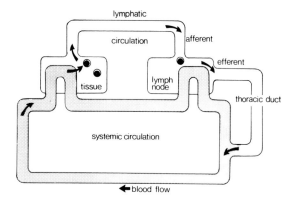

Fig. 6–7   Traffic and recirculation of lymphocytes. Blood-borne lymphocytes enter the tissues and lymph nodes and leave through the draining lymphatics. The efferent lymphatics finally emerging from the last node in each chain join to form the thoracic duct, which returns the lymphocytes to the blood stream where it empties into the left subclavian vein. (Adapted from Roitt, I.: *Essential Immunology*, 3rd Ed. Oxford, Blackwell Scientific Publications, 1977.)

p. 37). The synthesis of antibody is under genetic control.

At the time of primary sensitization by an antigen, the largest amount of antibody is produced in the lymphatic tissues, especially the lymph nodes. Simple experiments have demonstrated that an antigen injected into the foot stimulated the regional lymph nodes to change their cell population, and that antibody could be found in the lymphatic vessels draining the particular nodes following a suitable interval of time. When lymph nodes are enlarged and swollen (e.g., around the elbow or in the axilla of the arm that has an abscess of the hand), one should recognize that, in addition to serving as a filter, the nodes are actively producing antibody.

For a moment it may be useful to sketch the anatomy of the lymph node (Fig. 6–6) and to illustrate the traffic flow through the different areas that can be recognized (Fig. 6–7). The respective areas of the lymph node that are populated by B and T cells are illustrated.

ANTIBODY-ANTIGEN REACTIONS

When antibody and antigen interact, they form what is known as an immune complex, a large and complicated molecule or mass of molecules that is often composed of more than just the antigen and antibody (complement, for example). This material then triggers or initiates several mechanisms: agglutination, opsonization and complement fixation. If the antigen is a particular structure such as a bacteria, then antibody will result in agglutination of the antigen. This is due to the multivalent nature of antibody

CHEMOTAXIS
(polymorphs)

ANAPHYLATOXIN
(histamine release)

C3a   fragments   C5a

antibody=A C_1 C_4+C_2 C_3 C_{567} C_{89}

A → AC1 → AC142 → AC1423 → AC1423567 → AC142356789

membrane

IMMUNE ADHERENCE   CYTOLYSIS
(then phagocytosis)

Fig. 6–8 The sequence of complement activation. This sequence of biochemical interactions is much like a cascade. The immune complex activates C1, creating AC1, which activates C_4 and C_2, creating another active complex AC142. This activates C_3, yielding more active enzymes, and AC1423, which goes on to activate C567, and so on. The active fragments are important in the defense process; chemotactic substances attract phagocytic polymorphonuclear leukocytes, and histamine increases vascular permeability, allowing blood cells to flood into the area. (Adapted from Roitt, I.: *Essential Immunology*, 3rd Ed. Oxford, Blackwell Scientific Publications, 1977.)

molecules, each having two antigen binding sites. Agglutination facilitates trapping and phagocytosis of immune complexes by the scavenger cells of the reticuloendothelial system. Opsonization is the name given to the process of coating the bacteria with antibody. This process enables the polymorphonuclear leukocytes to ingest bacteria more easily. Opsonization and agglutination occur when the antigenic stimulus is cellular or attached to a cell. When the antigen is an unattached macromolecule, the antigen-antibody combination becomes a massive macromolecular complex also easily phagocytosed.

When antigen and IgG or IgM antibodies interact with antigens a series of reactions involving another set of serum proteins is triggered. These particular proteins are collectively called **complement** (Fig. 6–8). There are nine separate proteins in complement (C1-C9), which react sequentially. This results finally in the production of cytotoxic complex that is able to punch holes in cell membranes. The cell to which the immune complex is attached is unable to maintain its internal environment and collapses as does a balloon that lands on a thistle (Fig. 6–9).

Various by-products of these immunologic reactions are part of the inflammatory response. Some molecules are chemotactic and attract polymorphonu-

clear leukocytes and monocytes. Some cause histamine to be released from mast cells in the tissue; histamine then increases vascular permeability, which brings more cells and more antibody to the site. Other molecules make the surface of the antigenic cell stick to a phagocytic cell, which greatly increases the likelihood of the destruction of the antigenic cell.

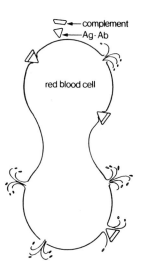

complement
Ag·Ab

red blood cell

Fig. 6–9 This figure shows a red blood cell being lysed by antigen-antibody complexes.

It is therefore apparent that the formation of immune complexes in vivo ultimately leads to inactivation of the antigen, or its lysis if it is cellular, and finally phagocytosis by scavenger cells.

It is also possible to form immune complexes artificially in vitro. This forms the basis of a large number of diagnostic serological tests detecting a circulating antigen in the patient's serum. For example, if a patient is suffering from an infection by an unknown biologic agent, tests can be performed on his serum to determine what antibodies are present. For example, if the infection is suspected to be one of four possible agents, the serum may be mixed with each of the four suspect antigens and then observed to see which provokes immune complex formation. The antigen that forms the complex must be specific for the patient's antibody. We conclude that this antigen is the likely cause of the infection.

Conversely, one can make the diagnosis of an infectious disease by testing the serum for the presence of an antibody that forms a complex with a purified antigen of the suspected microorganisms. For instance, this is the way AIDS serology is being performed.

CYTOKINES

Among the newest areas of development are substances secreted by cells which have been stimulated by some form of injury. These substances, which are principally polypeptides, function as molecular signals between cells and were once thought to be principally products of lymphocytes which had been activated. They were thus designated *lymphokines*, but are better called cytokines, since a broad range of cells is now known to produce such messengers. Cytokines relevant to the immune responses and the function of hematopoietic cells are called interleukins. We already alluded to interleukins 1 and 2 in the sections on lymphocytes and macrophages.

A list of the best known human cytokines with their designations and their biological properties is in Table 6–4.

Much current interest in cytokines is focused on the possibility that their growth-stimulating properties may be of value in treating patients with leukemia who have been given radiation and bone marrow transplantation, or victims of radiation accidents such as those exposed to radiocesium at Chernobyl in 1986, or Brazil in 1987. Other excitement focuses on the cytotoxic use of lymphokines in attempts to treat such tumors as malignant melanoma or renal cell tumors as mentioned in Chapter 11.

Interferon could be said to be the original cytokine, discovered in 1957 by Isaacs as a glycoprotein (molecular weight 20,000), produced by many types of cells, particularly lymphocytes after exposure to a virus. The substance interferon effectively prevented the

Table 6–4. Prominent Biologic Properties of Human Lymphokines

LYMPHOKINE	BIOLOGIC PROPERTIES
Interleukin-1 (alpha and beta)	Activates resting T cells; is cofactor for hematopoietic growth factors; induces fever, sleep, ACTH release, neutrophilia, and other systemic acute-phase responses; stimulates synthesis of lymphokines, collagen, and collagenases; activates endothelial and macrophagic cells; mediates inflammation, catabolic processes, and nonspecific resistance to infection.
Interleukin-2	Is growth factor for activated T-cells; induces the synthesis of other lymphokines; activates cytotoxic lymphocytes.
Interleukin-3	Supports the growth of pluripotent (multilineage) bone marrow stem cells; is growth factor for mast cells.
Colony-stimulating factor (CSF)	
Granulocyte-macrophage CSF	Promotes neutrophilic, eosinophilic, and macrophagic bone marrow colonies; activates mature granulocytes.
Granulocyte CSF	Promotes neutrophilic colonies.
Macrophage CSF	Promotes macrophagic colonies.
Interleukin-4 (B-cell stimulating factor-1)	Is growth factor for activated B cells; induces DR expression on B cells; is growth factor for resting T cells; enhances cytolytic activity of cytotoxic T cells; is mast-cell growth factor.
B-cell stimulating 2 (B-cell differentiating factor)	Induces the differentiation of activated B cells into immunoglobulin-secreting plasma cells; is identical with beta$_2$-interferon, plasmacytoma growth factor, and hepatocyte-stimulating factor.
Gamma-interferon	Induces Class I, Class II (DR), and other surface antigens on a variety of cells; activates macrophages and endothelial cells; augments or inhibits other lymphokine activities; augments natural-killer-cell activity; exerts antiviral activity.
Interferon (alpha and beta)	Exerts antiviral activity; induces Class I antigen expression; augments natural-killer-cell activity; has fever-inducing and antiproliferative properties.
Tumor necrosis factor (alpha and beta)	Is direct cytotoxin for some tumor cells; induces fever, sleep, and other systemic acute-phase responses; stimulates the synthesis of lymphokines, collagen, and collagenases; activates endothelial and macrophagic cells; mediates inflammation, catabolic processes, and septic shock.

multiplication of further viruses and was therefore deemed an antiviral agent which seemed to work by interfering with translation.

Interferon also enhances natural killer cell activity It is used in the treatment of Kaposi's sarcoma and an unusual form of leukemia.

In the immune response the most important cytokines are interleukins 1, 2 and 6. Their structure, as well as the structure of their receptors on the target cells, are known and most of their functions are well established. These are listed in Table 6–4. The secretion of interleukins in vivo is subjected to the activation of the various cells involved in the immune responses and, therefore, this has a regulatory effect on their cellular targets. Their coordinated functions and regulations lead us naturally to the comparison with hormones in the endocrine system. It remains to be established if it will have a widespread use in the treatment of immunological disorders, or, conversely, which ones could be specifically blocked for therapeutic purposes.

IMMUNITY

The beneficial and usual consequence of the immune response is called **immunity.** The immune host is resistant to particular diseases or poisons. Immunity comes about when the host is exposed to an antigen and, as a result of this exposure, acquires the capacity to recognize, react with, and neutralize the antigen the next time it is encountered. Anyone who has ever had diphtheria, even a mild, barely noticeable case, is immune for life. On every subsequent occasion that this person is exposed to diphtheria, immunologic memory mobilizes a response so fast that the toxin is neutralized before it produces the disease.

This accelerated immune response on second infection is called an **anamnestic response** (Greek *anamnesis,* memory). It occurs in about half the time it took to mobilize the first or primary response (Fig. 6–10). Lymphoid tissue contains greater numbers of plasma cells this time, and more cells produce more antibody. This process probably results from the presence of "memory" cells that developed at the time of initial exposure.

The anamnestic response will occur at any time during a person's life when there is exposure to antigen. However, the response does diminish slightly as time from the initial exposure passes. In vaccinations this diminished response can be overcome by giving repeated doses of antigen, known as "boosters," to reawaken waning immunity (Fig. 6–11).

Anergy is the opposite of the anamnestic response.

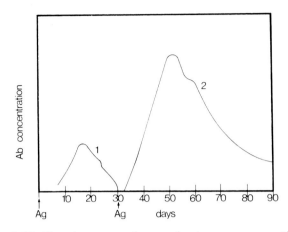

Fig. 6–10 The primary versus the secondary immune response. The secondary response is greater and more immediate because of the presence of memory cells formed during first exposure. (Adapted from Weiser, R.S., Myrvik, Q.N., and Pearsall, N.N.: *Fundamentals of Immunology.* Philadelphia, Lea & Febiger, 1969.)

The immune response may be either retarded or ineffective in elderly, debilitated, malnourished, and seriously ill patients, in persons with overwhelming infections or cancer, in patients with AIDS, or for reasons we do not understand. In these instances, the cellular immune mechanism seems paralyzed and unable to respond to the presence of normal antigen. The ineffective immune state (anergy) has become the focus of recent interest, and is used currently to define how ill a patient is. It has become evident that both acute and chronic illness may render someone anergic, and that acutely occurring anergy can be reversed by supportive measures such as hyperalimentation and successful management of shock.

Immunity can be either active or passive. Active immunity refers to the process of antibody formation in response to an antigen. This process can be induced naturally, by infection by the pathogenic organism, or artificially, by vaccination by either injection or ingestion of a particular antigen that has been rendered harmless but retains its antigenic properties. This process stimulates antibody production and hence produces active immunity without causing the disease. For example, bacteria and viruses may be killed in such a way that their antigenic components remain intact. The process of rendering someone resistant or immune (e.g., through vaccination) is called immunization.

Passive immunity means that the infected host does not form his own antibody, but is given injections of antibody from another (immune) person or animal. This procedure is useful in emergencies. However, it is only a temporary measure. The person who receives such passive antibody has no immunologic

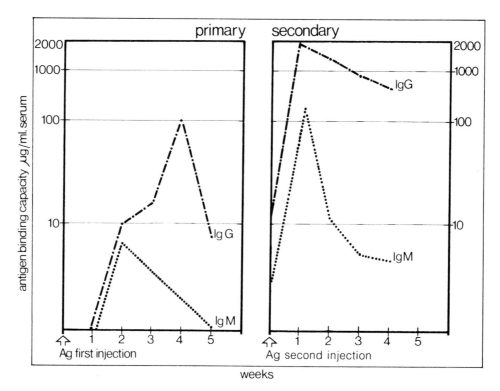

Fig. 6–11   The synthesis of antibodies in the mouse during primary and secondary responses to bovine serum albumin. The IgM response to a secondary challenge is not much greater than it was during first exposure. The secondary response is largely an IgG response produced by "memory" B cells. A secondary response elicited by a "booster" injection will literally "boost" immunity to a high level, as shown. (Adapted from Roitt, I.: *Essential Immunology*, 3rd Ed. Oxford, Blackwell Scientific Publications, 1977.)

memory of the infection, and copes no better with a second infection of the same organism. In addition, in cases of passive immunity antibody is soon metabolized and excreted by the host; actively immune hosts continually replace lost antibody. Passive immunity is also acquired naturally, before birth. Maternal antibodies are transferred across the placenta to the fetus. Thus there are 4 ways of acquiring immunity: (1) by being **exposed to infection** (active, natural); (2) **by inoculation of dead or harmless organisms** (active, artificial); (3) **by transfer of antibodies from mother to fetus** (passive, natural); and (4) **by transfer of antibodies from a previously immunized person or animal** (passive, artificial).

HYPERSENSITIVITY

The opposite side of the coin to anergy or tolerance can be thought of as hypersensitivity. This section discusses diseases caused by the immune response: diseases in which the immune system produces tissue damage and disordered function rather than immunity. In these diseases, immune complex formation and complement activation ultimately destroy the host's tissue.

The terms used to describe this type of phenomenon are confusing and misleading. Therefore, before describing the diseases themselves, we shall examine the terminology. The first term used to refer to disease of this nature was the word "allergy," which originally meant an "altered state of reactivity." In recent years, however, the word "allergy" has become a nonspecific term that can be applied equally to ragweed, to eggs, or to mothers-in-law. Efforts to find a more precise description of immune phenomena produced the term "hypersensitivity."

The notion of a hypersensitivity reaction or of a state of hypersensitivity has even passed into the jargon of the layman and is used casually to mean hypercritical. However, in biology and in the context of this chapter and book, the term refers to an altered state of reactivity. Thus all who have been immunized may be potentially hyperreactive should they encounter the appropriate antigen. The term best applies to those cases in which an untoward or destructive rather than a simple neutralizing or defensive reaction occurs. There are instances of this extraordinary inflammatory reaction in which edema and even death take place following exposure to an agent to which the person is allergic or **hypersensitive.**

Table 6–5. Atopic Conditions

CONDITION	COMMONLY ASSOCIATED ALLERGENS
Allergic rhinitis	Inhalants (spores, pollens, animal dander)
Extrinsic asthma	Mold spores
Atopic conjunctivitis	Inhalants (spores, pollens, animal dander)
Atopic dermatitis	Various food allergies
	Drug hypersensitivities: especially penicillins, sulfonamides, streptomycin
	Local anesthetics
	Heavy metals
	Reactive chemicals
Urticaria-angioedema	Insect bites
	Food allergies
Gastrointestinal allergy	Food allergies (cereals, milk, eggs, shellfish, fruit)
	Drug hypersensitivities
Serum sickness syndrome	Drugs, especially penicillin
Anaphylaxis	Heterologous antisera
	Vaccines
	Iodinated radiographic material

(Adapted from Bach, M. K.: Reagin allergy. In *Immunology*. Edited by B. A. Thomas. Scope Monograph Series. Kalamazoo, Michigan, Upjohn Co., 1975.)

Hypersensitivity can best be thought of as an increase in sensitivity to a particular antigen, or as an abnormal overreaction by an oversensitive immune system. Persons who experience such a reaction, be it to pollen, to metal, or to penicillin, may be considered to be more sensitive to that antigen than the rest of the human population, which does not normally react to that antigen. Hence, the former may be referred to as "hypersensitive individuals." In fact, they are really only "sensitive" to the antigen, whereas the rest of the population is "nonsensitive."

Familiar examples may help to express this idea. Ten percent of the North American population experiences hay fever; these persons are then described as hypersensitive to plant pollen, relative to the remaining 90% who produce no reaction to pollen. Most persons react to bee venom with pain, redness and swelling, but a few are truly hypersensitive and respond with a systemic, life-threatening reaction, and may die as a result of a bee sting.

In all attempts to define hypersensitivity, one thing must remain clear, that is, that in all hypersensitivity diseases, antigens, when introduced to the body, evoke immune processes that damage the host (Table 6–5). These processes involve the same basic pathways that lead to immunity on other occasions: antibody formation, immune complex formation, and complement activation, for example. When immunity is the result of the immune response, the invading antigen is neutralized, and on second exposure the defense is so successful that there is no evidence of disease. In the hypersensitivity state, second exposure leads to self-destructive reactions that can be catastrophic, such as the anaphylactic reaction to a bee sting.

All allergic or hypersensitivity reactions have been divided into 4 groups, 3 mediated by humoral antibody, and 1 mediated by T cells (see Table 6–6). Most of these reactions have features that are found in "normal" immune responses; it is only when there is exuberant, unregulated control of some features that

Table 6–6. 4 Types of Hypersensitivity Reactions

	ANAPHYLACTIC (TYPE I)	CYTOTOXIC (TYPE II)	COMPLEX-MEDIATED (TYPE III)	CELL-MEDIATED (TYPE IV)
Antibody-mediating reaction	IgE, mast cell binding	IgG or IgM	IgG	Receptor on T-lymphocyte
Antigen	Usually exogenous	Cell surface	Extracellular	Extracellular or cell-surface
Response to intradermal antigen:				
maximum reaction	30 min	—	3 to 8 hrs	24 to 48 hrs
appearance	Wheal and flare	—	Erythema and edema	Erythema and induration
histology	Degranulated mast cells, edema, eosinophils	—	Acute inflammatory reaction; predominant polymorphs	Perivascular inflammation: polymorphs migrate out, leaving predominantly mononuclear cells
Damaging agent	Biochemical mediators from IgE-sensitized cells produce tissue response	Complement may or may not be involved	Complement and polymorphs produce tissue damage	Lymphokines released from antigen-sensitized lymphocyte, reactions produce tissue damage
Transfer sensitivity to normal subject	←———————— Serum antibody ————————→			Lymphoid cells, transfer factor
Examples	Atopic allergy, e.g., hay fever	Hemolytic disease of newborn (Rh)	Serum sickness; complex glomerulonephritis	Tuberculin skin reaction; contact dermatitis

one can observe "hypersensitive" reactions leading to damage of the host's tissues.

Type I—Anaphylaxis

Everyone knows a person who, on a spring day, has a fit of sneezing and weeping even with wheezes, or someone who visits a house in which a family of cats has made its home for many years on the only available sofa, where the visitor sits, trying to make conversation as his eyes run and he itches furiously. This allergic reaction to contact with pollen or dander is mediated by IgE or reaginic antibody (Fig. 6–12). On first exposure, IgE antibody is formed; it binds to mast cells or tissue basophils, cells that contain granules of histamine and other vasoactive amines in the cytoplasm. On subsequent exposure to the same antigen, the binding of antigen to antibody causes degranulation of the mast cells and basophils, which results in a marked vasomotor, vascular and axonal response characteristic of inflammation. The substances released cause smooth muscle contraction and stimulate the nerve endings, in addition to increasing capillary permeability. This response leads to wheals, flare, and itching. The reaction occurs locally in some instances and systemically in others, for reasons that are not well understood.

Local anaphylactic-type reactions are seen in some persons who have an inherited tendency (idiosyncrasy or atopy) to overreact to normal environmental antigens. Such persons tend to form IgE in response to dust, cat fur, and plant pollen, for example. Ninety percent of the population do not react to the presence of these substances. The common reaction site is the mucus membranes of the nasal sinus. There histamine and the other amines cause local edema and other inflammatory responses.

Hay fever is one of the best-known examples of local Type I reaction. The attacks are strictly seasonal, occurring in spring, summer, or autumn, depending on whether the patient is hypersensitive to the spring pollens of trees, summer pollens of grasses, or that of fall plants such as ragweed. Symptoms of itching, congestion of the eyes, violent paroxysms of sneezing, and a profuse watery discharge from the nose (called rhinorrhea) are typical. The particular protein responsible can usually be identified by means of skin tests, i.e., scratching the arm and rubbing in the suspected protein; if an inflamed area or wheal is produced, the patient is hypersensitive to that protein. When the protein is identified, the patient may be desensitized against it by means of repeated small injections of the protein before the onset of the hay fever season. The aim of desensitization is to produce excess antibody in the person's blood, so that the antigen will be destroyed before it reaches the tissues. (It is in the tissues that the allergic reaction is triggered.) This procedure may render the sensitive person partially or totally insensitive.

Far more serious is systemic anaphylaxis, usually referred to simply as anaphylaxis (Greek *ana* [to reverse] and *phylaxis* [to guard]). The term describes the situation in which the expected or anticipated immunity does not follow exposure to a small dose of toxin, but instead an extraordinary susceptibility to small doses of antigen results.

The mechanisms involved in this reaction are basically the same as those of the local reaction: IgE is formed and attaches to mast cells and basophils. However, in this case, the site of the reaction is not limited to the nose; it occurs all over the body. The substances released by IgE-antigen complexes cause a massive generalized change in capillary permeability, leading to hypotension and shock. In different mammals there are different responses, but in man there frequently is smooth muscle contraction, particularly in the bronchial tree, which causes respiratory distress or asthma-like symptoms. Edema of the larynx may threaten to obstruct the airways and sometimes requires an immediate tracheostomy.

Anaphylaxis is often life-threatening, but if it is treated immediately with adrenalin and antihistamines, and if the airways are kept open, the patient will usually survive.

The foregoing are two kinds of Type I or anaphylactic sensitivity: atopic reactions usually limited to the

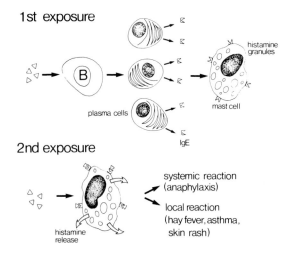

Fig. 6–12 This figure illustrates the Type I hypersensitivity reaction. On first exposure to antigen, B cells proliferate and differentiate into plasma cells that produce antibody. The antibody attaches to the surface of mast cells and basophils. On second exposure, the antigen combines with the antibody, which triggers degranulation of the attached cells.

mucus membranes of the upper respiratory tract, but sometimes also involving the skin and systemic reactions (anaphylaxis).

Type II—Cytotoxic

The second general type of hypersensitivity reaction is an antibody-dependent cytotoxic reaction, in which an antigen, when introduced to the body, binds to either red blood cells, leukocytes, or platelets. Antibody against these cells is formed, which subsequently complexes with antigen, complement is fixed, and the blood cells with immune complexes on their surfaces are lysed. Another mechanism of Type II cytotoxic hypersensitivity does not require complement; in this situation an antibody binds directly to a target cell and leukocytes bearing receptor for the Fc portion of the antibody are recruited. These leukocytes then lyse the target cells; the whole process is called antibody-dependent cell-mediated cytotoxicity (ADCC). The effect of this phenomenon depends on the type of cell being destroyed as well as on the severity of the allergic reaction. If the antibody is located on red cells, red cells will be destroyed, leading to hemolysis, jaundice, and anemia. If leukocytes are involved, the result may be an increased susceptibility to infection, whereas the result of antiplatelet antibodies will be thrombocytopenia and hemorrhagic manifestations (Fig. 6–13).

Cytotoxic reactions have been seen occasionally with penicillin therapy. The drug becomes attached to the red-cell membrane. Antibodies are formed that complex with the drug, complement is activated, and the red cell is destroyed.

The same principle is involved when a patient is given a transfusion of mismatched blood (this is not, strictly speaking, a hypersensitivity reaction; the immune system is merely acting normally to destroy foreign material). In a mismatched transfusion, the donated blood cells are recognized as foreign; they have antigens on the cell's surface against which the host has antibodies. For example, a person with Type A blood has A antigens and anti-B antibodies. If he is transfused with Type B blood, the anti-B antibodies will complex with B antigens on the surface of the donor's blood cells and will cause hemolysis of the donor's cells.

Symptoms of such a transfusion reaction are restlessness, anxiety, flushing, chest or lumbar pain, tachypnea (rapid breathing), tachycardia (rapid heart rate), and nausea. These symptoms may be shortly followed by shock and renal failure. The problems associated with blood group incompatibilities are discussed fully in Chapter 23.

There are other instances of this same type of reaction: Rh incompatibility (Fig. 6–14), autoimmune hemolytic anemia, and Goodpasture's syndrome, to mention some.

Type III—Immune Complex-Mediated Hypersensitivity

In this form of hypersensitivity, a soluble or particulate antigen elicits an antibody response resulting in the formation of an intravascular antigen/antibody immune complex. So far this obeys the normal laws of immunology and the process can be characterized as appropriate. However, complement often binds to the immune complex, and, for a set of documented or hypothetical reasons, the intravascular immune complex now becomes injurious to neighboring endothelial cells (Fig. 6–15). It is important to note that even though the most heavily damaged target is the endothelial cell, it is not the triggering antigen and participates only as an innocent bystander. You recall that, by contrast, in Type II reaction cytotoxicity is observed because the damaged cell carries an antigen which is the target of the antibody.

The mechanisms of Type III hypersensitivity rely on cells recruited by the immune complexes such as neutrophils. As expected, some of the complement components present in the immune complex participate actively in this recruitment.

The end result of immune complex-mediated hypersensitivity is fibrinoid necrosis of arteriole and cap-

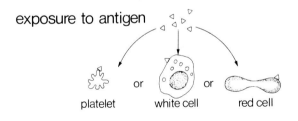

exposure to antigen

platelet   or   white cell   or   red cell

antibody formation

thrombocytopenia   leukopenia   anemia

Fig. 6–13 The cytotoxic reaction. In the Type II reaction only 1 exposure to the antigen is necessary. The antigen attaches itself to the surface of a circulating blood cell, then when antibody is formed and complexes with the antigen, complement is activated and the host cells are destroyed. Which type of disease results depends on the particular blood cells that are destroyed.

pregnancy 1

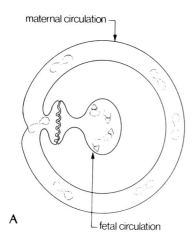

maternal circulation

fetal circulation

A

immediately after birth of first baby

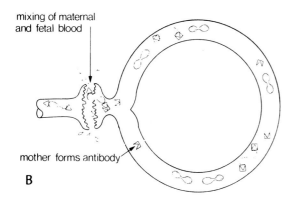

mixing of maternal
and fetal blood

mother forms antibody

B

births 2,3,4, etc.

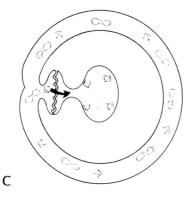

C

Fig. 6–14   *A,* An illustration of a Type II or cytotoxic immune reaction involving Rh antigens. In this disease, the mother is Rh negative (i.e., has no Rh antigen), and the father is Rh positive (i.e., his red blood cells have Rh antigen on the surface). The fetus has inherited the Rh antigen from his father. Normally, maternal and fetal blood do not mix; rather the placenta allows capillaries from both systems to come into close contact so that nutrients, oxygen and fetal wastes can pass across the capillary walls from one circulation to the other. Therefore, the fetal Rh antigen is contained within the fetal circulation. *B,* At birth, mixing of maternal and fetal blood may occur as the placenta breaks away. Should the Rh antigen enter the maternal system in this way, the mother will recognize the Rh antigen as foreign and will form anti-Rh-antibody, which will destroy any fetal red blood cells in her system. Her first child is safe, since he or she has already been born, because the full-blown maternal immune response does not occur until 2 weeks after childbirth. *C,* However, if her next child is also Rh positive, there will be problems. The mother will still have some anti-Rh-antibody in circulation, which she may continue to produce at a low rate. This antibody is small enough to cross through the placental capillary system and into the fetal circulation, where it will destroy fetal red blood cells. Thus the second child will be anemic at birth. The plight of the third child will be worse, because the maternal response increases every time. The fourth child may die *in utero.*

The treatment for this condition is simple. The mother and her baby are blood-typed when the baby is born. If Rh incompatibility is found, then the mother is given a dose of anti-Rh-antigens. This removes the Rh antigen from her system before she mobilizes her own immune response. A few weeks later, the donated Rh antibody is also cleared from the system. When the next child is conceived, the mother's immune system has no recollection of an Rh antigen, since she has never produced it herself.

illary walls. This consists of damage to the endothelial lining, deposition of fibrin in the wall of the blood vessel, microthrombosis, and local ischemia. The features of immune complex-mediated hypersensitivity are exemplified by an experiment named Arthus reaction (Fig. 6–15).

Maurice Arthus showed that rabbits that had been hyperimmunized and had developed high levels of precipitating antibody reacted violently to the **intradermal** injection of soluble antigen. This resulted in a large, red, swollen reaction that reached the maximum size about six hours after the injection. Histology of this area shows an intense infiltration with polymorphonuclear leukocytes. Special studies show antigen, antibody, and complement all within this lesion, which often is accompanied by thrombosis and necrosis of the vessel walls. This whole process can be blocked by removing complement or polymorphonuclear leukocytes from the serum of the experimental animal before the injection of the challenging antigen.

In humans, Type III immune injury is observed either systemically or locally. Systemic manifestations were seen when there was an abundant use in humans of serum containing animal-derived antibodies for passive immunization; this produced serum sickness disease (Fig. 6–16). The local manifestations can be observed most often in the kidney glomeruli, joints and skin. Chapter 20 describes the mechanisms of various types of glomerulonephritis that can be attributed to the deposition of immune complexes.

The characteristic common to most forms of Type III hypersensitivity is that it takes a few days to become clinically apparent. This is because, following exposure to the antigen, the host has to mount an antibody response. After a few days there is just the right proportion of secreted antibody and antigen still present in the circulation to form immune complexes with the right size and features to bind complement and attach to neighboring endothelium.

Type III hypersensitivity subsides once the antigen has cleared completely from the circulation, and the

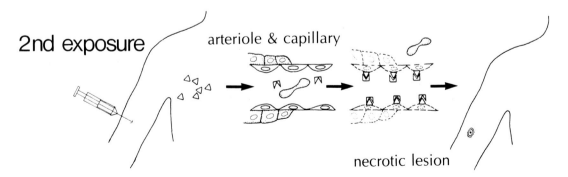

Fig. 6–15 This diagram illustrates an Arthus reaction. Antibodies are formed when a small amount of antigen is introduced into the body. The antibodies attach themselves to the capillary endothelium at the spot where the antigen was injected. The next exposure to antigen produces immune complexes that lead to the destruction of endothelial cells by the host's own immunologic defense.

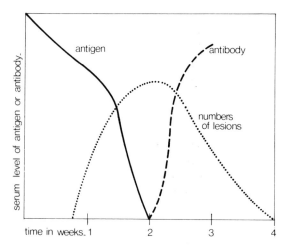

Fig. 6–16 This diagram illustrates the immune response to radioactively labeled antigen in immune AgAb complex disease. Circulating AgAb complexes can be measured about a week after injection of antigen. With the appearance of these immune complexes, the clinical and histologic manifestations of the disease develop.

When the number of immune complexes decreases, lesions begin to heal. This evidence, along with demonstration of the complexes in the lesions themselves, implicates immune complexes as a cause of Arthus reactions and of serum sickness. (Adapted from Sell, S.: Immunopathology (hypersensitivity diseases). In *Pathology*, 7th Ed. Edited by W. A. D. Anderson and J. M. Kissane. St. Louis, C. V. Mosby, 1977.)

circulatory immune complexes are trapped by the reticuloendothelial system. In some autoimmune diseases such as lupus, to be described in this chapter, there is a continuous release of antigenic material and, therefore, a more constant production of antibodies. In this case the immune injury persists as long as effective treatment is not initiated.

The antigen/antibody/complement complex is chemotactic to polymorphonuclear leukocytes and brings many of these cells to the site where the liberation of their enzymes triggers local tissue destruction. To aggravate the situation further, the immune complexes are able to trigger the coagulation factors that lead to the observed thrombosis.

Type IV—Cell-Mediated Reactions (Tuberculin Hypersensitivity)

The first three types of toxic immune reactions discussed are mediated by **soluble** antibody. The fourth type is mediated by the T lymphocytes and involves essentially the same mechanisms as the protective response of T cells. This reaction takes at least 12 hours to develop and is therefore called "delayed hypersensitivity." It is characterized by the presence of macrophages and lymphocytes rather than of polymorphonuclear leukocytes. Most lymphocytes present at the

reaction site belong to the CD4 positive, i.e. helper/inducer, population.

Poison ivy, contact dermatitis, eczema, and the tuberculin reaction are all examples of this type of allergy. Tuberculin is a lipoprotein extracted from the mycobacterium of human tuberculosis. Testing with patches containing the allergen usually defines the specific material to which one is sensitive because of the reddening, weeping, blisters, and hyperplasia of the epidermis that result after topical exposure (Fig. 6–17).

Hypersensitivity to plant poisons is a common affliction. Such plants as poison ivy, poison oak, and the genus *Primula* (primrose family) may set up a severe inflammation of the skin (*dermatitis venenata*) when the sensitive person touches the leaves. Even the smoke of burning poison ivy can bring about the same result. It often happens that florists develop hypersensitivity only after they have been handling plants of the genus *Primula* for many years, a fact that suggests induced rather than natural hypersensitivity.

Studies have shown that the cell-mediated delayed-type reactions depend on the intact thymus. Lymphocytes that arise in the paracortical area of the lymph node and migrate to various sites are responsible for this type of reaction. These are therefore T cells and, indeed, they are the predominant cell population at the site of cell-mediated hypersensitivity. They are activated and, together with macrophages that are also commonly present, secrete a number of interleukins. This type of immune reaction is also observed as a

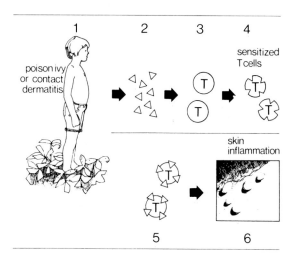

Fig. 6–17 This diagram illustrates cell-mediated hypersensitivity. Contact with poison ivy allows the antigen to enter the skin where it evokes a T-cell response. T cells are sensitized by the antigen, and then interact with it to cause dermatitis.

normal means of defense against the mycobacterium that causes tuberculosis, viruses, fungi and parasites.

Cell-mediated immunity is also an important determinant of transplant rejection which is discussed below.

Few classification schemes neatly contain every existing piece of biologic data, and the attempt to classify immunologic reactions presented here is no exception. Many clinical examples of hypersensitivity cannot be easily fitted into any one of these classes.

INHERITED FORMS OF IMMUNODEFICIENCY

The immune system can be defective from the early stages of development and this defect can involve the cellular or the humoral arm of immunity, or both. Inherited immunodeficiencies are rare. They are typically discovered in infants, signalled by an excessively high number of infectious diseases.

Anergic states occur in congenital immunologic deficiencies, or they may be acquired in a variety of conditions later in life. Congenital immunologic deficiencies can involve B cells, T cells, or both, depending on the disease. Such a disorder usually becomes apparent within the first 6 to 8 months of life.

Agammaglobulinemia is a relatively common condition in which B cells are either absent or are remarkably few in number. The infant makes little immunoglobulin on his own. However, he usually appears to be healthy for the first 5 or 6 months after birth because he is protected by maternal immunoglobulin (transferred through the placenta or in milk). Disease becomes evident as the maternal immunoglobulin disappears; the infant suffers from repeated infections. This condition is generally familial and sex-linked, being confined to males. The T cell system is unaffected in this disease.

T cell deficiencies result from hypoplasia of the thymus. Infants with this disorder have little thymus tissue and few, if any, T cells. Thus these children are vulnerable to viral and fungal infections as well as to some bacterial infections. B cells and serum immunoglobulins may be relatively unaffected, but because some types of T cells help B cells to produce antibody to some antigens, a defect in T cells may manifest itself as a defect in B cells as well. Diseases involving combined B and T cell deficiencies have been reported. They produce a syndrome designated severe combined immunodeficiency disease (SCID) which is particularly lethal.

B and T cells are not the only elements of the immune response that can be deficient. Any disorders in the complement of reticuloendothelial systems impair the host's ability to respond appropriately.

As a group, congenital immune deficiencies are rare compared with the acquired types of immune disorder.

ACQUIRED IMMUNE DEFICIENCY SYNDROME (AIDS)

AIDS is a viral disease characterized by a progressive destruction of the immune system. The first cases of AIDS were reported in 1981 in young homosexual men. In the western world, AIDS most often affects homosexual men and IV drug users, or their heterosexual sex partners. In Africa, where the disease spreads with alarming proportions, AIDS is found in the promiscuous heterosexual population.

The AIDS virus was identified by Luc Montagnier when he was able to show an increase in reverse transcriptase in the lymphocytes obtained from the lymph node of a patient with symptoms of AIDS. Montagnier and Gallo found the appropriate culture conditions to grow cells producing the viral particles. The virus is now called HIV, for **human immunodeficiency virus**. The most important type is HIV-1. Its genome is contained in RNA, and HIV functions as a retrovirus.

After HIV enters a target cell its RNA genetic material is converted into DNA by using reverse transcriptase. The DNA which is thus produced becomes integrated into the DNA of the target cell. Specific HIV genes exert a profound influence not only on viral replication but also on the integrity of the target cell.

HIV infects cells by binding to the CD4 molecule, a cell surface protein found mostly on helper/inducer T cells. This triggers a complex series of changes and the final outcome is a depletion of the CD4 lymphocytes. This has profound functional consequences because the CD4 lymphocytes are T cells which are involved in the recognition of foreign antigens on infected cells, and activation of B lymphocytes. B lymphocytes in turn produce antibodies. CD4 cells also mediate the activity of CD8 lymphocytes which are involved in the killing of infected cells. Finally, CD4 cells also influence monocytes and macrophages. Therefore the CD4 cell occupies a central part of the immunologic picture.

Other cells, besides the helper T cell, carry the CD4 antigen and, therefore, HIV can bind to them. Gallo has shown that HIV can infect not only CD4 lymphocytes but also monocytes/macrophages, which is consistent with the finding that 40% of monocytes and dendritic cells express CD4. It is important to note however that CD4 lymphocytes are killed by HIV whereas monocytes/macrophages are not. There is evidence suggesting that monocytes/macrophages could act as reservoirs for the virus.

Less clear is the mechanism of infection by HIV of brain and intestinal cells which are known to be devoid of a significant number of CD4 molecules on their surface, and yet can be infected. Whatever the cell to which the virus binds, there is a unique protein, called gp120, on the viral coat of HIV that interacts specifically with the CD4 molecule of the target. Following binding, the next step is the entry of the virus into the cell; this is probably done through direct fusion between the virus coat and the cell membrane.

Following the integration of HIV in the target cell genome, three different events can happen. First, persistent infection characterized by production of new viral particles and no, or little, cell death. Second, formation of syncytia cells which die shortly after formation. Syncytia are multinucleated giant cells. Third, rapid death of the target cells without the formation of syncytia.

The formation of syncytia is explained in the following way. They form because HIV infected cells manufacture the protein gp120 and carry it on their cell membrane. Then when an infected cell encounters an uninfected cell that carries the CD4 antigen, the gp120 of the infected cell can bind to the CD4 of the uninfected cell. Eventually the two cells join by direct fusion. These multinucleated cells have a limited life span and their death partly explains changes in the number of helper T cells that have contributed to their formation.

HIV replication and cell death increase when infected helper T cells become activated. The activation can be the result of various antigenic stimuli, such as infection by various microorganisms. HIV itself can act as an activating stimulus. Consequently, instead of being beneficial to the host, the activation of the immune system creates the condition of increased viral replication and, ultimately, cell death.

Overall the loss of CD4 lymphocytes decreases defense against viruses, fungi, parasites, and certain bacteria, including mycobacteria.

In the description of the clinical features of AIDS the focus should be on the full course of HIV infection not solely on AIDS.

In the initial definition of AIDS the diagnostic criteria were strict and included two common complications of AIDS: Kaposi's sarcoma or opportunistic infections, such as Pneumocystis carinii pneumonia. Kaposi's sarcoma is a slow growing cancer derived from the endothelial cells of blood vessels, and is found most often on the skin, and later in internal organs. Pneumocystis carinii is a protozoan present in most normal individuals, but causing a severe op-

portunistic pneumonia in AIDS patients. Now the definition of AIDS includes the full clinical spectrum of HIV infection.

According to a proposed classification, there are six clinical stages of HIV infection, based on the following criteria: CD4 lymphocyte count, CD4 cell function, lymphadenopathy, skin tests, and opportunistic infections. The various stages of decrease in CD4 lymphocyte are particularly important.

Stage 0 starts at the time of infection (IV needles, transfusion with infected blood, intercourse with infected individual, etc.). The infection is conveniently detected by the serological demonstration of anti-HIV antibodies in the serum. Following infection, it can take from six weeks to a year before the affected individual becomes seropositive.

Once the HIV test is positive patients are said to be in Stage I. Most people have no symptoms. Some patients develop a disease resembling infectious mononucleosis with fatigue, fever, and swollen lymph nodes. A rash can be present. Furthermore, various disorders of the central nervous system are sometimes present ranging from headaches to encephalitis. All these signs and symptoms usually disappear within a few weeks. However, HIV continues to replicate silently.

Stage II of the disease is characterized by the development of chronic lymphadenopathy, i.e., more than two months in duration. This enlargement of lymph nodes is due to the overstimulation of B cells. This is accompanied by hypergammaglobulinemia due to the production of many antibodies. However, these antibodies are not functional in antigen recognition. Stage II of HIV infection lasts from 3 to 5 years.

Stage III is characterized by a persistent drop of CD4 cell count to less than 400 per cubic millimeter.

Approximately 18 months later, patients enter Stage IV which is characterized by an impairment in cell mediated immunity as shown by the failure to respond to 3 out of 4 routine skin tests.

Transformation to Stage V is characterized by the development of anergy, i.e., total absence of delayed hypersensitivity. This is usually accompanied by thrush which is a fungal infection due to *candida albicans* involving the oral cavity. Other viral or fungal infections can be present as well. For instance, herpes simplex virus infection with persistent and painful sores in the skin surrounding the anus, the genital area, or the mouth. After one or two years following the beginning of Stage V, patients develop disseminated opportunistic infections in internal sites beyond the skin and the mucus membranes. This characterizes entry into Stage VI.

Stage VI is characterized by opportunistic infections

and an extremely low count of CD4 cells at 100 or less. Table 6-7 lists opportunistic infections associated with AIDS. Most patients die within two years. The most common infections associated with AIDS in the western world are due to Pneumocystis carinii causing pneumonia, toxoplasmosis which can infect the brain, and cryptosporidiosis causing chronic diarrhea. Patients can also develop meningitis due to cryptococcosis and disseminated histoplasmosis which is a common cause of chronic fevers in HIV infected patients. Among the viral infections, cytomegalovirus is often reactivated and causes pneumonia, encephalitis, blindness, and inflammation of the gastrointestinal tract.

The exact mechanism of the neurological complications of HIV infection are not fully understood. They can occur at two different times during the course of infection. In early HIV infection subtle alterations are present in cognitive function, i.e., memory and judgment. In the terminal stage of HIV infection one observes what is called AIDS dementia which is characterized by a gradual loss of precision in thought and motion.

HIV is sometimes associated with various types of cancers. The most common is Kaposi's sarcoma, as mentioned above, which produces tumors in the skin and the linings of internal organs. Some patients develop lymphomas and carcinoma of the rectum and the tongue. The lymphomas are usually B cell lymphomas and they can be observed early in the course of the disease.

Table 6-7. Opportunistic Infections Occurring Commonly in HIV-infected Patients, Listed By Microorganisms Affecting Each Organ System

Lungs
  Pneumocystis carinii
  Mycobacterium avium-intracellulare
  Cytomegalovirus

Gastrointestinal tract
  Candida
  Cytomegalovirus
  Cryptosporidium
  Giardia
  Salmonella
  Amoeba
  Herpes simplex

Lymph nodes
  Epstein-Barr virus
  Mycobacterium avium-intracellulare

Central nervous system
  Toxoplasma
  Cytomegalovirus
  Herpes simplex
  Papovavirus

Once infected it is thought that most patients progress to Stage VI of the disease and die prematurely.

Since the first consideration of AIDS in this text in 1984, the biology of this disease has unfolded at many levels in fascinating ways. It seems relevant to recount here some additional aspects of the disease.

Retrospective identification of cases of AIDS have become possible both from the patterns of unusual infections and tumors and by use of new technology such as the polymerase chain reaction and immunocytochemical tests on tissue and serum banked decades ago. It seems likely that the earliest positive cases date to the middle 1950s. Although there is no unanimity in accepting the origin of the HIV virus most evidence points to Africa as the geographical source, and sexual activity as the primary mode of transmission. Cultural changes, social upheavals, disturbances of population with increasing travel and promiscuity probably created traffic between Central and East Africa, facilitating the dissemination of HIV-1.

In the U.S., although blacks comprise only 18% of the population they constitute 40% of all reported cases. Homosexual and bisexual men account for 62%, and homosexual men who use IV drugs make up 7%. Only 4% of all AIDS cases are heterosexual. Recipients of transfusions constitute 3%, and 1% of the AIDS population are hemophiliacs. Most childhood cases are due to perinatal infections with HIV in utero, at birth, or in breast milk acquired from infected mothers.

Current estimates for the numbers of cases of AIDS in the U.S. and worldwide vary according to the source. As of October 31, 1988, 75,000 adult and adolescent cases and more than 1,000 children had been reported to the U.S. Centers for Disease Control with 43,000 deaths, a case fatality rate of 56% (Fig. 6-18). The states of New York, California, New Jersey, Florida and Texas accounted for two-thirds of all reported cases. It has been estimated by one source that there will be in excess of 80,000 cases in 1992.

Projections for the epidemic in the U.S. suggest a cumulative number of 365,000 HIV infections by December 31, 1992, with 263,000 deaths if these projections are not altered by some major factor. Other data offer back calculations which postulate as many as 500,000 persons in the U.S. infected with HIV in 1985. Global distributions of HIV infection, reported AIDS cases, and estimates of HIV prevalence are shown in Table 6-8. In addition, Table 6-9 shows the number of AIDS cases reported to NATO from Europe through December 1989. The estimates of the World Health Organization, based on two assumptions that there will be no effective vaccine or cure and that in given

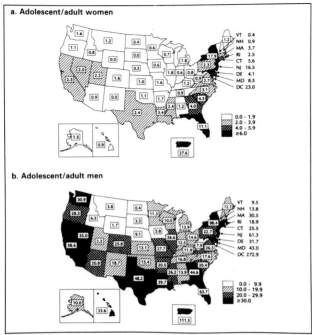

*Per 100,000 population.

Fig. 6–18 Rate of reported AIDS cases per 100,000 population among adolescents and adults, by sex and state of residence—United States, 1990. (From Centers for Disease Control, Morbidity and Mortality Weekly Report, 40(22):363, 1991.)

Table 6–8. Global Distributions of HIV Infections, Reported AIDS, and Estimated/Projected AIDS, December 1989

AREA	ESTIMATED HIV INFECTION PREVALENCE	CUMULATIVE AIDS CASES REPORTED	CUMULATIVE AIDS CASES ESTIMATED BY WHO
Africa	>3,000,000	36,486	320,000
Americas	2,000,000	131,250	220,000
Asia	100,000	481	1,000
Europe	500,000	28,247	36,000
Oceania	30,000	1,701	2,200
Total	>5,630,000	198,165	579,200

* Adapted from J. Chin, personal communication.

(From Braun, M.M., et al.: The global epidemiology of HIV infection and AIDS. Annu. Rev. Microbiol., 44:555, 1990.)

Table 6–9. AIDS Cases Reported to WHO from Europe Through December 1989

COUNTRY	CUMULATIVE CASES	RATE[a]
France	8,025	4.5
Italy	4,663	2.9
West Germany	4,093	1.9
Spain	3,965	3.9
United Kingdom	2,649	1.2
Switzerland	1,046	5.1
Netherlands	983	2.0
Belgium	563	1.2
Denmark	470	2.4
Sweden	346	1.0

[a] Cases per 100,000 in 1988.

(From Braun, M.M., et al.: The global epidemiology of HIV infection and AIDS. Annu. Rev. Microbiol., 44:555, 1990.)

geographic areas the modes of transmission remain constant, suggest that between 12.2 and 18.3 million people will be infected by HIV 1 in the year 2,000, assuming 5.1 million persons were infected in 1991.

Some other studies indicate that the number of cases is levelling off, particularly in selected areas, and that under constant conditions some countries (e.g., Norway) will not see an epidemic. Figure 6–19 shows projections for annual AIDS incidence in 1991–1995 for the entire U.S. and for four transmission groups. These projections are corrected 10% for under reporting.

At the present time, the most promising therapies for AIDS include AZT and dideoxycytidine. The current treatment of Kaposi's sarcoma uses alpha-interferon. No vaccine is available yet, but interesting results have recently been reported with vaccines developed in an experimental model of AIDS in monkeys.

We have to address the risk of contracting AIDS for health care workers. Puncture of the skin with needles contaminated with the blood of HIV infected people seems to be the predominant risk. The risk is relatively low, although not negligible, as shown by the fact that only 4 out of 870 healthy workers who had needle punctures contaminated with HIV developed a positive HIV antibody test. Two of these four, however, have developed AIDS-related symptoms. The overall lesson is to be as careful as we are with viral hepatitis in the manipulation of blood and tissues from AIDS patients.

In conclusion, the complications of HIV infection are multiple and usually follow a pattern which reflects the severity of the various stages of the disease. The pathogenesis of HIV infection has greatly benefited from the basic research on both the virus and the target cells. One might speculate that this will gener-

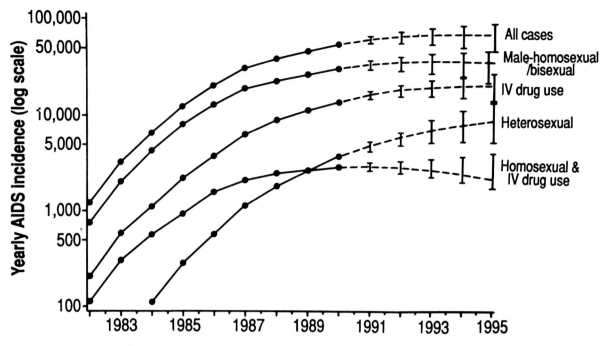

Fig. 6–19 Projections of annual AIDS incidence 1991 to 1995 (log scale) for the entire United States and four transmission groups. Projections corrected 10% for underreporting. Infections after April 1990 are assumed to occur at rate 10,000 per year among homosexuals, intravenous drugs users, and heterosexuals, and 30,000 per year overall. Ranges account for uncertainty in this infection rate and some uncertainty in the incubation period. (From Brookmeyer, R.: Reconstruction and future trends of the AIDS epidemic in the United States. Science, 253:37, 1991.)

ate tools helping to better understand and perhaps control this complex disease.

Besides AIDS, suppression of immune and inflammatory reactions occurs in several situations. One of the most common instances is a person who takes corticosteroids in substantial amounts. Severe injury, debilitating disease, and infections with virus or massive tuberculosis can also cause the anergic response, in injury and disease, by methods that are poorly understood, and, in the use of corticosteroids, by interfering presumably with the lymphocytes directly. Anergy also occurs in patients who have neoplastic diseases, particularly Hodgkin's disease. Conversely, it has been hypothesized that these debilitating neoplastic diseases emerge because of a failing immune system. Finally, anergy occurs sometimes in old age for reasons that are not clear.

TRANSPLANTATION

The replacement of a failed organ (kidney, liver, heart) by a donated new organ from another individual, formally called an allograft, has become a medical fact despite technical and immunologic barriers to its success. Each of us is so special that we normally rec-ognize and reject the tissues of another person when they are introduced into our body, except if this other person is an homozygous twin sister or brother. We refuse to accept the foreign tissue and usually produce antibodies against it. An inflammatory reaction rejects the transplant.

Many early insights resulted from P.B. Medawar's work arising from his interest in skin grafts of burned patients. He showed that whereas the first graft might be tolerated for a few weeks, a second graft was rejected in a much shorter time. Of course, this did not happen with grafts of the patient's own skin (autograft), but grafts from other species (xenografts) were always rejected, as well as grafts from other human beings.

The graft survives better if the donor and recipient are related. One study of renal transplants illustrated this fact by showing that 60% of kidneys donated by siblings, 50% of those donated by parents, and 30% of cadaver kidneys remained functional after five years.

A failed skin graft illustrates the rejection process. First the graft becomes vascularized as part of normal healing. Then it becomes heavily infiltrated with lymphocytes, macrophages, and plasma cells, so that within a week it becomes dark, hard, and thick. After two weeks the blood flow through the graft stops suddenly, resulting in thrombosis and necrosis. Finally it is shed as a dark, dry scab (Fig. 6–20).

There are two main types of mechanisms involved in human organ rejection. The first one is best described as cellular rejection and is attributable mostly to T cells which are found in aggregates in the interstitium of the graft. This may occur at any time after the few days that follow transplantation and is relatively easy to reverse using the appropriate therapy. The second mechanism of rejection is humoral and targets on the blood vessels of the graft. It accounts for a necrotizing inflammation of the blood vessels, i.e., a vasculitis. It is difficult to treat and tends to evolve slowly into a subacute and then a chronic form of vasculitis with marked narrowing of the blood vessel due to fibrosis of the wall. The final result is chronic ischemia of the graft with loss of function. Fortunately for clinical transplantation, not all grafts are rejected, and some are rejected less vigorously than others. The vigor with which a graft is rejected depends on the histocompatibility of the donor and the recipient (Fig.

6–21). This term refers to the degree of similarity of donor and recipient antigens, or to the literal compatibility of donor and recipient tissue.

There appear to be two antigen systems that play major roles in histocompatibility. The first is the ABO blood group system. Donor-recipient pairs must be matched for blood type in accordance with the usual rules for blood transfusions. The second group of antigens is called human leukocyte antigens (HLA antigens), and belongs to the major histocompatibility complex (MHC). MHC is itself composed of three classes of antigens, classes I to III, all found on human chromosome 6. The class I MHC molecules are present on all nucleated cells of the body and are recognized by the CD8 T lymphocytes of the graft recipient. The class II MHC molecules are normally restricted to B cells, dendritic cells and activated T cells, and are recognized by the CD4 lymphocytes. MHC III is not directly involved in transplantation rejection. It is important to note that the various MHC classes have other roles besides transplantation. In Chapter 2 we

FIRST SET REJECTION ──────────────────────

SECOND SET REJECTION ──────────────────────────

Fig. 6–20 Skin graft rejection. When skin from A mouse is grafted onto B mouse, B rejects the tissue within 10 to 20 days. The next time skin is grafted from A to B, rejection occurs in half the time, which shows that memory of the first contact has been retained. (Adapted from Barrett, J.T.: *Basic Immunology and Its Medical Application.* St. Louis, C. V. Mosby, 1976.)

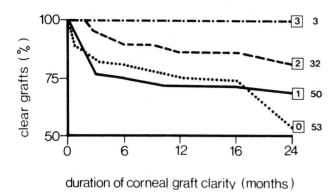

duration of corneal graft clarity (months)

Fig. 6–21 This figure shows the influence of HLA (human leukocyte antigens) matching on duration of corneal graft success. The boxed numbers represent the numbers of HLA antigens shared by both donor and recipient. The numbers of patients studied are shown in unenclosed numerals to the right of the boxes. When a corneal graft is rejected, it becomes cloudy. The grafts where HLA antigens are in common are most successful, whereas those grafts in which no HLA matching exists, or where only one HLA antigen is shared, show a different failure rate than those where 2 or more HLA antigens are shared. (From Morris, P.J., Batchelor, J.R., and Festenstein, H.: Matching for HLA in transplantation. Br. Med. Bull., 34:259, 1978.)

explained that some MHC types are associated with an increased risk or a resistance to some diseases.

Much tissue transplantation between different persons is considered to be of questionable value because of the problem of rejection. It is probably obvious from the preceding discussion that the limitation of transplantation is not so much the performance of the surgical grafting but the maintenance of a partially compatible organ in an immune competent receiver. Recent use of the drug cyclosporin has vastly improved the rate of success in transplantation. However, the other side of the coin shows that cyclosporin is toxic to the kidney above a certain dose. Another potential problem with drugs used to prevent and treat rejection is linked to their non-specific immunosuppressive effects. Consequently, the risk for the recipient is that ordinary bacteria and fungi, which are normally successfully handled by the body, may cause infection. Such infections are referred to as opportunistic, since they have seized the chance to gain access to the weakened host. In addition, the long-term follow-up of transplant patients shows that they are more likely to have certain forms of cancer, such as cancer of the cervix and lymphoma.

In many instances, transplantation has proved to be invaluable. Autogenous transplants in man are of course most desirable, and these are used in skin grafts. Allogenic transplants (i.e., transplants between two individuals who are not monozygous twins) have proved to be of great use, not only for

end-stage liver, heart, lung and kidney diseases, but also in diseases of bone, fascia, nerves, blood vessels, and the cornea of the eye.

A problem, associated mostly with bone marrow transplantation, is graft-versus-host (GVH) disease. It is caused by lymphocytes in the graft which recognize the host cells as foreign, producing severe skin, liver and intestinal changes. This often fatal complication is more likely to occur in cases of suboptimal MHC matching.

AUTOIMMUNE DISORDERS

The idea of being allergic to oneself seems strange, and yet the idea that the body may react to certain of its own tissues in an adverse way has been clearly demonstrated. A fundamental issue is to decide whether the patient is reacting against unmodified cell or tissue components. Immunologists have suggested that during intrauterine development our lymphocytes go through a selection process in the thymus. Those that are potentially reacting against self constituents are eliminated. Other lymphocytes are left to migrate to distant lymphoid tissues where they will be able to react against nonself constituents when the need arises. In other words, we normally become tolerant to our self during this process of maturation. Consequently, if this process of lymphocyte elimination is defective, we can potentially develop an autoimmune reaction later in life.

Another completely different possibility is that the so-called autoantigen has been previously damaged by some injury that has changed its structure from self to "slightly nonself." Autoimmune diseases may be defined as **diseases that result from antibodies or immune cells produced by the host that react with some of the host's own antigens.** The antigens may be in the serum or in the cells of a particular tissue, such as the thyroid gland. Criteria to establish that a particular disease is of autoimmune etiology have been proposed:

Criteria for Autoimmune Disease

1. The antigen in question should be present in the affected tissues, and the lesions should show inflammatory mononuclear cells and/or immunoglobulins in the affected tissue.
2. Antibodies that react with these antigens should be present in all cases of this disease.
3. The disease should have a clinical presentation usually associated with immune disorders and

Table 6–10. Some Autoimmune Diseases

DISEASE	ANTIGEN	LESION
Autoimmune hemolytic anemia	Red blood cells	Erythrocyte destruction
Hashimoto's thyroiditis	Thyroglobin	Infiltration of thyroid by lymphocytes and plasma cells, destruction of follicular cells
Pernicious anemia	Intrinsic factor	Blocking antibody prevents binding of vitamin B_{12} to intrinsic factor. B_{12} is necessary for red blood cell maturation (see Chap. 3)
Systemic lupus erythematosus	DNA, nucleoproteins, blood clotting factors	Systemic disease. Widespread lesions of connective tissue in skin, kidney glomeruli, joints, serous membranes, and blood vessels
Myasthenia gravis	Skeletal and heart muscle acetylcholine receptor	Blocks neuromuscular transmission leading to muscle weakness
Rheumatoid arthritis	IgG	Inflammation of synovial tissues leading eventually to joint destruction

should respond to anti-inflammatory drugs such as corticosteroids.

Some examples of autoimmune diseases are given in Table 6–10 and are fully discussed in various chapters.

To summarize, we have outlined the features of the immune system and have discussed some disorders that are clearly of allergic rather than of infectious or other etiology. Currently, the pendulum has swung far in the direction of explaining many additional diseases of the reticuloendothelial system, the endocrine glands, the bowel, the liver, and central nervous system as being disorders of the immune system. In some instances, there are good grounds for this designation (Hashimoto's disease), whereas in others, the evidence is at most scanty (Crohn's disease). For those who are hearing about disease for the first time, listen with a critical ear to the claims that a particular disease of uncertain cause is of an immunologic etiology.

The most important message of this chapter is that not all inflammation is caused by physical, chemical, or biologic (in the sense of bacterial, viral, or protozoal, for example) injury, but rather that the interaction of antigen and antibody can serve as a potent agent for tissue destruction.

SYNOPSIS

Response to antigen depends on macrophages, which are nonspecific, and lymphocytes, which react specifically with an antigen.

Lymphocytes are of two types: B cells, which secrete antibody, and T cells. Macrophages and lymphocytes secrete mediators named interkeukins.

Passive transfer of maternal immunity to fetus occurs in utero and lasts for a short time after birth.

Antigen and antibody combine to form immune complexes. This triggers several mechanisms, one of which is complement fixation.

After a single exposure to an antigen, the host recognizes and destroys it faster the next time. This is the anamnestic response.

Hypersensitivity refers to the altered state of reactivity that is destructive rather than defensive.

Systemic anaphylaxis is a massive allergic response that involves widespread change in capillary permeability that leads to shock and respiratory distress.

A cytotoxic allergic reaction causes destruction of cells in the blood or tissue.

Immune complex disease involves thrombosis and necrosis of small blood vessel walls either locally or systemically.

Cell-mediated hypersensitivity is a delayed allergic reaction in which T cells interact with antigen to cause inflammatory lesions.

Immunodeficiency can be congenital or acquired, such as in AIDS. The basic mechanism of AIDS is the destruction of the T lymphocytes by HIV.

Autoimmune diseases, such as systemic lupus, are due to the attack of the immune system against self-constituents.

Terms

Immunity	*Interleukin*	*Cytotoxicity*
Sensitization	*Immune complex*	*Delayed hypersensitivity*
Tolerance	*Complement*	*Transplantation*
Autoimmunity	*Anamnestic response*	*Rejection*
T cells	*Active/passive immunization*	*Immunosuppression*
B cells	*Anergy*	*AIDS*
Antigen	*Anaphylaxis*	*HIV*
Antibody	*Atopy*	*Arthus reaction*
MHC		

FURTHER READING

Akira, S., Hirano, T., Taga, T., and Kishimoto, T.: Biology of multifunctional cytokines: IL 6 and related molecules (IL 1 and TNF). FASEB J., 4:2860, 1990.

Anderson, R.M., et al.: The spread of HIV-1 in Africa: sexual contact patterns and the predicted demographic impact of AIDS. Nature, 352:581, 1991.

Arai, K., Lee, F., Miyajima, A., et al.: Cytokines: Coordinators of immune and inflammatory responses. Annu. Rev. Biochem., 59:783, 1990.

Austen, W.G.: Heart transplantation after ten years. N. Engl. J. Med., 298:682, 1978.

Baisch, J.M., Weeks, T., Giles, R., et al.: Analysis of HLA-DQ genotypes and susceptibility in insulin-dependent diabetes mellitus. N. Engl. J. Med., 322:1836, 1990.

Baltimore, D., and Feinberg, M.B.: HIV revealed: Toward a natural history of the infection. N. Engl. J. Med., 321:1673, 1989.

Beer, A.E., and Billingham, R.E.: Transplantation in nature. Perspect. Biol. Med., 22:155, 1979.

Bochner, B.S.: Current concepts: Anaphylaxis. N. Engl. J. Med., 324:1785, 1991.

Braun, M.M., Heward, W.L., and Curran, J.W.: The global epidemiology of HIV infection and AIDS. Annu. Rev. Microbiol., 44:555, 1990.

Brookmeyer, R.: Reconstruction and future trends of the AIDS epidemic in the United States. Science, 253:37, 1991.

Cooper, M.D.: Current Concepts: B Lymphocytes: Normal development and function. N. Engl. J. Med., 317:1452, 1987.

Davis, M.M.: T-cell antigen receptor genes and T-cell recognition. Nature, 334:395, 1988.

Ferrara, J.L.M., and Deeg, H.J.: Mechanisms of disease: Graft-versus-host disease. N. Engl. J. Med., 324:667, 1991.

Gayle, H.D., Keeling, R.P., Garcia-Tunon, M., et al.: Prevalence of the human immunodeficiency virus among university students. N. Engl. J. Med., 323:1538, 1990.

Giesecke, J., Scalia-Tomba, G., Håkansson, C., et al.: Incubation time of AIDS: progression of disease in a cohort of HIV-infected homo- and bisexual men with known dates of infection. Scand. J. Infect. Dis., 22:407, 1990.

Greene, W.C.: The molecular biology of human immunodeficiency virus type 1 infection. N. Engl. J. Med., 324:308, 1991.

Guttman, R.D.: Renal transplantation. N. Engl. J. Med., 301:975, 1038, 1979.

Hansen, J.A., and Nelson, J.L.: Autoimmune diseases and HLA. Crit. Rev. Immunol., 10:307, 1990.

Harris, E.D., Jr.: Mechanisms of disease: Rheumatoid arthritis—Pathophysiology and implications for therapy. N. Engl. J. Med., 322:1277, 1990.

Hong, R.: Update on the immunodeficiency diseases. AJDC, 144:983, 1990.

Jaffe, H.W.: AIDS: Epidemiologic features. J. Am. Acad. Dermatol., 22:1167, 1990.

James, L.P., Jr., and Austen, K.F.: Fatal systemic anaphylaxis in man. N. Engl. J. Med., 270:597, 1964.

Kelly, K.A., Rouse, I.L., Roberts, M., and Sesnan, K.T.: Measuring the HIV epidemic: the Western Australian experience. Med. J. Australia, 153:394, 1990.

Kotloff, K.L., Tacket, C.O., Clemens, J.D., et al.: Assessment of the prevalence and risk factors for human immunodeficiency virus Type 1 (HIV-1) infection among college students using three survey methods. Am. J. Epidemiol., 133:2, 1991.

Lafferty, W.E., Glidden, D., and Hopkins, S.G.: Survival trends of people with AIDS in Washington State. Am. J. Public Health, 81:215, 1991.

McCune, J.M.: HIV-1: the infective process in vivo. Cell, 64:351, 1991.

McDermott, M.R., Befus, A.D., and Bienenstock, J.: The structural basis for immunity in the respiratory tract. In *International Review of Experimental Pathology*. Edited by G.W. Richter. New York, Academic Press, 1981.

Milstein, C.: From antibody diversity to monoclonal antibodies. Eur. J. Biochem., 118:429, 1981.

Mizel, S.B.: The interleukins. FASEB J., 3:2379, 1989.

Mygland, A., Tysnes, O.B., and Aarli, J.A., et al.: Myasthenia Gravis patients with a thymoma have antibodies against a high molecular weight protein in sarcoplasmic reticulum. J. Neuroimmunol., 37:1, 1992.

Nossal, G.J.V.: The basic components of the immune system. N. Engl. J. Med., 316:1320, 1987.

Oldham, R.K.: Natural killer cells: history, relevance, and clinical applications. Nat. Immun. Cell Growth Regul., 9:297, 1990.

Patterson, R., Zeiss, C.R., and Kelly, J.K.: Classification of hypersensitivity reactions. N. Engl. J. Med., 295:277, 1976.

Pedersen, C., Gerstoft, J., Tauris, P., et al.: Trends in survival of Danish AIDS patients from 1981 to 1989. AIDS 4:1111, 1990.

Peters, B.S., Beck, E.J., Coleman, D.G., et al.: Changing disease patterns in patients with AIDS in a referral centre in the United Kingdom: the changing face of AIDS. Br. Med. J., 302:203, 1991.

Prud'homme, G., and Parfrey, N.: Role of T helper lymphocytes in autoimmune diseases. Lab. Investig., 59:158, 1988.

Rennie, J.: The body against itself. Sci. Am., Dec:106, 1990.

Revillard, J.P.: Iatrogenic immunodeficiencies. Curr. Opin. Immunol., 2:445, 1991.

Roitt, I.: *Essential Immunology*, 4th Ed. Oxford, Blackwell Scientific Publications, 1988.

Rose, N.R.: The discovery of thyroid autoimmunity. Immunol. Today, 12:167, 1991.

Rosenberg, P.S., Biggar, R.J., Goedert, J.J., and Gail, M.H.: Backcalculation of the number with human immunodeficiency virus infection in the United States. Am. J. Epidemiol., 133:276, 1991.

Sen, G.C., and Lengyel, P.: The interferon system—a bird's eye view of its biochemistry. J. Biol. Chem., 267:5017, 1992.

Stigum, H., Grønnesby, Magnus, P., et al.: The potential for spread of HIV in the heterosexual population in Norway: a model study. Stats. Med., 10:1003, 1991.

Smith, K.A.: Interleukin-2. Sci. Am., 262:50, 1990.

Taylor, J.M.G., Kuo, J.-M., and Detels, R.: Is the incubation period of AIDS lengthening? J. AIDS, 4:69, 1991.

Torres, C.G., Turner, M.E., Harkess, J.R., and Istre, G.R.: Security measures for AIDS and HIV. Am. J. Public Health, 81:208, 1991.

Van Boehmer, H., and Kisielow, P.: How the immune system learns about self. Sci. Am., 265:74, 1991.

Van Snick, J.: Interleukin-6: An overview. Annu. Rev. Immunol., 8:253, 1990.

Wilson, M.E., Fordham von Reyn, C., and Fineberg, H.V.: Infections in HIV-infected travelers; risks and prevention. Ann. Intern. Med., 114:582, 1991.

7

BACTERIAL INFECTIONS

The bacterium is nothing; the soil is everything.—PASTEUR

GENERAL PRINCIPLES

One bacterium gives rise to hundreds of millions in the course of 24 hours, provided conditions are suitable, i.e., food, moisture, and temperature. This enormous increase is possible under laboratory conditions because reproduction is not a complicated process; one bacterium simply divides into two. Bacteria are so small they cannot be seen with the naked eye, but only with the oil immersion lens of the light microscope. When stained with chemical dyes they can be seen to vary in size and shape, and have been divided into three groups: **cocci,** which are round, **bacilli,** which are rod-shaped, and **spirilla,** which are, as the name implies, spiral.

Typically, pneumonia is caused by a coccus, tuberculosis by a bacillus, and syphilis by a spirillum. Diplococci grow in pairs, staphylococci in clusters like grapes, streptococci in long or short chains. Bacteria are named according to the disease they produce, but new and more complex nomenclatures have replaced the old. What was once called *Bacillus tuberculosis* is now known as *Mycobacterium tuberculosis; Bacillus typhosus* is now called *Salmonella typhi.* New names have been attributed to the cultural requirements of the organisms, or to the appearances of the organisms in culture media. Fortunately, some bacteria (staphylococci, streptococci) have escaped this renaming process. For our purposes, we shall use the common and important names.

When a microorganism invades tissues or a host, one of three things may happen: (1) The bacterial invader may die, which is most likely. (2) The microorganism may survive without giving rise to disease, but may cause an immune reaction in the host, which abbreviates subsequent infections. (3) Exceptionally, the microorganism survives, multiplies, and produces clinically apparent disease that may prove fatal not only to the host, but often, necessarily, to the microorganism.

Although bacteria may be the living form responsible for many of man's afflictions, these small organisms are also responsible for many good things in our lives. Bacteria derive their sustenance from already dead materials, whether plant or animal. Their role is to return the complex elements of living forms to a simpler, elemental nature. Thus the floor of the forest, littered with leaves, is rendered to humus by millions of bacteria. Other bacteria play more specific roles, such as those that are able to capture nitrogen in its gaseous form and affix it in an organic form, from which it can be converted eventually into protein. We use different terms to define the different roles of bacteria. Bacteria that live on dead materials are called saprophytes, whereas those that live on living material are known as parasites.

Physicians tend to be preoccupied with disease-producing (pathogenic) bacteria and are apt to forget that most bacteria are harmless, if not beneficial. We can go so far as to say that without bacteria life would long ago have ceased on this planet, for they keep the building blocks of metabolism in circulation. Bacteria prepare the substrate for plants, which in turn are eaten by animals. Without bacteria, the nitrogen cycle would come to a full stop and the existence of all higher forms of life would be impossible. It used to be thought that life in animals and in man was impossible without the presence of bacteria, particularly those in the bowel. We now know this is not true because various forms of life (birds and mammals) have been raised in germ-free environments. It is interesting, in the light of the previous chapter, to remark on what happens to animals brought from a germ-free to a normal environment. All guinea pigs die of overwhelming infection within 48 hours; 50% of mice also die, but rats and chickens show no ill effects.

Many regions of the body are normally inhabited by bacteria (see Table 7–1). Occasionally, when a host's defenses are weakened, or when these bacteria leave

155

Table 7–1. Predominant Microbial Species Found in Various Human Anatomic Regions

REGION	MICROORGANISM	% INCIDENCE
Skin	*Staphylococcus epidermidis*	85 to 100
	Staphylococcus aureus	5 to 25
	Propionibacterium acnes	45 to 100
Nose and nasopharynx	*Staphylococcus epidermidis*	90
	Staphylococcus aureus	20 to 85
	Hemophilus influenzae	12
Mouth and tooth surfaces	*Staphylococcus epidermidis*	75 to 100
	Staphylococcus aureus	Common
	Streptococcus mitis and other	100
	alpha-hemolytic streptococci	95
	Lactobacillus	Common
	Actinomyces israeli	25 to 100
	Hemophilus influenzae	Common
	Bacteroides fragilis	15 to 90
	Fusobacterium nucleatum	6 to 50
	Candida albicans	Common
	Borrelia vincentii	
Ileum	Distal portion may have small numbers of Enterobacteriaceae and anaerobic gram-negative bacteria	
Large intestine	Gram-negative bacilli:	100
	Bacteroides fragilis	
	Fusobacterium nucleatum	
	Gram-positive bacilli:	
	Lactobacillus	20 to 60
	Clostridium perfringens	25 to 35
	Enterococcus (group D streptococcus)	100
	Escherichia coli	100
	Klebsiella spp.	40 to 80
	Enterobacteriaceae	40 to 80
	Proteus spp.	5 to 55
	Candida albicans	15 to 30
	Bacteroides spp.	60 to 80
Vagina and uterine cervix	*Clostridium* spp.	15 to 30
	Staphylococcus epidermidis	35 to 80
	Candida albicans	30 to 50
	Trichomonas vaginalis	10 to 25

(Adapted from Pelczar, M., Jr., et al.: *Microbiology*, 4th Ed. New York, McGraw-Hill, 1977.)

their natural habitat and migrate to another part of the body, where they are less welcome, disease develops. These bacteria are called opportunistic microorganisms, because they cause trouble only when the opportunity arises. Table 7–2 shows the types of opportunistic and other infections known to occur when host resistance is compromised.

Outside the body it is easy enough to kill bacteria by means of agents that are capable of denaturing their protein, or of interfering with their metabolism. It is much more difficult to do so in the living body because substances, such as carbolic acid, that kill the bacteria are injurious to body cells. Specific treatment that attacks bacteria without injuring body cells has been developed only in the last 65 years. Modern antibiotics such as penicillin and streptomycin have been prepared from fungi in the soil and can kill bacteria in vitro with startling rapidity. In the living body they may not do this directly, but they prevent bacteria from multiplying, thus giving the defenses of the body time to mobilize and attack the invaders. We speak of **bacteriostatic** agents and of other antibiotics that are **bacteriocidal.** It is true, in addition, that antibiotics that kill unwanted bacteria may also kill those useful inhabitants of the intestine. Bacterial overgrowth by more pathogenic organisms may lead to greater complications.

The effects of bacteria are achieved principally by enzymes directly secreted into the immediate bacterial environment. Bacterial enzymes break down complex food materials—whether protein, carbohydrate, or fat—into amino acids or peptides and short chains of carbon and acetic acid. These substances can be assimilated and used by the bacteria. The enzymatic activity in the intestine results in the decomposition of the organic material that has been ingested. As we have said, decomposition returns to the soil those elements that can be used in the next cycle of growth. Intestinal bacteria have been called nature's fertilizer factory. Bacteria serve also outside the body to purify sewage and to make it inoffensive, as in a compost heap. Many essential vitamins such as the B complex are formed by the bacteria in the large intestine of man, and are then used by him.

The activity of bacteria is manifest in various ways. Fermentation of carbohydrates results in the production of gas and acid, which are used by the professional microbiologist to identify certain bacteria, and by the industrialist in the manufacture of alcohol, vinegar, cheese and many good things. Pasteur was first drawn to the study of bacteria by his work on the fermentation of wine. The breakdown of proteins (proteolysis) into simpler substances, some of which smell foul, is achieved by the enzymes of anaerobic bacteria. The decomposition of dead tissue is an example of proteolysis. Toxin production varies from bacteria to bacteria. Comparatively few bacteria produce exotoxins, that is, poisons secreted by the living bacteria. Diphtheria bacillus and the clostridia group of spore-bearing, gram-positive bacilli are examples. The organisms of tetanus, gas gangrene, and botulism, three members of the clostridia group, illustrate the variation in action and types of exotoxin. Tetanus bacilli grow under anaerobic conditions (without air) in dead tissue, and there produce an exotoxin that

Table 7–2. Infections in the Compromised Host

	MAJOR DEFECTS	ETIOLOGIC AGENTS	INFECTIONS
Burns	Tissue necrosis, loss of epithelial barrier, lymphocytopenia	*Streptococcus pyogenes* *Staphylococcus aureus* *Pseudomonas*	Cellulitis Bacteremia Pneumonia
Diabetes	Reduced vascular supply, decreased leukocyte chemotaxis	*Staphylococcus aureus* *Candida* Enteric bacilli *Mycobacterium tuberculosis*	Cellulitis Urinary tract infection Bacteremia
Thermolytic disease	Reduced monocyte-macrophage function	*Salmonella* *Streptococcus pneumoniae*	Bacteremia Pneumonia Osteomyelitis Meningitis
Cystic fibrosis	Bronchial obstruction by hyperviscous mucus	*Staphylococcus aureus* *Pseudomonas*	Bronchitis Pneumonia

(From Thorn, G.W., et al. (Eds.): *Harrison's Principles of Internal Medicine*, 8th Ed. New York, McGraw-Hill, 1977.)

causes no local inflammatory reaction, but rather passes along the course of the peripheral nerves to the central nervous system. There it causes catastrophic clinical results, but still without apparent tissue damage. The organisms of gas gangrene, on the other hand, produce profound and widespread local damage in wounds by means of their enzymes. Finally, the bacilli of botulism do not need to live in the tissues of the host, but proliferate in insufficiently sterilized canned goods. There they elaborate one of the most deadly poisons known, which kills swiftly when ingested. When an exotoxin is treated with formaldehyde, it no longer causes disease when injected, but confers immunity. Such a modified toxin is called a **toxoid.** Toxoids are used more particularly for protection against diphtheria and tetanus. Practically all bacteria contain endotoxins, which are liberated when the bacteria die and disintegrate. Examples are the gram-negative intestinal bacilli.

Spread of Infection. Different pathogenic or disease-producing bacteria have different portals of entry to the body. Some may be introduced through the skin, but most enter through natural passages. Some prefer the respiratory passages, others the alimentary or the genitourinary tracts. Some are discharged from the body in feces and urine, others by the mouth, nose, respiratory tract, saliva, and even the blood by means of insect bites. Knowledge and appreciation of these routes are necessary if the spread of infection is to be prevented. When an infection is transmitted intentionally through a series of laboratory animals, the **virulence** is likely to be increased, probably because the bacteria adapt themselves to the environment. The same thing is seen in human epidemics, in which virulence increases until a peak is reached, followed by a decline, perhaps be-

cause only the resistant members of the community remain to be infected. There are four principal methods of spread: (1) physical contact, (2) air, (3) food and water, and (4) insects or other vectors (Fig. 7–1).

Physical Contact. The contact may be direct, the infecting bacteria not surviving outside the body; the classic example is venereal disease (Table 7–3). The contact may also be indirect, through **fomites,** that is to say, clothing, utensils, and other possessions of the patient, the bacteria surviving for some time outside the body.

Airborne Infection. Bacterial and viral infections of the respiratory tract are transmitted through the air by dust or droplets. Dust infection comes from bacteria in dried sputum that become attached to dust particles; this is particularly true of tuberculosis. Droplet infection is the basis of epidemics of upper respiratory disease. It is estimated that 20,000 droplets containing possible pathogens may be expelled by one sneeze (Fig. 7–2), and the droplets 1 mm in diameter may pass over a distance of 5 meters. Were it not for natural and acquired defenses we might all be ill.

Food-borne Infection. This constitutes an important public health problem (Fig. 7–3). The possibility of infection by food or water must be considered in every major epidemic of intestinal disease. Epidemics of typhoid, dysentery and cholera are due to infection of food or water.

Insect-borne Infection. Insects are important conveyors of infection, not only bacterial, but also viral and protozoal. Thus plague is spread from the rat to man by the rat-flea, typhus by lice, and yellow fever virus and the malaria parasite by mosquitoes. It is obvious how necessary is a knowledge of the spread of infection by insects if some of the great scourges of the tropics are to be controlled.

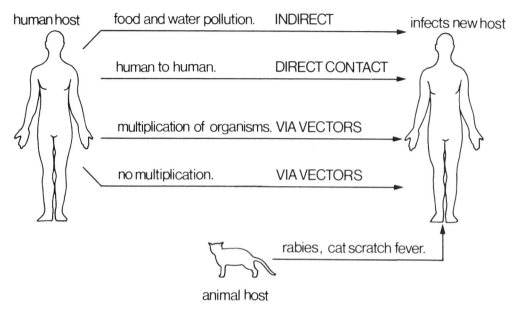

human host

food and water pollution.   INDIRECT   infects new host

human to human.   DIRECT CONTACT

multiplication of organisms. VIA VECTORS

no multiplication.   VIA VECTORS

rabies, cat scratch fever.

animal host

Fig. 7–1   Transmission of pathogenic microorganisms from person to person occurs in a variety of ways, ranging from direct contact, to fomites, and by intermediate vectors. Animals may also transmit pathogens to humans. (From Pelczar, M., Jr., et al.: *Microbiology*, 4th Ed. New York, McGraw-Hill, 1977.)

Diagnostic Methods. It might be thought that it would be a simple matter to determine the bacterial agent causing a given disease. In some cases this is easy, but in others it may be extremely difficult. Robert Koch established the criteria necessary to justify the assumption of an etiologic relationship in 1881. These four criteria have long been known as **Koch's postulates.**

Koch's Postulates
1. The suspected organism must always be present in the lesions.
2. It must be grown in pure culture on laboratory media.
3. It must cause the same disease when injected into a susceptible animal.
4. It must be recovered from the experimental animal.

The most notable of the many contributions that

Table 7–3.   Agents of Sexually Transmitted Diseases

Viruses	*Mycoplasmas*
Herpes simplex	Mycoplasma hominis
Cytomegalovirus	Ureaplasma urealyticum*
Molluscum contagiosum (poxvirus)	*Chlamydiae*
Epstein-Barr	Chlamydia trachomatis*
Hepatitis A and B*	*Fungi*
Bacteria	Candida species
Neisseria gonorrhoeae*	Histoplasma capsulatum?
Neisseria meningitidis	*Endoparasites*
Treponema pallidum*	Entamoeba histolytica*
Haemophilus ducreyi*	Trichomonas vaginalis*
Shigella species	Giardia lamblia*
Group B streptococci?	*Ectoparasites*
Gardnerella vaginalis*	Phthirus pubis*
Listeria monocytogenes?	Sarcoptes scabiei*
Calymmatobacterium granulomatis*	
Campylobacter fetus	

* Epidemiologic treatment probably appropriate

(From Rein, M.F.: Therapeutic decisions in the treatment of sexually transmitted diseases: An overview. Sexually Transmitted Diseases, 8:93, 181.)

Fig. 7–2   The microorganisms that cause many respiratory diseases can be spread from one person to another in aerosols generated by sneezing, coughing, or even conversation. (From the American Society for Microbiology, Washington, D.C.)

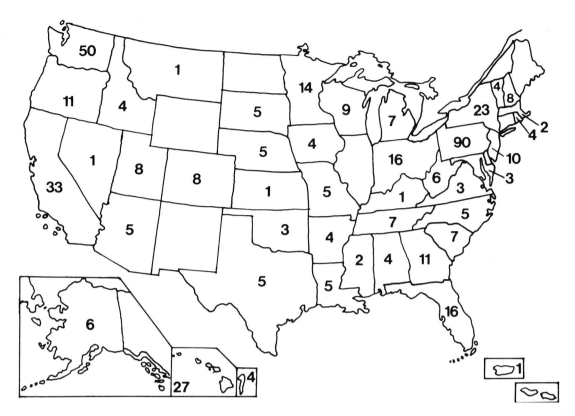

Fig. 7–3 This map shows the reported food-borne and water-borne disease outbreaks in 1974. (Insets illustrate, left to right, Alaska, Hawaii, Guam, Puerto Rico, and Virgin Islands.) These outbreaks affected 15,489 persons in 44 states, Puerto Rico, the District of Columbia, and Guam. The numbers are the numbers of such outbreaks in each state. (Adapted from Centers for Disease Control: Foodborne and waterborne disease outbreaks, annual summary, 1974. Atlanta, United States Public Health Service, 1976.)

Koch made to bacteriology was his demonstration of the true cause of tuberculosis, for in the space of a year he demonstrated the tubercle bacillus in the lesions by special staining, grew the bacilli on a medium that he invented, reproduced the disease by injecting the culture into suitable laboratory animals, and recovered tubercle bacilli from these animals. Such conclusive proof of the bacteriologic cause of disease is not always possible, but it serves as a model for outlining the causal relationships in any disease. Thus Koch outlined a philosophically sound basis for establishing the etiology of any disease.

In summary of the diagnostic aspects of bacterial infections, we may say that an immediate laboratory diagnosis of the nature of the infective agent is of prime importance, so that appropriate antibiotic therapy may be started at the earliest possible moment. The first step is gram-staining of the smears, which allows a preliminary classification before the final culture and sensitivity tests become available. An exact bacteriologic diagnosis is necessary because microorganisms respond so differently to different chemotherapeutic agents. For further reading on special

stains and cultural characteristics of bacteria see the Appendix, p. 186.

Host Reactions to Bacteria. Different bacterial pathogens produce different lesions. Some are focal, others diffuse; some evoke acute inflammatory response, others are granulomatous, and so on. A general idea of the types of the infecting agent may be gathered from a consideration of the character and histologic appearance of the lesions (Table 7–4), but absolute certainty can only come from such bacteriologic techniques as staining the organisms in smears or tissue, growing them in culture, reproducing the disease in an animal, or demonstrating the presence of antibodies by appropriate serologic methods.

Suppurative lesions are produced in most cases by one or another of the pus-forming (pyogenic) cocci. When the suppuration remains localized, the lesion forms an abscess, with necrosis of tissue and collections of polymorphonuclear leukocytes. **Granulomatous inflammation** is characterized by a reaction composed of both round cells and giant cells. The classic example is, of course, tuberculosis.

Changing Picture of Infection. Under normal condi-

Table 7–4. The Syndrome Approach to Infection

TYPE OF INFECTION	COMMON ETIOLOGIC AGENT
Skin and subcutaneous tissue	*Staphylococcus aureus*
Sinusitis	*Streptococcus pneumoniae*
	Staphylococcus aureus
Pneumonitis	*Streptococcus pneumoniae,*
	Mycoplasma pneumoniae
	Mycobacterium tuberculosis
Bacterial endocarditis	*Streptococcus viridans*
	Staphylococcus aureus
Gastroenteritis	*Salmonella, Shigella*
	Enteric viruses
Peritonitis, cholangitis, intra-abdominal abscess	*Escherichia coli,* enterococcus
	Bacteroides, anaerobic streptococcus
Urinary infection	*Escherichia coli, Klebsiella-* Enterobacter
	Proteus, enterococcus
Meninges	*Streptococcus pneumoniae*
	Hemophilus influenzae
	Neisseria meningitidis
	Various viruses

(Adapted from Thorn, G.W., et al. (Eds): *Harrison's Principles of Internal Medicine*, 8th Ed. New York, McGraw-Hill, 1977.)

tions, life in the bacterial world is a constant competition for survival. If the local environment becomes unfavorable, the power to mutate or to bring latent enzyme systems into play becomes apparent. The widespread and often unnecessary use of antibiotics have greatly exaggerated this tendency. In the Toronto General Hospital, resistant strains of *Staphylococcus aureus* rose from 6% in 1947 to 60% four years later. Antibiotic-resistant strains were present in the nose and throat of both patients and staff, and the distance between the nose of a surgeon and a surgical wound is very short. The incidence of penicillin-resistant staphylococci was much higher in hospital inpa-

tients than in outpatients, and it was still lower in the general population (Table 7–5).

A chemotherapeutic agent can displace the normal harmless flora of the throat, which is soon replaced by intestinal bacteria, also harmless in their proper habitat. In the new environment, however, they may cause serious local infections and may even invade the blood stream. It is indeed a paradox that the more an antibiotic is used (or abused) in a hospital community, the less valuable it becomes. The widespread use of antibiotics in animal food is another important source of resistant organisms that can spread to man.

We must not suppose that this changing picture of bacterial infection is a new thing. The incidence, character, and severity of microbial diseases change from one generation to another, owing to changing environmental conditions, to the development of immunity in the population, or to the introduction of prophylactic measures, such as vaccination against smallpox and toxoid inoculation against diphtheria. In such cases we may turn for an explanation to the natural tendency to mutation in the rapidly recurring generations of bacteria. *The Andromeda Strain*, Michael Crichton's science fiction novel, is based on this premise. Leprosy practically disappeared in England during the sixteenth century. Long before the modern era of chemotherapy, syphilis had changed its character profoundly, and the mortality rate from tuberculosis has fallen steadily since 1945. It would appear that the changing picture of infection, although partly man-made, is also partly natural. We must admit, however, that the majority of fatal infections used to be produced by streptococci, staphylococci, and tubercle bacilli, originating in apparently healthy persons outside a hospital. Now common culprits are gram-negative bacilli, staphylococci, viruses, and fungi.

Lest the picture presented in the foregoing para-

Table 7–5. Infections in Compromised Host: Iatrogenic

	MAJOR DEFECTS	ETIOLOGIC AGENTS	INFECTIONS
Glucocorticosteroids	Decreased cellular immunity	*Staphylococcus aureus*	Cellulitis
	Decreased chemotaxis	Enteric bacilli	Bacteremia
		Some viruses	Pneumonia
		Candida	
Cytotoxic drugs	Neutropenia	Enteric bacillic	Bacteremia
	Monocytopenia	*Candida*	
	Lymphopenia	*Pseudomonas*	
Antibiotics	Colonization by resistant bacteria	*Staphylococcus aureus*	Superinfections
		Pseudomonas	
		Serratia	
Prosthetic devices	Foreign body	*Staphylococcus aureus*	Abscesses
		Enteric bacilli	Bacteremia
		Candida	

(From Thorn, G.W., et al. (Eds.): *Harrison's Principles of Internal Medicine*, 8th Ed. New York, McGraw-Hill, 1977.)

graph be too depressing, we may recall that of the children born in London between 1762 and 1771, two-thirds died before the age of 5 years. This was in the century called the Age of Reason! There was certainly no danger of an exploding population. At the same period and in the same country, Queen Anne had 12 pregnancies, but not one child survived. Improved living conditions and, in particular, improved sanitation altered this picture significantly. (Until the mid-nineteenth century the water supply to the city of Vienna ran through the municipal cemetery.) Modern antibacterial therapy has also contributed greatly to human survival.

GRAM-POSITIVE COCCI

Pathogenic gram-positive cocci are often called pyogenic cocci because their reaction in the body produces pus. The most important of these are staphylococci and streptococci. (Their general characteristics are reviewed in the Appendix p. 186.)

The Staphylococci

These are small, spherical bacteria which usually grow in small clusters like a bunch of grapes (Fig. 7–4). They are nonmotile and grow easily in culture. When grown on blood agar (a culture medium containing blood) they produce colonies of characteristic colors varying from golden to white. The three principal species are S. aureus, S. epidermidis, and S. saprophyticus.

S. aureus is the most pathogenic species of the staphylococci. Coagulase-negative staph are largely regarded as nonpathogenic. However, S. saprophyticus is now known to cause urinary tract infections in children and young women. S. epidermidis has been known to colonize indwelling vascular catheters and prosthetic devices like artificial heart valves and ventricular shunts used for the relief of hydrocephalus. Infected patients may develop bacterial endocarditis or abscesses. The first rule in the treatment of such infections is "remove the foreign body."

S. aureus is the cause of multiple problems. The chief lesion may be external or internal. External lesions occur in the following places: (1) **Skin pimples** are staphylococcal infections in the surface layer of the skin; **boils** are in the deeper layer; and a **carbuncle** is a large collection of pus in the subcutaneous tissue that communicates with the surface by several openings. **Infected wounds and stitch abscesses** are caused by staphylococci. (2) Boils on the upper lip and nose are of especial importance, as the infection is apt to pass back along the facial vein (which has no

Fig. 7–4 The morphologic changes in *Staphylococcus aureus* produced by the antibiotic cephalothin. *(A)* Normal cells of S. aureus. *(B)* S. aureus cells after exposure to cephalothin. Note enlarged spheroplasts—cells without walls. (From Lilly Research Laboratories, Eli Lilly & Co., Indianapolis, Indiana.)

valves) into the cavernous venous sinus in the base of the skull, with a resulting **thrombophlebitis.** (3) On the eyelid, staphylococci may cause a **stye.** Internal lesions take the form of abscesses principally in the bones (osteomyelitis) and kidneys. Some persons are subject to repeated staphylococcal infections, particularly boils. Recurrent infections suggest that there may be some lack of normal defense mechanisms. S. aureus endocarditis has also been reported in intravenous drug users.

Certain strains of staphylococci produce toxins. Some of these, called enterotoxins A, B, C, and D, are the most common important causes of food poisoning in the western world. A classic case of this disease is illustrated in Figure 7–5. Enterotoxin F is associated with a disease called **toxic shock syndrome,** which includes such symptoms as high fever, low blood pressure, rash and disturbances in kidney function. This syndrome made newspaper headlines in 1980 when an outbreak occurred in young women using a new brand of tampon. The symptoms appeared in the first three days of menses, in women using tampons. Staphylococci producing enterotoxin F were isolated from the vaginal secretions of almost 90% of patients. The precise role of the tampon remains unclear; how-

Fig. 7–5 An outbreak of staphylococcus food poisoning on an international jet flight. *A,* A cook preparing ham and omelet breakfasts for an international flight has blisters on 2 fingers that are infected with staphylococci. The cook handles at least 205 portions of ham, which are kept at room temperature for 6 hours during preparation of the food trays. *B* and *C,* The contaminated food trays are stored overnight at 50°. Staphylococci multiply at temperatures over 40°, and as they multiply they produce a toxin that is a common cause of food poisoning. *D* and *E,* The food trays are loaded onto the plane. In 6 to 7 hours, they are heated in 300° ovens for 15 minutes, treatment that cannot inactivate the toxin. *F,* The passengers are served. From 2 to 6 hours later, those who ate the contaminated food begin to experience staph food-poisoning symptoms: nausea, vomiting, cramps, and diarrhea.

ever, once the suspect brand was taken off the market the number of cases declined. Toxic shock syndrome is not limited to this circumstance but may occur in any patient infected with staphylococci whether a premature infant or aged grandparent.

Penicillin is the drug of choice for all S. aureus bacteria that are sensitive to penicillin. Today, when a bacterium is isolated from an infection its sensitivity spectrum is tested, i.e., several different antibiotic tablets are placed on the bacterial culture plate and those which inhibit growth are noted. Methicillin or oxacillin may be used in penicillin-resistant S. aureus infections.

The Streptococci

The streptococcus is a gram-positive organism identical in appearance with the staphylococcus except that it grows in chains of varying length instead of in clusters. It is more difficult to grow than the staphylo-

coccus, and flourishes best on media enriched with blood (blood agar).

Viridans streptococci. The hemolytic group causes more acute and virulent infections than the viridans group. Nevertheless, *Streptococcus viridans* is an important cause of disease. It gives rise to focal or limited infection in the tonsils, at the roots of teeth, in the sinuses of the nose and face, and in the valves of the heart, where it causes bacterial endocarditis, a condition that used to be uniformly fatal.

Hemolytic streptococci. These are further classified according to carbohydrate antigens on the bacterial cell surface. This classification is called the Lancefield scheme, and it separates the streptococci into groups labeled A, B, C, etc. The most important pathogens are groups A, B and D. Group A contains only one species, S. pyogenes, which has long been a major cause of human suffering. Group B also contains a single species and it is an important cause of meningitis in the newborn. Group D contains two species and several strains, not all of which are hemolytic on blood agar. These may infect the bloodstream, the urinary tract or the meninges. We will now leave these last two groups and turn to one of the most important subjects of this chapter.

Infections Caused by Group A Streptococci. These bacteria are the cause of many different diseases which may be local or invasive, or the bacterial products may evoke an immunologic response that produces tissue damage. Recently there have been new epidemics (among military recruits) of severe streptococcal infections and a subsequent recurrence of rheumatic fever, as well as toxic shock-like syndromes, all traceable to newly virulent type A streptococci. There was, in addition, a nationwide outbreak of infections due to similar streptococci in Norway in 1987–88 which included 84 cases of bacteremia with septicemia and shock leading to a 25% fatality. This three-fold rise in streptococcal infections, particularly in infants and the elderly, in a modern nation underscores the continuing evolution of bacteria in the face of antibiotic treatments.

Local Infections. The most common infection due to group A streptococci is the streptococcal sore throat. In infants the infection may spread to the middle ear or meninges. In adults and older children the disease is characterized by intense inflammation of the nasal cavity, throat and tonsils, with swollen lymph nodes in the neck and usually a high fever. If the infecting bacterium produces an erythrogenic toxin (literally meaning red-making), the patient also gets a bright red rash which gives the disease the name **scarlet fever.** Some people have immunity against the erythrogenic toxin and get all of the symptoms but no rash. Impetigo is another local streptococcal disease; it is an infection of the skin which is highly contagious in children. (The staphylococcus also can produce a form of impetigo.)

Invasive Infections. Streptococcus pyogenes used to be a common cause of puerperal sepsis, the frequently fatal infection that used to follow childbirth. Erysipelas is an acute, spreading inflammation of the lymphatics of the skin caused by hemolytic streptococci with marked rash-producing power. The usual site is the face or scalp, the bacteria probably entering from the nose. The inflamed skin is of a bright red color and curiously firm. Like other streptococcal and staphylococcal infections, erysipelas is accompanied by fever and leukocytosis. The clinical picture of erysipelas may also be produced by Staphylococcus aureus, although this is not common.

Poststreptococcal Diseases. Two important diseases appear to be caused not by the bacterium directly but by a hypersensitivity response that follows the streptococcal insult. These are glomerulonephritis and rheumatic fever, and they tend to appear about 1 to 4 weeks after the streptococcal infection. Nephritis is more commonly preceded by impetigo, whereas rheumatic fever tends to follow an upper respiratory infection. Glomerulonephritis will be discussed in connection with diseases of the kidney.

Rheumatic Fever. This acute inflammation principally affects the joints and the heart. It may be regarded as a complication of infection with group A hemolytic streptococci, usually located in the throat or tonsils. These bacteria are not found in the organs attacked by rheumatic fever, such as the joints and the heart. Because high antibody titer to a surface antigen of streptococcus (ASO) can be shown in the serum, we believe that **these organs have become hypersensitive or allergic to the streptococci or its product.** It is not clear why the heart and serous membranes of the joints or blood vessels in the brain are the targets of injury, and it is even more mysterious why the heart valves (mitral and aortic) should become scarred 20 years after the acute episode.

The most striking and obvious **clinical feature** in rheumatic fever is acute inflammation of the **joints,** which become tender; the slightest movement of the joint produces excruciating pain. The inflammation is not a suppurative one; there is little destruction of tissue, and when the infection subsides the joints return to their normal condition. The acute joint symptoms such as swelling and pain are greatly relieved by the use of anti-inflammatory salicylates, which are practically a specific remedy for this infection.

The same is not true, however, of the **heart.** During the acute illness there may be no evidence of any cardiac lesion, but months or years later symptoms of these lesions may make their appearance. Both the heart valves and the heart muscle are attacked, but the lesions need not be described here in detail, as they will be considered in connection with diseases of the heart. The characteristic microscopic lesion is the Aschoff body, marked by fibrinoid necrosis and collections of large chronic inflammatory cells. It is evident that the heart lesions of rheumatic fever are much more serious than the joint lesions, although it is the latter that first claim the attention of the patient and the doctor. For this reason, an important element in the treatment of rheumatic fever is bed rest, so that the affected heart may have every chance of recovering to the greatest extent possible. Moreover, in some persons, particularly in children, the inflammation in the joints may be so slight that the disease is not diagnosed as rheumatic fever, yet the heart may be seriously affected. Patients with rheumatic heart disease

Fig. 7–6   Group A beta-hemolytic streptococcal bacteremia cases in a hospital—Denver, Colorado, January 1987-September 1989. (From Centers for Disease Control, Morbidity and Mortality Weekly Report, 39(1):4, 1990.)

may therefore give a history of repeated sore throats, but not of the acute joint pains. For all this the truth of the saying becomes apparent that **"rheumatic fever licks the joints, but bites the heart."** Fortunately, with early treatment of streptococcal sore throats, acute rheumatic fever and its long-term complications, mitral and aortic valve disease, are less common than in the 1950s but there have recently been new epidemics in many parts of the world (Colorado, Norway) (Fig. 7–6).

Streptococcus Pneumoniae

S. pneumoniae, more commonly referred to as the pneumococcus, differs from the other streptococci in that it usually exists in pairs, or diplococci. It is surrounded by a polysaccharide capsule which protects it from phagocytosis. Antigens in the capsule are the stimulus for long-lasting immunity. Unfortunately, however, there are many different capsular types and infection with one type produces immunity only to that type.

The pneumococcus produces hemolysis on blood agar, but it can be easily distinguished from the viridans group by simple biochemical tests.

This bacterium is a normal inhabitant of the nasopharynx. In children it is a common cause of ear infections (otitis media) from which it may spread to the sinuses and meninges. In adults the chief lesion produced is lobar pneumonia.

A vaccine is available which provides some immunity to 14 different capsular types of S. pneumoniae. Unfortunately it appears to have no effect on the very young. Most pneumococci are sensitive to penicillin, although resistance to this antibiotic appears to be growing.

ENTEROCOCCI

Microscopic bacteria occurring in the colon, vagina, and urethra, are commonly seen in pairs or short chains, and were classified until recently as Group D streptococci. They have recently been given status as a separate genus and are called enterococci, distinct from streptococci, because they differ in many respects. They are important causes of endocarditis, neonatal infections, bacteremia, urinary tract infections, pelvic infections, and are often associated with other bacteria.

GRAM-NEGATIVE COCCI: THE NEISSERIAE

We now turn to the gram-negative neisseria. The two members of the group that concern us are *Neisseria meningitidis* and *Neisseria gonorrhoeae*. They resemble each other morphologically as closely as the proverbial two peas. In addition to being gram-negative, they are bean-shaped diplococci with the convex surfaces opposed. Both the meningococcus and the gonococcus are found in large numbers within the polymorphonuclear leukocytes of pus, an environment in which, unfortunately, they seem to flourish. They grow only in enriched media.

Neisseria Meningitidis

The **meningococcus** is a normal inhabitant (commensal) of the nasopharynx, and in times of epidemic, 90% of persons in a crowded army camp may be carriers. Children between the age of 3 months and 5 years are at greatest risk of acquiring invasive infection, which may take the form of meningitis or septicemia, or both. In the adult (over 13 years) overwhelming meningococcal infections may occur with alarming outcomes. While the infections are generally rare in adults the mortality will exceed 50% with most deaths occurring in the first 48 hours from irreversible shock and multiple organ failure. In one study the female to male ratio was 3:1, and shock was the outstanding clinical problem.

Bacteriologic diagnosis of meningococcal meningitis is made by examining the **cerebrospinal fluid,** obtained by lumbar puncture, for the tell-tale gram-negative intracellular diplococci. The cerebrospinal fluid bathes the central nervous system and therefore shares any inflammation of the superficial layers. The disease used to be frequently fatal, but modern antibiotic therapy has entirely altered the prognosis. The meningococcus used to be highly sensitive to sulfonamides, but in the mid-1960s resistance appeared. Fortunately, no resistance has ever been shown to penicillin. Lesions and clinical features of meningococcal meningitis are described in the chapter on the nervous system.

Neisseria Gonorrhoea

In physical appearance and staining characters, the gonococcus is identical with the meningococcus. It is harder to grow in culture than the meningococcus. If allowed to dry, it dies immediately when removed from the body. The gonococcus is a complete parasite living on a human host; it does not live in the body as a harmless commensal. With these facts in mind, it is surprising that the gonococcus manages to hold its place in the natural world, but that it does succeed is only too evident.

Gonococcal infection is a venereal disease. The gonococcus is highly adapted to survival on the mucus membranes of the cervix, urethra, anus, and pharynx. Virulent organisms have pili (proteinaceous strands which project from the cell) which mediate attachment to the mucosa and increase resistance to phagocytosis. Some gonococci also secrete enzymes which degrade the IgA molecules that normally constitute an important part of defense on the mucosal surfaces of the body. This may contribute to the ability of the gonococcus to produce repeated infections. Once the gonococcus reaches the male or female genital tract, it makes itself at home. The initial process is an acute suppuration developing a few days after infection, with a copious discharge of pus loaded with intracellular gonococci. If prompt and effective treatment is given, the discharge disappears like magic and the infection clears up.

The untreated case is a different matter. The inflammation may become chronic, spreading upward, and followed by fibrosis. This can lead to stricture of the urethra and stenosis of the vas deferens in men, causing sterility, whereas in women the fallopian tubes may be converted into bags of pus, with sterility again a frequent result. It is not clear how many of those infected actually get the serious consequences listed above. It now appears that many gonococcal infections may be asymptomatic. In up to 20% of males and 30 to 50% of females with gonococcal infections no symptoms are apparent, but such individuals carry and spread the organism for several months.

Gonococcal infection may also be passed from mothers to infants during delivery, causing a severe purulent conjunctivitis. Currently, all newborns are treated prophylactically at birth.

The treatment of gonorrhea is an important public health problem (Figs. 7–7, 7–8). When the sulfonamides were first introduced, the gonococcus proved to be so susceptible that it seemed as if the disease might be completely eliminated, especially since the

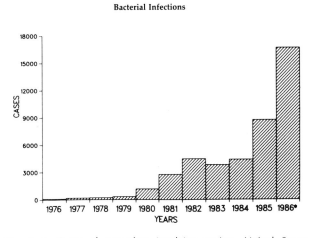

Bacterial Infections

Fig. 7–7　Cases of gonorrhea involving strains—United States, 1976–1986. (From Centers for Disease Control, Morbidity and Mortality Weekly Report, 36(12):174, 1987.)

*1986 projected
†1990 objective

Fig. 7–8 Incidence of gonorrhea by year—United States, 1970–1990. (From Centers for Disease Control, Morbidity and Mortality Weekly Report, 36(12):173, 1987.)

organism is unable to live outside the body. Soon, however, most strains became resistant. Penicillin took the place of sulfonamides with complete success, but again the sad story of resistant strains was repeated. Then came streptomycin, but the gonococci proved as resourceful as ever. Yet they had once again become sensitive to the sulfonamides. And so the battle of attack and defense continues with varying fortunes (Fig. 7–9).

THE ENTERIC GRAM-NEGATIVE BACILLI

The enteric bacilli are bacteria which are either normal or pathogenic inhabitants of the gastrointestinal tract, that is, they either live there normally and produce disease elsewhere in the body, or they live outside the body and produce disease when they visit the G.I. tract. They constitute a large heterogeneous group; they are all short rods, facultative anaerobes (growing with or without oxygen) and have varying degrees of motility. They are identified in the laboratory by growth on selective media, by their ability or inability to ferment a variety of sugars, in particular lactose, by their ability to produce hydrogen sulfide, and many other tests. The group includes the salmonellae, one of which causes typhoid, the shigellae which produce dysentery, vibrios, one of which is the cause of cholera, and Escherichia coli and related

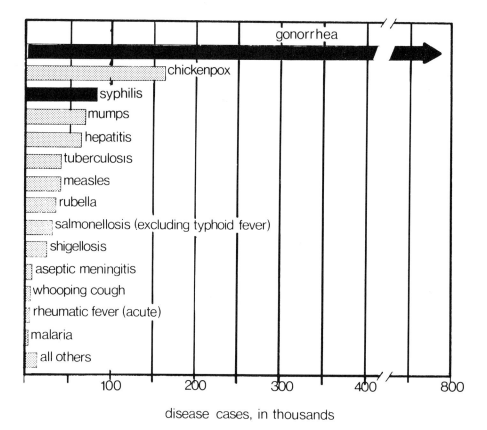

disease cases, in thousands

Fig. 7–9 The striking importance, in numbers of cases, of sexually transmitted diseases as compared with other communicable diseases is illustrated in this chart published by the United States Public Health Service. About 800,000 cases of gonococcal infections were reported in 1973 in the United States. (From United States Public Health Service.)

organisms, which may produce diarrhea but may also infect other organs of the body.

As may be surmised from this list, diarrhea is the chief symptom associated with enteric bacilli infections. There are two mechanisms involved, both of which are diarrheagenic. First, bacteria can produce diarrhea by invading the bowel wall, as in the case of salmonella and shigella and some strains of E. coli. Second, the bacteria may float comfortably in the bowel lumen and secrete a toxin (Table 7–6). The toxin is absorbed by the epithelial cells, where it stimulates these cells to secrete massive amounts of water and electrolytes. The gut lumen becomes filled with fluid and diarrhea results. The diarrhea of cholera is produced this way. Some strains of E. coli can also elaborate such toxins.

Toxins produced by enteric bacilli fall into two groups: exotoxins, which the bacterium secretes into the surrounding medium, as described for Vibrio cholerae, and endotoxins, substances which are liberated only when the organism disintegrates. Endotoxins are very important in the pathogenesis of disease. Some are responsible for producing fever, some give rise to bacteremia and may cause peripheral vasodilatation and increased vascular permeability, leading to a fall in cardiac output, impaired tissue perfusion and the phenomenon of **endotoxic** or **septic** shock.

Before delving further into the unsavory habits of enteric bacilli let us remember that most of our contact with bacteria is on friendly terms. The intestine is the natural home of myriads of gram-negative, motile bacilli, most of which are not only harmless, but serve a useful purpose, such as synthesizing vitamin K and members of the B complex, so that we must beware of banishing them too completely by overenthusiastic antibiotic therapy.

Salmonella

The genus Salmonellae acquired its name not from the fish, but from Daniel Salmon, an American veteri-

Table 7–6. Characteristics of Enteropathogenic Bacterial Infections*

	DIARRHEA†/ DYSENTERY‡	SITE OF DISEASE	MODE OF INTERACTION	ENTEROTOXIN	EXTRAINTESTINAL MANIFESTATIONS
Salmonella *Salmonella typhi*	0/±		Penetrates mucosal cells, carried throughout body of macrophages	0(?)	Fever-bacteremia
Salmonella enteritidis var. *typhimurium*	±/±	Small intestine Large intestine	Penetrates mucosal cells Septicemia	0(?)	Fever, focal infection
Shigella *Shigella dysenteriae* *Shigella flexneri* *Shigella boydii* *Shigella sonnei*	+/+ ±/+ ±/+	Small intestine Large intestine	Penetrates mucosal cells. Bacteria multiply within and kill epithelial cells; cause ulceration, acute inflammatory reaction. Enterotoxin may have effect on small intestine	+§	Seizures; meningismus
Cholera *Vibrio cholerae*	+/0	Small intestine	Bacteria attach to mucosal cells; rarely penetrate; multiply on epithelial cell surface. Induce disease by producing enterotoxin	+	Dehydration, shock Hypokalemic nephropathy
Enteropathogenic *Escherichia coli*	+/0 0/+	Small or large intestine	Depending on strain, may cause dysentery or diarrhea syndromes. Individual strains may cause one or other syndrome but not both	+	Dehydration, shock

* (Adapted from Grady, G.F., and Keusch, G.T.: Pathogenesis of bacterial diarrheas. N. Engl. J. Med. 285:831, 1971; and Savage, D.C.: Survival on mucosal epithelia, epithelial penetration and growth tissues of pathogenic bacteria. *In* Smith, H., and Pearce, J.H. (eds.): *Microbial Pathogenicity in Man and Animals.* New York, Cambridge University Press, 1972. Reproduced from Youmans, G.P., Paterson, P.Y., and Sommers, H.M.: *The Biologic and Clinical Basis of Diseases,* 2nd ed. Philadelphia, W.B. Saunders Co., 1980.)

† Diarrhea—profuse, watery diarrhea—no inflammatory cells.
‡ Dysentery—abdominal cramps, tenesmus, pus, blood in stools.
§ *Shigella dysenteriae* I only.

narian who first isolated the bacterium from hogs with diarrhea. Salmonellae are gram-negative, motile rods, which derive their motility from numerous flagellae. The major species are S. enteritidis, a cause of gastroenteritis, S. typhi and S. paratyphi, the causative agents of typhoid and paratyphoid. The largest reservoir of salmonellae is in animals (Fig. 7–10) such as ducks, chickens and reptiles.

Salmonella typhi. Typhoid fever is spread from a person with typhoid bacilli in his digestive tract. Such a person may be a patient with clinically apparent disease, or he may be a **carrier.** A carrier is one who has had an attack of the disease, sometimes so mild that it fails to be diagnosed, but who continues to harbor the bacilli after recovery. Commonly, the bacilli live in the gallbladder of the carrier, from which they pass into the intestine and are excreted in the feces.

The infecting agent has to be swallowed to produce the disease, and the bacilli may be conveyed by infected water, milk or food, or by direct contagion. Water infection is generally due to fecal contamination. Food and milk infection may be caused by the contaminated fingers of a nurse who has been looking after a typhoid patient, by a cook or dairy farmer (usually a carrier), or by flies. A most famous example of the danger of a cook's being a carrier is that of Typhoid Mary, a cook in New York, who was responsible for at least 50 cases of typhoid fever, many of whom died, before she was finally tracked down. Oysters grown in shallow water at the mouths of infected streams occasionally have been

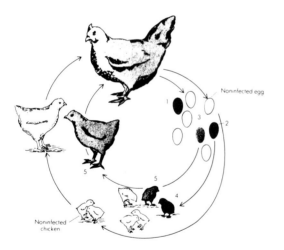

Fig. 7–10 Cycle of *Salmonella enteritidis* var. *typhimurium* infection in chickens. (1) Badly infected egg (addled) which produces no chick; (2) moderately infected egg which gives rise to an infected chick (4) which dies; (3) lightly infected egg from which an infected chick (5) is hatched, which survives and grows into a bird which may continue to excrete salmonellas. (From Marthedal, H.E.: The occurrence of salmonellosis in poultry in Denmark 1935–1975, and the controlling programme established. International Symposium on Salmonella and Prospects for Control. Ontario, June, 1977.)

Although carriers and sick people may contaminate food or drink, the greatest source of salmonellosis is the reservoir of salmonellas in lower animals. Many species of *Salmonella* occur naturally in chickens, turkeys, ducks, rodents, cats, dogs, turtles and many other animals.

responsible for outbreaks. Apart from water- and milk-borne epidemics, the important causes of infections are the fouling of food by fingers and by the feet of fecal-feeding flies. Typhoid is no longer a common disease in our society due to vastly improved sanitation.

Lesions. In typhoid, lesions are in the lymphoid tissue of the intestine, the spleen, the abdominal lymph nodes, and the bone marrow. The intestinal lesions are most marked at the lower end of the small intestine. Here the lymphoid tissue is collected into small masses in the deeper part of the mucus membrane that are called Peyer's patches. The bacilli, which have been swallowed, lodge in these masses and cause an inflammatory reaction with accompanying swelling of the patches. By the end of a week, the mucus membrane covering the patches is shed and the underlying lymphoid tissue becomes necrotic, disintegrates, and is lost, so that many ulcers of varying depths are formed. As a rule, the ulcers heal by the end of the third week, but one or more of the ulcers may extend deeply, just as in the case of a gastric ulcer, until finally perforation may occur into the abdominal cavity.

Symptoms. These are partly general, partly intestinal, and partly related to the blood and blood-forming organs.

The general symptoms are fever, headache, malaise, lethargy, and a clouding of the mind, which gives the name to the disease (Greek, *typhos*, a cloud). The **fever** usually lasts about three weeks, but sometimes considerably longer. About the end of the first week small red patches appear on the abdominal wall; these are known as **rose spots.** Bronchitis and nosebleeds are early symptoms. The center of the tongue is heavily furred. The fever, headache, and lethargy are due to the toxins of the bacilli in the blood stream. The rose spots are caused by clumps of bacilli lodging in the capillaries of the skin.

The intestinal symptoms are abdominal discomfort, and constipation or diarrhea. With diarrhea, the feces may have an appearance described by the unpleasantly vivid term "pea-soup" stools. **Hemorrhage** from the bowel may take place owing to an ulcer's having opened into a blood vessel.

The diagnosis of typhoid fever may be made using four tests: (1) blood culture, (2) stool culture, (3) urine culture, and (4) agglutination tests, which used to be referred to as the Widal test. Blood culture is the most useful test for patients in the first two weeks with active disease.

Typhoid fever may be treated with ampicillin or chloramphenicol, although resistance to both these drugs has been reported. Other antibiotics are available for resistant strains.

Other Salmonellae. A clinical picture resembling typhoid fever but milder in type may be caused by other members of the salmonella group, more particularly *Salmonella paratyphi* A and B. Paratyphoid A infection is more common in Asia; paratyphoid B, usually due to dairy products, occurs in Britain and North America. Its prevalence in the United States is shown in Figure 7–11 and Table 7–7. The vaccine used for protection against typhoid is known as TAB; this label indicates that it contains all three types of organisms. Other more common types of the salmonella bacteria cause gastroenteritis (*Salmonella enteritidis*), particularly in children under the age of 5 years. The incidence pattern of these and other salmonella diseases is seasonal.

Fig. 7–11 Isolated rate per 100,000 population of *Salmonella enteritidis*, by region—United States, 1976–1989. (From Centers for Disease Control, Morbidity and Mortality Weekly Report, 39(50):911, 1990.)

Shigella

The Shigella species, named for the Japanese bacteriologist Shiga, are nonmotile gram-negative aerobic rods. There are several species: *S. flexneri* and *S. sonnei* are the causative agents of most shigellosis in the United States (Fig. 7–12). *S. dysenteriae*, more prevalent in Central America, produces more severe disease.

The major illness caused by shigella is dysentery, an acute colitis characterized by diarrhea, with blood, pus, and mucus in the stools. Two entirely different diseases are known by this name as the result of ancient usage; they are bacillary dysentery and amebic dysentery, only the first of which will be considered here.

The shigella bacterium damages the bowel in two ways, first by invasion of the wall itself, and second, by secreting a powerful exotoxin which irritates the bowel wall. Infection

Table 7–7. Number of Reported Outbreaks and Associated Cases and Deaths Caused by *Salmonella Enteritidis*, by Year—United States, 1985–1990

YEAR	OUTBREAKS	CASES	DEATHS
1985	26	1,166	1
1986	48	1,539	6
1987	53	2,498	15
1988	40	1,010	8
1989	77	2,394	14
1990*	49	1,646	2
Total	293	10,253	46

* Through October 31.

(From Centers for Disease Control, Morbidity and Mortality Weekly Report, 39(50):911, 1990.)

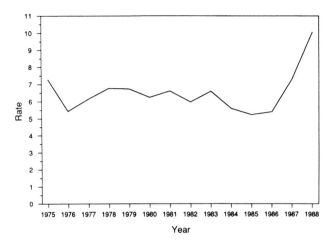

Fig. 7–12 *Shigella* isolation rates per 100,000 population by year—United States, 1975–1988. (From Centers for Disease Control, Morbidity and Mortality Weekly Report, 39(30):509, 1990.)

is acquired through the ingestion of contaminated food and water, just as in the case of typhoid. The infection may come from a patient suffering from the disease or from a carrier. Like amebic dysentery, the disease is prevalent in the tropics, but it also may occur in temperate zones, especially when persons are crowded together under poor hygienic conditions. In the past it has been a great destroyer of armies in the field. It is prevalent in large mental hospitals, and it is an important cause of acute diarrhea associated with the passage of pus and blood in children, especially in hot weather.

Like salmonella, most, but not all, shigella bacteria are sensitive to ampicillin.

Escherichia Coli and Coliforms

Escherichia coli. This gram-negative, motile bacillus (Fig. 7–13), is generally a harmless inhabitant of the bowel, but it is a common cause of acute and chronic inflammation elsewhere, especially when supported by other organisms. It can cause acute inflammation in the appendix and gallbladder, as well as in the pelvis of the kidney and the urinary bladder in cases of obstruction to the outflow of urine. Its toxins (endotoxin) are an important cause of shock. It is in children, in the aged, and in surgical cases that infection with E. coli is most to be feared.

E. coli may also cause diarrhea either by invasion of the bowel wall or by producing toxins which stimulate the mucosal cells to secrete water and electrolytes. The second of these two methods is the more important. "Traveller's diarrhea" or "Montezuma's revenge" is probably caused by toxin-producing strains of E. coli much of the time.

Coliforms. These are a large and heterogeneous group of gram-negative rods which resemble E. coli. They include such organisms as Klebsiella, Enterobacter, Serratia and others. They may cause a wide variety of infectious diseases, especially in patients with diminished resistance.

Proteus and Pseudomonas

These two groups of motile gram-negative intestinal bacilli have come to assume increased importance because of

Fig. 7–13 The morphologic changes, which occur in *E. coli* as a result of exposure to penicillin, shown in this illustration, provide visual evidence that this antibiotic acts upon the cell wall. *(A) Normal cells of E. coli. (B) E. coli cells after exposure to penicillin.* Enlarged (bulged) defect indicates alteration of cell wall. (From Lilly Research Laboratories, Eli Lilly & Co., Indianapolis, Indiana.)

Fig. 7–14 *Proteus vulgaris.* Electron micrograph of the actively motile bacterium. Note flagella all over bacterial cell. (Courtesy of Roerig Division, Inc., New York.)

their extreme resistance to antibiotics, so that they tend to supplant other bacteria when such therapy is long-continued. The proteus group (Fig. 7–14) ferments carbohydrates; the pseudomonas group does not, but produces a distinctive blue-green pigment (*Bacillus pyocyaneus*). Both groups only become dangerous invaders when general resistance is lowered or when local tissues are damaged. The urinary tract is most frequently involved. Pseudomonas infections are common in burns.

Vibrio Species

Asiatic cholera is a disease that I trust the reader will never encounter, but he or she ought to know something about it. There are recent outbreaks in South America and Iraq, associated with war and civil unrest, which involve thousands of people (Table 7–8). It is caused by a motile, gram-negative bacillus shaped like a comma, and therefore easily distinguished from the ordinary gram-negative bacilli seen in the stools. It is called *Vibrio cholerae*, and the disease is known as Asiatic cholera because the lower basin of the Ganges is the area where the disease is endemic and from which fearful epidemics spread across the world before it was known that infection was due to drinking water polluted by fecal discharge.

The vibrio does not invade the bowel wall (Fig. 7–15); it produces diarrhea by its toxins: it secretes a very powerful exotoxin which induces the mucosal cells of the small intestine to churn out vast amounts of fluid into the lumen and then out in the stools. So much fluid may be excreted that 20% of the body weight may be lost in 24 hours, and the result is a **dehydration** so profound that it used to kill the patient in 75% of untreated cases. The vibrios proliferate in the watery fluid as in a culture, so that the "rice-water stools" are intensely infective and can contaminate wells, streams, and other sources of drinking water. Before this was known, 50,000 persons died of cholera in England in 1831 (Fig. 7–16).

Treatment consists of restoring fluid and electrolytes to the blood at the earliest possible moment. Prophylactic inoc-

Table 7–8. Cholera—Western Hemisphere, 1991

COUNTRY	NO. CASES*	NO. HOSPITALIZED	NO. DEATHS	DATE OF REPORT
Peru	223,564	86,954	2,163	June 22
Ecuador	30,535	22,623	501	July 6
Colombia	3,196	1,970	31	June 22
Chile	41	NR†	2	June 22
Mexico	27	7	0	July 3
Brazil	22	8	0	July 15
United States	14	7	0	June 19
Total	257,399	111,569	2,697	

* Probable and confirmed cases.
† Not reported.

(From Centers for Disease Control, Morbidity and Mortality Weekly Report, 40(30):517, 1991.)

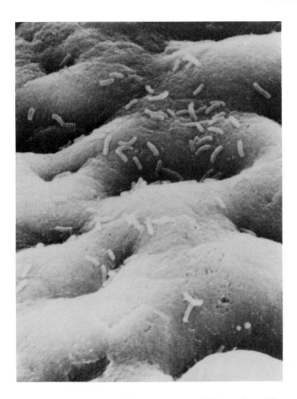

Fig. 7–15 Cholera vibrios adherent to mucosal lining of small bowel. (Scanning electron micrograph.) (From Smith, A.L.: *Microbiology and Pathology*, 12th Ed. St. Louis, C.V. Mosby Co., 1980. Courtesy of Dr. Richard Finklestein, Dr. Edward T. Nelson, and Bob Fenley, Director, Office of Medical Information, The University of Texas Health Science Center at Dallas.)

ulation is of value, but ensuring a pure water supply is infinitely more important. Today, treatment by replacement of fluid and electrolyte loss by mouth saves thousands of lives annually. Tetracycline is effective in killing the bacterium but is not as important as fluid replacement. A vaccine

Fig. 7–16 A cholera cot, used in the treatment of cholera patients in Bangladesh. The patients' stools are collected in the bucket so that the amount of fluid lost can be measured. If the patient drinks the same volume of fluid as he loses he stands a good chance of recovery. (Courtesy of Dr. Robert Oseasohn, School of Public Health, San Antonio, Texas.)

is available, but it only protects 50% of those vaccinated, and then only lasts for 3 to 6 months. It therefore has limited use.

FOOD POISONING

This term denotes acute gastroenteritis (with the exception of botulism) caused by bacterial contamination of food or drink. The condition is a toxemia rather than a bacterial invasion. There are two distinct forms of different origin, but with a similar clinical picture: (1) the **infection type,** in which bacteria in the contaminated food multiply and produce their toxins in the bowel (an example is traveller's diarrhea caused by E. coli), and (2) the **toxin type,** in which toxins are produced in the food before ingestion (an example is staph poisoning—see Fig. 7–5). Both forms are marked by violent vomiting and diarrhea accompanied by severe prostration. The symptoms usually begin 6 to 12 hours after the infected food has been eaten, being naturally earlier in the toxin type, and perhaps delayed for 24 hours in the infection type.

The infection type is usually caused by one of the Salmonella group (although not by the typhoid bacillus itself), sometimes by one of the Shigella (dysentery) group. The food (animals or game birds) usually has stood for 2 or 3 days, but it does not smell nor does it look bad. The outbreak is likely to involve all the members of a family or the guests at a large social gathering or picnic where there is a common food supply, probably imperfectly cooked or shielded from infection. In the toxin type, the poison is formed in the food before it is eaten, so that the onset is early, sometimes within an hour. Typically, the food may be pastry or cream sauce. The bacteriology is obscure. It is known that some strains of *Staphylococcus aureus* and some *Proteus* strains can produce a powerful enterotoxin in decomposing meat. The different problem of botulism must be mentioned here, although it is discussed in relation to the anaerobic spore-bearing clostridia. The spores of *Clostridia botulinum* can survive boiling for hours and, if they develop in canned goods, they produce one of the most powerful poisons known. (One gram of the toxin would kill 33 million mice!) The symptoms are due to the action of the toxin on autonomic nerve endings.

SMALL GRAM-NEGATIVE RODS

Hemophilus Influenzae

H. influenzae is a small gram-negative coccobacillus. The name *hemophilus* means blood-loving, which refers to the fact that these bacteria require various factors normally found in blood in order to grow.

There are several species of hemophilus, but H. influenzae is the most important pathogen. The H. influenzae species received its name in the influenza epidemic of 1890, when it was thought to be the cause. We now know that influenza is caused by a virus, although H. influenzae and other bacteria frequently give rise to superinfection.

There are two forms of H. influenzae, those with capsules and those without. The encapsulated form is divided into six groups (a–f), based on different polysaccharide antigens in the capsule. Type b is responsible for most infections.

H. influenzae is a major cause of nasopharyngitis, meningitis and otitis media (middle ear infections) in children. Most adults are immune. A vaccine containing the capsular antigen is available, but, unfortunately, infants do not react to it.

A most dangerous infection caused by H. influenzae is acute epiglottitis, in which the epiglottis swells and may even block the airway. Although this disease is more frequent in children, it is thought to have been the cause of George Washington's demise.

H. influenzae infections may be treated with chloramphenicol or ampicillin. Since resistance to each of these is fairly common, serious infections should be treated with both drugs.

Bordatella Pertussis (Whooping Cough)

B. pertussis is a minute gram-negative bacillus, which is found in great masses entangled in the cilia of the bronchial mucosa. Like H. influenzae, it cannot grow without blood in the culture medium. It causes whooping cough, which has largely disappeared in North America today owing to the universal practice of immunization with **DPT** or diphtheria, pertussis, and tetanus vaccine. However, a small amount of mild pertussis still exists in every community. It is never recognized because it is so mild, producing only a persistent cough. B. pertussis may also cause bronchitis or pneumonia without whoops.

Yersinia

We will consider two Yersinia species, *Yersinia pestis* and *Yersinia enterocolitica*.

Yersinia pestis (Plague). Plague is caused by the pest bacillus (*Yersinia pestis*), a small, gram-negative, extremely virulent organism. There is no more terrifying chapter in the story of disease than that of plague. The great plagues of the Middle Ages were worse than any wars. The Black Death came the nearest to exterminating the human race, for it killed 25 million people in Europe at a time when the population of that continent was very small (Fig. 7–17). Zinsser, in his de-

Spread of Black Death in Europe.

Fig. 7–17 This figure illustrates the spread of the plague, or Black Death, as it was called, through Europe in the mid-fourteenth century. This disease was brought to Europe from the East, probably by Mongol armies and commercial caravans, who began to travel vast distances after the founding of the Mongol Empire by Genghis Khan (1162 to 1227). (Adapted from Carpentier, E.: Au tour de la peste noire: famines et épidémies dans l'histoire dû XIVe siècle. Annales—Économies, Sociétés, Civilisations, 6:1062, 1962.)

lightfully written *Rats, Lice and History*, refers to plague and typhus as "those two calamities sharing with human ferocity the greatest responsibility of wholesale sorrow, suffering, and death throughout the ages." This disease is being reported more frequently now in the United States (Fig. 7–18).

The bacillus usually enters the body through the skin by means of the bite of a flea, which carries the infection from the rat to man. Indeed, plague is primarily a disease of rats. A human epidemic is accompanied or preceded by a rat epidemic. When a rat dies, the infected fleas leave it and go in search of a new and preferably human victim. A patient with plague is not infective unless fleas carry the infection from him to others.

There is no inflammation at the site of the flea bite, but the nearest lymph nodes become swollen and acutely inflamed, forming masses called buboes. It is these masses that give the disease its name of bubonic plague. The bacilli then invade the blood stream and are found in enormous numbers in the internal organs. The patient dies of overwhelming septicemia before there is time for marked lesions to develop. The mortality is extremely high, and the patient may be dead in less than 24 hours.

Sometimes an epidemic takes a pneumonic form, in which the infection is spread by droplets of sputum. Pneumonic plague is one of the most deadly and rapidly fatal of all infections.

The control of plague consists of exterminating rats and preventing them from leaving a ship that comes from a country in which plague is prevalent. This is

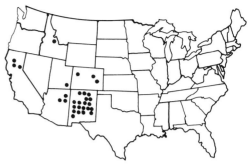

Fig. 7–19   This map shows the incidence and distribution of plague in the United States from 1965 to 1970. Each dot represents one case. (From Gilbert, E.F., and Huntington, R.W.: *An Introduction to Pathology*. New York, Oxford University Press, 1978.)

Fig. 7–18   Since 1925, all human plague cases in the United States have occurred singly or in small common-source clusters. The usual source of infection has been wild rodents or their fleas. At times, pet dogs and cats have served as the link between wild rodent plague sources and humans, either by transporting infected wild rodent fleas, or in the case of cats, serving as a direct-contact source of plague infection. In at least 1 case a cat probably transmitted plague organisms by the airborne route to its owner. Whether or not the increase in human cases observed since 1965 is due to increased animal plague activity, increased human population in enzootic areas, or other factors is not clear. The first 2 factors are not entirely unrelated: the development of lands for housing in enzootic areas sometimes increases the harborage of hosts of the vector and thus the number of cases of animal plague and the degree of human exposure. Surveillance, health education, preventive vector control, and awareness of plague activity among the medical community have been effective in preventing cases and reducing mortality. (From Centers for Disease Control: Annual summary, 1981: Reported morbidity and mortality in the United States. Morbidity and Mortality Weekly Report, 30(54):67, 1982.)

done by placing large discs on the ship's cables which prevent the rats from running down the ropes. The problem of the flea is met with insecticides. This dreaded disease has not been entirely wiped out, and a few cases are occasionally reported in the United States (Fig. 7–19). Y. pestis infections are treated with streptomycin.

Yersinia enterocolitica. Human illness caused by *Yersinia enterocolitica* was first described in New York State in 1933. It has since been reported in Northern Europe, in Japan, and in Canada. In 1976, an outbreak of yersiniosis in New York was found to be due to contaminated chocolate milk that children were drinking at school. The predominant symptoms were acute abdominal pain and fever.

Francisella Tularensis (Tularemia)

Tularemia is a plague-like disease which affects animals principally, but it may spread from them to man.

It is caused by another organism, *Francisella tularensis*. Ground squirrels and jack rabbits are the animals most often affected. The name comes from Tulare County in California, where an epidemic of the disease killed many ground squirrels. Infection is carried from animals to man (1) by biting fleas, (2) by ticks, and (3) most often by contact with skins of infected rabbits. It is seen, therefore, in farmers, hunters, butchers, housewives, and others who are likely to skin rabbits. In man the disease is fortunately not nearly so fatal as in animals.

The bacteria enter through cuts and cracks in the skin, and an ulcer develops at the site of infection. In this respect the disease differs from plague. The regional lymph nodes are swollen and tender, as in plague. There is prolonged fever and prostration. Recovery is the rule, but convalescence may take some months. In fatal cases, areas of necrosis are found in the internal organs.

Brucella (Undulant Fever)

Undulant fever is caused by a small organism midway in form between a coccus and a bacillus. For this reason it is called neither, but is given the name of its discoverer, Sir David Bruce, and is known as brucella. Infection with brucella (**brucellosis**) is essentially an animal disease, attacking particularly cattle and goats. Brucellosis is said to be the most common illness conveyed to human beings from animals. In North America, the only infecting agent that need be considered is *Brucella abortus*.

The disease is extraordinarily prevalent in cattle. In some parts of the eastern states, 90% of the herds are infected. Most of the persons who drink infected cows' milk show no sign of the disease, although they may have agglutinins in the blood, indicating that they have been infected. However, the disease undoubtedly used to be much more common than is usually thought. Its importance lies in the possibility of confusion with such long-continued fevers as typhoid, miliary tuberculosis, and subacute bacterial endocarditis. These are all serious diseases, whereas in undulant fever the mortality rate is less than 2% (Fig. 7–20).

The disease begins insidiously with an evening rise of temperature, and the patient may be ill for some time without knowing that he has any fever. The fever may come in waves, hence the name undulant fever, although this feature is often absent. Its most striking characteristic is its remarkable persistence; three months is an average duration, but it may last for years. Persistent weakness, muscle pains, joint pains, and marked perspiration with a sweet sickly odor to the sweat are some of the common features and may easily pass unrecognized. The patient may feel extraordinarily miserable, and a doctor remarked on recovering from the disease: "If the cows felt as miserable as I did, I do not blame them for aborting." Strange to say, there are no characteristic lesions, merely those of any septicemia.

The most reliable means of diagnosis is the test for agglutinins in the blood against *Brucella abortus*, a test identical to the Widal test for typhoid. The most satisfactory antibiotic treatment is with tetracycline, which seems to be specific for undulant fever and prevents relapses.

Fig. 7–20   Human brucellosis, United States, 1947 to 1975. (From Centers for Disease Control, Morbidity and Mortality Weekly Report, 25, 1976.)

GRAM-POSITIVE RODS

Bacillus Anthracis (Anthrax)

Bacillus anthracis is a large, square-ended, gram-positive bacillus, which forms spores outside the body. The spores are resistant to chemical disinfectants and also to heat. They may remain alive in the soil for many years, and when they finally enter the body again, they develop into bacilli. The organisms grow readily in culture. They are aerobic, in marked contrast to the anaerobic spore-bearers to be considered.

Anthrax is a disease of animals, principally cattle and sheep. It is prevalent in European animals, but is uncommon in North America, so that in this country the human disease is correspondingly rare.

Man is infected from animal material, not from other persons, usually from the hides of cattle or from the wool of sheep. The skin is the common site of infection, but the disease may be acquired by those using infected shaving brushes, or working with the hides of diseased cattle. The spores may be inhaled into the lungs, usually in the process of the "carding" of wool; the pulmonary form is known as "woolsorters' disease." There was an epidemic of human anthrax in Russia in the late 1960's during a period of famine. Animal carcass by-products were mixed with grain to feed beef cattle and this preparation was improperly processed. Beef infected with anthrax was sold on the black market and over 60 humans died from anthrax.

The skin lesion is called a malignant pustule and is easily recognized. A pimple appears on the surface of the hand, forearm, or face, which develops into a boil and then a pustule containing blood-stained fluid swarming with anthrax bacilli. The surface turns black, and then presents a highly characteristic appearance. If it is recognized and promptly excised, recovery follows. If not, the blood stream is invaded, the bacilli multiply with great rapidity, filling the capillaries of all the organs, and death soon results. A specific antiserum gives good results when used in conjunction with early excision of the lesion. The pulmonary form is almost always fatal. Penicillin and tetracycline have been used with beneficial results in anthrax infections in recent years.

Corynebacterium Diphtheriae (Diphtheria)

The diphtheria of Klebs-Löfler bacillus (*Corynebacterium diphtheriae*) is a thin gram-positive bacillus, often slightly curved. It stains irregularly with methylene blue, some parts appearing dark while others remain light; for this reason the bacilli may have a granular appearance. There is apt to be pleomorphism, i.e., variation in structure, and some of the bacilli may have an expanded end, giving an Indian-club appearance. The bacilli are easily stained and easily grown in culture within 24 hours. Löfler's blood serum (solid) is the standard medium for this purpose. Under the microscope the bacilli present an arrangement that suggests a spilled box of matches.

Unlike many of the other pathogenic bacteria, the diphtheria bacillus does not invade the tissues of the patient. It remains on the surface of the mucus membrane of the throat and produces a powerful exotoxin, which kills the cells with which it comes in contact. It also excites a plentiful production of fibrin. The dead or necrosed cells are not shed, but are bound together by the threads of fibrin to form a tough, leathery layer known as the false or **pseudo membrane,** so called because it is not a natural or true membrane of the body (Fig. 7–21). The name diphtheria is from the Greek meaning leather.

The danger to the patient is twofold: (1) he may die of suffocation owing to the false membrane's obstruct-ing the air-passages, especially the glottis; (2) the toxin may be absorbed into the blood and cause damage to either the heart or the peripheral nerves.

Infection may be spread directly from person to person, or indirectly by infected articles such as cups, handkerchiefs, and even books. Direct infection may be from a patient, but often it is from a healthy carrier, i.e., a person carrying diphtheria bacilli in the throat, but not suffering from the disease; often, indeed, he has never had a previous clinical attack, but has established a complete immunity, presumably from a subclinical infection.

Immunity against diphtheria may be natural or artificial. About 85% of nursing babies have natural immunity which comes from the mother. This immunity disappears after 8 months. Most children are therefore susceptible, and 80% of the deaths used to occur in children under 5 years of age. Susceptible children can be immunized by means of diphtheria **toxoid.** This diphtheria toxin has been rendered harmless by the addition of formalin. The immunity is of variable duration, but usually lasts for several years. These procedures are of value both for persons who have been exposed to infection and for children during an outbreak of diphtheria.

Outbreaks of diphtheria still occur in the United States in groups of non-immunized people.

Clostridia

All the bacteria considered so far are able to live and multiply in air, or rather in oxygen. They are aerobes. We now come to a group that cannot do so, and in particular, the genus *Clostridium*, composed of many members that live in the soil, where they take part in the process of putrefaction, so that they are readily ingested in vegetables. All the clostridia are large gram-positive bacilli that produce spores that can survive in dry earth for years and are extremely resistant to heat and antiseptics. The three important pathogens of the group are: (1) *Clostridium perfringens*, causing gas gangrene, (2) *Clostridium tetani*, causing tetanus, and (3) *Clostridium botulinum*, causing botulism.

Gas Gangrene. The common cause of gas gangrene is *Clostridium perfringens*, although other members of the clostridia group are sometimes responsible. It occurs in the intestinal tract of men and animals, where it does no harm, but wounds may become infected either by soil containing animal manure or by contaminated clothing. The bacillus is short, plump, gram-positive, produces spores, and is surrounded by a capsule that gives it a characteristic appearance.

The chief characteristic of *Clostridium perfringens* is

Fig. 7–21 This photograph shows the membrane (at arrow) lining the trachea and bronchus in a case of diphtheria. This membrane is composed of fibrin and polymorphonuclear leukocytes and is sufficiently large to obstruct the airways. Today, immunization against diphtheria makes such a lesion exceedingly rare. (McGill University, Department of Pathology Museum.)

that it produces gas from the muscle sugars, so that it is commonly called the "gas bacillus," and the disease itself is known as gas gangrene. The gas is the result of fermentation, which may be defined as the splitting of a complex organic compound (in this case, muscle sugar) into simpler elements. The gas spreads along the muscle sheaths, separating these from the muscles, and bubbles of foul-smelling gas and blood-stained fluid can be pressed up and down the length of the muscle. This fluid is highly toxic, so that it kills the muscle fibers, which are then invaded by the bacteria. The process is one of putrefaction or breaking down of muscle, and is marked by a terrible odor. A toxin is also produced, which poisons the patient. Against this toxin an antitoxin has been prepared.

The most important part of the **treatment** of gas gangrene is to reduce the likelihood of anaerobic environment for the organisms by adequate surgical treatment to remove dead tissue and blood clots. The use of antiserums and large doses of penicillin are also effective in controlling this type of infection in wounds.

Tetanus. *Clostridium tetani*, the tetanus bacillus, is a slender anaerobic organism with a spore at one end, giving it a characteristic, drumstick-like appearance. It lives in the intestine of horses and occurs in about 15% of horses' feces, so that it is found in soil that has been fertilized with manure.

This bacillus causes a dangerous wound infection, which results when infected soil or the dirt of streets gains entrance to a wound. The spores can live in dust for long periods.

The organism remains localized in the wound and does not invade the tissues. In this respect it is the exact opposite to the clostridia causing gas gangrene. As it is anaerobic, it grows best when other bacteria are present that kill the tissue so that the supply of oxygen diminishes (Fig. 7–22).

The tetanus bacillus is dangerous because it produces one of the most powerful toxins known, far more virulent than the most deadly snake venom. The toxin gradually passes along the nerves from the wound to the spinal cord. There it becomes anchored to the motor nerve cells, which it stimulates (Fig. 7–23), so that the muscles become rigid and the patient is thrown into terrible convulsions. The jaw muscles are involved early by stiffness, and the mouth cannot be opened. Hence the common name of the disease is lockjaw.

The incubation period, i.e., the time between infection and the first appearance of symptoms, is long, for the toxin travels along the nerves slowly. The average time is 7 to 10 days. In wounds of the face it is shorter, as there is less distance for the toxin to travel. In other cases it may be several weeks. This long incubation period is fortunate, because it makes preventive inoculation possible. When the possibility of tetanus is suspected, and this should be the case in all street

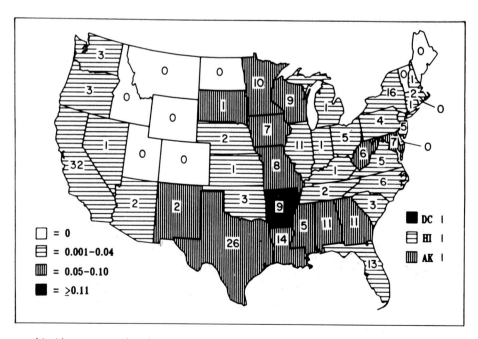

Fig. 7–22 Average annual incidence rates and total cases of tetanus, by state—United States, 1982–1984, per 100,000 total population using July 1, 1982, population estimate. (From Centers for Disease Control, Morbidity and Mortality Weekly Report, 34(39):607, 1985.)

NORMAL   BOTULISM   TETANUS

BRAIN

SPINAL
CORD

TRICEPS   BICEPS

Fig. 7–23 Nervous control of muscles that raise and lower the forearm is diagrammed schematically. In a normal individual (left) impulses from the brain can excite a motoneuron (1) to cause the biceps to contract, stretching the triceps. A stretch-sensitive receptor (2) in the triceps would thereupon cause a triceps motoneuron (3) to fire and oppose the stretching—except that this firing is inhibited by impulses from an inhibitory nerve (4). In botulism (center) the neuromuscular junction is blocked (5), causing flaccid paralysis. In tetanus (right) the inhibitory impulses to the triceps motoneuron are blocked (6); both muscles contract, causing a spasm. (From van Heyningen, W.E.: Tetanus. Scientific American, 218:69, 1968.)

accidents or contaminated wounds, a prophylactic injection of tetanus antitoxin is given (Fig. 7–24). This neutralizes the toxin before it has time to reach the nerve cells in the spinal cord. After that it is usually too late to do much good, as the toxin is irreversibly bound to the nerve cells.

Botulism. *Clostridium botulinum* is primarily a soil bacterium, but it is also found in the intestine of domestic animals. This anaerobic bacillus is entirely different in its action from anything so far considered. In adults we are not concerned with the organism itself, for it does not grow in the adult body. However, it does grow in spoiled sausage (Latin *botulus*, a sausage), preserved meat, canned vegetables and ripe olives. Its spores are resistant, and if the temperature employed in home canning is insufficient, the bacilli will produce a potent toxin which, if taken even in tiny amounts, may cause death. The condition is called botulism. The toxin does not produce any in-

flammation in the stomach or intestine, but is absorbed and acts on the neuromuscular junction, inhibiting the transmission of signal from nerve to muscle (Fig. 7–23). Gradually the muscles of the body become paralyzed, starting with the small muscles of the eye and eventually terminating with respiratory muscle paralysis. Mechanical ventilation may be life-saving.

Prevention is the best treatment, and this means proper attention to detail in home canning, or boiling home canned goods for at least 10 minutes prior to eating.

In infants, botulism can have a different pathogenesis. It appears that infants may eat the C. botulinum spores themselves (in food, or perhaps from sucking on dirty fingers), after which they grow and produce toxin in the intestine. The toxin is absorbed, producing a mild form of the syndrome described above, resulting in a "floppy infant." This may be one cause of the sudden infant death syndrome (SIDS) in which

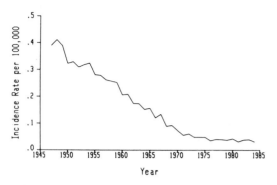

Fig. 7–24 The relative absence of tetanus among persons 5–19 years of age reflects the success of the U.S. childhood vaccination program. Forty-seven states and the District of Columbia require primary immunization against tetanus for entry into school. Annual nationwide surveys indicate over 95% of children entering school since 1980 had received a primary series of tetanus immunizations. However, immunity levels in older populations are lower. In particular, serosurveys done since 1977 indicated that 49%–66% of persons 60 years of age or older lacked protective levels of circulating antitoxin antibody against tetanus. Expanded efforts to ensure that vaccination against tetanus is up-to-date in individuals of all ages could reduce further the remaining burden of tetanus in the United States. (From Centers for Disease Control, Morbidity and Mortality Weekly Report, 34(39):610, 1985)

infants die suddenly without signs of antecedent illness, and without explanation after autopsy.

Diagnosis of infant botulism is made by finding both C. botulinum and its toxin in the stool. Adult botulism is diagnosed upon finding the toxin (not the bacterium) in the patient's serum.

SPIROCHETES

Spirochetes are motile bacteria that have a slender spiral shape. Many of them are pathogenic, but only one will be discussed here, that is *Treponema pallidum*, the causative agent of syphilis.

Syphilis is a sexually transmitted disease (STD). It is acquired by contact with a syphilitic lesion in a patient suffering from the disease, usually during sexual intercourse, so that the first lesions to appear are on the genital organs. Sometimes, however, the primary lesion may appear on the fingers as in the case of a doctor examining a syphilitic patient, or on the lips or mouth from contact with an infected area. Its appearance epidemiologically coincides with large populations (Figs. 7–25 and 7–26).

The spirochete resembles the gonococcus in that it cannot survive outside the body. It cannot be grown on any of the ordinary culture media nor stained by ordinary staining methods. It is best demonstrated by the dark-field method, in which a special attachment to the microscope enables the organisms to be seen as bright white threads against a dark background. The early lesions, both on the genital organs and in the mouth, contain enormous numbers of treponemata so that these lesions are highly infectious.

Natural History of the Disease. Syphilis seems to have lost much of its virulence since it was first introduced into Europe by the sailors of Christopher Columbus returning from the New World. It was spread from the sailors to their prostitutes who helped spread it all over Portugal and Spain. With the help of the army of Charles VIII of France, syphilis swept through Italy like a plague, so that it came to be called *lues* (plague), a name still occasionally used today.

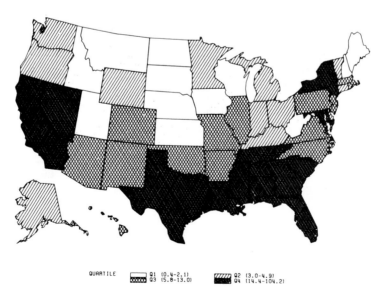

Fig. 7–25 Syphilis (primary and secondary)—reported cases in civilians per 100,000 population, by state, United States, 1981. (From Centers for Disease Control: Annual summary, 1981: Reported morbidity and mortality in the United States. Morbidity and Mortality Weekly Report, 30(54):83, 1982.)

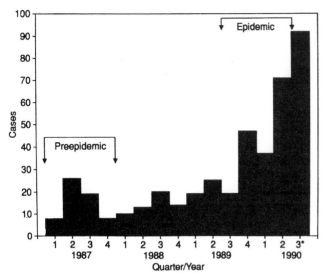

* July and August only

Fig. 7–26 Early syphilis cases, by quarter of report—Escambia County, Florida, 1987–1990. (From Centers for Disease Control, Morbidity and Mortality Weekly Report, 40(19):324, 1991.)

Following the defeat of Charles VIII in Naples, the army disbanded and carried the "great pox" to all the corners of Europe. By 1498, the speedy spirochete had reached England, and within the next 7 years the disease appeared in India, the Philippines and China, courtesy of European exploration.

Syphilis plagues both prince and pauper. King Henry VIII of England (1491–1547), who was infected before his first marriage, searched industriously for a non-infected wife. His children were undoubtedly syphilitic and many attribute the deaths of Mary (Bloody Mary, died at age 42) and Edward VI (died at age 16) to the congenital form of this venereal disease.

The natural history of the disease is peculiar and highly interesting, and can be divided into three stages known as primary, secondary, and tertiary. For 3 or 4 weeks after infection, the person feels well and shows no evidence of the disease. Then a lesion known as the primary sore or chancre appears at the site of infection. It takes the form of a curiously hard nodule, quite painless, which may become ulcerated, enormous numbers of spirochetes being discharged from the raw surface. The lesion consists of masses of chronic inflammatory cells, with no sign of acute inflammation. In the course of a few weeks it heals and may or may not leave a tell-tale scar. The regional lymph nodes, i.e., those that drain the part, are enlarged and hard in the primary stage. Usually these are the nodes in the groin, but if the primary lesion is on the lip the nodes below the jaw may be involved. At the end of the primary stage, the patient appears to have recovered, but the reaction to a serologic test on the blood has now become positive, and shows

that, although the patient seems to be so well, he is really suffering from active syphilis.

The secondary lesions appear after 2 or 3 months, and are due to the spirochetes' having been carried far and wide throughout the body by the blood stream from the primary lesion. The skin, mucus membranes, and lymph nodes are principally affected. A variety of **skin rashes** may appear, which may easily be mistaken for some other skin disease. White patches develop on the mucus membrane lining the mouth, tongue, and tonsils; they are called **mucus patches,** and as they discharge countless spirochetes they are highly infective. The **lymph nodes** all over the body become slightly enlarged. All of these secondary lesions finally disappear without leaving any trace, and the patient again appears to be well, although results of serologic tests are still positive. It is not clear why the secondary lesions occur. Many recent reports have hypothesized that this secondary exacerbation results from immunosuppression of host responses by the spirochete.

In about one-quarter of all untreated cases, late complications (tertiary lesions) occur. The tertiary lesions appear after an interval of many years, with something of the inevitability of a Greek tragedy.

Tertiary syphilis may involve the central nervous system, the spinal cord, or the cardiovascular system. In addition, there used to be a further complication in which the loss of proprioception due to dorsal column disease resulted in a knee or ankle joint that became generally unusable. Today, fortunately, tertiary syphilis is extremely rare.

The diffuse lesions are of three types: (1) **cardiovascular,** (2) **central nervous system,** and (3) **spinal cord lesions.** They are essentially destructive, and even if they do heal they leave the organ damaged and badly scarred. Syphilis frequently attacks the arteries; in the brain, the small arteries become thickened and narrowed so that thrombosis is apt to develop; in the main arteries such as the aorta, the wall becomes so weakened that the diseased part of the vessel dilates and forms a bulging known as an **aneurysm.** The most serious of all the tertiary lesions are those in the nervous system, which may develop many years after the original infection. The spinal cord may be involved by tabes dorsalis, also known as locomotor ataxia, or the chief lesions may be in the brain, causing general paresis, also known as general paralysis of the insane. We do not know why only about one-quarter of those affected with primary syphilis go on to develop any of the tertiary complications.

How does the treponema destroy these organs? One current explanation is that the organism produces an enzyme that breaks down mucopolysaccharide ground substance. This is the cement that holds cells together. The treponema does this because it needs certain components of the mucopolysaccharide for the synthesis of its capsule. It is thought that the capsule is highly water soluble and is constantly dissolving into the fluid of tissues. Since this capsule appears to be vital to the survival of the treponema, it must be constantly rebuilt, requiring a constant supply of building materials.

Diagnosis. The diagnosis of syphilis depends on different techniques at different stages of the disease. In the primary stage, the chancre is teeming with organisms and these may be seen on dark field microscopy. After the primary stage has passed, most patients have produced antibody which may be tested serologically. Two tests are used: first, the VDRL (Venereal Disease Research Laboratory) test which contains an antigen (cardiolipin) that reacts with an antibody in syphilitic serum. The VDRL test is simple and inexpensive, and therefore makes a good screening test. However, it is not specific; not only does it react with syphilitic serum, but also with antibodies from many patients with viral diseases. So when the VDRL test is positive, another test specific for T. pallidum is necessary. This is the treponema pallidum hemagglutination test (TPHA).

Treatment. Today, syphilis is treated with penicillin and resistance to this drug is as yet unknown. It is important to note, however, that reinfection is very common after treatment. We do develop immunity to T. pallidum, but it evolves very slowly over time, and if the course of infection is interrupted by penicillin, the immune response will not be sufficient to prevent disease on the next exposure to treponemes. The immune response to T. pallidum is complicated and not well understood.

An investigation of the natural history of syphilis was conducted by the United States Public Health Service in Macon County, Alabama, from 1932–1972. When published, this study, called the Tuskegee Study, became the subject of great moral debate because the experimenters had denied medical treatment to a poor, uneducated, black, male population. When the study was begun in 1930, the only pertinent literature on syphilis suggested that the disease ran a benign course, and that the available treatment was of questionable effectiveness. Under these circumstances, a study on natural history seemed desirable. In 1943, penicillin was recognized to be an efficient treatment in the early stages of syphilis. However, use of this treatment in the later stages of the disease was not fully accepted until a decade later, by which time such treatment would have had little therapeutic effect on the subjects of the study.

According to some authorities, criticism of this study uses modern ethical standards (like informed consent) to judge events that occurred in a different intellectual climate. Others are horrified by what was obviously experimentation with human life, and argue that there was no reason for withholding a drug once proven to be beneficial at any stage of the illness. Experimentation with human life is an on-going, vital part of medical progress, controlled very carefully today by hospital ethics committees and other agencies, which screen all proposed studies. The lives of our future patients who might benefit from such studies are worth no more or no less than the lives of our current patients.

Congenital Syphilis. A child infected with syphilis, which may be congenital (from the mother before birth), does not necessarily show signs of the disease at birth. Indeed, with regard to congenital syphilis, there are three possibilities: (1) The child may be born dead, usually showing well-marked evidence of syphilis. The disease used to be an important cause of stillbirth. (2) The child may be born alive with external evidence of syphilis. The skin shows inflammatory patches on the buttocks, the spleen is enlarged, and the mucus membrane of the nose is ulcerated with subsequent destruction of the bridge of the nose (saddle nose of congenital syphilis). (3) The child may appear healthy at birth, but lesions appear later. These lesions are on the whole similar to those of acquired syphilis, but in addition, the teeth may be small and peg-shaped, and the cornea of the eye may become hazy and opaque.

Lyme Disease

Lyme disease is another disorder caused by a spirochete. Lyme disease has become a fashionable diagnosis in the last two years to explain rashes, headaches, or arthritis unexplainable by other means or undiagnosed by conventional tests. This newly-recognized tick-borne disease, caused by a spirochete, was rediscovered in 1975 when about 60 cases were identified in Lyme, Connecticut. Fifteen years later more than 3,000 cases have been reported in the United States and Great Britain (Fig. 7–27).

Because of the epidemiologic pattern of the early cases which showed clusters of patients, predominantly children, with unusual arthritis occurring in the summer, it was thought that the disease could be caused by rickettsia. The breakthrough in discovering the etiology and transmission of the disease came when some patients with the rash remembered being bitten by a tick. This tick was identified as different from a dog tick (dermacentor variabilis). Subsequently, spirochetes (now named borrelia burgdorferi) were cultured from the blood, skin, and cerebrospinal fluid of patients with Lyme disease as well as from the ticks. The spirochetes may involve the nervous system of patients just as the spirochetes of

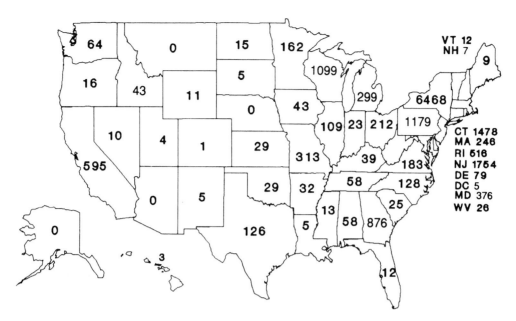

Fig. 7–27   Reported Lyme disease cases—United States, 1989–1990. (From Centers for Disease Control, Morbidity and Mortality Weekly Report, 40(25):417, 1991.)

syphilis do. But there are attacks of arthritis in most cases of patients who are not treated early in the disease. The arthritis usually involves knees and other large joints.

It is interesting that the symptoms of the disease are out of proportion to the number of organisms present which has led investigators to postulate that the bacterium triggers release of interleukin. This agent then acts as a pathogen. Thus, the affected joints may be bacteriologically sterile while appearing markedly inflamed. The treatment of Lyme disease is easy since most broad spectrum antibiotics are effective.

Campylobacter

A family of organisms now called campylobacter (formerly vibrio) are being identified more and more frequently as a cause of acute diarrhea, particularly in young adults. In any instance of acute diarrhea *Giardia lamblia* may be the agent, particularly when the episode is traced to camping or some waterborne source. Campylobacter, however, is the second most common cause of such episodes often traceable to water from streams contaminated by the feces or urine of wild or domestic animals. One such episode was reported in Northern Norway in 1990; others have been investigated in England, Israel, Sweden and Vermont.

The cause of the enterocolitis is a cholera-like enterotoxin, as well as cytotoxins which cause a severe, acute abdominal pain with acute diarrhea, lasting

about a week after a 3–4 day incubation period. As well as water-borne infections, campylobacter infections have been reported from handling wild birds, domestic birds (principally chickens), puppies, kittens, and meat such as beef, veal, pork and lamb. Campylobacter is also common in raw milk. Various species of campylobacter such as C-jejuni, coli, fetus, pylorii have been identified as causing other diseases.

Helicobacter (campylobacter) is a member of the same family which has recently been given its own status. It is also a curved or S-shaped gram negative bacilli with several long flagella. Interest in this organism stems from the mounting evidence that it plays a role in acute inflammations of the stomach often accompanied by ulceration.

A number of enzymes, particularly peptidases, and a potent urease have been identified as the products of this campylobacter. Its ability to survive in the acidic hostile gastric environment through, its microaerophilic adaptation, and adherence factors seem to be unique. It also appears to secrete an inhibitor of acid secretion as well as produce an extracellular protease which degrades gastric mucin. In the absence of mucin the gastric mucosa is much more susceptible to cytotoxins, and the effects of ammonia produced by the urease of the helicobacter organism. Whether this organism is truly the etiologic agent of all gastric ulcers and disease remains to be determined, but its identification, and an awareness of its potential to cause disease, are a new chapter in the search for an understanding of gastritis.

MYCOBACTERIA

Mycobacteria are rod-shaped bacteria which do not stain reliably by the gram method. However, once the stain is taken up, the cells resist decolorization by acid or alcohol and are therefore called "acid-fast" bacilli. The most important pathogens are M. tuberculosis and M. bovis, which cause tuberculosis, and M. leprae, the cause of leprosy. There are other pathogenic mycobacteria but they produce disease less often. These have been called "atypical" mycobacteria.

Mycobacterium Tuberculosis

M. tuberculosis is a thin, curved rod with a waxy coat that does not grow on ordinary culture media. It can be stained in a specific way, being colored red by carbol fuchsin and retaining the color after treatment by acid, which removes the color from other bacteria. Tuberculosis is usually caused by M. tuberculosis, but it may also result from M. bovis infection. Pathogens that produce tuberculosis are called tubercle bacilli. On account of its waxy sheath the tubercle bacillus is an exceptionally hardy organism. It may live outside the body for months.

Tuberculosis used to head the list of the killing diseases, so that Osler called it the "Captain of the Men of Death." In the 19th century the disease was called consumption because it appeared literally to consume its victims. In 1900 it was the leading cause of death in the United States; the death rate from this disease was then higher than the present death rate from cancer (see Fig. 2–15). Today there are about 30,000 cases of tuberculosis reported yearly in the United States, and about 3,000 in Canada. Much of the rest of the world has not seen such improvement; tuberculosis

remains a leading worldwide cause of death. Its prevalence in the United States in 1978–80 is shown in Figure 7–28. Observed and expected cases of TB in the United States in 1981–88 are shown in Figure 7–29.

Tuberculosis is particularly prevalent among peoples who live under crowded conditions in which droplet infection is facilitated, and in people who are debilitated through malnutrition or other causes. Large city slums provide the right conditions and these continue to act as depots of infection. Chronic alcoholics are also at high risk.

In the 19th century, tuberculosis primarily affected children and young adults. The tragedy of the young dying of consumption abounds in the literature and opera of the period. In North America today, the disease is most frequently seen in the elderly, particularly in non-white males.

Humans have a considerable natural resistance to tuberculosis. Although only 30,000 cases of disease are reported annually, it is estimated that there are 15 million Americans infected with the bacillus (Fig. 7–30). Probably only 5% will ever develop clinical disease. That one may harbor the bacillus in the body but be clinically healthy is an important concept in the understanding of tuberculosis, as will be seen later. When the natural defense is broken down by malnutrition, steroid therapy, debilitating illness or other stress, the tubercle bacillus seizes the opportunity to come out of hiding.

Tuberculosis spreads mainly by droplets in the air. The bacilli may be inhaled from sputum that has dried and has been changed into dust. The bacilli are soon killed by sunlight, but may survive a long time in the dark. When a patient with pulmonary tuberculosis coughs, he infects the air in the immediate neighbor-

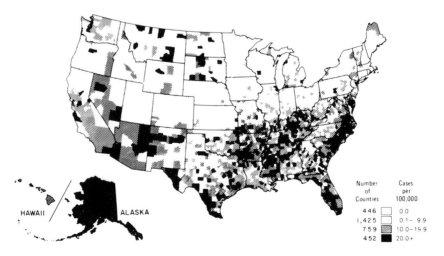

Fig. 7–28 Tuberculosis—reported average cases per 100,000 population, by county, United States, 1978–1980. (From Centers for Disease Control: Annual summary, 1981: Reported morbidity and mortality in the United States. Morbidity and Mortality Weekly Report, 30(54):91, 1982.)

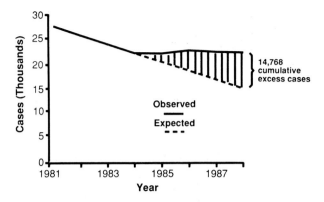

Fig. 7–29 Observed and expected tuberculosis cases—United States, 1981–1988. (From Centers for Disease Control, Morbidity and Mortality Weekly Report, 39(10):154, 1990.)

hood with millions of tubercle bacilli contained in tiny drops of moisture. It has been estimated that a moderately advanced case may expel from 2 to 4 billion bacilli in 24 hours. However, only organisms deposited in the small airways produce infection; thus only the very fine droplets are contagious. Probably 20% of the contacts of a newly diagnosed patient have acquired infection, and approximately 1% of contacts will develop disease. The infected but not diseased individual does not spread the bacillus. The diseased and treated individual does not spread the disease once his sputum has been cleared of bacilli.

There are two other ways of acquiring tubercular infection, both of which are infrequent. M. bovis infection may be acquired by drinking infected cows' milk. Pasteurization and disease detection in cattle

have reduced the rate of bovine tuberculosis to very low levels. Direct inoculation may rarely transmit tuberculosis; this is an occupational hazard to surgeons, pathologists, morticians and lab technicians. The reader is referred to the section on the pathogenesis of tuberculosis in the Appendix, p. 186.

Diagnosis. Tuberculous infection is easily detected by the tuberculin test, which is a purified protein derivative of the tubercle bacilli. This is injected into the skin and the injection site is examined 48 to 72 hours later. If during this time 10 mm of visible and palpable swelling has occurred, the individual must harbor tubercle bacilli (or an "atypical" mycobacterium). If there is no such reaction, the individual is either free of tubercle bacilli, or is anergic (immunologically nonreacting). Anergy may be produced in a variety of illnesses, including active tuberculosis.

It is important to note that the tuberculin test is only a test of infection. Diagnosis of tuberculous disease requires isolation of M. tuberculosis from sputum or other suspected material, which is examined using the acid fast stain. Contaminated fluids may also be cultured, although the culture medium must be incubated for 6 to 8 weeks due to the slow growth of the organism. Guinea pigs may be injected with cultured material and later autopsied and examined for evidence of tuberculosis.

Chest x-rays are valuable in diagnosis, as is the tuberculin test, which is helpful, particularly if the patient is known to have previously been tuberculin negative. It is recommended that all health personnel be tested with tuberculin so that their status may be recorded for future reference.

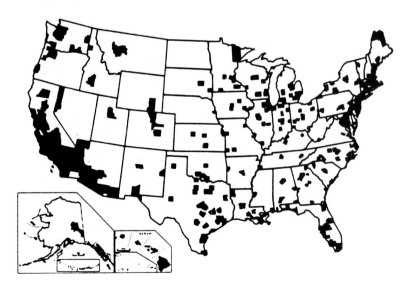

Fig. 7–30 Counties reporting tuberculosis among Asians/Pacific Islanders-United States, 1985. (From Centers for Disease Control, Morbidity and Mortality Weekly Report, 36(21):332, 1987.)

In spite of these diagnostic aids, many cases of tuberculosis are first diagnosed at autopsy.

Treatment. Today, tuberculosis is treated with a combination of drugs, because there are always bacteria present which are resistant to one individual drug but never resistant to three. The most commonly used regimen includes isoniazid, rifampin, and ethambutol. These drugs must be taken for 9 months in order to completely eradicate the tubercle bacilli.

Prevention. Isoniazid may be given to close long-term contacts of tuberculous patients. This does not include hospital personnel.

There is a vaccine for M. tuberculosis called the **BCG** (Bacille Calmette-Guérin). It uses a live strain of tubercle bacilli rendered avirulent by prolonged culture on special media. It does not produce disease but it does convert most individuals who receive it from tuberculin negative to tuberculin positive. Whether or not it actually prevents disease is a matter of current debate. Some recommend that all individuals at risk, including health personnel, be vaccinated. Others dispute the effectiveness of the vaccine arguing that there is no definite proof that it prevents disease. Because it prevents use of the tuberculin test in diagnosis (all vaccinated persons are positive regardless of whether they are actually protected against the disease or not), some argue that the BCG should not be used for health professionals (Fig. 7–31).

Mycobacterium Leprae

Leprosy was significant in medieval Europe, until the Black Death killed so many infected persons that leprosy almost disappeared. At that time, "leprosy" was used to describe a number of different infections

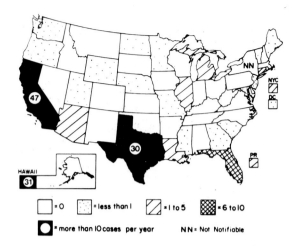

Fig. 7–32 Leprosy—average annual reported cases, 1970–1972. (From Centers for Disease Control, Morbidity and Mortality Weekly Report, Annual supplements. Summaries. Vols. 19–21, 1970–1972.)

that affected the skin in conspicuous and horrible ways. The disease as we know it today is caused by a rod-shaped bacillus, *Mycobacterium leprae*, first identified in 1873 by a Norwegian doctor, Armauer Hansen. Like its relative, the *Mycobacterium tuberculosis*, *Mycobacterium leprae* is acid-fast. It has never been cultivated in vitro, and only recently has it been possible to grow it on animal tissue.

At present there are probably 10 to 20 million people with leprosy in the world, many of them living in tropical countries where the disease is more common. In the United States, 419 cases were reported between 1971 and 1973, mostly in California, Texas, and Hawaii (Figure 7–32).

Leprosy is classified into three types: lepromatous, tuberculoid, and borderline. Lepromatous leprosy involves extensive skin lesions, nasal symptoms (stuffiness) and, in males, infiltration and scarring of the testes, which leads to sterility. In addition, there is some neurologic involvement. Tuberculoid leprosy is characterized by fewer skin lesions and by pronounced nerve involvement, leading to muscle atrophy, crippling, and blindness when the facial nerve is involved. Borderline leprosy is a combination of the other two types.

Effective chemotherapy is available, and many of the deformities of the advanced disease can be prevented by proper attention.

MISCELLANEOUS BACTERIA

Some bacteria cannot be considered in the broad categories we have already discussed, but they are nonetheless important and must be included.

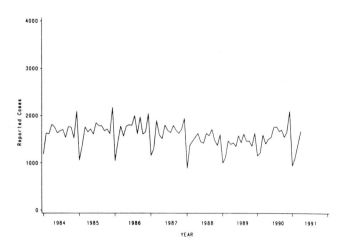

Fig. 7–31 Tuberculosis cases by 4 week period of report—United States, 1984–1991. (From Centers for Disease Control, Morbidity and Mortality Weekly Report, 40(16):273, 1991.)

Legionella Pneumophila

This pneumonia of current interest came into prominence during the summer of 1976 when many persons who were attending a convention of the American Legion in Philadelphia were stricken by a serious and frequently fatal (15%) respiratory illness. Epidemiologic work since the outbreak has identified the organism responsible, a previously unidentified gram-negative bacillus that can be propagated in embryonated egg yolk sacs, and has been designated *Legionella pneumophila* (Fig. 7–33).

This organism seems to thrive in warm, damp places; the current and previous outbreaks occurred between June and November in the northern hemisphere, and have been traced to cooling towers or evaporative condensers, or to exposure to cleaning such equipment. Although there are different types of *Legionella pneumophila*, the availability of serologic diagnostic methods has made it possible to diagnose other epidemics of respiratory illness retrospectively. An epidemic of a 2- to 5-day acute febrile illness in Pontiac, Michigan, of 144 people who worked, paradoxically, in a county health department building, was shown to be due to this organism. Two other similar outbreaks, one in St. Elizabeth's Hospital, Washington, D.C., and another in Spain, were both so identified.

Clinical Pattern. The disease has an incubation period of 2 to 10 days and appears with malaise, headache, and muscular aches and pains, without previous upper respiratory tract illness. A nonproductive cough, with chest pain and sometimes vomiting, diarrhea, and delirium are often present. Patients have ranged in age from 10 to 84 years, with a median age of 55 years. Males seem to outnumber females 3:1. Chest films show patchy, multilobar involvement with consolidation, and pleural effusions are frequent. Fortunately, erythromycin seems to be effective in treating the disease.

Mycoplasmas

Mycoplasmas are the smallest and simplest living things that are capable of independent existence. They are smaller than all other bacteria but larger than viruses. Because of their small size, and their lack of the typical bacterial cell wall, there has been much confusion as to how they should be classified. In the past they were referred to as "pleuropneumonia-like organisms" (PPLO). Today they are considered to be bacteria.

The mycoplasma cell is bounded only by a cell membrane and contains the minimum organelles necessary for growth and reproduction. Without a cell wall, they are highly pleomorphic (variable in shape) and also completely resistant to penicillin, which acts by disrupting cell wall synthesis. Fortunately, the mycoplasmas are quite sensitive to other antibiotics.

Some species of mycoplasmas belong to the normal flora of the body, but most are pathogenic. *Myco-*

Fig. 7–33 Scanning electron micrograph of the Legionnaires' disease bacterium, *Legionella pneumophila* (x16,200). (From Ourth, D.D.: Legionnaires' disease bacterium. Am. J. Clin. Pathol., 73:121, 1980.)

plasma pneumoniae is the most important pathogen; it is the most common cause of pneumonia in school age children and young adults. Two other species, *Mycoplasma hominis* and *Ureaplasma urealyticum*, are commonly cultured from the genitourinary tract; they can produce urethritis and pelvic inflammatory disease. Their role in the pathogenesis of other urinary tract diseases is currently under study.

Mycoplasma pneumonia is described in the chapter on the respiratory tract.

SYNOPSIS

Bacteria as a biologic form are utilitarian, and higher organisms depend on them.

Bacterial infections may be local or systemic diseases.

Bacterial endotoxins and enzymes are causes of injury.

Antibodies to bacterial antigens are aids to diagnosis.

Hypersensitivity to bacterial antigens is a cause of tissue injury.

Koch's postulates are a paradigm for the germ theory of disease.

Tuberculosis is a model of infectious disease in which tissue destruction, immunity, and hypersensitivity all exist.

The carrier state, as in typhoid fever, is an important complication of infectious disease.

Spores of bacteria represent an important factor in the spread of disease.

Terms

Bacteriostatic	*Staphylococci*	*Cholera*
Bacteriocidal	*Streptococci*	*Plague*
Virulence	*Scarlet fever*	*Tetanus*
Fomites	*Pneumococcus*	*Incubation period*
Vectors	*Diphtheria*	*Spores*
Gram stain	*Tuberculosis*	*Mycoplasma*
		Lyme disease

FURTHER READING

Amyes, S.G.B., Gemmell, C.G., and Smith, J.T.: Antibiotic resistance in bacteria. J. Med. Microbiol., 36:4, 1992.

Baker, C.J.: Group B streptococcal infection in newborns: prevention at last? N. Engl. J. Med., 314:1702, 1986.

Barnes, A.M.: Surveillance and control of bubonic plague in the United States. Symp. Zool. Soc. Lond., 50:237, 1982.

Bartlett, J.G.: Infant botulism in adults. N. Engl. J. Med., 315:254, 1986.

Bartlett, J.G.: Virulence factors of anaerobic bacteria. Johns Hopkins Med. J., 151:1, 1982.

Benedek, T.G.: The "Tuskegee Study" of syphilis: analysis of moral versus methodologic aspects. J. Chronic Dis., 31:35, 1978.

Black, R.E., et al.: Epidemic yersinia enterocolitica infection due to contaminated chocolate milk. N. Engl. J. Med., 298:76, 1978.

Blake, P.A., et al.: Cholera—a possible endemic focus in the United States. N. Engl. J. Med., 302:305, 1980.

Burnet, F.M.: *Natural History of Infectious Disease*, 2nd Ed. Cambridge, Cambridge University Press, 1953.

Davos, D.E., et al.: Outbreak of brucellosis at a South-Australian abattoir. 2. Epidemiological investigations. Med. J. Aust., 2:657, 1981.

Denny, F.W.: The streptococcus saga continues. N. Engl. J. Med., 325:127, 1991.

Dick, J.D.: Helicobacter (campylobacter) pylori: A new twist to an old disease. Annu. Rev. Microbiol., 44:249, 1990.

Dondero, T.J., et al.: An outbreak of Legionnaires' disease associated with a contaminated air conditioning cooling tower. N. Engl. J. Med., 302:365, 1980.

Dudley, M.N.: Overview of gram-negative sepsis. Am. J. Hosp. Pharm., 47(Suppl.3):S3, 1990.

Fraser, D.W.: Legionnaires' disease: four summers' harvest. Am. J. Med., 68:1, 1980.

Gemmell, C.G.: The staphylococcus—new features 100 years after its discovery. J. Infection, 4:5, 1982.

Giraud, T., et al.: Adult overwhelming meningococcal purpura. Arch. Int. Med., 151:310, 1991.

Hook, F.W., III, and Marra, C.M.: Acquired syphilis in adults. N. Engl. J. Med., 326:1060, 1992.

Huppertz, H.-I.: Childhood Lyme borreliosis in Europe. Eur. J. Pediatr., 149:814, 1990.

Hutchinson, C.M., and Hook E.W., III: Syphilis in adults. Med. Clin. N.A., 74:1389, 1990.

Judson, F.N.: Gonorrhea. Med. Clin. N.A., 74:1353, 1990.

Lew, J.F., Swerdlow, D.L., Dance, M.E., et al.: An outbreak of shigellosis aboard a cruise ship caused by a multiple-antibiotic-resistant strain of shigella-flexneri. Am. J. Epidemiol., 134:413, 1991.

Lewis, C.M., and Zervos, M.J.: Clinical manifestations of enterococcal infection. Eur. J. Clin. Microbiol. Infect. Dis., 9:111, 1990.

Mackowiak, P.A.: Microbial synergism in human infections. N. Engl. J. Med., 298:21, 1978.

McDonald, K.L., Osterholm, M.T., et al.: Toxic shock syndrome. J.A.M.A., 257:1053, 1987.

McEvedy, C.: The bubonic plague. Sci. Am., 258:118, 1988.

Martin, D.H.: Chlamydial infections. Med. Clin. N.A., 74:1367, 1990.

Martin, P.R., and Hoiby, E.A.: Streptococcal serogroup A epidemic in Norway 1987–1988. Scand. J. Infect. Dis., 22:421, 1990.

Melby, K., Dahl, O.P., Crisp, L., and Penner, J.L.: Clinical and serological manifestations in patients during a waterborne epidemic due to *Campylobacter jejuni*. J. Infect., 21:309, 1990.

Moellering, R.C., Jr.: The enterococcus: a classic example of the impact of antimicrobial resistance on therapeutic options. J. Antimicrobial Chemotherapy 28:1, 1991.

Muhlemann, M.F., and Wright, D.J.M.: Emerging pattern of Lyme disease in the United Kingdom. Lancet, 260:8527, 1987.

Ojajärvi, J.: Effectiveness of hand washing and disinfection methods in removing transient bacteria after patient nursing. J. Hyg., Camb., 85:193, 1980.

Pelczar, M., Jr., et al.: *Microbiology*, 4th ed. New York, McGraw-Hill Book Co., 1977.

Rappuoli, R., Perugini, M., and Falsen, E.: Molecular epidemiology of the 1984–1986 outbreak of diphtheria in Sweden. N. Engl. J. Med., 319:393, 1988.

Rein, M.F.: Therapeutic decisions in the treatment of sexually transmitted diseases: an overview. Sexually Transmitted Dis., 8:93, 1981.

Riley, R.L.: Disease transmission and contagion control. Am Rev. Respir. Dis., 125:16, 1982.

Rolfs, R.T., and Nakashima, A.K.: Epidemiology of primary and secondary syphilis in the United States, 1981 through 1989. J.A.M.A., 264:1432, 1990.

Schachter, J., and Dawson, C.R.: Chlamydial infections, a worldwide problem: epidemiology and implications for trachoma therapy. Sexually Transmitted Dis., 8:167, 1981.

Schwartz, B., Facklam, R.R., and Breiman, R.F.: Changing epidemiology of group A streptococcal infection in the USA. Lancet, 336:1167, 1990.

Sheagren, J.N.: Staphylococcus aureus, the persistent pathogen. N. Engl. J. Med., 310:1368, 1984.

Skirrow, M.B.: Campylobacter. Lancet, 336:921, 1990.

Special Symposium on Hansen's Disease: Advances in clinical and experimental research. Am. J. Trop. Med. Hyg., Vol. 44(4), April 1991.

Snider, D.E., Jr., and Roper, W.L.: The new tuberculosis. N. Engl. J. Med., 326:703, 1992.

Stenius-Aarniala, B., and Tukiainen, P.: Miliary tuberculosis. Acta Med. Scand., 206:417, 1979.

Steere, A.C., Syndman, D., et al.: Historical perspective of disease. Zentralblatt fur Bakteriologie 263:3, 1986.

Swerdlow, D.L., and Ries, A.A.: Cholera in the Americas—Guidelines for the clinician. J.A.M.A., 267:1495, 1992.

APPENDIX

General Notes on Bacteria

Special stains and cultural characteristics are of value in recognizing and classifying certain bacteria. The aniline dye, methylene blue, will stain most bacteria satisfactorily, but two special methods are invaluable. The first of these is **Gram's stain,** in which the film is stained with gentian violet followed by iodine, and then decolorized with alcohol and counterstained. Bacteria that resist the decolorization and so remain stained blue are said to be **gram-positive;** those that are decolorized by the alcohol, but are shown up by a counterstain of a different color, are said to be **gram-negative.** This method is indispensable in routine laboratory work, for it separates bacteria, both cocci and bacilli, into two great groups. The second method is **acid-fast staining.** The term "fast" is taken from a German word meaning resistant. Bacilli that resist decoloration with acid after being stained red with hot carbol fuchsin are said to be acid-fast. The reader will appreciate that acid-fast corresponds to gram-positive; in the former, acid is used as the decolorizing agent, in the latter, alcohol. The only important members of the acid-fast group are the bacilli of tuberculosis and of leprosy. There are many other special stains, but these two are mentioned because we refer frequently to acid-fast ba-

cilli and to gram-positive and gram-negative organisms in the course of this chapter.

Cultural characteristics are also important in determining the nature of an infection. The four requirements for successful culture are food, temperature, moisture, and oxygen. Some media suit some types of bacteria; other media, such as those containing hemoglobin, are better for other types. Moisture is essential, because water is as vital to bacteria as to all other forms of life. It is for this reason that a swab of infective material must never be allowed to dry out in its passage from the bedside to the laboratory by being left lying around. The temperature best suited for pathogenic bacteria is usually that of the body to which they are accustomed, so that the incubator in which the media are placed is kept at 37°C (98.4°F). Oxygen is required for growth by most bacteria; they are said to be aerobic. An important group are peculiar enough to demand absence of air for continued growth; they are called anaerobic bacteria or anaerobes, and the laboratory technique must be regulated accordingly. To this group belong the spore-bearing bacilli that live in soil that has been fertilized by manure and infect wounds contaminated with such soil, the most important being the bacillus of tetanus and the bacilli that cause gas gangrene. Finally, there are some that can survive both in the presence and absence of oxygen, as the circumstances dictate. These are called facultative anaerobes.

The Staphylococci

Usually S. aureus produces yellow colonies (*aurum*, Latin for gold) as opposed to the other two which are white. However, some S. aureus strains grow white colonies, and for this reason, white colonies must always be tested for coagulase, an enzyme which S. aureus alone produces. This enzyme causes a marked formation of fibrin from the fibrinogen of plasma. Coagulase-positive organisms are more virulent, because the film of fibrin protects them from the action of antibodies and antibiotics. The presence of this enzyme is a reliable criterion of virulence. It must be admitted that the fibrin tends to limit the spread by blocking paths of dissemination. Some strains of staphylococci produce a "spreading factor," hyaluronidase. This enzyme digests hyaluronic acid, the mucopolysaccharide of ground substance that forms a natural obstacle in the interstitial compartment. Hyaluronidase breaks down this cement that holds the cells together, increasing the permeability of the tissues to bacteria.

In addition to these enzymes, various strains of S. aureus can also produce a large number of toxins which are secreted into the tissues and are thought to be important in the pathogenesis of some disease states. These will be discussed below.

The natural habitat of the staphylococcus includes the skin and mucus membranes. Virtually all humans carry S. epidermidis on their skin (hence the name), and most harbor S. aureus at one time or another. However, hospital personnel, especially doctors and nurses, are much more frequent carriers of S. aureus. Once again the importance of hand washing must be stressed.

The staphylococci are hardy creatures; they are resistant to heat, drying and chemicals. They may live for weeks in dried pus. Many strains are resistant to penicillin and other antibiotics.

Bacteriological diagnosis of a staphylococcal infection is

easily made with the gram stain, culture and coagulase tests. For some purposes it is necessary to go further than this, and to determine the exact strain of S. aureus responsible. In outbreaks of S. aureus infections in hospitals, this must be determined in order to locate the source. In this case, bacteriophage typing is used. Bacteriophages are viruses that attack bacteria, and they are highly specific; that is, only certain phages will attack a specific strain of staphylococcus. Bacteria are typed according to the number of the phage that attacks and lyses it.

The staphylococcus is a pyogenic organism, a pus-producer, and is a common cause of acute inflammation. It enters the body through cracks in the skin, often as a result of local irritation. The mere pricking of a pimple may start the infection. In contrast to streptococci, the staphylococcus usually produces inflammation that remains localized. We must always remember that staphylococci are normal inhabitants of the body. They have been called the jackals of the microbial parasitic world, usually unable to mount an attack against the healthy body, but ready to invade the tissues when resistance is lowered by other disease states.

The Streptococci

Some species of streptococci are natural inhabitants of the mouth and intestinal tract, but the most frequent pathogen, S. pyogenes, is not normally found in the body. We acquire S. pyogenes infections only from other infected individuals who may be clinically ill or may be healthy carriers. In this case, spread is via droplets from the respiratory tract or skin.

Like the staphylococci, streptococci may acquire resistance to antibiotics. Penicillin resistance is less common, although the streptococcus readily becomes resistant to other antibiotics, especially tetracycline. Penicillin is the drug of choice, or erythromycin for patients who are allergic to penicillin.

The streptococcus tends to produce spreading inflammation that extends widely throughout the tissues in comparison with the circumscribed lesions caused by the staphylococcus. This power of infiltration seems to depend largely on the power to produce fibrinolysin and hyaluronidase. **Fibrinolysin** prevents the formation of fibrin and tends to dissolve any that has formed, thus eliminating the fibrin barrier to the spread of infection.

There are many different species of streptococci and their classification is based on a number of factors, the most important being (1) action on red blood cells (or blood agar), and (2) antigenic testing. Streptococci can be divided into three groups depending on their reaction on blood agar, called alpha, beta, and gamma. The beta group, also called the **hemolytic streptococci,** cause hemolysis or breaking down of blood in the medium, so that colonies are surrounded by a colorless halo. The alpha group, also called the **viridans streptococci,** do not completely hemolyse the blood, leaving a green halo. The gamma group produce no hemolysis at all and no color change. As these are mostly non-pathogenic they will not be considered further.

Pathogenesis of Tuberculosis

Pathogenesis. The tubercle bacillus may invade the blood stream. The infection may spread in three ways: (1) **Through the tissues.** In the organ infected, unless the defense forces gain mastery, the disease gradually spreads until the greater part of that organ is destroyed. (2) **By the lymphatics.** The bacilli tend to spread from the site of infection along the lymphatic vessels to the lymph nodes that drain the part, where they set up tuberculous disease. Thus the nodes in the neck are infected from the tonsil, the nodes in the chest from the lung, the abdominal nodes from the bowel. (3) **By the blood stream.** A tuberculous lesion may perforate the wall of a vessel and discharge millions of bacilli into the blood stream. These are arrested in every organ in the body, where they cause the formation of numberless minute lesions the size of a pin's head; these are called miliary tubercles and the condition is known as generalized miliary tuberculosis. In addition to this massive infection, occasional bacilli may enter the blood stream and set up a single tuberculous focus in one organ such as the kidney or bone, causing collapse.

Lesions. Tuberculosis is a chronic inflammation. The characteristic cell of the inflammatory exudate is the macrophage, which becomes changed in character so that it has a swollen, pale body and indefinite outlines. These characteristics are due to the fact that the fatty envelope of the bacillus is dissolved and taken up by the cells, which in their new form are called **epithelioid cells** (epithelial-like) and are the most characteristic single feature of the tuberculous reaction (see Chapter 5). The bacilli are surrounded by a mass of these cells, which are actively phagocytic. Sometimes a number of epithelioid cells fuse together to form a large **giant cell,** with as many nuclei as there are cells in its formation. Further out there is a zone of **lymphocytes,** also called small round cells. There is none of the dilation of blood vessels nor exudation of serum that is so characteristic of acute inflammation, and for this reason the heat and redness of acute inflammation are also absent.

The collection of inflammatory cells around the clump of tubercle bacilli forms a little mass that becomes visible to the naked eye and is called a **tubercle** or **miliary tubercle** (Latin *milium*, a millet seed). This is the standard lesion of tuberculosis, and is found in whichever organ the disease occurs, be it lung, kidney, or brain. Indeed, it is the tubercle that originally gave the disease its name. As the bacilli spread throughout the organ, large numbers of tubercles are formed, and these grow ever larger, fuse together, and thus come to form extensive tuberculous areas.

Meanwhile, a further change takes place in the center of the tubercle. The cells are killed by the bacilli, undergo necrosis, and finally lose all vestige of structure and fuse together to form a cheesy mass, which is called caseous (cheesy) material, the process being known as **caseation.** In the course of time the caseous material may become liquefied, so that a cavity or cavities are formed in the organ, or the material may calcify.

Any organ of the body may be involved by tuberculosis. It is exceptional, however, for more than one or two organs to be attacked at the same time, except in miliary tuberculosis. Although a bone such as the femur must necessarily be infected from the blood stream, it is nevertheless unusual for other bones to be involved in the same case. It is difficult to give a satisfactory explanation for this behavior.

The lungs and pleura are most frequently attacked, and pulmonary disease accounts for 85 to 90% of all deaths from tuberculosis. Lymph nodes come next, most often those in the hilum of the lung, less frequently the abdominal nodes.

Possible Outcome. Tuberculosis is a fight in which the forces of attack and defense, of destruction and defense, of destruction and conservation, are usually evenly balanced.

The outcome depends on two main factors: the resistance of the tissues and the size of dose of the bacilli. If the resistance is good and the dose small, there is a proliferation of fibrous tissue around the tubercle that limits the spread of the infection and eventually invades the tubercle and converts it into a mass of scar tissue known as a healed tubercle. This process of encapsulation and scarring is seen particularly well in the lung, and may occur even when the tuberculous area is of considerable size. Tuberculous scars are commonly found at the apex of the lung, and these scars often contain calcium, which is deposited in the caseous material as healing occurs, and which can be detected by radiology. Healing of the tuberculous lesion is by far the most common outcome.

When the dose of bacilli is larger, or the resistance of the patient is lowered, the disease tends to progress slowly, but fibrous tissue is continually forming, so that the destruction of tissue is gradual, and the process may be halted after it has lasted for a long time. Halting, however, is not synonymous with recovery, and unless the patient pays strict attention to the rules of hygiene, the process may light up again, with recurrence of the severe symptoms. The patient is metaphorically sitting on a barrel of gunpowder and he must not forget that fact.

Finally, the infection may be overwhelming and resistance may be at a minimum. In these cases there is almost

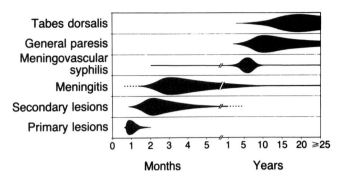

Fig. A7–2 Approximate time course of the clinical manifestations of early syphilis and neurosyphilis. Shaded areas corresponding to each syndrome represent the approximate proportion of patients with the syndrome specified and do not indicate the proportion of all patients with syphilis who have that syndrome. (From: Hook, III, F.W., and Marra, C.M.: Acquired syphilis in adults. N. Engl. J. Med., 326:1060, 1992.)

pure destruction with practically no attempt at limitation; the disease rages like a fire throughout the lung, huge cavities are formed, and the patient dies in the course of a few weeks or months. These are the cases that used to be popularly and justifiably known as galloping consumption. The fatal outcome of pulmonary tuberculosis was often due to rupture of the lesion into a vein or artery and hemorrhage into the lung. The tragic heroine Camille of A. Dumas died in such a way, and many Victorian tragediennes faded away with pulmonary tuberculosis.

Syphilis

As with tuberculosis, the changing population of our cities, and the changing mores of our population have led to a new epidemic of syphilis. Figure A7–1 shows the changing number of primary and secondary syphilis cases between 1956 and 1990, in both men and women. This epidemic rise is linked to epidemics of illegal drug use because of inner city activities, particularly in "crack houses." It is worthwhile noting that this population is generally underserved medically and reluctant to help with tracing exposures. The time course of the clinical manifestations of syphilis is shown in Figure A7–2, and we can expect a recrudescence of tabes and general paresis in the early years of the next century.

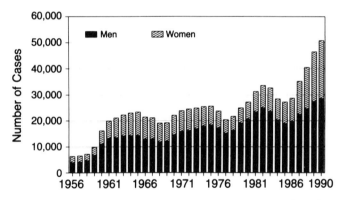

Fig. A7–1 Number of cases of primary and secondary syphilis in the United States, according to sex, 1956 to 1990. (From: Hook, III, F.W., and Marra, C.M.: Acquired syphilis in adults. N. Engl. J. Med., 326:1060, 1992.)

8

VIRUSES AND OTHER INTRACELLULAR PARASITES

Repetition is the only form of permanence nature can achieve.—SANTAYANA

We come now to viruses, a class of small but powerful life forms. Viruses are intracellular parasites, dependent on a phase of intracellular growth. In between cycles of intracellular replication, the virus exists as a free particle known as a virion, which contains the viral chromosome and a variable number of enzymes within a stabilizing structure. Viruses infect organisms as diverse as bacteria, plants and human beings, and are as varied in their structure and their biologic impact as this universality suggests. The role of viruses as disease-causing agents is well known, but viruses have also been invaluable tools for experimental biologists in unraveling the basic mechanisms of nucleic acid replication, regulated gene expression, protein synthesis and processing, and the assembly of protein and membrane complexes. Many viruses can be studied *in vitro* in cell culture. Their streamlined life cycles have facilitated analysis of the molecular mechanisms of biological processes. Because they are generally haploid, viral mutants whose altered behavior aids in understanding normal function have been generated with relative ease. Because they can be grown to high titer, many viruses have been available in significant amounts as a relatively pure source of material for biochemical analysis. From viruses we have been able to learn much about the regulatory and mechanistic aspects of a broad spectrum of biological processes.

The history of virology and viral diseases is remarkable. More than 100 years ago, Pasteur showed that disease could be produced by agents too small to be seen with the microscope, so minute that they were not held back by the finest filter. Unlike bacteria, they would not multiply when grown on defined culture media. These unknown agents were called viruses. It is amazing to learn that he was able to immunize persons suspected of being exposed to a viral infection, namely rabies. Equally remarkable was Jenner's success in 1796, when he immunized people against the ravages of smallpox, which we now know to be a viral disease. The first virus to be actually demonstrated was the causative agent of a plant disease, tobacco mosaic virus. In 1898, the first definitive linkage of an animal disease with a virus was achieved for foot-and-mouth disease of cattle. In 1901 came the proof of the first viral disease in man, namely yellow fever. But it is in the last 40 years that the most dazzling progress has been made. This acceleration has largely been due to the discovery that viruses can be grown outside the body in tissue culture. Culture was first achieved in the yolk sac of a hen's egg (the living embryo), and more recently in tissue cultures derived from somatic cells of primates or rodents. For pioneering this work, Enders and his associates were awarded the Nobel prize. Tissue culture technology has been instrumental in the development of viral vaccine strains and the testing of anti-viral drugs. Not so long ago the public had never heard of viruses, but now everyone diagnoses his or her own complaints as being due to a virus.

VIRAL STRUCTURE AND FUNCTION

The general anatomy of a virus is a nucleic acid core within a well-structured protein coat, which may or may not be surrounded by a lipid envelope. The nucleic acid may be RNA or DNA; it directs the replication of many new viral genomes, and codes for various viral proteins. Some of these proteins are the structural components of the virion; some are enzymes that facilitate the replication and growth of the virus in the cell. The host provides the energy, the substrates, and the synthetic machinery for viral growth (Fig. 8–1). A virus is an elegant, elementary, extraordinary parasite.

The nature of the virus-host relationship varies enormously, ranging from relatively benign coexistence, similar to a stowaway on a ship, to massive destructive takeover, as a hijacker redirects and can ultimately destroy his target. A virus may enter a cell and neither change its cellular structure nor disturb its function. This phenomenon is seen in some enteroviruses (cultured from the stools of infected persons who therefore act as carriers), such as the Coxsackie

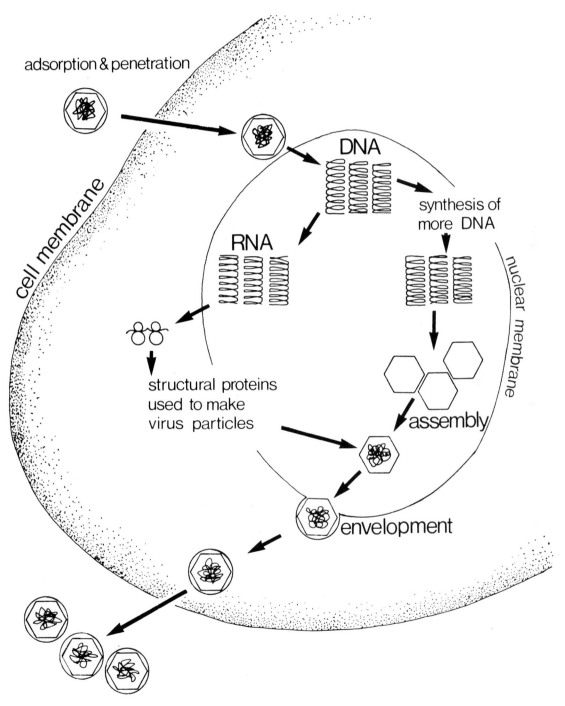

Fig. 8–1   This diagram shows the various steps in the entry, development, assembly, and formation of viral particles. The virus shown in the upper left with its coat must gain access to the nucleic acids of the cell, where new synthesis of viral particles takes place. Subsequently, assembly of the viral particles occurs. The cell is usually destroyed in the process. (Adapted from S. Dales.)

viruses, for example. At the other extreme we have the explosive effects of the yellow fever virus on the liver cells, and the poliomyelitis virus on the anterior horn (motor) cells of the spinal cord. There is thus a world of difference between viral infection and viral disease. In viral infection, which is much more common than viral disease, the virus may sojourn indefinitely in the comfortable surroundings of the cell. It may simply be a boarder, as in some cases where viral genes remain in the cell but are not expressed. At some later time, this genome may become active and its effects may become apparent. Alternatively, the sojourning virus particle may become one of the family, and multiplication of the virus proceeds without damage to the cell. Various circumstances such as age, stress, or nutritional or hormonal imbalance may upset the harmony and may convert the latent virus into a virulent one. Bacterial infection may also spark this conversion, one of the best examples being the well-known relation between herpes simplex ("cold sore") and pneumococcal infection. In viral disease, the normal functions of the cell may be rapidly shut off, as the virus directs cell machinery to manufacture virus particles. The cell may be blown to pieces by the explosive proliferation of the virus, but evidence of cellular degeneration, known as the cytopathic effect of the virus, is much more common.

Viruses pose an interesting evolutionary dilemma. The rules of natural selection and survival of the fittest apply to viruses as well as to the rest of the biologic world. Any genetic change that increases the efficiency of viral proliferation enhances the ability of that virus strain to survive. However, more efficient proliferation may result in rapid elimination of the host. Viruses need their hosts in order to multiply; destroying the host during infection is obviously counterproductive. This parasitic dependence leads to a modulation of virulence in the wild, so that virus and host may coexist. Therefore, many viral infections are productive but inapparent. Our concept of viruses as agents of disease comes from those cases where the effects of infection are apparent or perhaps even fatal.

The viral life cycle involves several stages. A virus must find susceptible cells. These may be restricted to a single species of animal, or to a particular type of tissue. Susceptibility is usually determined by the presence of appropriate receptors on the cell membrane which are recognized by proteins on the surface of the virus. The cellular protein exists to perform a normal physiological role; its function as a viral receptor is secondary to the host but essential to the virus. This is an example of the fine-tuned coevolution of a virus and its host. A virus binds to the receptors of the cell and penetrates the cell (by fusion to the membrane or endocytosis), where it is uncoated and initiates the cycle of nucleic acid transcription and translation. The result is the synthesis of viral proteins and the replication of new viral genomes. The nature of these processes, along with the virion structure, is the basis of contemporary viral classification. DNA viruses have a DNA genome, as do their hosts. The replication of DNA from DNA, and the transcription of DNA to RNA to protein is thus similar to normal cell function. Host enzymes may play vital, accessory or no roles in these functions. Viruses may use all of the existing cell machinery, or they may bring about their own modifications. The more complex the virus (the greater the number of its components and the functional proteins it encodes), the more "independence" it has in its intracellular cycle. By providing their own polymerases and/or other replication machinery, viruses can grow in nondividing cells, in the cytoplasm rather than in the nucleus, or they can shift the net effect of synthesis to viral functions and away from those of the host.

RNA viruses are the only living forms to have solely RNA as their genomic information. Since cells do not normally copy RNA from RNA, viruses must bring along their own enzymes. RNA viruses may have single-stranded or double-stranded genomes, contained in one or multiple segments. Single-stranded RNA is classified as follows: + RNA functions directly as mRNA (messenger RNA), that is, it is translated into proteins. − RNA must first be copied, and the complementary + RNA serves as the mRNA. In + strand viruses, the encapsidated RNA of the virion may be translated directly into proteins. Replication is accomplished by synthesizing a complementary − RNA, and then by making many new + virion RNAs from this template. In − strand viruses, complementary + RNA must be made first, for use as mRNA and as the template for virion − RNA synthesis.

The viral mRNAs must then be translated into proteins on host ribosomes with the aid of the host translational machinery. Lytic viruses have evolved several mechanisms to mediate the preferential synthesis of their own proteins at the expense of the host's proteins. They may inactivate co-factors which are required for host mRNA translation (such as cap-binding proteins) but are dispensable for the translation of viral mRNAs which have evolved to be independent of these factors. They may rely on numerical superiority (many viral mRNAs are synthesized at high levels) or on competitive advantage (the viral mRNAs may have a greater affinity for the components of the translational machinery than do host mRNAs).

Once the replication and protein synthetic pathways have been accomplished (with or without an accompanying cessation of host functions), the new virions must be assembled and released. In some cases, viruses accumulate and cell lysis causes their dispersion. In other cases, the new virions assemble at the cell membrane, bud out, and finally pinch off without disrupting the cell. Released viruses are then "inert" particles until they encounter new host cells and begin the cycle again. Some virions are highly stable, ensuring the survival of infectious viruses even when a susceptible host is not encountered immediately. Other virions are fragile, rendering the survival of these viruses dependent on a ready pool of susceptible hosts. Thus, the nature of the virion plays a role in the epidemiology of the infection.

In addition to causing cell death, other adverse effects are exerted by viruses. Viruses are capable of transforming and augmenting the growth potential of cells. Infected cells may become immortal, their growth may be rendered independent of the usual regulatory growth signals, or they may be converted to a full-blown neoplastic state. Thus, some viral infections are linked to the development of cancer. Viruses may also establish a latent, or nearly silent infection, and then re-emerge as more cytolytic agents at a later time. Finally, viruses may persist in the host, causing chronic infections.

As well as the direct effects of viral infection on target cells, many symptoms of disease are related to the host's reaction to viral growth. Viral infections often cause fever, which is accompanied by many common symptoms. Viruses and virally infected cells are also often highly antigenic and mobilize the immune system. Reactions of virus and circulating antibodies are often responsible for the rashes associated with viral disease. Inflammation and tissue damage result from mobilized cellular immunity; the release of previously inaccessible cellular components is responsible for the damage associated with viral infections involving the central nervous system. In these cases it is the host-virus interaction, rather than the virus itself, which causes the damage. Finally, viral infections often heighten an individual's susceptibility to bacterial infections for reasons that are not always clear; this susceptibility is responsible for many fatalities in viral-associated diseases. For example, influenza virus destroys the epithelial cells lining the respiratory tract. This epithelium is a primary barrier against bacterial invaders, and, once it is compromised, a bacterial pneumonia may easily invade and overcome an elderly or weakened person.

IMMUNITY AND RESISTANCE

The immune response of the host is often part of the evolution of disease in viral infections; nevertheless, it is certainly an essential defense that limits viral disease. Viruses elicit circulating antibodies (IgG and IgM) and evoke localized antibodies present in body secretions (IgA). These antibodies may either curtail the viral infection or prevent its spread to secondary target tissues. It is often during the secondary spread of infection that the most serious complications of viral infection arise. In addition to stimulating antibody production, viruses elicit cell-mediated immunity (T-cell response). Moreover, a "memory" of viral infection endures in the immune system; if the same pathogen is encountered again, this "memory" triggers a rapid and effective response which often protects the patient from re-infection.

This protective immune response is the key to the success of vaccination. **Vaccination is the process by which the host is rendered immune to a pathologic organism without suffering through the disease itself.** As Pasteur and Jenner discovered, there are 2 ways of producing immunity without producing disease. One is to use killed virus, the other is to use live virus of reduced pathogenicity. Killed virus is inactivated in such a way (e.g., by heat) that it can no longer replicate, but its antigenicity is preserved. The dead virus stimulates production of antibodies in the bloodstream without causing disease. Vaccination with dead virus is quite safe, but may not provide adequate protection, because non-replicating virus cannot stimulate production of tissue-specific antibodies (IgA) or antibodies to viral proteins which are not encapsidated in virions. Vaccination with attenuated, live virus usually causes a fuller immune response. We owe this method to the English physician Jenner, at that time a country practitioner, who observed that milkmaids who contracted cowpox were immune to smallpox. He then used the living cowpox virus, which causes a mild disease in humans, to prevent smallpox infection. (The word vaccination is derived from this experience, Latin *vacca* meaning cow). Today, viruses can be attenuated by repeated replication in a laboratory culture, where, deprived of normal host conditions, they lose their virulence. Attenuated strains can also be generated using techniques of modern recombinant DNA technology. When attenuated virus is used in vaccination, a normal infection is mimicked and tissue antibodies are produced as well as circulating antibodies. Replication of the attenuated virus, and therefore development of the desired immunity, can sometimes be blocked by inapparent, but concurrent, infections in the host. The greater potential of attenuated vaccines is also accompanied by several disadvantages. There are usually more disease-like symptoms after live vaccination, and occasionally there are other contaminants in live vaccine preparations. Live virus will be released from vaccinees, which may present a danger to nonimmune individuals in their environment. Finally, the attenuated virus can on occasion regain its potency, posing a danger to vaccinees and their contacts.

There has been tremendous debate over the relative merits and dangers of the 2 types of vaccine: dead or live attenuated virus. The controversy surrounding the use of the Sabin polio vaccine (attenuated) or the Salk vaccine (dead) provides the best example. For viruses which are not easily attenuated, or which can establish latency or increase the chance of developing neoplasias, live vaccines are untenable.

New approaches to vaccination are being developed as a result of modern biotechnology. Recombinant DNA technology has allowed biologists to study isolated viral genes and to learn about immunogenic viral peptides in depth. These techniques—as well as very exciting advances in the science of synthesizing specific peptides—are allowing scientists to produce antigens in bulk. These may well be a major source of vaccination material in the future. Finally, scientists are splicing genes for the proteins of one virus into the chromosome of another virus. Genes of dangerous and poorly understood pathogens—herpes simplex and hepatitis viruses—have been introduced into the vaccinia genome, where they are integrally expressed during the vaccinia life cycle. Since vaccinia was used successfully in world-wide eradication of

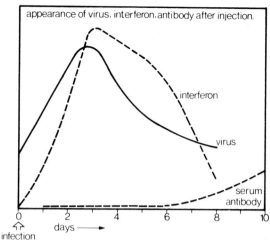

Fig. 8–2 This graph shows the temporal sequence between the appearance of virus, the appearance of interferon, and the appearance of serum antibodies following infection. (Adapted from Roitt, I.: *Essential Immunology*, 3rd Ed. Oxford, Blackwell Scientific Publications, 1977.)

smallpox, its potential as a vehicle for eliciting multiple immunities is promising and exciting. In animal studies, these recombinant vaccinia viruses have been used to establish immunity to influenza, herpes simplex I and II, and hepatitis B infection. Although much work remains to be done, new options for vaccination are clearly emerging.

Some viral diseases do not lend themselves well to

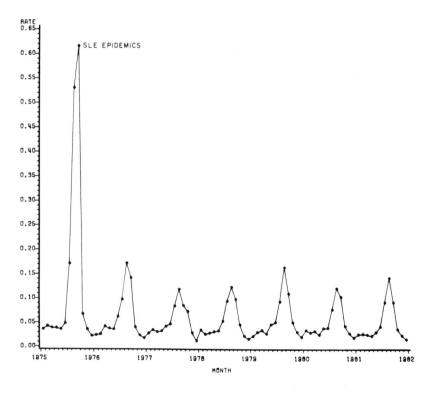

Fig. 8–3 Encephalitis reporting for 1981 was typical of years without major arbovirus epidemics. The most recent year with major arboviral epidemics was 1975 when St. Louis encephalitis outbreaks appeared in several large geographic areas of the United States. The seasonal increase in incidence probably reflects a composite of increased arboviral and enteroviral activity during the warmer months. (From Centers for Disease Control: Morbidity and Mortality Weekly Report, 30(54):33, 1982.)

Table 8–1. The Taxonomy of the Major Viruses Associated with Human Disease

FAMILY	GENERA	EXAMPLES
RNA VIRUSES		
+ strand genome		
Picornaviruses	Entero- Rhino-	Poliovirus, Cocksackievirus, Hepatitis A Rhinoviruses (common cold)
Caliciviruses	Calici-	Norwalk agent, Hepatitis E
Coronaviruses	Corona-	Coronovirus (common cold)
Togaviruses	Alpha- Rubi-	Eastern, Western, Venezuelan encephalitis Rubella virus
Flaviviruses	Flavi- ?	Yellow fever, Dengue fever (arboviruses) Hepatitis C
Retroviruses	Onco- Lenti-	HTLV I and II HIV I and II (AIDS)
– strand genome		
Rhabdoviruses	Vesiculo- Lyssa-	 Rabies virus
Filoviruses		Marburg virus, Ebola virus
Paramyxoviruses	Paramyxo- Morbilli- Pneumo-	Parainfluenza, mumps viruses Measles virus Respiratory syncytial virus
– strand segmented *genome*		
Orthomyxoviruses	Influenza- Type C	Influenza types A, B Influenza type C
Arenaviruses	Arena-	Lassa fever

Bunyaviruses	Bunya-
	Phlebo-
	Nairi
	Hanta-
		California encephalitis,
		  LaCrosse virus
		Sandfly fever, Rift valley
		  fever
		Crimean-Congo hemorrhagic
		  fever
		Hantavirus disease

double-stranded *genome*		
Reoviruses	Reo- Orbi- Rota-	 Colorado tick fever Non-bacterial infantile diarrhea viruses
DNA VIRUSES		
Hepadnaviruses		Hepatitis B virus
Papovaviruses	Polyoma Papilloma	JC, BKV Human Papilloma Viruses (HPV-16)
Parvoviruses	Dependo- Parvo-	Adeno-associated virus (AAV) B19
Adenoviruses		Adenoviruses (respiratory diseases)
Herpesviruses	Alpha-	Herpes simplex I and II, Varicella zoster

vaccination. These are diseases that result from many viral serotypes. The term serotype refers to the different antigenic properties that members of a virus species may possess. For example, there are 3 serotypes of poliovirus identical in all respects except for the surface markers (proteins) that serve as antigenic stimuli to the host immune system. Vaccination with 1 polio serotype provides no protection against the other 2, hence poliomyelitis vaccines contain all 3 types. The host who has formed all 3 antibody types for polio is immune to the disease. Poliomyelitis does not present a big vaccination problem. However, in the case of influenza, or of the "common cold," the number of serotypes is much greater, and it is impractical to protect against the large numbers of strains occurring in the wild. Similarly, natural immunity from an infection does not protect against later bouts with different serotypes. Hence we all contract many colds, but only one case of measles.

Since viruses must have a host, they have had to evolve along with host defenses such as immunity. Some viruses, such as influenza, have established mechanisms for frequent change, so that immunity as a result of prior infection does not block their infection. Other viruses can survive only in large populations, where the introduction of new preimmune hosts is frequent enough to provide for maintenance of the virus. The childhood diseases of mumps and measles fit this pattern. Other viruses persist in the host and are reactivated years later. Still others are maintained in an animal reservoir, in which breeding is sufficiently rapid that there are always new hosts, although each infection may kill or may induce lifelong immunity.

In addition to the host's immune response, there is another general, antiviral defense mechanism. Cells that have been infected with virus produce and secrete proteins capable of inhibiting or interfering with the growth of many viruses, the stimulus for this probably being viral nucleic acid. These proteins, named the **interferons**, seem to have many of the properties of a viral antibiotic. Interferon spreads to other cells in which it creates an antiviral state that renders those cells unable to support viral replication. The antiviral state may also be produced in the original infected cell and may modify the on-going infection cycle. This defense mechanism is different from the immune system. Immune antibodies are specific, differing for each disease and each infecting organism. Interferons show no specificity with respect to the infecting organism, but different classes of interferons are specifically produced by different cell types. In addition, interferons show species specificity and are relatively inactive when tested on foreign cell types. Antibodies only begin to make their appearance relatively late in the disease, whereas interferon is found in large quantities often during early stages of infection (Fig. 8–2).

E.coli
2μ

chlamydia
3000Å

herpes
variola
vaccinia
2000-3000Å

mumps
1200Å

influenza
800Å

adenovirus
700Å

yellow fever
220Å

poliomyelitis
100Å

red blood cell 8μ

Fig. 8–4 This illustration shows the relative sizes of a red blood cell, half of which is shown in a silhouette the length of the figure, and a bacterium (E. coli), which is shown in the upper part of the field. Chlamydia, herpes, mumps, and the smaller viruses are also indicated. (Adapted from Pelczar, M., Jr., et al.: *Microbiology*, 4th Ed. New York, McGraw-Hill, 1977.)

Because viruses insinuate themselves so thoroughly into the workings of the host cell, development of antiviral "antibiotics" has been difficult. However, as our knowledge of the unique features of each virus increases, drugs targeted at specific viral enzymes have been developed. Most antiviral agents are directed at inhibition of viral polymerases; many are nucleoside analogues. Acyclovir (used to treat

Herpes simplex I and II), gancyclovir (used to treat herpesviruses, especially cytomegalovirus), vidarabine (used to treat Herpes simplex I and varicella zoster), ribavirin (used to treat respiratory syncytial virus), and amantadine (effective against influenza A) are promising examples of modern antiviral therapeutics. Zidovudine (AZT) is another anti-viral agent of current importance, having shown some therapeutic efficacy in treating HIV (the etiologic agent of AIDS) infections.

TRANSMISSION

The usual routes of transmission of viral infections are through the respiratory or gastrointestinal tracts. Unhygienic conditions and crowded environments are key factors in viral spread and control. Viruses may also spread by direct skin contact, as in animal or insect bites. **Arboviruses** (*arthropod-borne*) are transmitted by insect vectors. The insect is not a passive carrier; arboviruses are capable of productive growth in insects although no disease is present. In temperate climates the presence of disease coincides with the distribution of the insects (Fig. 8–3). Insects then transmit the viruses to a plentiful reservoir of animal hosts, where disease results. Arboviruses are not endemic to human populations, but rather they become significant after migrations into new environments. These infections are among the most virulent and lethal of human diseases, yellow fever or encephalitis, for example.

Viruses have been classified historically by the tissue they infect, by their size or shape, and more recently by their nucleic acid and enzymatic characteristics. Table 8–1 outlines a contemporary catalog of viruses (Fig. 8–4).

RNA VIRUSES

These are viruses whose genome is composed of RNA. We shall consider first the smallest and simplest of the RNA viruses.

Picornaviruses

These viruses (Italian *pico*, small, and *rna*) fall into two general subdivisions: enteroviruses (polio-, coxsackie, echo-) and rhinoviruses.

They are nonenveloped viruses that have within their icosahedral shells a single + strand RNA genome of approximately 7.5 kilobases. This RNA directs the synthesis of one long polypeptide which is subsequently cleaved to the mature proteins. In addition to 4 structural proteins, these viruses encode a protease(s) involved in polyprotein processing, a replicase, and a protein linked to the genomic terminus which plays a role in viral repliation. Replication of the RNA through a double-stranded intermediate supplies a pool of virion RNA. Replication, translation, and assembly of the virus occur in the cytoplasm. Shutdown of host RNA and protein synthesis is rapid and dramatic. Picornaviruses have evolved an effective means of ensuring that only viral proteins are translated. The mRNA cap-binding complex of the cell is inactivated, rendering capped host mRNAs untranslatable. Viral mRNAs possess a 5' sequence which ensures efficient translation in the absence of a cap or a cap-binding complex. At the completion of the infectious cycle after approximately 8 hours, newly assembled virions are released by lysis of the infected cell.

Enteroviruses. These are unusually acid- and bile-resistant. In light of their transmission by ingestion and their intestinal site for multiplication this resistance is teleologically understandable. They can be grown in tissue culture with striking cytocidal effects.

Poliovirus exists in three serotypes that are infectious only for primate cells. Interestingly, most (90–95%) poliovirus infections are inapparent. Of those that are clinical, many cause a mild disease with headache, nausea, and fever. A few cases progress to aseptic meningitis, with pains in the back and neck, ending in rapid and complete recovery. In less than 2% of total cases, poliovirus infection causes flaccid paralysis, frequently with loss of anterior horn cells and the consequent loss of muscle innervation, which may be prolonged and is often irreversible. Poliomyelitis has existed since ancient times, was documented as early as the late 1700s, and continues as an important clinical problem today in developing countries.

After ingestion of the virus, there is a 1- to 2-week incubation period with viral multiplication in the lymphoid tissues of the pharynx and gut. This period may be followed by viremia and distribution of the virus to secondary target organs. Recent studies suggest that skeletal muscle may be an important target tissue. Poliovirus replicates preferentially at this stage in the anterior horn cells of the spinal cord and causes the characteristic paralysis. (Greek *polios* [gray] refers to the gray matter of the spinal cord.)

Environmental factors that increase the likelihood of paralysis have been discussed and described, such as pregnancy, fatigue, vigorous exercise concurrent with infection, and tonsillectomy. Early in the 20th century, with poorer sanitation, poliovirus was endemic. Most people suffered inapparent or mild infections at a young age. As hygiene improved, this widespread (herd) immunity changed. People were more likely to be exposed later in childhood, when the chances of serious complications are higher. There were also significant numbers of susceptible nonimmune persons, and the virus usually spread in an epidemic fashion when it appeared. Poliomyelitis has declined dramatically with the advent of the Salk (killed) and Sabin (live) vaccines. In 1952, just before the Salk vaccine became generally available in the United States, there were 3,145 deaths and 21,269 cases of paralysis, whereas in 1969 there were only 19 cases of paralytic polio and not a single death (Fig. 8–5). An average of 12 cases of poliomyelitis are recorded annually in the United States, and many of these arise following vaccination with live, attenuated virus. In the developing countries of the world, poliovirus remains a major clinical problem which causes significant morbidity and mortality.

Molecular and genetic analysis of poliovirus has flourished in the last few years since the synthesis of an infectious cDNA (complementary DNA) copy of the virus with recombinant DNA methodologies. The availability of a DNA copy of the genome has permitted scientists to introduce subtle and dramatic alterations into the viral genes and to identify regions which

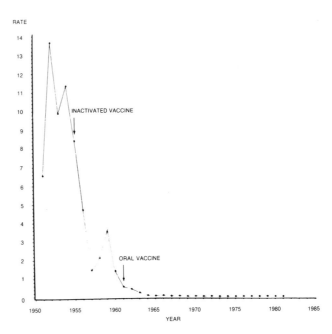

Fig. 8–5 Poliomyelitis (paralytic)—reported cases per 100,000 population, by year, United States, 1951–1981. (From Centers for Disease Control: Morbidity and Mortality Weekly Report, 30(54):69, 1982.)

play important roles in determining infectivity, neurovirulence, receptor-attachment, etc. The cellular receptor for poliovirus has been identified and cloned; it is an integral membrane protein present on the outer surfaces of many human cells. Transgenic mice which express the receptor for human poliovirus have been generated, and these mice are susceptible to poliovirus infection and to the associated paralytic disease. This is a tremendous breakthrough which will allow scientists to understand how poliovirus spreads through the body, which tissues permit viral growth, how paralysis develops, and how vaccines and/or antiviral therapies can be used to block disease. Finally, the crystal structure of poliovirus has been solved, and this structural information in conjunction with the precise knowledge of specific mutations which decrease viral infectivity is allowing a picture of virus-cell interaction to be drawn in increasing detail. These advances should allow the development of safe attenuated vaccines and raise hopes that worldwide control of poliovirus infection is a reasonable goal.

Coxsackieviruses and **echoviruses** have similar life cycles and are responsible for many illnesses. These include febrile abdominal illnesses, rashes, upper respiratory tract infections, meningitis, and myocardiopathy. There are far too many serotypes to make vaccines a sensible or practical possibility. Persistent infection with **Coxsackie B** virus has also been implicated in the etiology of the recently recognized **post-viral fatigue syndrome** (PVFS) (also known as chronic fatigue syndrome, myalgic encephalomyelitis [ME]). This poorly defined syndrome is associated with significant skeletal muscle fatigue, and patients complain of recurrent headache and decreased concentration. The illness can persist for weeks or months, and often follows from an acute "viral" illness. The syndrome has been seen with increasing frequency, and cases fall into both sporadic and epidemic classes.

Hepatitis A. The disease known as hepatitis is actually a group of similar diseases with distinct viral etiologies. Hepatitis A (previously known as infectious hepatitis) is caused by an enterovirus with a particle size of 27 nm and the characteristic positive-strand RNA genome. The virion possesses the acid-resistance common to the enterovirus family; HAV virions are unusually temperature-resistant as well. HAV is generally transmitted by the fecal-oral route. Contaminated water systems and food supplies have often been incriminated: unsanitary conditions and polluted shellfish are the suspected causes of most outbreaks. Transmission via intravenous drug use is an increasing problem, and sexual contact as a mode of infection is now also recognized. Person-to-person

spread is especially troublesome because non-symptomatic individuals shed virus during the incubation period, making quarantine or prophylactic treatment of contacts difficult. The virus is endemic in developing countries, and most adults are immune. There is only one recognizable serotype. The distribution of Hepatitis A in the United States is shown in Figure 8–6, its incidence in Figure 8–7.

The disease begins abruptly with a preicteric stage following an average incubation period of 30 days. This phase is characterized by fever, nausea, anorexia, and abdominal discomfort. Laboratory tests reveal elevated enzyme levels characteristic of liver dysfunction. A week later the icteric stage follows with the onset of jaundice, although this diagnostic hallmark is frequently absent in children. Jaundice recedes after roughly 2 weeks, and 90% of infected individuals experience full recovery. The hepatic pathology is probably not a reflection of the direct cytopathic effects of the virus, but is rather a consequence of the immune response of activated T-lymphocytes. Seropositivity against the virus is usually detectable by the onset of clinical symptoms, and immunity is thought to be life-long. Until recently, the only effective prophylactic measure has been the administration of immune globulin (IG) to exposed contacts. When given before or within 2 weeks of exposure, illness is prevented in 80 to 90% of individuals. The ubiquity of hepatitis A infection, and the increasing severity of the disease as the average age of affected individuals increases with improved hygiene, are ample incentives to develop an effective vaccine. The presence of only one viral serotype and the longevity of anti-hepatitis A immunity suggest that this is a feasible goal. Killed-virus vaccines have been prepared and shown to be safe and effective in animal trials; promising clinical studies which address the vaccine's safety and immunogenicity in man are underway. Efforts at developing live attenuated vaccine strains have also been reported, although it is more likely that the killed-virus vaccine will be licensed and available in the near future.

Rhinoviruses. Although they are more acid-labile, these viruses are similar to the enteroviruses. They have a clear preference for growth in vitro at 33°C. This preference is consistent with their localization in the nasal passages, which are cooler than the core body temperature. Rhinoviruses are the causative agents of many of our "common colds." Experimental work has shown that nasal entry is the most efficient mode of infection, and that virus shedding starts as soon as 24 hours after entry and can continue for weeks. Edema of mucus membranes, fluid exudation, increased secretory activity of submucosal glands,

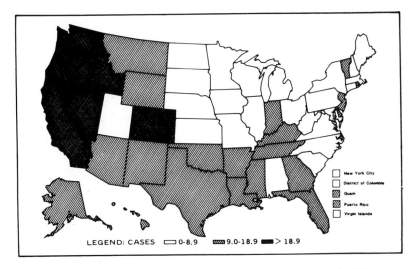

Fig. 8–6   Reported hepatitis A cases/100,000 population, by state, United States, 1981. (From Centers for Disease Control: Morbidity and Mortality Weekly Report, 32(2SS):24SS, 1983.)

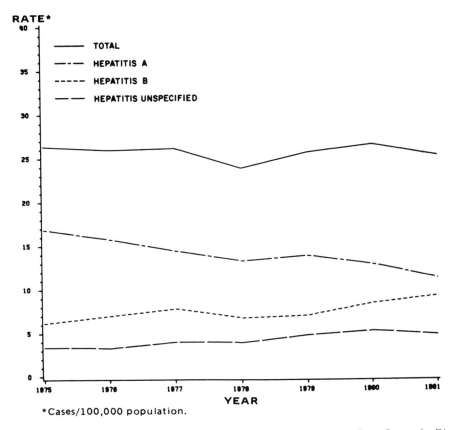

Fig. 8–7   Reported incidence of viral hepatitis, by type and year, United States, 1975–1981. (From Centers for Disease Control: Morbidity and Mortality Weekly Report, 32(2SS):24SS, 1983.)

and coughing are at their peak 2 to 3 days after infection. This continues for about a week. The virus titer is highest in nasal secretions rather than in saliva. Sneezes are contagious. The primary route of infection is thought to be by contamination of the contactee's hands followed by transfer to the nose or mouth. Antibodies are stimulated by rhinovirus infection; whether clinical improvement is a function of antibody intervention or of interferon induction is debatable. The cellular receptor for rhinoviruses has recently been identified as **ICAM-1**, an integral membrane protein whose normal function pertains to cellular adhesion. The potential for development of antiviral therapies based on interference with virus-receptor interactions is of obvious interest. The number of rhinovirus serotypes is enormous, and so any thoughts of classical virus-based vaccines are not productive.

Caliciviruses

These spherical viruses have a diameter of approximately 33 nm; the faces and apices of the icosahedral surface are characterized by cup-shaped hollows. One major polypeptide of 66 kDa comprises the viral capsid, within which is contained the 9 kb, + sense RNA genome. Detailed analysis of these viruses has been impaired by an inability to establish productive infections in tissue culture, but their association with acute outbreaks of vomiting and diarrhea is clear.

Norwalk Agent. Although the definitive molecular comparisons remain to be completed, this etiological agent of viral gastroenteritis is thought to be a member of the **calicivirus** family. Epidemic outbreaks occur during all seasons and have affected families, camps, schools, nursing homes, cruise ships and restaurants. Person-to-person spread and waterborne transmission are the primary routes of spread.

After an incubation period of 18 to 48 hours, the illness is marked by diarrhea and vomiting of 24 to 48 hours' duration. Recovery is then rapid and full. The virus appears to induce characteristic lesions in the proximal small intestine of infected individuals. Immunity following recovery is short-lived and susceptibility returns after 27 to 42 months. Interestingly, one third of volunteers fed the virus remained well, although no evidence of pre-existing antibody was found. These individuals showed a consistent resistance on re-challenge, suggesting that some unknown non-immune factors may play a role in determining susceptibility to Norwalk infection.

Hepatitis E virus. The Hepatitis E virus is the etiologic agent of enterically transmitted non-A, non-B hepatitis. It has recently been isolated and appears to be most closely related to the **calicivirus** family. This form of hepatitis is associated with outbreaks which can affect tens of thousands of individuals; these outbreaks affect developing countries and are particularly common in the Indian subcontinent. Fecally contaminated water is the culprit in transmission of Hepatitis E. Following exposure, a 6 week incubation period is typical, followed by development of a self-limiting hepatitis. Transmission to secondary contacts is inefficient, perhaps because of the observed lability of the Hepatitis E virion. Young adults appear to be most suceptible; an unusually high mortality rate (20%) is associated with infection of pregnant women.

Togaviruses

These viruses are composed of an RNA genome inside a capsid, which in turn is surrounded by a membranous envelope (hence Latin *toga*, cloak). The genomes of togaviruses (alphaviruses and rubiviruses are the genera of medical importance) are composed of single-stranded RNA of + polarity and are approximately 9 (rubiviruses) to 12 (alphaviruses) kilobases in length.

Togaviruses multiply in the cytoplasm and replicate much as do picornaviruses. Host protein synthesis shuts off rapidly; RNA synthesis stops late in infection. During their assembly, viral cores line up at the cell membrane under patches in which viral glycoproteins have become embedded. The virions then bud off, surrounded by a lipid and glycoprotein envelope. Virion budding leaves the cell intact. The single segment of the togavirus genome is transcribed into more than 1 mRNA species, which in turn are translated into viral proteins. This is a first step towards increasing genetic complexity, and probably allows more evolutionary or adaptive flexibility than the simple system employed by picornaviruses. With 2 mRNAs, the timing and relative quantities of protein synthesis can differ.

Alphaviruses. This genus contains numerous human pathogens, including several which induce encaphalitis and others which cause fever, rash and polyarthritis. All of these viruses are *arboviruses*, referring to their mode of transmission (*ar*thropod-*bo*rne). Birds, rodents or equines serve as natural animal reservoirs for these viruses, and mosquitos are the major means of transmission. The animal population supplies new susceptible hosts through breeding; the high virus titers in the animal blood during the viremic phase provide a rich source for viral passage by the blood-sucking insects. The virus replicates efficiently within the insects without cytopathic effects. In vitro, arboviruses have been shown to infect both insect and vertebrate cell cultures, demonstrating their flexibility with respect to the host environment. The ability of the same virus to replicate effectively in insects and in a variety of birds and mammals provided irrefutable support for the universality of the genetic code.

Alphaviruses cause significant morbidity and mortality in the United States and elsewhere in the world today. **Eastern equine encephalitis virus** (EEE) (Fig. 8–8), for example, causes sporadic but severe problems in swampy areas of the eastern United States, such as Massachusetts. The disease is spread to horses and humans through the bite of infected mosquitoes, and causes an encephalitis which frequently progresses to coma and death. Survivors may have severe neurological sequelae. A less virulent encephalitis is caused by **Western equine encephalitis virus** (WEE), another mosquito-borne alphavirus. **Venezuelan equine encephalitis** (VEE) virus causes a febrile, influenza-like illness which rarely culminates in encephalitis. For all of these viruses, prevention of infection is of highest importance and is accomplished by avoidance of insect bites. Monitoring and control of the animal reservoir species is also essential; for most of these viruses, man is an incidental host.

Chikungunya virus, O'nyong-nyong virus, Sindbis virus, Mayaro virus, and Ross river virus are examples of alphaviruses which induce an acute febrile illness with characteristic arthralgia and myalgia in infected patients. These viruses are endemic or cause sporadic epidemics in various parts of South-east Asia, India, East Africa, South America, Australia and the South Pacific. Outbreaks are associated with climatic conditions which amplify the insect vector population; during explosive epidemics, the virus can be spread directly from one viremic individual to another by insect bites.

Rubiviruses. The sole member of this genus is the **rubella**, or German measles, virus. This is a non-arthropod-borne togavirus that is transmitted by inhalation, after which it multiplies in the upper respiratory tract and passes into the blood stream by means of the cervical lymph nodes. It causes a trivial rash, which involves the face and is probably due to localized antigen-antibody reactions. There is one serotype, man is the only known natural host, and immunity is long-lasting.

The importance of rubella is that it affects the fetus of pregnant women in the first trimester. It exerts teratogenic effects on the fetus which can cause blindness, deafness, heart defects, and retardation. The mechanism responsible for this pathology is unknown, but it is likely that infected fetal cells survive but divide too slowly or abnormally. The virus spreads through contiguous cells of the fetus. This renders maternal antibody inefficient in halting the infection. Thus organs derived from infected cells are often improperly developed. Clearly, exposure of pregnant, nonimmune women to rubella virus may have serious consequences. Immunization with attenuated viral strains was introduced in 1969, and the incidence of infection has been drastically reduced (Figs. 8–9, 8–10).

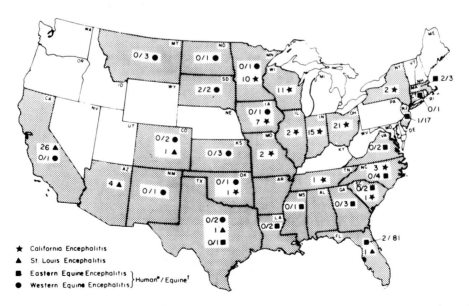

Fig. 8–8 Arboviral infections of the central nervous system—United States, 1984. (From Centers for Disease Control, Morbidity and Mortality Weekly Report, 34(20):284, 1985.)

Fig. 8–9 Incidence rates of reported rubella and congenital rubella syndrome—United States, 1966–1990. (From Centers for Disease Control: Morbidity and Mortality Weekly Report, 40(6):93, 1991.)

Flaviviruses

The flaviviruses were previously classified as a genus of the togavirus family, but have recently been given status as an independent virus family. Like togaviruses, these arboviruses are enveloped, spherical viruses with a single-stranded RNA genome of + polarity. However, the flavivirus genome is not polyadenylated, only a single mRNA species is thought to be transcribed, and no evidence of polyprotein precursors has been found. Finally, virion assembly is thought to involve budding of the virions into intra-

cellular cisternae rather than from the plasma membrane.

The members of the flavivirus family include numerous human pathogens. Tick- and mosquito-borne viruses cause a variety of encephalitides; other flaviviruses cause general or hemorrhagic febrile illnesses such as yellow fever or dengue fever. Finally, the Hepatitis C virus responsible for inducing blood-borne non-A non-B hepatitis has recently been identified and is distantly related to the flaviviruses.

The **St. Louis Encephalitis** virus (SLE) causes the most important arboviral disease in North America. The disease may be asymptomatic, especially in children, or may be accompanied by febrile disease associated with severe headache, aseptic meningitis, or encephalitis. **Japanese encephalitis** was a major health concern in Asia; vector control and the introduction of a killed-virus vaccine have led to a remarkable reduction in the incidence of the disease.

Yellow Fever. Few arbovirus infections have been of such broad economic and political significance to man as the agent responsible for yellow fever. The real interest, indeed romance, of yellow fever is not so much the virus that causes it as the means by which the virus is transmitted. Until 1900, it was believed that the disease was due to unsanitary conditions, that the infection was probably conveyed from the sick to the healthy by intestinal discharges. In that year, the American Yellow Fever Commission under Walter Reed determined to put to the test the theory that a mosquito might carry the infection, as had al-

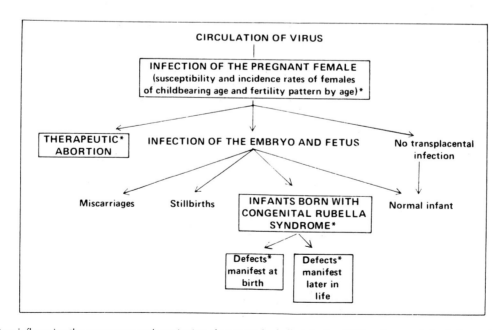

Fig. 8–10 Factors influencing the occurrence and monitoring of congenital rubella infection (CRI) and congenital rubella syndrome (CRS). (From Centers for Disease Control, Morbidity and Mortality Weekly Report, 33(4SS):1SS, 1983.)

ready been shown to be the case with malaria. At that time no animal was known to be susceptible to the disease, so human volunteers had to be used. These persons allowed themselves to be bitten by mosquitoes that had already fed on yellow fever patients. One member of the Commission, Dr. Carroll, developed yellow fever and nearly died; a second, Dr. Lazear, became even more desperately ill and finally did die.

The centuries-old problem of yellow fever had at last been solved. The disease was transmitted by a mosquito, the female *Stegomyia* (different variety from the *Anopheles* that carries malaria). If the *Stegomyia* could be destroyed, the scourge of the tropics could be eradicated. The successful control of yellow fever opened up South and Central America, made Rio de Janeiro habitable, and made the Panama Canal possible.

These arthropod-borne viruses are injected into the capillaries of the host with saliva when the insect bites. The viruses multiply in the vascular endothelium and the reticular cells of lymph nodes, liver, and spleen. This phase is characterized by viremia, and may represent the full course of the disease. Flaviviruses are potent stimulators of interferon. Progress of the infection may cause arthralgia and rashes. In the case of yellow fever, the virus attacks the capillaries and causes hemorrhaging, particularly in the liver and the kidneys. The most characteristic lesions are in the liver, which shows areas of necrosis, inclusion bodies, and rupture of the biliary passages with escape of bile into the blood. The chief symptoms are fever, vomiting, diarrhea, and intense jaundice, so that the skin turns yellow. In epidemics there is a mortality rate of 80%. Because of the extensive viremia accompanying these viral diseases, survivors have a life-long, type-specific immunity. There is now an effective yellow fever vaccine that employs a lab-attenuated strain.

Dengue virus (Fig. 8–11), another flavivirus, causes frequent outbreaks in Southeast Asia. Infection is followed by headache, myalgia, arthralgia, nausea, and vomiting. Fever is intense and often follows a saddleback curve. A rash may follow; full recovery is usual. The same virus, however, may also cause dengue hemorrhagic fever, a far more serious disease with high fevers, shock, and hemorrhagic diathesis. As in all of these arbovirus-induced fevers, control of the insect virus population is the primary means of disease prevention.

Hepatitis C virus. The identity of the agent(s) causing non-A non-B hepatitis eluded virologists for many years. Recently, investigators concentrated the particulate fraction from plasma of chronically infected chimpanzees and purified all of the nucleic acids contained within this pellet. Molecular clones of all of the nucleic acid sequences (both RNA and DNA) were generated in vitro and propagated in a bacteriophage library. Host bacteria were directed to synthesize the

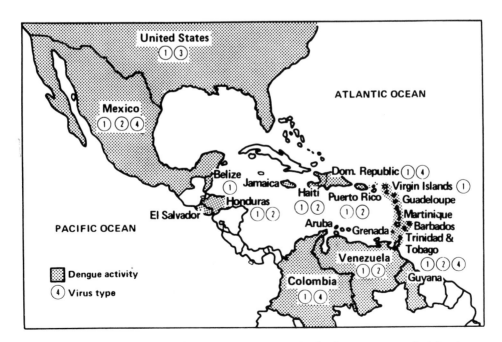

Fig. 8–11 Dengue has been endemic in the Americas for over 200 years. Recently, the disease appears to be following a pattern similar to that in Southeast Asia 30 years ago, where many countries began to report increased occurrence of sporadic cases of DHF in association with increased incidence of dengue infection. (From Centers for Disease Control, Morbidity and Mortality Weekly Report, 35(4):57, 1986.)

proteins encoded by these nucleic acid fragments, and filters containing these proteins were screened with antisera from chronically infected patients. This technique identified fragments of the Hepatitis C genome encoding viral antigens and allowed the complete RNA molecule to be identified and analyzed. The genome is a single + strand RNA molecule of 10 kb which encodes a polyprotein containing both structural and non-structural components. The organization and sequence of the proteins shows some similarity (although distant) to other flaviviruses, and has been tentatively assigned to a new genus within this family.

HCV transmission can occur via transfusion or from contaminated needles; however, a large number of cases seem unlinked to either of these routes of transmission. Sexual transmission of the virus is a distinct possibility. Many cases are asymptomatic, and the acute hepatitis which does occur is generally mild. However, relapsing or chronic hepatitis are frequent outcomes. Cirrhosis of the liver is associated with 20% of chronic infections. An association of viral infection with the development of hepatocellular carcinoma has also been found. The identification of the etiologic agent has opened the way for screening of blood banks, a preventative measure which will reduce transfusion-related HCV infection.

Coronaviruses

These enveloped viruses contain a single-stranded RNA genome of approximately 12 kb. The capped, polyadenylated genome is of + polarity; within the infected cell, a cRNA of − polarity is synthesized which serves as the template for the transcription of six subgenomic mRNAs. The viral proteins subsequently synthesized include four components of the virion itself. The 80–120 nm virions mature by budding into the endoplasmic reticulum of the infected cell; the glycoprotein peplomers which project from the surface of the virion form the characteristic "corona" observed in the electron microscope.

Human coronavirus infection is associated with respiratory tract illness. The most common presentation is an acute "common cold" of a week's duration; approximately 10% of acute respiratory tract illness in children is ascribed to coronavirus etiology. A role for coronaviruses in the etiology of gastroenteritis and diarrheal illness has also been proposed.

Rhabdoviruses

The rhabdoviruses are bullet-shaped, enveloped viruses with a 12 kb genome consisting of a single segment of − strand RNA. Viral proteins include a nucleocapsid protein, a surface glycoprotein, a matrix protein, and putative polymerase proteins. The glycoprotein spikes of the virus have hemagglutinating activity. The proteins are translated from multiple mRNAs (each coding for 1 protein) derived from the single genomic RNA, and thus can vary in the timing and level of their synthesis. In some cases host functions are shut off completely; in other instances infected cells continue to produce virus persistently. The virus enters cells by membrane fusion or phagocytosis. Newly produced virions leave the cell by budding. Frequently, characteristic acidophilic inclusions known as Negri bodies appear in the cytoplasm of infected cells. These are ribonucleoprotein complexes that persist in the cells but are not released and not infective.

Rabies Virus. This rhabdovirus infects most warm-blooded animals. Bats are thought to be asymptomatic carriers. Their urine, which they spray when flying, contains the virus, and even the air of densely populated bat caves may be dangerous to breathe. In other hosts, the disease is violent and usually fatal. A characteristic behavior of rabid animals is the frenzied biting of other animals. Since the virus is present in saliva, it is spread effectively. Rabies infection is zoonotic; infection of humans is incidental and results from exposure to infected animals, both wild (raccoons, foxes, skunks, bats) and domesticated (dogs) (Fig. 8–12).

Symptomatic rabies occurs in roughly one-half of exposed cases; the incubation time, usually 1 to 3 months, may range from 1 week to 1 year. The disease begins with general malaise and hyperesthesia in the wound. The principal symptoms, whether in animal or in man, are terrific cerebral excitement and rage, spasm of the muscles of the pharynx, especially at the sight of water, so that the patient is unable to drink, and generalized convulsions. It is one of the most terrible of all diseases, and when symptoms have developed, is almost always fatal. The virus does not spread from the wound by means of the blood stream, but rather along the neurons. Amputation of the infected area can halt the disease. The lesions are entirely microscopic, for the brain appears normal to the naked eye. Microscopically, there is degeneration of the nerve cells and collars of inflammatory cells around the small vessels, but the pathognomonic feature is the presence of Negri bodies. When a dog suspected of rabies has bitten a person, it must be killed and its brain examined for Negri bodies. After exposure to the disease, persons are usually given immune serum, followed by rabies vaccine. This procedure is

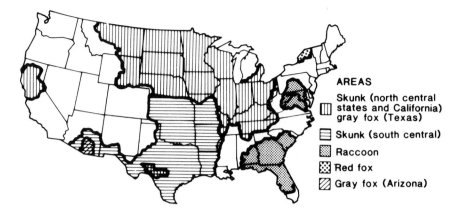

Fig. 8–12 Distribution of five antigenically distinct rabies virus strains and the predominant wildlife species affected contiguous United States. (From Centers for Disease Control, Morbidity and Mortality Weekly Report, 35(35):555, 1986.)

generally effective because of the long incubation period of the disease. It is remarkable that the modern treatment of rabies was introduced by Pasteur, who knew nothing of filterable viruses. He found that the spinal cord of rabbits infected with the disease was rich in the infective agent, as shown by the results of animal inoculation. He also found that he could lower the virulence by drying the spinal cord; the longer the drying, the lower the virulence. Pasteur then used the material of low virulence as a vaccine, with which he repeatedly inoculated the person bitten by the rabid animal. By this means the patient built up resistance to the virus, so that by the time it reached the spinal cord some 2 months later, he had become immune. If the Pasteur treatment was commenced immediately after the bite, there was complete prevention in every case. Surely this was a stroke of pure genius in the earliest days of microbiology!

Control of rabid animals, vaccination of dogs, and effective treatment protocols have greatly reduced the frequency of symptomatic rabies. The incidence of rabies in the United States for the last several decades is shown in Figure 8–9. For exposed individuals, post-exposure prophylactic treatment should be undertaken immediately. Thorough irrigation of the wound and administration of immune globulin and rabies vaccine are recommended. Since symptomatic rabies is almost always fatal, these measures are of the greatest importance. The vaccine currently in use, a killed virus vaccine which was introduced in 1978 (human diploid cell vaccine), shows significant utility in preventing rabies in exposed patients. For the future, the technologies of recombinant DNA have opened up the potential for engineering more effective and safer rabies vaccines. Efforts aimed at using recombinant poxviruses encoding immunogenic rabies virus pro-

teins to immunize animals of key reservoir species are already underway. Elimination of rabies in foxes and raccoons would be of tremendous help in preventing human infection.

Filoviruses

The virion of this family of enveloped viruses is filamentous and pleiomorphic; it has a diameter of 80 nm, but the length of the particle is highly variable. Infectivity co-purifies with rod-like virions of approximately 1000 nm in length; within the outer envelope is a helical nucleocapsid. These viruses were previously thought to be indistinguishable from rhabdoviruses, but are now considered an independent family. The genome is contained in a single, 12 kb RNA strand of − polarity from which six polyadenylated mRNAs are transcribed. The virus can be grown in primate cell lines; infection leads to vigorous production of virions which are released by budding. The virus is highly cytopathic and infected cells lyse eventually. Filoviruses, which are human pathogens, include **Marburg virus** (MBO) and two distinct forms of **Ebola virus** (EBO). These viruses cause sporadic outbreaks which initiate from contact with infected monkeys or their tissues (blood, organs, cell cultures). Secondary spread is usually to medical or household contacts, mediated by contact with secretions or utilization of unsterilized needles. Because human-human transmission is inefficient, the outbreaks are usually transient. The disease, whose occurrence has largely been limited to sub-Saharan Africa, is characterized by an acute febrile illness accompanied by myalgia, anorexia, abdominal pain, rash and gastrointestinal bleeding. Recovery begins at the end of the first week in those rare non-fatal cases. Fatality is the most common outcome, with severe shock following generalized hemorrhage. Spread of filoviruses to other parts of the world has recently been confirmed and is associated with export of (infected) monkeys for vaccine production or research.

Paramyxoviruses

This family includes the genera *paramyxovirus, morbillivirus, and pneumovirus* which include **parainfluenza** and **mumps** viruses, **measles** virus and **respiratory syncytial** virus, respectively.

These enveloped viruses possess a genome of a single strand of −polarity RNA of approximately 18 kb. They can be grown in culture without extensive cell destruction. Cytologic characteristics are acidophilic inclusions and the frequent fusion of infected cells to form giant syncytia (multinucleate masses of cytoplasm produced by the merging of cells). Viruses multiply in the cytoplasm, using a viral transcriptase, and are released by budding through the cell membrane. Proteins are translated from multiple messages, and precursor proteins are cleaved during maturation. These processing steps probably involve host functions and are often essential in producing fully infectious virions. Proteins include nucleocapsid, matrix, and glycoprotein; glycoprotein spikes most often have hemagglutinating activities, and sometimes hemolysin and fusion potentiation as well. There is no dramatic shutdown of host cell functions.

Parainfluenza Viruses. Infecting the epithelia of the upper respiratory tract, symptomatic after a 2- to 6-day incubation period, these viruses may cause fever, pharyngitis, and bronchitis. In infants, lower respiratory tract involvement is common; one of the best-known complications is croup, an acute laryngotracheobronchitis caused primarily by parainfluenza 1. These viruses replicate locally in the respiratory epithelium and are highly contagious. Reinfection with similar serotypes is common, since the relevant antibody is tissue IgA, which is neither abundant nor long-lived. Even in the presence of circulating antibody, the disease progresses unchecked. These viruses occur worldwide and are typically endemic.

Mumps Virus. Upon infection of tissue culture cells, this virus produces characteristic inclusions in both the cytoplasmic and nuclear compartments, and induces the formation of giant syncytia. Its glycoproteins possess hemagglutinin, hemolysin, fusion and neuraminidase activity. Natural infection is limited to humans. Clinical infection shows seasonal variability, and one-half of mumps infections are inapparent. There is on average an 18-day incubation period. Virus multiplication is concentrated in the upper respiratory tract and lymph nodes, with 3 to 5 days of subsequent viremia. Prodromal symptoms include malaise, decreased appetite, fever and myalgia. The virus may then spread to characteristic target organs. The most common symptom by far is swelling of the parotid (salivary) gland(s). In postpubescent males, orchitis with or without resultant sterility is frequent. Meningitis follows in roughly 10% of the cases. Infection stimulates interferon and antibody production. Antibodies to the hemagglutinin antigen are thought to be the most long-lived and relevant to immunity. An effective mumps vaccine was licensed in 1967; as the prevalence of vaccination has increased, the incidence of mumps has shown a corresponding decline. The attenuated mumps vaccine is usually administered as part of a trivalent inoculum which also contains vaccines directed against rubella and measles. The incidence of mumps in the United States during the last 2 decades is shown in Figure 8–13.

Measles Virus. Epidemic measles infections have been a worldwide health problem for centuries. Severe epidemics accompanied immigration of infected patients to naive communities; with the increased mobility and mixing of communities epidemics became milder and more frequent. The availability of an attenuated virus vaccine has dramatically changed the appearance of measles in the western world and has made elimination of measles as an endemic childhood disease a possibility. In recent years, budgetary and administrative restrictions have hampered vaccination campaigns in cities such as New York, where episodic waves of measles infection remain a public health problem (Fig. 8–14).

Transmission is usually via inhalation. The virus then multiplies in the epithelia of the upper respiratory tract prior to spread to lymph nodes and secondary lymphoid tissues. T lymphocytes are important target cells for virus multiplication. In 9 to 12 days, antibody levels rise in the blood and the characteristic rash appears, commencing with Koplik's spots (red ulcerations inside the cheek). The rash is probably due to an antigen-antibody reaction. Other symptoms include fever, cough and conjunctivitis. Recovery is usually rapid and complete, and immunity is lifelong. Patients with compromised cell-mediated immunity suffer more severe infections.

In a few cases, encephalomyelitis may develop as a result of delayed hypersensitivity, when lymphocytes infiltrate infected neural tissue, sometimes causing demyelination. Even more rarely, a slow neurologic disease, SSPE (subacute sclerosing panencephalitis) is found in older children with a previous history of measles. SSPE patients have high levels of antibodies to most measles antigens, and tissue of the central

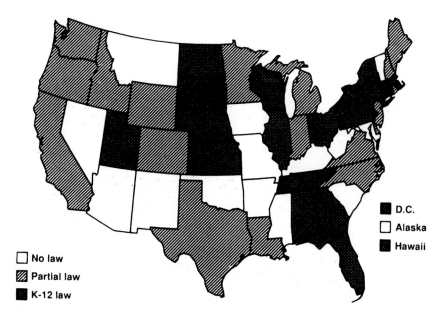

No law
Partial law
K-12 law

D.C.
Alaska
Hawaii

Fig. 8–13 Mumps school immunization laws, by reporting area— United States, December 31, 1988. (From Centers for Disease Control, Morbidity and Mortality Weekly Report, 38(7):105, 1989.)

nervous system contains a measles-like virus. Virus recovered from SSPE patients lacks the ability to produce the M, or matrix, protein. This protein is required for assembly and release of virions. Infection in the absence of the M protein is thought to induce a chronic infection in which virus remains cell-associated and spreads via cell-cell fusion. Under these circumstances, the absence of free extracellular virus would retard immune clearance, whereas infected cells bearing viral antigens on their plasma membranes might be a target for immune attack. Another variant of measles infection is atypical measles, a febrile disease associated with rash and pneumonia. This syndrome was associated with prior administration of a killed-virus vaccine; administration of this vaccine has obviously been halted and replaced with the current attenuated virus vaccine.

Fig. 8–14 Reported measles cases, United States, 1950–1984. (From Centers for Disease Control, Morbidity and Mortality Weekly Report, 34(21):309, 1985.)

Respiratory syncytial virus (RSV). This *pneumovirus* contains a 15 kb – strand RNA genome which is transcribed to ten mRNAs encoding ten viral proteins. Unlike the other genera of paramyxoviruses, the RSV virion does not have hemagglutination or hemolytic activities. The characteristic features of infection in culture or within the affected individual are the presence of cytoplasmic inclusions and the formation of giant multicellular syncytia.

In adults, RSV causes upper respiratory infections that are indistinguishable from colds. In infants, it can cause serious lower respiratory tract infections, in which secondary bacterial infection is the rule. These infections reach epidemic proportions annually in urban centers. Associated pathologies include bronchiolitis and pneumonia. Ribavirin, a nucleoside analogue, is an effective anti-viral agent recommended for therapeutic treatment of infants suffering from RSV infection. It is administered as an aerosol. Although immunity in recovered patients is not long-lived and does not prevent reinfection, the severity of subsequent infections is reduced. Significant efforts have been focused on the development of safe and effective RSV vaccines, but to date none of the results have been satisfactory.

Orthomyxoviruses

This family includes two genera of influenza viruses, one encompassing the etiologic agents responsible for types A and B, the other the virus causing type C.

These are enveloped viruses with roughly 550 glycoprotein spikes per virion. Their glycoproteins have hemagglutinin and neuraminidase activities. The A and B types are distinguished by the nucleoprotein antigen; within these types, strains are characterized by glycoprotein antigenic variations. The genome of the virus occurs as 8 (types A, B) or 7 (type C) distinct pieces of − strand RNA, which range from 0.9 to 2.4 kb. Each segment is transcribed into an mRNA copy which directs protein synthesis. The segmentation of the genome not only allows for multiple mRNAs that permit translational control, but also for high levels of recombination (segment shuffling) among the different influenza genes. This recombination is probably responsible for the extensive antigenic changes that influenza virus undergoes rapidly.

After inhalation, influenza virus establishes an upper respiratory infection with a 1- to 2-day incubation period. The cellular receptor to which the virus binds is sialic acid. The first phase of infection is characterized by constitutional symptoms of fever, chills, and aches. A more obvious respiratory infection follows, with cough, coryza, and rhinorrhea. High titers of virus are released in nasal secretions. To establish infection, influenza virus must bypass any local IgA present from previous influenza infections. In addition, there are glycoprotein inhibitors of viral attachment in the nasal mucus that are attacked by the viral neuraminidase. This interaction causes the runny fluid exudate of influenza respiratory disease. Although influenza virus can be grown in cell cultures with no cytopathic effects, the result of patient infection is necrosis and shedding of the respiratory epithelium. This epithelium is the first line of defense against bacterial infection, which occurs with great ease when the infected epithelium is destroyed. The raw surface of the trachea and respiratory tree are then exposed and subject to invasion and attack by normal bacterial inhabitants of the upper airways. A secondary or superinfection can result in pneumonia, which is the cause of high fatality rates in influenza epidemics.

Because the main obstacle to the establishment of influenza is a relatively small amount of tissue IgA, any antigenic changes that allow the virus to bypass this line of defense are strongly selected. Changes in the viral hemagglutinin and neuraminidase (surface glycoproteins and convenient antigenic markers) are the primary mode of antigenic drift, by which a new, slightly different strain of influenza appears and is more successful in establishing infection and in spreading among a population. This evolution is rapid in influenza A viruses, and one variant tends to dominate at any given time. The evolutionary drift in Hepatitis C viruses is slower, and several variants co-exist in the circulating population. At intervals of roughly 10 to 15 years, a dramatically different strain appears, a so-called antigenic shift. We believe this results from the recombination of a human influenza virus with a virus from a different species of animal host, perhaps by an exchange of 1 of the 8 genomic pieces. This new strain can find a large pool of susceptible hosts, and it causes the great influenza epidemics that have been disastrous in recent medical history. Serologic studies of persons of all ages have allowed the sketching of a profile of influenza antigenic drift and shift for the last hundred years.

Amantadine and ribavirin are antiviral agents which show some therapeutic benefit in treating influenza A and B infections, respectively. Influenza vaccines containing killed-virus preparations of the viral strains that predominated during the previous season are currently available. They are recommended prophylactically for elderly patients and other individuals with sensitive or compromised respiratory tracts.

Arenaviruses

These round or pleomorphic enveloped viruses contain characteristic electron-dense granules which are now known to be host ribosomes. Their genome appears as 2 pieces of single-stranded RNA (designated L, 9 kb and S, 4.8 kb); the virions also package host rRNA species. The genomic strands are highly unusual in that they are "ambisense"—for example, one gene on the S strand is found in the + polarity, whereas the other gene is present in the − polarity and cannot be expressed until the infecting genome is replicated. This unusual arrangement ensures a temporal regulation of gene expression.

Arenaviruses are natural viruses of rodents; humans are at risk when they enter locales in which chronic infection of rodents is endemic. Arenaviruses associated with human pathogenesis include **Lymphocytic choriomeningitis virus (LCMV), Lassa fever virus, Junin virus** (Argentine hemorrhagic fever) and **Machupo virus** (Bolivan hemorrhagic fever).

Lassa Fever Virus. This virus is transmitted by the respiratory or alimentary route and an incubation period of two weeks is typical. It replicates in lymph nodes and invades reticuloendothelial tissue, inhibiting the effects of immune-related cells. Symptoms include fever and associated myalgia as well as vomiting, abdominal pain, dizziness, and weakness. Capillary damage is usual and may be evidenced by swelling of the face and neck as well as by bleeding. The febrile stage usually recedes after a few weeks unless the disease progresses to severe shock and death. Fifteen percent of hospitalized cases are fatal. The prognosis is especially poor when pregnant women are affected. This rare disease is seen primarily in Africa, where the endemic zoonoses exist.

Bunyaviruses

Five genera contribute to this abundant family of viruses. Most isolates come from Africa or Latin America, where a complex ecologic environment contributes to the availability of insect vectors and animal reservoirs associated with these viruses. Most of these agents induce febrile diseases which may be accompanied by rash and/or hemorrhagic fever. Bunyaviruses are spherical, enveloped viruses of approximately 100 nm in diameter. Particles mature in infected cells by budding into cisternae of the Golgi apparatus and are shed from the cell by exocytosis or upon cell lysis. The viral proteins are encoded in a tri-segmented RNA genome (designated L, M and S). The evolution of new viruses by segment shuffling in chronically infected insect vectors has been proposed. Like arenaviruses, some of these genomic segments are of ambisense polarity (some genes are present in the + polarity, others in the—polarity). The most important bunyaviruses associated with human disease include: **La Crosse** virus, a member of the *bunyavirus* genus associated with encephalitis; **sandfly fever** and **Rift valley fever** (hemorrhagic) viruses, members of the *phlebovirus* genus associated with endemic and epidemic fevers; **Crimean-Congo hemorrhagic fever** virus, a member of the *nairovirus* genus; and **Hantaan** virus, a member of the *hantavirus* genus asociated with a hemorrhagic fever accompanied by a renal syndrome. All but the last virus are arboviruses. The *hantaviruses* are transmitted directly by infected rodent species.

Reoviruses

Reoviruses are unique in possessing a genome of segmented double-stranded RNA. Although these viruses have been of great interest to biologists, their role in human disease was unclear until recently. In the last decade, the *rotavirus* genus of reoviruses has been identified as one of the major causes of viral gastroenteritis. The 75 nm particles have 11 genomic segments and derive their name from their wheel-like appearance in electron micrographs. Virus infection is world-wide, with a peak incidence in children from 6 months to 2 years of age, and a seasonal predominance in temperate climates of fall and winter (Fig. 8–15).

The virus infects the epithelial cells of the intestinal villi. After an incubation period of a few days, infec-

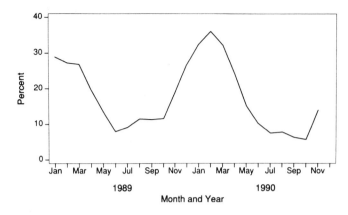

Fig. 8–15 Percentage of laboratory tests positive for rotavirus—United States, January 1989-November 1990. Number of specimens tested each month ranged from 1410 (September 1990) to 3275 (January 1990). (From Centers for Disease Control, Morbidity and Mortality Weekly Report, 40(5):81, 1991.)

tion is followed by vomiting, diarrhea and fever. Evidence of upper respiratory infection is not infrequent. After 7 days, symptoms usually subside with no sequelae. Rotavirus infection is followed by strong but short-lived humoral immunity. IgA has been shown in clinical tests to be important in elevating resistance to symptomatic rotavirus infection. There is also good evidence that neonates are protected by maternal antibody; breast-feeding is arguably implicated in providing IgA-mediated immunity to nursing infants. Because rotavirus infection causes extensive world-wide morbidity, the feasibility of a vaccine is being investigated. Oral attenuated vaccines are currently thought the most promising.

Retroviruses

These are a unique class of enveloped viruses. Their genome consists of 2 identical + strand RNAs of approximately 9 kb each. When infection takes place, RNA is transcribed to DNA by the viral reverse transcriptase. The DNA is made double-stranded and then integrates permanently into the host genome. From this integrated copy, virion RNA and viral messages may be transcribed, proteins may be synthesized, and virions may be assembled at the cell membrane. Most retroviruses are not cytolytic and may be expressed indefinitely. Many of these viruses, members of the *oncovirus* genus, have been shown to be natural causes of cancer in a range of animal species. In some cases, these viruses have inserted themselves into the germ line DNA and are inherited as cellular genes by all members of an animal population.

Recently, the first examples of human retroviruses were documented. Human T-cell leukemia virus I

(HTLV I) (genus *oncovirus*), is associated with adult T-cell leukemia (ATL). The virus and disease are prevalent in localized geographic areas in Japan, Africa, and in the Caribbean. Transmission is by sexual contact, transfusion, sharing of needles, and intrauterine infection. Infection is now on the rise in urban areas of the United States. The virus has a tropism for lymphocytes bearing the CD4 surface antigen; infection leads to integration of a DNA copy of the genome into the host chromosome. The virus can immortalize infected cells and transform them into precancerous cells in culture. In addition to containing the basic genes of all known retroviruses, HTLV I (and a related virus, **HTLV II**) contain additional genes which are thought to be essential to its role in causing leukemia. In some as yet unknown manner, the presence of the virus disturbs normal cellular behavior and growth control and eventually causes cancer. The incubation time before ATL development is estimated to be 15–20 years. HTLV II was isolated from an individual with hairy cell leukemia; its tissue tropism and biological properties resemble those of HTLV I. The scope of its association with human disease, and indeed the extent of its presence worldwide, remain unknown.

Within the last few years, another human retrovirus has been isolated and identified as the etiologic agent of **Acquired Immune Deficiency Syndrome**, or AIDS. This disease is arguably the greatest world health cri-

sis in the twentieth century. AIDS is a progressive disease that affects previously healthy individuals. The syndrome commences with an ill-defined period of malaise, weight loss, lymphadenopathy, and possibly fever. The next and most characteristic phase is the appearance of one or more opportunistic infections or malignancies. Pneumonia caused by *Pneumocystis carinii*, candidiasis, fungal infections, and a rare malignancy known as Kaposi's sarcoma are typical. The outbreak of infections and malignancies considered rare in otherwise healthy young patients suggests that AIDS represents a severe immune deficiency. In fact, patients have been shown to have T-lymphocyte depletion, defective natural killer-cell activity and decreased lymphocyte proliferative response. The opportunistic infections that follow this immune deficit, unfortunately, lead to fatality in greater than 70% of AIDS patients. Recently, an effect of viral infection on central nervous system functions has also been documented.

A striking feature about AIDS is the rapidity with which it has appeared and spread. The disease was first recognized in the United States in 1981, and infection is now known to be world-wide, affecting millions of people (Figs. 8–16, 8–17). High-risk individuals in the western world are primarily intravenous drug users and their sexual partners, and sexually active male homosexuals. Infected women transmit the

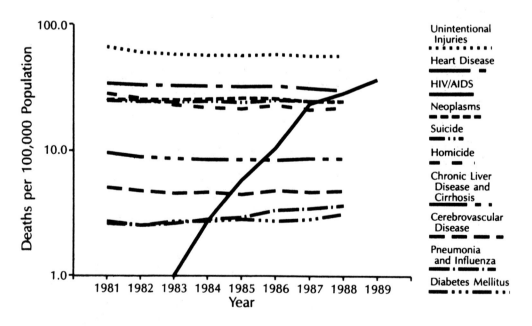

* National vital statistics. Final data for 1981–1988; provisional data for HIV infection/AIDS for 1989.

Fig. 8–16A Leading causes of death among men 25–44 years of age—United States, 1981–1989. (From Centers for Disease Control, Morbidity and Mortality Weekly Report, 40(3):42, 1991.)

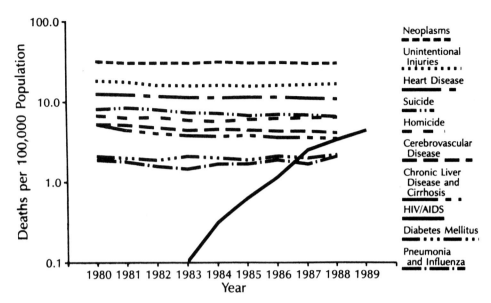

Fig. 8–16*B* Leading causes of death among women 25–44 years of age—United States, 1980–1989. National vital statistics. Final data for 1980–1988; provisional data for HIV infection/AIDS for 1989. (From Centers for Disease Control, Morbidity and Mortality Weekly Report, 40(3):42, 1991.)

AIDS virus to 33% of fetuses *in utero*. Until recently, hemophiliacs receiving clotting factors from pooled blood donations and patients requiring blood transfusions were also at risk. Identification of the causative agent, and development of good diagnostic tests, have rendered the blood supply essentially safe. It is now well established that the disease is not spread by casual contact, but requires extensive and intimate exposure to bodily fluids or their direct introduction into the bloodstream. In Africa, the disease has

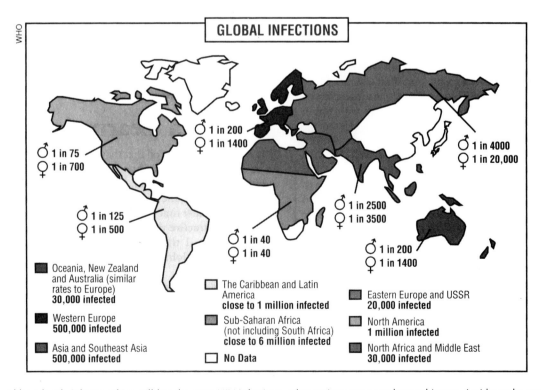

Fig. 8–17 Although sub-Saharan Africa still has the most HIV infections, other regions appear to be catching up. Incidence by sex is for adults aged 15 to 49. (World Health Organization.)

reached epidemic proportions, and has spread by heterosexual intercourse and pregnancy throughout the population. The severity of the morbidity and mortality cannot be stated strongly enough. If measures to treat or prevent the disease are not forthcoming, a shocking portion of the population may die from this new and ruthless disease.

Another striking feature of the natural history of this disease is the long incubation period. Indeed, onset of symptoms may not occur until 7 years following exposure to the virus. Because the infectious agent is a retrovirus, it is believed that this long latent period represents a time in which the virus is stably carried by infected cells, but during which period viral functions are repressed. The variation in the onset and severity of symptoms in individuals which are known to have been exposed to the virus is unexplained. Diagnosis of infection is made by monitoring patients' sera for antibodies to the infecting virus. Although this test is quite accurate and sensitive, it provides no clue as to the time of viral infection, the current state of transmissibility of the virus, or the likelihood of the onset of disease symptoms.

The retrovirus identified as the etiologic agent of this disease is known as **HIV**—human immunodeficiency virus (genus *lentivirus*). As a classic retrovirus, it has an RNA genome which is copied into DNA by the viral reverse transcriptase upon entry into infected cells. This complementary DNA can be inserted into the cellular chromosome and carried indefinitely by the infected host cells. The cellular receptor for HIV is the CD4 surface antigen present on T-helper lymphocytes and certain other cell lines. Recently, it has been discovered that the virus will also infect cells of the macrophage lineage. Infection may lead to a latent state in which cytopathic effect is minimal, or to a highly explosive and lytic infectious cycle. In addition to containing the classic retroviral genes necessary for replication and maturation, HIV contains several novel genes which permit complex and sensitive regulation of viral growth. The *tat* protein is a trans-activator which interacts with cellular components to activate viral genes. A variety of cellular transcription factors known to respond to extracellular stimuli must also be present for viral gene expression to occur. When and if sufficient levels of *tat*-stimulated gene expression are reached, a second viral protein known as *rev* accumulates. *Rev* activates a switch which turns on the production of the structural proteins which will form progeny HIV virions. It is thought that the observed behaviors of alternate latent or lytic infection are thus carefully modulated in response to the state of immune reactivity of the infected lymphocytes and environmental conditions within the infected patient.

Because of the severity of AIDS, extensive research is ongoing to develop therapeutic drugs and preventive vaccines. The antiviral research has been focused on agents which inhibit the viral reverse transcriptase, such as zidovudine (AZT). Vaccine development has been hampered by the high degree of variation exhibited among different viral isolates. The surface viral glycoprotein, which would be a good candidate as an immunogen, is unfortunately quite variable. Attempts to produce vaccines from isolated viral proteins or peptides, or by incorporating single HIV genes into vectors such as the safe vaccinia virus, are underway. Successful defense against this disease is probably the major challenge confronting virologists and infectious disease specialists today.

DNA VIRUSES

Since these viruses have a DNA genome, as does the host, life-cycle pathways of replication and transcription can rely to a greater extent on the normal cellular enzymatic machinery. Some simple DNA viruses use only host enzymes. With increasing complexity, DNA viruses bring in their own polymerases. These viruses are bigger and more complicated than RNA viruses, and they can replicate in a greater variety of cells. Some stimulate resting cells to grow, others replicate independently of the host genome. Perhaps because of this potential for control of DNA replication and growth in cells, many DNA viruses have been shown to have oncogenic potential in animals. As we shall discuss, there is a growing evidence for the association of viruses with the development of some human cancers. The importance of latent and persistent infections with DNA viruses will also become apparent.

Hepadnaviruses

Hepatitis B, previously known as serum hepatitis, is caused by a novel type of DNA virus (HBV). The spherical 42 nm virion, known as the Dane particle (Fig. 8–18), carries on its surface the diagnostic HbsAg surface antigen. Within the envelope of the virion is a 28 nm core which contains at least a viral DNA polymerase and the genomic DNA. This DNA is a gapped circular duplex of 3.2 kb with varying degrees of single-strandedness. The particle-associated polymerase will repair these gaps. It has recently been demonstrated that intracellular HBV DNA replication proceeds via an RNA intermediate: like retroviruses, a DNA strand is synthesized from this RNA template. In the case of HBV, however, the packaged nucleic acid (the genome) is the DNA species.

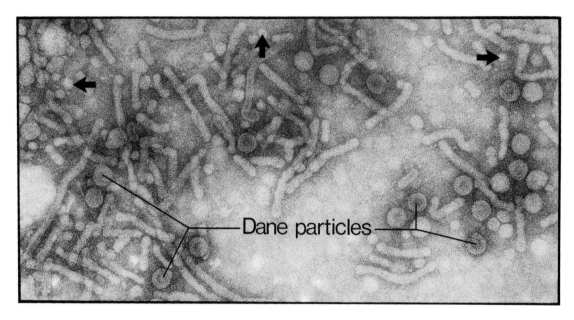

Fig. 8–18 This electron micrograph shows the Dane particle and HB antigen particles (arrows) in a negatively stained preparation. x155,000 (Courtesy of Dr. S. N. Huang, Pathology Institute, McGill University.)

Table 8–2. Epidemiologic and Clinical Characteristics of Reported Cases of Viral Hepatitis by Serologic Type, 1981

EPIDEMIOLOGIC CHARACTERISTICS	HEPATITIS A N = 4,151		HEPATITIS B N = 9,130		HEPATITIS NON-A NON-B N = 1,591	
	NO.	(%)	NO.	(%)	NO.	(%)
Child/employee in day-care center	247	(6)	57	(*)	41	(3)
Household contact of child/employee in day-care center	381	(9)	161	(2)	71	(4)
Personal contact with hepatitis A	1,054	(25)	189	(2)	85	(5)
Employed as a food handler	274	(7)	476	(5)	71	(4)
Association with food-borne or water-borne outbreak	164	(4)	87	(1)	19	(1)
International travel	207	(5)	126	(1)	35	(2)
Personal contact with hepatitis B	77	(2)	1,323	(14)	80	(5)
Employed in medical/dental field	103	(3)	683	(8)	113	(7)
Association with dialysis/transplant unit	12	(*)	202	(2)	29	(2)
Patient	7		92		12	
Employee	2		44		7	
Contact or patient/employee	2		49		7	
Blood transfusion	45	(1)	370	(4)	170	(11)
Hospitalized prior to illness	189	(5)	1,295	(14)	344	(22)
Surgery	81	(2)	617	(7)	180	(11)
Dental work	206	(5)	1,287	(14)	216	(14)
Drug abuse	79	(2)	1,133	(12)	131	(8)
Homosexual activity	93	(2)	512	(6)	32	(2)
Other percutaneous exposures	166	(4)	1,333	(15)	202	(13)
Clinical characteristics						
Jaundice	3,161	(76)	6,262	(69)	1,025	(64)
Hospitalized for hepatitis	1,703	(41)	4,259	(47)	852	(54)
Death as a result of hepatitis	27	(*)	113	(1)	41	(3)

* <1%.

(From Centers for Disease Control: Morbidity and Mortality Weekly Report, 32(2SS):29SS, 1983.)

HBV transmission is primarily by parenteral means: blood transfusions, needle-sticks, infection of open cuts or mucous membranes. Medical personnel, intravenous drug users, male homosexuals, hemodialysis patients and hemophiliacs receiving clotting factors are populations at high risk for HBV infection (Table 8–2).

The primary site of HBV replication within the body is unknown, and no tissue culture system has been found to fully support the cultivation of HBV. The onset of hepatitis B symptoms occurs gradually after an average incubation period of 60 to 90 days. The diagnostic feature of HBV infection is the presence of high levels of circulating viral antigens prior to any signs of liver dysfunction. The cases in the United States in 1981 are shown in Figure 8–19. The HbsAg is found in 22 nm aggregates known as the "Australia antigen." Jaundice and increased enzyme levels signaling liver disease follow this period of viral replication. Symptoms are often prolonged, and although full recovery is usual, it may be slow. In some cases hepatitis may become chronic, leading to conditions of variable severity.

A key feature of hepatitis B infection is that as many as 10% of affected individuals remain chronic carriers of the virus. Antiviral therapy with agents known to inhibit the viral polymerase and/or with alpha-interferons have been found to decrease the levels of replicating virus found in the heptocytes of affected patients. Treatment of chronic infections is of obvious advantage to carriers; moreover, the continued shedding of virus from chronically infected patients represents a source of infection to others. Immune globulin (IG) or hepatitis immune globulin (HBIG) is used prophylactically to treat exposed individuals. Moreover, a hepatitis B vaccine has recently been developed and tested in clinical trials. The vaccine, composed of inactivated HbsAg particles purified from asymptomatic chronic carriers, is administered in three doses. It appears to be effective and is currently available to high-risk populations.

Another feature of HBV infection is the association with the **delta virus (HDV)**. This associated pathogen is composed of a single-stranded 1.7 kb RNA molecule of − polarity which encodes a single polypeptide (HDV antigen). The RNA has a high degree of self-complementarity, reminiscent of the viroids associated with plant pathology. The RNA molecule has catalytic properties which play a role in its replication. Persistence of HDV requires HBV infection; the structural protein comprising the HDV particle is in fact the HBV surface antigen. Thus, HDV is a "satellite" of HBV infection. Co-infection with hepatitis B and delta viruses results in a more severe (and sometimes fulminant) acute hepatitis; superinfection of HBV carriers with the delta virus is associated with development of chronic hepatitis. The molecular basis for this increased pathogenicity is as yet unknown.

A final feature of HBV infection is its possible link to the etiology of hepatoma. Epidemiologic evidence has suggested that hepatoma patients present a higher than average incidence of HbsAg expression. Animal studies of hepatitis viruses analogous to HBV (for example, the woodchuck system) indicate that viral infection leads often to the development of hepatoma as well as hepatitis. A recent prospective study of 22,707 Taiwanese men makes this correlation clearer. After following these men for several years, the authors report that the incidence of primary hepatocellular carcinoma is 223-fold higher among HbsAg carriers than among noncarriers. This and other factors in the study support the conclusion that HBV

Reported hepatitis B cases/100,000 population, by state, United States, 1981

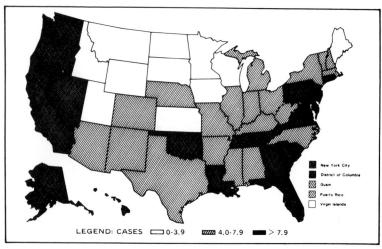

Fig. 8–19 Reported hepatitis B cases/100,000 population, by state, United States, 1981. (From Centers for Disease Control: Morbidity and Mortality Weekly Report, 32(2SS):25SS, 1983.)

infection plays an important etiologic role in the development of hepatoma.

Papovaviruses

This family contains two genera, *polyomaviruses* and *papillomaviruses*. These viruses contain a double-stranded, closed circular genome which is enclosed in an icosahedral virion. Polyomaviruses have been of great value to molecular virologists in studying gene expression and oncogenic transformation. The **JC** *(polyomavirus)* virus has been recovered from the brains of patients suffering from progressive multifocal leukoencephalopathy (PML), a demyelinating disease. **BKV** *(polyomavirus)* was first recovered from a renal transplant patient. Both are now known to be ubiquitous, with infection thought to be common before adolescence. Seroconversion to BKV positivity is usually not accompanied by any apparent symptoms of infection, although virus is frequently recovered from the tonsils removed from children with recurrent respiratory infections. JC virus is considered the cause of PML; no other symptoms associated with the vast majority of childhood JC infections have been found.

Papillomaviruses are associated with a variety of warts and other proliferative lesions of the skin and mucosal surfaces of the oral cavity and anogenital tract. The genome can either replicate within the nuclei of infected cells as an extrachromosomal plasmid, or can integrate into the host chromosome. Papilloma infections are associated with a spectrum of epithelial lesions which range from benign to dysplastic or malignant. The most clinically significant feature of papilloma infections pertains to their role as sexually transmitted diseases. Human papilloma virus (predominantly HPV-16) is associated with perhaps 90% of cervical cancers: whether or not these viruses are the direct cause of the cancers, some role in promoting their development cannot be overlooked. As well, carcinomas of the penis and vulva appear to develop in pre-existing condylomata, the result of enduring papilloma infections. Vaccination of high-risk populations against HPV-16 and other serotypes would be worthwhile, and efforts are underway to investigate such a possibility.

Parvoviruses

These small icosahedral viruses contain single-stranded DNA genomes which have unusual hairpin termini. The genus *dependoviruses* includes adeno-associated virus, a virus detected in human tissues but not associated with any pathogenic effect. **B19** virus, a member of the genus *parvovirus*, is causally associated with development of aplastic crises in patients with chronic hemolytic anemias and is more frequently the cause of "fifth disease," erythema infectiosum (EI). The prodromal phase of EI is characterized by the appearance of mild "flu-like" symptoms. Diagnosis can be made by the subsequent development of a facial rash which has a "slapped cheek" appearance; a maculopapular rash on the trunk and limbs follows. The most common complication, especially in adult patients, is joint involvement which may progress to frank arthritis. Recovery is usually complete.

Adenoviruses

These icosahedral viruses have a 30 kb double-stranded genome packaged within a capsid containing at least 14 proteins. Virions are relatively stable and suited to survival outside the host. After entry into susceptible cells, multiple mRNAs are synthesized in the nucleus, copying different regions along both strands of the DNA at different times. Significant RNA processing is involved in the temporal control of the viral protein synthesis. Shortly after infection, host DNA synthesis is stimulated, perhaps to ready the cell for virus replication. Later in infection, host DNA, RNA, and protein synthesis are inhibited. Viral DNA is replicated in the nucleus; levels of adenovirus DNA reach that of total uninfected cell DNA. Particles are assembled in the nucleus, where they form characteristic crystalline arrays. They are released on disruption of the infected cell.

There are at least 31 serotypes of human *adenoviruses*. These are endemic, and only some 50% of childhood infections cause symptomatic disease. The common adenovirus disease is an acute respiratory infection with the pharynx as the site of viral multiplication, and an incubation period of 5 to 7 days. The frequent recovery of adenovirus from tonsils of patients who do not have an adenovirus-like disease suggests frequent inapparent and chronic infections. Virus shedding usually outlasts the duration of the disease. Transmission is usually through respiration or by the fecal-oral route. Adenovirus accounts for about 5% of viral respiratory disease. There are a few examples of more serious adenovirus complaints, one of which, ARD (acute respiratory disease), is a disabling respiratory ailment prevalent among new military recruits. Adenoviruses have also been shown to have oncogenic potential in animals.

Herpesviruses

Herpesviruses are among the most widely distributed viruses in the general population. Contributing to this ubiquity are the diversity of herpesviruses, their generally high contagiousness, and their ability to endure in infected individuals in a latent and/or recurrent state after the initial infection. The herpes viruses are large, with a double-stranded linear DNA genome of approximately 150 kb. The DNA is associated with proteins in a barbell formation, and is surrounded by a protein capsid, outside of which is a lipid envelope. The virions are acid-labile. Their DNA codes for approximately 70 proteins, including numerous virion components. There are 162 capsomers in the icosahedral capsid. The lipid envelope is thought to be derived largely from the nuclear envelope.

The herpesvirus genomes are known to encode several enzymes involved in DNA synthesis, including a DNA polymerase, precursor biosynthetic enzymes, various nucleases, and proteins involved in the initiation of replication at the viral origin. Replication occurs in the nucleus. The virus also encodes proteins which regulate sequential phases of gene expression. After mRNA transcription and cytoplasmic protein synthesis, the proteins are returned to the nucleus where virion assembly occurs. The envelope is acquired during the process of budding out. The cytopathic effect, and the degree to which host functions are interrupted, varies among the different types of herpesviruses and the cell type infected. Infections vary from latent to lytic. The particular strains of herpesviruses will be discussed in the context of their various diseases. Genera include *alphaherpesviruses,* containing **herpes simplex 1 and 2** and **varicella zoster**; *betaherpesviruses,* represented by **cytomegalovirus** and **human herpesvirus 6**; and *gammaherpesviruses,* including **Epstein-Barr virus**.

Herpes Simplex, 1 and 2. These 2 related viruses cause primary infections during childhood that are usually inapparent. Although they can each establish infection anywhere on the body, type 1 is usually transmitted orally and causes infections of the upper body, primarily of the mouth, and type 2 is transmitted genitally and causes infections of the lower body. When apparent, symptoms appear after about a week, appearing as sores that result from lytic viral replication. Complications are more serious when babies are infected during birth with vaginal HSV-2. Because women can be asymptomatically infected with HSV, any women who have had sexual partners infected with herpes simplex should be concerned about this potential problem. In cases where cervical or vaginal herpes infection is documented near term, caesarian delivery is indicated.

The real significance of herpes simplex virus (HSV) is not in its primary infection, but in its persistence in a latent state following infection. Fever, radiation, sunlight, and other stresses can activate herpes. The most common presentation of HSV-1 reactivation is the "coldsore," or "fever blister" on the lip. Experimental evidence suggests that the virus remains in a latent state in the sensory nerve ganglia, and travels in times of stress to the epidermis, where it can replicate freely. Circulating anti-HSV antibodies do not halt this reactivation. The evolutionary advantage of such persistent infections for the virus is obvious; the prevalence of anti-HSV antibodies in primitive societies suggests an early origin and widespread prevalence of these viruses.

Because herpes simplex 2 is transmitted sexually, and because it recurs repeatedly in affected individuals, herpes virus became the venereal disease of the 1980s. The virus has become widespread among young, sexually active adults, and caused psychological trauma more significant than the physical discomfort involved. Education about the virus, and the adoption of some precautions, should relieve some of the socially negative ramifications of HSV infection. Sexual habits, such as oral sex, have resulted in the appearance of HSV-2 in facial areas and of HSV-1 around the genitalia. Recurrences of viral expression in men are usually apparent, and sexual contact should be avoided during these times. However, women can often be asymptomatic carriers, and men can shed virus even when viral blisters are not developed. Obviously, a good deal of work is underway to develop antiviral drugs and vaccines. Since natural humoral immunity seems ineffective in preventing viral persistence, any future vaccine may only be effective for individuals with no prior exposure to the virus. Antiviral drugs, such as acyclovir and vidarabine, are being tested as topical and/or oral treatments. They are effective, but the ease with which drug-resistant viral mutants arise limits their value as widespread therapies.

Herpes infection can also cause serious infections in the conjunctiva of the eye, with possible resultant blindness. Luckily, herpes-induced keratitis infections are responsive to topical application of antiviral agents that interfere with DNA metabolism.

Varicella-Zoster Virus. In primary infection this herpesvirus is responsible for *chickenpox* (varicella). The virus is thought to enter through the oropharynx, the upper respiratory tract, conjunctiva, or perhaps through the skin. The virus replicates by spreading through contiguous cells. Infected cells display ballooning and develop intranuclear inclusions. Virus circulates in the blood and lymph, stimulating an immune response. After a week, the immune response is overpowered, viremia increases, and systemic symptoms of fever and malaise appear. There are successive crops of skin vesicles, red macules with a centrally placed vesicle of clear fluid ("dewdrop"). Different stages of macule, pustule, and scab can be seen simultaneously; the lesions occur centripetally, primarily on the trunk. Virus is present in these lesions for less than one week. The disease is normally mild, although highly contagious; immunity to exogenous infection is lifelong, and there is only one known serotype. A disease of greater severity, accompanied by pneumonia and encephalitis, can arise in immune-compromised children; varicella infection is also more severe in adults, in whom accompanying pneumonia is common. Various vaccines have been developed, but none is licensed for use in the United States. It is not clear that the risks and costs are justified in a disease that is usually so mild.

After varicella infection, the virus is thought to persist in dorsal root or cranial nerve ganglia. Various stresses may cause a reactivation of the virus, causing it to travel down a sensory nerve with accompanying pain. Blisters develop on the area supplied by the nerve; the lesions are unilateral and terminate abruptly at the midline. This is zoster ("girdle") or shingles, an illness plaguing .3 to .5% of the population per year. More than one-half of those affected are over 50 years of age. The virus in the zoster lesions is identical to that in chickenpox; one may contract chickenpox from a person who has zoster lesions. This again underlines the selective advantages of such reactivatable latent infections.

Cytomegalovirus. This ubiquitous herpesvirus is associated with a variety of syndromes which range from mild to severe. Inapparent infections are common; chronic and recurring infections are also characteristic. When disease does develop, symptoms can include pneumonia, hepatitis, mononucleosis, and arthritis. Transmission is by the oropharyngeal or genital route, as well as transplacentally to the fetus. Individuals with CMV infection excrete virus in their saliva and urine, and sexual transmission is also strongly suspected. CMV can also be transmitted by transfusion or organ transplantation. Latent infections are frequently re-activated in individuals undergoing immunosuppressive therapy, often inducing an interstitial pneumonia. Induction appears to increase the degree of immunosuppression, causing a heightened susceptibility to opportunistic infections. Graft rejection is also more frequent in CMV-infected transplant patients. Transplacental infection can be fatal to the fetus, or it may leave a child mentally retarded. The clinical importance of CMV infections has risen due to its prevalence in patients in-

fected with HIV, the causative agent of AIDS. CMV infection in these patients is associated with increased morbidity and mortality.

Human herpesvirus 6 (HHV 6). This herpesvirus has recently been identified as the primary cause of roseola infantum, also known as sixth disease or exanthem subitum. Roseola is a syndrome of infants which is characterized by a generalized rash appearing after three or four days of high fever. The disease is widespread among infants from 6 months to 2 years; its ubiquity is underscored by the finding that more than 50% of adults are seropositive for antibodies to HHV 6. The rash usually fades in a few days, and recovery is rapid and complete. In culture, the tissue tropism of HHV 6 is for T lymphocytes. Recently, a herpesvirus which is probably HHV 6 has also been isolated from lymphocytes of AIDS patients—the role of HHV 6 in contributing to diseases other than roseola infantum needs to be determined.

Epstein-Barr Virus. The agent of infectious mononucleosis, this is a ubiquitous virus that causes many inapparent infections, especially when contact occurs in childhood. Transmission can be respiratory or through the mouth, frequently through the salivary exchange of kissing. In 4 to 7 days, malaise and lethargy appear, accompanied by pharyngitis and enlargement of cervical and axillary lymph nodes. Fever and chills may occur, and the spleen may become enlarged. The disease usually runs its course in 1 to 2 weeks, but prolonged discomfort can occur. When the Epstein-Barr virus (EBV) enters the host's mouth, it probably first replicates in the epithelia of the mouth and throat. The virus is spread through the blood and lymph and infects B lymphocytes. Various changes in the lymphocyte population occur, with a characteristic appearance of atypical T lymphocytes. Some but not all infected B cells are killed. Recently, the profile of the immune response has been studied. IgM and then IgG antibodies to the virus capsid antigen (VCA) first appear, followed by transient IgG antibodies to D, a diffuse viral antigen found in nuclei and cytoplasm of infected cells. Finally, lifelong antibodies appear to Epstein-Barr nuclear antigen, which is virally induced. Heterophil antibodies arise and are diagnostic for the disease (Fig. 8–20).

EBV is not a simple lytic virus. The virus can induce either lytic or latent infections. Lytic infections lead to the productive release of progeny virions. EBV infection, however, can also immortalize B lymphocytes. The proliferation of these cells is somehow kept in check by the immune system. When latent virus is induced from a subset of cells, the released virus can establish new latent infections in fresh target cells.

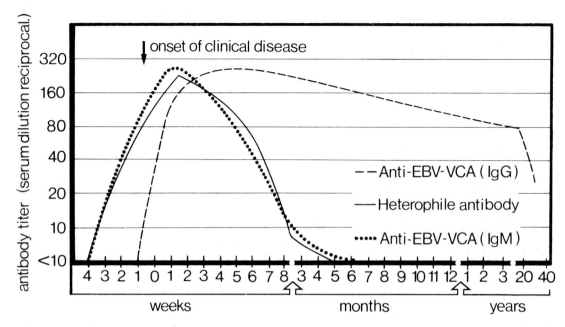

Fig. 8–20 The relative antibody titers during the evolution of infectious mononucleosis are shown in the accompanying graphs. The onset of clinical disease appears within one week of infection. The life-long immunity to anti-EB virus is shown in the top line. (From Schleupner, C.J., and Overall, J.C., Jr.: Infectious mononucleosis and Epstein-Barr virus. I. Epidemiology, pathogenesis, immune response. Postgrad. Med., 65:83, 1979.)

Cells latently infected with EBV express the EBNA antigen, and it appears that transformation reflects the presence of integrated EBV DNA. Although B cells from EBV⁻ individuals die after a short period in culture, a minority of B cells from EBV⁺ individuals are immortalized and grow indefinitely in culture.

It is likely that EBV persists in a latent form in B cells of infected persons, and that the disease is a cytolytic, self-limiting leukemia kept in check by the immune system. A syndrome of chronic EBV, with recurring bouts of malaise and lymphadenopathy, has recently been recognized.

EBV is intimately associated with two human cancers, Burkitt's lymphoma and nasopharyngeal carcinoma. *Burkitt's lymphoma* affects 1 in 10,000 children per year, primarily aged 6 to 8 years, in the warm, wet lowlands of Africa. It is a rapidly growing lymphoma of the neck and jaw. EBV is endemic in the locale of incidence, and infection usually occurs early in childhood. Patients with Burkitt's lymphoma (BL) have roughly 10-fold higher titers of anti-EBV antibodies than the normal African child. Ninety-eight per cent of monoclonal BL tissue contains EBV DNA, whereas it is not found in other lymphomas. The clinical prognosis of the disease correlates with anti-EBV antibody profiles (Fig. 8–21). Where therapy results in a decrease in the anti-R antibody (an early EBV antigen) titer, recovery is likely; persistence or increase in the anti-R titer after therapy usually implies a fatal recurrence. It is unlikely that all the monoclonal

tumors would arise in the small number of EBV-infected lymphocytes by chance. It seems probable that EBV infection or transformation is necessary but not sufficient for the onset of BL. Since the area of BL prevalence is coincident with that of malaria, the possibility of malaria as a cofactor has been suggested. Malaria is thought to weaken the immune response and to enhance lymphocyte proliferation. The seasonal variation in BL onset implies that the cofactor is environmental. It is also true that BL tissue has a chromosomal translocation involving segments of chromosomes 8 and 14; similar rearrangements have been observed in other lymphomas.

Nasopharyngeal carcinoma occurs in several limited geographic locales and racial groups. Genetic factors and chemical carcinogens have been suggested as etiologic agents. All biopsies have revealed EBV DNA in the carcinoma tissue. Patients have high titers of anti-EBV antibodies, especially to the D antigen; uniquely, IgA is frequently present in these cases. Patterns of antibodies to VCA and D antigens parallel tumor enlargement and regression after treatment, and also foreshadow tumor reappearance. Although causation has not been proven, experimental and epidemiologic data point to EBV, and perhaps to other herpesviruses, as human tumor viruses.

Poxviruses

This family contains the largest, most complex DNA viruses. The most famous poxviruses are **variola**

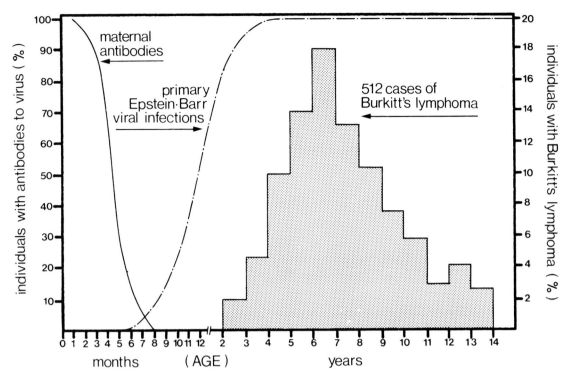

Fig. 8–21 This graph shows the relationships among maternal antibodies, primary infections with Epstein-Barr (EB) viral infections, and 512 cases of Burkitt's lymphoma. The Burkitt's lymphoma cases were preceded by infections with EB virus. (From Henle, W., Henle, G., and Lennette, E.T.: The Epstein-Barr virus. Sci. Am., 241:48, 1979.)

major, the causative agent of smallpox, and **vaccinia**, the related virus used in the successful vaccination campaign to eradicate smallpox. Historically, a number of important diseases were informally categorized as "poxes." The name is derived from the vesicopustular skin eruptions that characterize these diseases. We now know that "chickenpox" is indeed a herpesvirus disease, and the "great pox," syphilis, is not viral in nature.

Smallpox was one of the most virulent of infectious diseases. It has afflicted man for thousands of years. All races of men were susceptible, and no one from childhood to old age was exempt. Actual contact, direct or indirect, with a patient was not necessary for transmission. It swept through the country with the speed of a prairie fire. (Other virus diseases, such as influenza, may travel with the same terrifying speed.) Small wonder, then, that in bygone years nearly everyone, high or low, rich or poor, bore the marks of "the pox" on his or her face. The picture in 17th-century England is drawn thus by the vivid pen of Macaulay: "The smallpox was always present, filling the churchyards with corpses, tormenting with constant fears all whom it had not stricken, leaving on those whose lives it spared the hideous traces of its power, turning the babe into a changeling at which

the mother shuddered, and making the eyes and cheeks of a betrothed maiden objects of horror to the lover." Now almost no doctor living in countries where this book is likely to be read has ever seen a case of smallpox (Fig. 8–22).

The prototypic poxvirus for biochemical and genetic study has been **vaccinia**. This virus emerged during Jenner's historical efforts at developing a "vaccine" from cowpox which would protect people from subsequent contact with smallpox. Vaccinia and variola are closely related viruses—although one causes a mild or inapparent disease in humans and the other a terrible disease with a fatality rate that approaches 35%. There are more than 50 proteins in the brick-shaped virion, within which is a 190 kb double-stranded genome. After absorption onto specific receptors, the virus undergoes sequential uncoating steps. Early gene expression occurs in the cytoplasm within a membrane-bound viral core, and is accomplished entirely by enzymes brought in with the virion. Viral DNA replication also ensues in the cytoplasm, a feature which is unique among the DNA viruses. The enzymes involved in directing DNA synthesis are also encoded by the virus. The foci of cytoplasmic replication are known as factories, virosomes, or Guarnieri bodies (for variola). Following the late

Fig. 8–22   The value of vaccination. Three of a family exposed to smallpox; the child in the middle unvaccinated, the others vaccinated 1 year before (Schamberg and Kolmer).

phases of mRNA and protein synthesis, hundreds of new virions are released from the disintegrating cells as rapidly as 12 hours after infection. Poxviruses are now known to encode many proteins which moderate the immune response of the cell and prolong the production of viral progeny. These include proteins which interact with the host's complement cascade. A viral growth factor is also produced; upon secretion from infected cells, the metabolic readiness of neighboring cells is increased in order to facilitate the spread and productivity of the virus. This is truly an example of virus evolution!

Fig. 8–23   This caricature by Gillray (1802) illustrated the ridicule to which Jenner's discovery of vaccination was subjected. (From a print in the Wellcome Institute for the History of Medicine.)

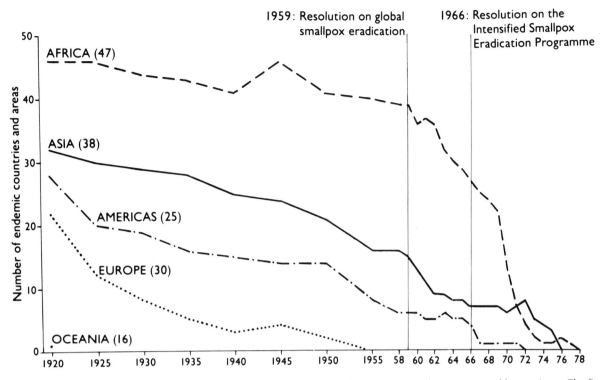

Fig. 8–24 Numbers of countries and territories in which smallpox was endemic between 1920 and 1978, arranged by continent. The figures in brackets indicate the numbers of countries and territories involved. (Fenner, F., Henderson, D.A., Arita, I., et al.: *Smallpox and Its Eradication.* Geneva, World Health Organization, 1988, p.171.)

The smallpox virus entered a susceptible host through the respiratory route, multiplying for 1 to 2 weeks in the lymph nodes and lungs. Cell lysis was typical. Two days of febrile viremia followed. During this circulatory phase, virus localized in the skin and grew in nodules. These were most frequent on the extremities, perhaps because high temperature inhibited viral growth, and the extremities remained cooler than the trunk. The nodules were at first solid papules, but in a few days they converted to pustules that might cover the face and the entire body. Swelling and "ballooning" of the epithelial cells occurred, with subsequent liquefaction of the cells; this was often followed by streptococcal superinfection. Scabs formed over the pustules; dried scabs covered with virus were cast off. From this description it will be seen how important the problem of nursing was, especially in a community that had not been adequately vaccinated. As the pustules healed, scars of varying depth were left in the skin. Thus the dangers of smallpox are twofold: (1) death, and (2) disfigurement.

Vaccinia virus has always been in the foreground of vaccine research. It was first found that the related cowpox virus would induce only a mild disease in human beings but would stimulate lasting immunity to the more severe smallpox virus (Fig. 8–23). Vaccinia emerged as the accepted vaccine strain, and the comprehensive campaign mounted by the World Health Organization led to the worldwide eradication of smallpox (Fig. 8–24). Smallpox was amenable to such an attack for several reasons: the absence of an animal reservoir, the presence of only one serotype, the ability to easily identify nonimmune individuals because of the characteristic scars left by infection, the life-long immunity which followed infection, the lytic nature of the virus which did not induce any latent or persistent infections, and the effectiveness, stability, and inexpense of the vaccine. As described above in the introductory sections, the effectiveness of vaccinia virus as a vaccine has led to current efforts to create recombinant vaccines in which the virus carries key genes of pathogens such as rabies, herpes, hepatitis, etc.

The poxviruses which cause human disease today are **molluscum contagiosum**, a virus which causes benign cutaneous papules, and **monkeypox**, which can be spread from rodents, squirrels or monkeys to humans and induces a disease which is far milder than smallpox but follows a similar course. Other poxviruses of animals are also transmitted to humans in rare cases.

UNCONVENTIONAL VIRUSES

Several slow neurologic diseases have been associated with "unconventional" viruses. These viruses are by definition filterable, but they are thermostable and ultraviolet-sensitive. No nucleic acid component has been found. No apparent immune response or inflammatory lesions accompany their infections. They induce slow degenerative diseases known as subacute spongiform virus encephalopathies. Similar diseases in animals include scrapie (sheep) and bovine spongiform encephalopathy (BSE) (cattle).

Kuru is one such disease found only among a single ethnic group in New Guinea. The "virus" is present in diseased brain tissue and can be passed to primates. It appears that the virus was spread by contact with and ingestion of infected brain tissue. Cannibalism as a mourning tribute was prevalent from 1920 until 1950; with its cessation, the disease has effectively disappeared. Apparently, the virus slowly accumulates in the central nervous system and gradually destroys tissue. Eventually neurologic symptoms appear, with tremors progressing to motor incapacity and death.

Creutzfeldt-Jakob disease (CJD) is nearly indistinguishable from kuru, and biopsies yield infectious material that produces analogous disease upon inoculation into primates. The symptoms are diffuse mental disorientation proceeding to dementia, mutism, rigidity, and death. This rare disease appears worldwide; there is a familial form which is heritable, and a transmissible form which is spread primarily via neurosurgical procedures, corneal transplants, and in pituitary-derived growth hormone preparations. Finally, the inherited Gerstmann-Straussler-Scheinker syndrome (GSS), is characterized by similar symptoms and biopsy material can also induce the disease in animals.

Significant progress has been made recently on developing a unifying hypothesis for these diseases. The particles associated with inducing disease are known as **prions**; these particles contain insoluble aggregates of a protein whose primary sequence is indistinguishable from that encoded by a normal cellular gene. Somehow, upon injection of the particulate, protease-insensitive form of the protein found in diseased brains, the endogenous protein is induced to adapt the altered morphology and behavior of the "infectious" prion. Recruitment of the host's protein amplifies the number of prions, and so an increase in the titer of transmissible prions occurs. The pathology of prion "infection" is related to the deposition of aggregated prion deposits, which disrupts the normal envi-

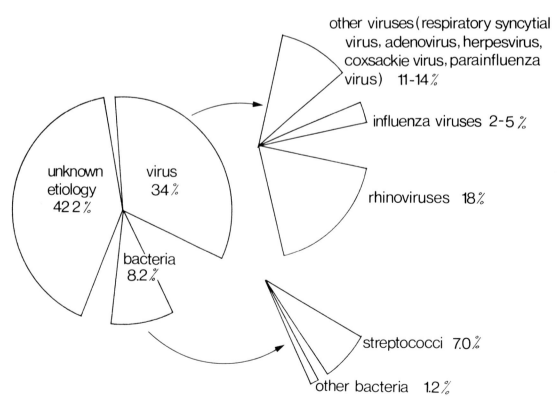

Fig. 8–25 This diagram shows the relative importance of different viruses and bacteria in causing respiratory tract infections. (After *Patterns of Diseases*, Morris Plains, N.J., Parke, Davis and Company, 1961.)

ronment and functioning of the surrounding brain tissue. The inherited GSS syndrome involves a mutation in a single amino acid of the endogenous prion protein. Transgenic mice which carry this altered gene have been shown to develop a comparable neurological disease, suggesting that the mutation may confer a tendency for the protein to spontaneously assemble into pathogenic prions.

PREVALENCE OF VIRAL INFECTIONS

It is important to keep some perspective in understanding the place of viruses as agents that cause disease in general. The accompanying diagram (Fig. 8–25) shows the proportions of respiratory tract infections caused by different viruses and bacteria. Of the unknown causes, one could estimate that half at least may be caused by viruses, leading to a grand total of 50% of all respiratory tract ailments, one of man's most common afflictions, being of viral etiology. Viruses are important causative agents of gastroenteritis, central nervous system disorders, immune deficiencies, hepatitis, and cancers. The value of gaining further insight into their life cycles and their varied modes of pathogenesis cannot be underestimated.

CHLAMYDIA AND RICKETTSIA

Chlamydia and Rickettsia are not viruses, although they have classically been grouped with viruses during discussions such as these, and their diagnosis is accomplished in virus laboratories. Unlike most bacteria, chlamydia and rickettsia cannot grow on inanimate media, but are obligate intracellular pathogens. Visible with the light microscope, they are larger than viruses but smaller than typical bacteria; they are sensitive to antibiotics such as tetracycline and erythromycin. They possess DNA genomes and messenger RNA, and replicate intracellularly by binary fission. Typically, transmission to human hosts is via arthropod vectors, and their persistence in nature often relies on a zoonosis, an animal reservoir.

Chlamydia

Several important human diseases are caused by C. trachomatis and C. psittaci. C. trachomatis is the leading cause of sexually transmitted non-gonoccocal urethritis. Women who develop resultant cervicitis can infect newborn infants during birth. Such infection most often causes neonatal opthalmia, a mucopurulent conjunctivitis of the eye, although pneumonia may also be a complication. C. trachomatis can also cause inclusion conjunctivitis in children and adults; transmission is thought to result from indirect contact

with secretions from genital infections, a fact reflected in the common term "swimming pool conjunctivitis."

Trachoma. This disease, endemic in tropical climates and caused by another serotype of C. trachomatis, is the most common world-wide cause of blindness. Most common in North Africa, sub-Sahara Africa, the Middle East, and southeast Asia, infection is spread by personal contact, flies, and infected fomites. The term trachoma was coined by a Sicilian physician in 69 A.D., but the disease has been described as early as 1500 B.C. in the Ebers papyrus. It was widespread in early times, as now, and afflicted both Cicero and Horace. It was introduced to Europe by returning crusaders and by Napoleon's troops coming from Egypt. The disease is still a problem in the United States where it exists in Indian reservations of the southwest. It has been found to be a disease of families, with the agent passing from child to child, sparing none under 2 years of age. The agent causes a severe follicular conjunctivitis, and invasion of the cornea with blood vessels is frequent. Corneal scarring prevents transmission of light to the retina, causing blindness. However, infection responds well to tetracycline and severe sequelae can be averted.

Psittacosis. Another disease caused by these agents is the acute febrile illness in which fever, headaches, muscle aches, and dry cough with interstitial pneumonia can be identified. This acute illness has been reported in pigeon breeders, people who have pet budgies, finches, or parrots, chicken or turkey farmers, poultry processors, and pet store personnel, or in children (Fig. 8–26). Since we now know that the organism (C. psittaci) can be passed from birds to man, this is called a zoonosis, a disease harbored by

Fig. 8–26 Confirmed psittacosis cases in poultry plant employees, by date of onset—North Carolina, October 1989. (From Centers for Disease Control, Morbidity and Mortality Weekly Report, 39(27):461, 1990.)

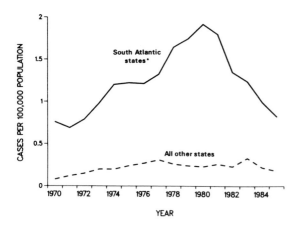

Fig. 8–27 Reported cases of Rocky Mountain spotted fever by year—South Atlantic states and all other states, 1970–1985. (From Centers for Disease Control: Morbidity and Mortality Weekly Report, 35(15): 249, 1986.)

an animal vector and transmitted on occasion to the human being. Psittacosis responds to tetracyclines, if the correct diagnosis is made. A rare but more serious outcome of infection is endocarditis.

Rickettsia

These bacteria, despite possessing the capacity for extensive metabolic independence, require an intracellular environment for growth. All rickettsiae are transmitted by arthropod vectors. They were first ob-

served in 1909 by H.T. Ricketts in the blood of patients with Rocky Mountain spotted fever, and in the tick that carried the disease. The next year, Ricketts found similar organisms in the intestine of lice that had fed on a patient with typhus. It is appropriate that these organisms should be named after Ricketts, since he died of infection with these agents during his studies.

Typhus. This acute infectious fever, historically a world scourge of epidemic proportions, is transmitted to man by the bites of infected ticks and lice, or by contamination of open scratches by their feces. This mode of transmission is reflected in the historic association of typhus epidemics with war, famines, and wretchedness. The reservoir of infection which maintains R. prowazekii during interepidemic periods was found to be the domestic rat, transmission from animal to animal being through the agency of the rat flea. If the rat dies and the rat flea is hard put to find a new host, he may bite man. Any lice in contact with the infected individual may now spread the disease to others in the community. Any reader who may wish to know more about the fascinating story of typhus in war and history should turn to Zinsser's delightful and entertaining *Rats, Lice and History*.

The onset of the disease is acute, with high fever, great weakness and prostration, a hemorrhagic rash, and mental apathy passing into stupor. The characteristic microscopic lesion is a swelling of the vascular endothelium throughout the body, including the skin

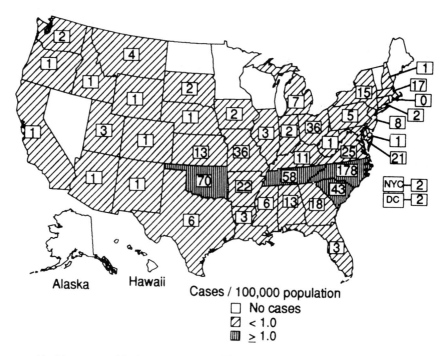

Fig. 8–28 Reported cases and incidence rates of Rocky Mountain spotted fever, by state—United States, 1990. (From Centers for Disease Control, Morbidity and Mortality Weekly Report, 40(27):452, 1991.)

and the central nervous system, the cytoplasm of the cells being crowded with rickettsiae. This is accompanied by thrombosis and hemorrhage that account for the symptoms. Curiously enough, in the louse the organisms are confined to the epithelial cells lining the gut, so that the excreta are swarming with rickettsiae which, when deposited on the skin, may enter through scratches and abrasions.

Five other diseases are known to be caused by rickettsiae. These will merely be mentioned. (1) Tsutugamushi fever is a typhus-like infection, also known as *scrub typhus*. It is endemic in Japan, Malaysia, and the East Indies, and the infection is transmitted by the bite of the infected larva of certain mites that live in rotting vegetation and tall grass, hence the name scrub typhus. (2) *Rocky Mountain spotted fever* bears a remarkable resemblance to typhus fever in regard to symptoms, lesions, and bacteriology. It used to be thought that the disease was confined to the Rocky Mountain region of the United States, but it is now known that the infection may be acquired over a considerable part of the United States and in southern Canada (Figs. 8–27, 8–28). The disease is conveyed by a wood tick. As in the case of typhus, laboratory workers may acquire the disease without being bitten by the tick. (3) *Trench fever* is so-called because it was the commonest of all the diseases affecting the troops in France during the trench warfare period of World War I. Infection was carried by the body louse. The mortality was so low that nothing is known of the lesions in man. (4) *Rickettsial pox* is a new rickettsial disease recognized in New York in 1946. The name is due to an eruption not unlike that of chickenpox. Infection is caused by the bite of a tick. The prognosis is uniformly favorable. (5) *Q fever* is a rickettsial disease carried by rodents and spread by ticks. The remarkable feature of the disease, which is widespread throughout the world, is the absence of any relation between the lesions, which take the form of pneumonic patches in the lungs, and the clinical picture, which is that of a typhoid-like state with a complete absence of respiratory symptoms. The mortality rate is low.

SYNOPSIS

Viruses are obligate intracellular parasites.

Viruses do not reproduce by dividing, but by directing the synthesis and export of a large number of like progeny.

Viruses can be classified by size, tissue specificity, and nucleic acid content.

Viruses may lyse cells, or they may alter their morphology or growth patterns.

Many viral infections are inapparent.

Viruses have been shown to be among the causes of cancer in animals.

Viral infections stimulate an immune response. In addition to curbing infection, the immune response can cause severe complications.

Viruses can exist in latent forms.

Viruses may be spread by droplet, blood, sewage, and insect vectors.

Terms

AIDS	*Immunity*	*Tissue tropism*
Arbovirus	*Interferon*	*Transformation*
Attenuated	*Latency*	*Vaccine*
Carrier	*Persistence*	*Viremia*
Cytopathic effect	*Syncytium*	*Virulent*

FURTHER READING

Baron, S.: The interferon system. ASM News 45:358, 1979.

Beasley, R.P., et al.: Hepatocellular carcinoma and hepatitis B virus. Lancet 2:1129, 1981.

Belshe, R.B.: *Textbook of Human Virology*, 2nd ed. Mosby Year Book, St. Louis 1991.

Bradley, D.W.: Enterically-transmitted non-A, non-B hepatitis. in *Viral Hepatitis*, A.J. Zuckerman, ed. British Medical Bulletin 46:442–462, 1990.

Choo, Q-L. et al.: Hepatis C virus: the major causative agent of viral non-A, non-B hepatitis. in *Viral Hepatitis*, A.J. Zuckerman, ed. British Medical Bulletin 46:423–442, 1990.

Cukor, G. and Blacklow, N.R.: Human viral gastroenteritis. Microbiological Reviews 48:157–179. 1974.

Cullen, B.R.: Regulation of HIV-1 gene expression. FASEB J.. 5:2361–2369. 1991.

Dolin, R., Treanor, J.J., and Madore, H.P.: Novel agents of viral enteritis in humans. J. Infect. Dis. 155:365–376, 1987.

Foege, W.H.: Should the smallpox virus be allowed to survive? N. Engl. J. Med. 300:670, 1979.

Haseltine, W.A.: Molecular biology of the human immunodeficiency virus type 1. FASEB J.. 5:2349–2361, 1991.

Henle, W., Henle, G., and Lennette, E.T.: The Epstein-Barr virus. Scientific American 241:48, 1979.

Kilbourne, E.D.: *Molecular Epidemiology—Influenza as Archetype.* (Harvey Lectures, Series 73.) New York, Academic Press, 1979.

Racaniello, V.: *Virus-receptor interaction in poliovirus entry and pathogenesis.* Harvey Society Lecture. Academic Press, New York, 1991.

Razin, S., and Jacobs, E.: Mycoplasma adhesion. J. Gen. Microbiol., 138:407, 1992.

Rosenberg, Z.F. and Fauci, A.S.: Immunopathogenesis of HIV infection. FASEB J.. 5:2382–2391, 1991.

Schachter, J.: Chlamydial infections. N. Engl. J. Med. 298:428, 1978.

Shulman, S.T.: What's new in infectious diseases? Current Problems in Pediatrics 21:3–7, 1991.

Sixbey, J. and Pagano, J.S.: New perspectives on the Epstein-Barr virus in the pathogenesis of lymphoproliferative disorders. In

Remington, J.S. and Swartz, M.N. (Eds)., *Current Clinical Topics in Infectious Diseases*, Vol. 5, McGraw-Hill, New York, 1984.

Stahl, N. and Prusiner, S.B.: Prions and prion proteins. FASEB J. 5:2799–2807, 1991.

Vanmiddelkoop, A., Vanwyk, J.E., Kustner, H.G.V., et al.: Poliomyelitis outbreak in Natal/Kwazulu, South Africa, 1987–1988. 1. Epidemiology. Trans. Roy. Soc. Trop. Med. Hyg., 86:80, 1992.

Westwood, J.C.N.: *The Hazard from Dangerous Exotic Diseases.* London, MacMillan Press Ltd., 1980.

Zuckerman, A.J., Banatvala, J.E. and Pattison, J.R. *Principles and Practice of Clinical Virology.* 2nd edition, J. Wiley & Sons, Chichester, UK 1991.

zur Hausen, H.: Human papillomaviruses in the pathogenesis of anogenital cancer (minireview). Virology 184:9–13, 1991.

9

FUNGAL INFECTIONS

Infectious disease is merely a disagreeable instance of a widely prevalent tendency of all living creatures to save themselves the bother of building the things they require.—ZINSSER

Fungi represent another type of organism than bacteria; unlike plants, they lack pigments necessary to manufacture their own food and therefore depend on other forms of life. Fungi may assume different appearances during their life cycle, and can exist as microscopic forms (yeast), or in large colonies (mushrooms). Historically, many diseases of medical importance caused by fungi (histoplasmosis, coccidioidomycosis), have been mistaken for those caused by protozoa, and other diseases once classified as fungal are now considered to be bacterial (nocardiosis, actinomycosis). Regardless of how they are classified, fungi are assuming greater importance than ever, because we now successfully treat most bacterial diseases and keep people safe longer from the traditional infectious agents by various techniques.

Fungi are omnipresent in the air, so that they are apt to contaminate culture media, to grow as molds on food, and to be generally troublesome. Fortunately, few are pathogenic. For growth they require a high humidity, warmth, and a free supply of oxygen. Any gardener trying to grow roses and prevent "black spot" knows this. The warmth and humidity of the tropics are particularly favorable for their multiplication, so it is natural that fungal diseases should be much more common in tropical countries and in the southern United States. Some reproduce only by budding, but others bud with failure to separate, giving rise to long branching filaments known as hyphae, which form masses called mycelia. A fungus causing an infection can be grown on culture media or demonstrated in the tissue, preferably with special stains such as PAS (periodic acid-Schiff) and silver methenamine.

The subject of fungal infections, known as the mycoses or mycotic disease, is acquiring a new importance by reason of the use and abuse of multiple antibiotics. These wipe out the harmless bacteria with which the fungi are accustomed to live and that restrain fungal growth. With elimination of the bacteria, the fungi occupy the field, to multiply without restraint, and to assume the role of pathogens. Damage to the tissues is not caused by toxins but is the result of allergic necrosis due to sensitization to the proteins of the fungi. Skin tests for hypersensitivity to these foreign antigens are of great value in many instances. Fungi are more resistant than bacteria to drying and to the action of antibiotics, which, after all, are derived primarily from fungi. With modern medical treatment involving many people in chemotherapy for cancer, immunosuppressive therapy for transplantation, and antibiotic therapy for common bacterial infections, we see greatly increased numbers of hospital patients who succumb to fungal diseases such as candidiasis, aspergillus infections, and mucormycosis. Because these fungi normally cannot infect a human being but are successful in the debilitated or immunologically deprived patient, such fungal diseases are called **opportunistic** infections. The fungi that cause superficial infections spread from animals to man, whereas those that cause systemic infections seem to come from the soil, vegetation, and bird droppings. Only a few of the pathogenic fungi will be considered in this text.

HISTOPLASMOSIS

This disease has an extraordinary history. The causal organism, named at that time *Histoplasma capsulatum*, was first demonstrated in 3 fatal cases in the Panama Canal Zone in 1906 and was believed from its appearance to be a protozoon animal parasite. The disease was believed to be confined to the tropics and to be uniformly fatal. Some 30 years later, the organism was cultured and shown to be a fungus, not a protozoon. This discovery proved to be the break-

HISTOPLASMIN
H-42 1:100

PERCENTAGE
REACTIONS 6+ M M
☐ 0 — 2
▨ 2 — 10
▨ 10 — 30
▨ 30 — 60
■ 60 — 80
■ 80 — 100

185,000 NAVY RECRUITS 1958-1962
white males 17 - 21 years
LIFETIME ONE COUNTY RESIDENTS

Fig. 9–1 This map of the United States shows the histoplasmin positive skin tests for 185,000 navy recruits between 1958 and 1962, illustrating their lifetime residence. The Mississippi River valley is the location of most of the fungal infections caused by this organism. (From Comstock, G. W.: In *Maxcy-Rosenau Preventive Medicine and Public Health,* 10th Ed. Edited by P. E. Sartwell. New York, Appleton-Century-Crofts, 1973.)

through, for the culture of the fungus was used as the antigen for a histoplasmin skin sensitivity reaction, to be followed shortly by a complement fixation test. These procedures proved to be revolutionary, for they showed that infection with the fungus was prevalent in the northeastern and central parts of the United States, the central Mississippi Valley in particular, and that to a much lesser degree, it was worldwide in distribution (Fig. 9–1). From the skin tests it soon became apparent that there were two different forms of the disease: one mild, localized, and common; the other severe, disseminated, rare, and nearly always fatal. In endemic areas, histoplasmin tests show that up to 75% of the population may be infected by the fungus without any clinical evidence of disease. The infection does not appear to be transmitted directly from person to person, but to be inhaled in the dust from the soil, where the fungus can be demonstrated. Many domestic animals are susceptible to infection, and several epidemics have been associated with contamination of the soil by animal excreta, especially that of pigeons and chickens.

Typically the epidemic will be a small group of persons involved in demolition or in cleaning out old silos or chicken coops, who become ill after an incuba-

tion of 1 to 2 weeks. Attack rates may reach 100% and cough, fever, and prostration are the typical symptoms in the illness, which lasts 1 to 3 weeks. This mild form is a benign inhalation infection of the lungs. At least 95% of cases are asymptomatic. It is startling to find radiologic evidence of extensive infiltration in the lungs with no symptoms or physical signs. The lymph nodes at the hilus of the lung are nearly always en-

Fig. 9–2 Cells of the lymph node packed with *Histoplasma capsulatum.* (From a section by Dr. W. A. D. Anderson. In Boyd, W.: *Textbook of Pathology.* Philadelphia, Lea & Febiger.)

Table 9–1.   Clinical Characteristics of Infected and Reinfected Persons in an Outbreak of Histoplasmosis at an Arkansas Courthouse In July, 1975

SYMPTOM	FREQUENCY IN 50 SEROLOGICALLY CONFIRMED CASES (%)
Fever	100*
Chills	76
Weight loss	44†
Cough	72
Headache	72
Myalgia	78
Chest pain	74
Arthritis	26
Mouth ulcerations (size unknown)	12
Erythema nodosum (red swelling on legs)	18

* Average 39.1°C (102.6°F)
† 1.8 kg to 5.6 kg

(From Dean, A.G., et al.: An outbreak of histoplasmosis at an Arkansas courthouse, with five cases of probable reinfection. Am. J. Epidemiol., 108:36, 1978.)

larged. A few patients have cough, fever, and loss of strength (Table 9–1).

The rare progressive form is an entirely different story, with a nearly always fatal finish. Acute disseminated histoplasmosis is generally the result of a heavy infection with the fungus or of poor resistance in young children and debilitated elderly persons. Tubercle-like nodules and necrotic foci are found in the lungs, liver, spleen, and kidneys, together with ulcerating lesions of the mouth, larynx, and intestine in many cases. Microscopically the reticuloendothelial cells are crowded with the organisms, which bear a remarkable resemblance to the protozoa causing leishmaniasis (Fig. 9–2).

COCCIDIOIDOMYCOSIS

Approximately 100,000 new cases of coccidioidomycosis occur per year in the United States, with about 70 deaths. It is said to be as common as chickenpox in some areas, and the medical interest lies both in the morbidity it causes and in the rarer, but often fatal, fulminant case. The disease is commonly called San Joaquin Valley fever and came into prominence during the early days of World War II when large numbers of recruits were stationed in that area, and later prisoners of war as well. These military men often became symptomatic, with a first diagnosis being made of pulmonary tuberculosis. Skin testing 35 years ago showed the distribution of positive reactors (Fig. 9–3).

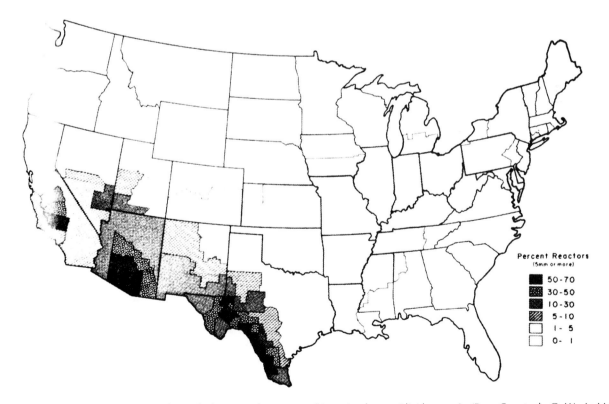

Fig. 9–3   This map of the United States shows the location of reactors to skin testing for coccidioidomycosis. (From Comstock, G. W.: In *Maxcy-Rosenau Preventive Medicine and Public Health,* 10th Ed. Edited by P. E. Sartwell, New York, Appleton-Century-Crofts, 1973.)

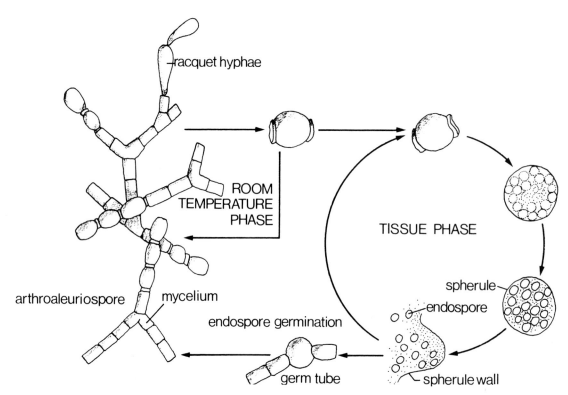

Fig. 9–4   This drawing illustrates the appearance of the fungus coccidioidomycosis. The hyphae of the fungus are shown on the left. An intermediate form between the hyphae and the microspheres appears at the top (between the arrows). The tissue phase (endospores) is shown on the right. (From Drutz, D. J., and Catanzaro, A.: Coccidioidomycosis. Am. Rev. Respir. Dis., 117:559, 1978.)

The causative agent is a dimorphic fungus (Fig. 9–4) that grows naturally and on media as a mold, but in man or in laboratory animals it may appear as spherules that contain endospores. The endemic region for the organism is the southwest, where the fungi sur-

Table 9–2. Frequency of Symptoms in 27 Archeology Students with Laboratory-Confirmed Coccidioidomycosis

SYMPTOM	FREQUENCY (%)
Cough	89
Fever	82
Headache	74
Chest pain	70
Chills	67
Shortness of breath	63
Malaise	59
Myalgia	52
Rash	52
Night sweats	44
Phlegm	30
Erythema nodosum	15
Meningismus	15
Weight loss	11

(From Drutz, D.J., and Catanzaro, A.: Coccidioidomycosis. Part II. Am. Rev. Respir. Dis., 117:727, 1978.)

vive in rodents' burrows and in the sandy soil. The fungus infects swine, cattle, and sheep, but they, like man, are largely resistant to infection. It has been reported in dogs, in horses, and even in tigers.

The disease is acquired by inhalation of the spores, therefore the dustier, drier, and richer the soil is with the agent, the better the chance for exposure. An unusual example of an epidemic was traced to a windstorm. The weather pattern and the cases related to the windstorm are illustrated in Figure 9–5.

The clinical symptoms are outlined in Table 9–2.

CRYPTOCOCCOSIS (TORULOSIS)

A subacute or chronic infection caused by *Cryptococcus neoformans* (*Torula histolytica*), cryptococcosis or torulosis may involve the lungs, skin, and other parts, but it has a special predilection for the meninges and brain, so that it is always dangerous (Fig. 9–6). In the lungs, the smaller lesions are easily mistaken for tubercles, but sometimes they are as large as an orange. The infection favors tissue weakened by reason of infancy, before resistance has had time to be established, of old age, of chronic debilitating illness,

Fig. 9–5 *A*, Map of the dust storm. Numbers represent surface pressures in millibars. The arrow indicates the direction of movement of soil dust, and the stippled area the area affected by settling dust. *B*, Reported cases of coccidioidomycosis according to week, in California. The upper portion shows the cumulative number; the hatched area represents the range of values, and the dotted line within the hatched area, the mean value. The lower portion shows the number reported each week; the hatched bars represent the mean for 1968 to 1977, and the open bars, the values for 1978. (*A* and *B* from Flynn, N.M., et al.: An unusual outbreak of windborne coccidioidomycosis. N. Engl. J. Med., 301:358, 1979. Reprinted by permission of the New England Journal of Medicine.)

Fig. 9–6 *Cryptococcus neoformans* shown in Alcian blue stain. The thick capsules of the organisms have been preserved by mounting in glycerin jelly. (Kindness of Dr. R. W. Mowry. In Boyd, W.: *Pathology for the Physician.*)

or of the displacement of the normal friendly bacterial inhabitants by antibiotics, so the balance is tilted still more decisively from health to disease.

BLASTOMYCOSIS

This is a chronic granuloma caused by a yeast-like fungus known as *Blastomyces*. The organisms are spherical, 2 or 3 times the diameter of a red blood cell, and show 2 characteristic features: (1) a clear double contour, and (2) budding yeast-like cells. The disease and the fungus that causes it occur in different forms in different parts of the world. Thus there is North American, South American, and European blastomycosis. The last is better named cryptococcosis, described in the foregoing section.

The North American form may be cutaneous or systemic. In the cutaneous (the common) variety, skin papules, which later ulcerate, develop especially on the face, the back of the hand, and the front of the leg. The disease spreads over the surface, so that a large area may be involved. In the systemic and naturally much more dangerous variety, infection spreads by the blood stream throughout the body, setting up nodules and abscesses usually in the lungs, but any organ may be involved.

South American blastomycosis, a chronic granulomatous disease of the skin, viscera, and lymph nodes that is most common in Brazil, is caused by a much larger fungus with numerous buds. The most characteristic feature is enlargement of the lymph nodes, particularly those of the neck, present in practically every case.

CANDIDIASIS

Candida, a saprophytic, dimorphic fungus, is commonly present on mucus membranes (oral cavity, genitalia), and in the gastrointestinal tract of man. Normally, the organism does not cause disease, but it has become increasingly a serious threat to life when there is prolonged therapy with antibiotics, corticosteroids, or immunosuppressive drugs, or in the presence of uremia, leukemia, hyperalimentation, or intravenous catheters.

The organism normally thrives in conditions of moisture and will appear as white patches involving the vagina, axillary folds, or mouth. When these patches occur in the mouth, they are known as *thrush*, and consist of growing mycelia, branching mycelial filaments with budding yeastlike cells that have thin walls. Normally, the infection is limited to the surface epithelia, but more cases of fungemia (blood stream infection) are being reported, often similar to and difficult to distinguish from endocarditis caused by other organisms.

Antibodies are made to the fungus and, in suspected cases, a serum agglutinating antibody titer can be done. It is also helpful to examine the buffy coat to see if the yeast-like organisms can be stained within the white blood cells. Tissue diagnosis by histologic examination is often diagnostic. Amphotericin B is the modern drug of choice, but its administration carries risks and it is wise to be certain of the diagnosis before beginning therapy.

MUCORMYCOSIS (PHYCOMYCOSIS)

This is another example of a disease caused by aerobic saprophytic fungi that are normally not pathogenic for man, but reside in soil and decaying matter. Again, in the debilitated host, someone with another illness such as diabetes mellitus, uremia, acidosis, burns, or cancer, or who has been receiving steroids, radiotherapy, chemotherapy, or antibiotics, these fungi may grow, prosper, and cause disease.

The organism normally grows as hyphae with a wide angle of branching and typically invades and obstructs blood vessels, leading to thrombosis and infarction, particularly in the lung in man. The organisms may involve branches of the retinal or cerebral vessels, sometimes arising in a sinus infection, or they may penetrate the gastrointestinal tract and compromise the circulation to the liver. These organisms may also cause weakening of the arterial wall, leading to the particular type of aneurysm called mycotic.

Diagnosis can be established by staining the suspected tissue, or by growing the organism from the sputum or blood. Mucormycosis is to be suspected in all instances in which the patient's defenses are compromised. It is best regarded as a complication of other disease, a true example of opportunistic infection.

DERMATOMYCOSES

This in common language is ringworm, which suggests that all dermatomycoses have the same etiology, and implies that the treatment may be the same. The dermatomycoses resemble each other in that areas of redness occur in patches on the skin of the head, groin, between the fingers and toes, or in the axilla, but the specific fungi are different. Because they are highly contagious, they are often difficult to treat in crowded living conditions or in those areas where facilities for personal hygiene are not available. These infections are communicated by means of contaminated clothing and structures such as the floors of rooms. Although not dangerous, dermatomycoses are notoriously difficult to treat. The following are some common forms.

Ringworm of the Scalp. This disease is also known as tinea (not to be confused with taenia or tapeworm). For some reason it affects only children. It is contagious, and in schools and institutions it may assume epidemic proportions. The fungus, known as *Trichophyton* (Greek *thrix*, hair and *phyton*, plant) invades and lives in the hair and in the roots of the hair; this explains why it attacks the scalp, why it produces bald patches, and why it is so difficult to eradicate.

Ringworm of the Groin. The causal fungus invades the epidermis, and is therefore known as an *Epidermophyton*. It frequently occurs in schools and among young athletes.

Interdigital Ringworm. This form occurs between the fingers and toes, and has become common because of the increased use of gymnasiums, locker rooms, showers, swimming pools, and the like. The frequency of the disease has in places been enormous. The association of the disease with various sports is the reason for its common name, "athlete's foot." The fungus usually responsible is *Epidermophyton*.

To put fungal infections in some perspective, of 1,251 cases seen in hospital between 1972 and 1974, 102 were candidal, 44 were aspergillus, 9 were mucormycoid, and the remainder were minor dermatomycoid infections.

SYNOPSIS

Biologic factors in fungal growth limit its infectivity.
Opportunistic infections are the most serious fungal threat to human life.
Superficial fungal infections are common; deep infections are rare.

Terms

Mycelia   *Hyphae*   *Epidermophyton*
Yeast   *Mycoses*

FURTHER READING

Conant, N.F., et al.: *Manual of Clinical Mycology*, 3rd Ed. Philadelphia, W.B. Saunders Co., 1971.
Dean, A.G., et al.: An outbreak of histoplasmosis in an Arkansas courthouse with five cases of probable reinfection. Am. J. Epidemiol., 108:36, 1978.
Drutz, D.J., and Catanzaro, A.: Coccidioidomycosis. Am. Rev. Respir. Dis., 117:559, 1978.
Ellis, D.H., and Pfeiffer, T.J.: Ecology, life cycle, and infectious propagule of *Cryptococcus neoformans*. Lancet, 336:923, 1990.
Flynn, N.M., et al.: An unusual outbreak of windborne coccidioidomycosis. N. Engl. J. Med., 301:358, 1979.
Goldstein, E., and Hoeprich, P.D.: Problems in the diagnosis and treatment of systemic candidiasis. J. Infect. Dis., 125:190, 1972.

Gustafson, T.L., et al.: Outbreak of acute pulmonary histoplasmosis in members of a wagon train. Am. J. Med., 71:759, 1981.
Hilton, E., Isenberg, J.D., Alperstein, P., et al.: Ingestion of yogurt containing lactobacillus-acidophilus as prophylaxis for candidal vaginiitis. Ann. Intern. Med., 116:353, 1992.
Kong, N.C.T., Shaariah, W., Morad, Z., et al.: Cryptococcosis in a renal unit. Aust. NZ J. Med., 20:645, 1990.
Medoff, G., and Kobazaski, G.S.: Pulmonary mucormycosis. N. Engl. J. Med., 286:86, 1972.
Rubenstein, E., et al.: Fungal endocarditis. Medicine, 54:331, 1975.
Sekhon, A.S., Isaac-Renton, J., Dixon, J.M.S., et al: Review of human and animal cases of coccidioidomycosis diagnosed in Canada. Mycopathologia, 113:1, 1991.

10

ANIMAL PARASITES

Nature is a labyrinth in which the very haste you move with will make you lose your way.—Bacon

An animal parasite is a member of the animal kingdom that has acquired the power of living in the body of another animal. The parasite may or may not produce disease in the host. Here we are concerned only with the human host and with pathogenic (disease-producing) parasites. Most parasites have developed a remarkable habit; they spend a part of their life cycle in one host (man) and another part of the cycle in another host (an animal). The second host may be of any size, from a cow to a mosquito, but each parasite has its own particular animal host; the cow and the mosquito are not interchangeable. Moreover, the second host is a necessity, not a luxury; unless it can be found, that particular parasite will die. It is evident that knowledge of this dependence places a powerful weapon in the hands of persons involved in the prevention of parasitic diseases. Finally, the second host may be responsible for conveying the disease to man, as in the case of the mosquito and malaria.

One of the most remarkable features of a parasite's life cycle is that the eggs produced in the body of an animal or man do not develop in the same animal. They may develop into larvae in the soil, but usually they must be ingested by another host and develop there. The **definitive host** is the host of the adult parasite (sexual cycle), and the **intermediate host** is the host of the embryo (asexual cycle). Man is the definitive host of the common tapeworms, but the intermediate host of the malaria parasite.

We can agree that animal parasites have evolved a remarkable and perilous method of completing their life cycles, for unless the appropriate intermediate host comes along, the family of the parasite is doomed, as the eggs cannot develop in the definitive host. To meet this hazard, parasites have learned to produce eggs in numbers that in some instances are astronomic. The fish tapeworm of man lays several million eggs daily and lives for several years, whereas the stomach worm of the sheep lays an egg every 10

to 20 seconds. The problem of reproduction has been simplified in some tapeworms by the male's being dispensed with entirely!

Before discussing various animal parasites, we might look at the question of parasitism from the point of view of the parasite. When an animal decides to adopt this way of life, it must be prepared to make certain sacrifices. The host provides the parasite with all the comforts of life, so that organs of locomotion and those of special sense required for hunting prey or avoiding enemies disappear. The parasite does not necessarily damage the host; they may live in harmony for many years. Indeed the successful parasite does not jeopardize the survival of the host, because in so doing it jeopardizes its own survival. However, the pathogenic parasites must occupy our attention. These occur commonly even in temperate climates, and, when tropical parasites are included, we meet some of the most important diseases of mankind. Only a few of the more serious will be considered here. Disease-producing parasites belong to two great groups: protozoa, or unicellular organisms, and worms, which fall under the category of metazoa. The worms are divided into roundworms, tapeworms, and flukes.

PROTOZOA

Amebiasis. This condition is commonly the cause of dysentery, an inflammation of the colon. The danger of dysentery, apart from the inconvenience, is dehydration, electrolyte loss, and loss of blood in the acute stages. With more chronic disease, perforation, peritonitis, and abscesses may occur. The clinical pattern of infections other than dysentery depends on the organs involved. Apart from the bowel, liver abscess is most common, and spread from there to the lungs may also occur. Symptoms of these infections are nonspecific and heralded by fever and malaise. To make the diagnosis, one must suspect the presence of such abscesses, which may be identified today by technetium-sulfur colloid liver scans, or by gallium citrate studies. Ultrasound studies may also reveal a hollow cavity with internal echoes (Fig. 10–1), but, of course, none of these techniques identifies the causal organism, only the presence of a lesion. In order to make the diagnosis, it is necessary to identify the ameba with the microscope.

The ameba is a single, large cell, recognized by its motility in a fresh specimen of feces. It often contains ingested red blood cells. In chronic cases of amebiasis, such as are seen in temperate climates, the ameba becomes globular and is converted into a cyst with a thick outer capsular layer. The cysts are the infective form of the parasite, for the active form is killed by the gastric juice as it passes through the stomach. Multiplication in this simplest of all animals is by direct division; there is no sexual stage.

Infection is usually the result of fecal contamination of water supply or food. The chief danger is from a carrier rather than from a patient suffering from the active form of the disease. Two reasons for this are: In the first place, the danger from the patient is obvious, and precautions can be taken to prevent the spread of the infection, whereas the carrier is unsuspected. The second reason is that the parasites discharged from the carrier in the form of cysts are much more resistant to the action of the gastric juice than are those from the patient with the active disease. For this reason, the amebas are able to pass through the stomach and to reach the large bowel, where they set up fresh lesions of the disease.

Recently, another amebic infection in man has been identified in which free-living aquatic amebas are able to infect man and to cause meningitis, most frequently from swimming areas.

The diagnosis is made by finding the amebas in the stools, but in order that they may be recognized, they must be living and moving. On being passed from the body, they soon lose their power of movement, especially when they are chilled. A specimen of stool (a tiny amount is required) should be placed in a warm receptacle, which is then wrapped so as to prevent chilling, and immediately dispatched to the laboratory, where it should be delivered directly to the pathologist, and not merely laid down on a table, where it may be overlooked for some time. Unless these precautions are taken, it will be impossible to detect the amebas.

Malaria. This disease is caused by a minute unicellular parasite, known as a plasmodium. Part of the life cycle is spent in man and part in the anopheles mosquito. Destruction of this type of mosquito will be followed by the disappearance of malaria. The disease is the most widespread serious malady affecting the human race, although necessarily confined to those parts of the world infested by the anopheles mosquito. Greece, a land of heroes, fell in a few centuries to be a land of slaves, largely because of malaria. The disease still constitutes the greatest public health problem in the world (Fig. 10–2). In certain tropical

Fig. 10–1 *A,* This ultrasound scan of the liver shows a multiloculated cystic mass in the inferior portion of the liver. The dense white line at the top indicates the position of the diaphragm. *B,* The drawing illustrates the position of the multicystic mass, which is typical of an echinococcal cyst.

Fig. 10–2   Locations of three malaria outbreaks—northern San Diego County, California, August 1988 and July and August 1989. (From Centers for Disease Control, Morbidity and Mortality Weekly Report, 39(6):92, 1990.)

regions, everyone is infected with malaria from early infancy until death. Such persons never know for a single day the feeling of perfect health. Malaria is responsible, either directly or indirectly, by weakening resistance, for about 2 million deaths every year in India alone, and it is estimated that about 100 million suffer annually from the disease in that country.

When an infected mosquito bites man, it injects the parasites into the blood stream. Each parasite enters a red blood corpuscle and multiplies inside it until it destroys the corpuscle, which then bursts and liberates the new parasites into the blood. These attack new red corpuscles, multiply inside them and destroy them. It is obvious that in this way billions of parasites may be produced, and billions of red blood corpuscles may be destroyed, so that the patient will develop a profound anemia. The time taken by the parasites to multiply in the blood cells is always the same, so that the billions of blood cells all burst at the same time and liberate the new parasites into the blood stream at the same time. This massive discharge of parasites into the blood produces sudden high fever and an attack of shivering known as a rigor. The temperature rapidly falls, and may remain normal until the next batch of parasites is liberated. One form of parasite completes this part of its life cycle every 48 hours, and so the fever and chills occur every other day; as this is every third day (counting the day of the attack), this form of the disease is known as tertian malaria. In another form, the life cycle occupies 72 hours; the attack of fever occurs on the fourth day (counting the

day of the attack), so that the disease is known as quartan malaria.

The human part of the life cycle is asexual, i.e., two sexes are not necessary for reproduction. However, this asexuality can continue for a certain time only. Unless rejuvenation of the parasite occurs by sexual reproduction, for which the mosquito is necessary, the parasite will die. Sexual forms, male and female, are present in human blood, but they are unable to unite. Their chance comes when the mosquito bites a malarial patient and sucks his or her blood into her stomach (it is only the female of the species that does the biting). The male and female forms now unite, and the fruit of the union is a fresh brood of rejuvenated parasites, which make their way to the mosquito's proboscis and wait to enter the blood of the next person the insect happens to bite. Thus the mosquito not only carries on the life cycle of a parasite, but conveys it from person to person. The complete life cycle of the parasite is illustrated in Figure 10–3.

The diagnosis of malaria is suggested by the chills and regular repeated attacks of fever, but it can only be made with certainty by finding the parasites in the red cells in a smear of the patient's blood. The best time to make the blood examination is just before the onset of a chill. The spleen is large, and in acute cases it is soft, but in chronic cases it becomes hard.

The control of malaria in the districts of the world in which it is common has been aided by intensive campaigns against the mosquito by measures such as drainage of marshes and the treatment of stagnant water with oil or DDT to kill the larvae of the mosquito. It is of interest to recall the original meaning of the word malaria. It means bad air (Italian *malo*, bad, and *aria*, air) and is a reminder of the days when the disease was thought to be transmitted by the miasmic vapors of marshes. It was the mosquitoes, not the miasmas, that lived in the marshes.

Many drugs are used in the treatment of a patient with malaria, and these have been improved greatly during recent years. The common drugs in use are quinine, chloroquine, pentaquine, mepacrine, and pamaquine. An important advance has been the introduction of mepacrine and chloroquine as means of suppression of the disease during times of exposure in malarial countries.

The drugs are effective in treating malaria because they kill the immature forms of the protozoa by interfering with the oxidation of glucose and lactate and by inhibiting oxygen consumption. The difficulty in treating any disease is to find an agent that is toxic to the parasite but harmless to the host, and in cases where the parasite has a complex life cycle, it is fortun-

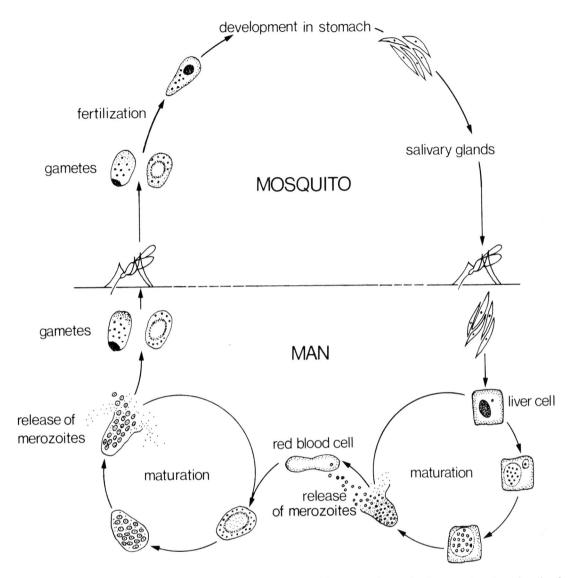

Fig. 10–3 This diagram shows the life cycle of the malaria parasite. The sexual forms are taken up by the mosquito where they develop and are subsequently reinfected into man, where the infectious agent is liberated from the liver. It then inhabits the red blood cell, where it develops again.

ate if any drug can be found to be effective for more than one stage of the parasite's cycle.

Sleeping Sickness. Trypanosomes are spindle-shaped protozoan parasites characterized by a macro-nucleus in the center, a micronucleus at one end, an undulating membrane, and a flagellum (Fig. 10–4). Sexual development occurs in an invertebrate host, the tsetse fly, which transmits the infection from one person to another. Asexual reproduction occurs in the blood of the intermediate host, namely man and many wild animals. There are many varieties of trypano-somes and many tsetse flies. Trypanosomiasis is confined to tropical Africa, since this region is the habitat of the tsetse fly.

Human trypanosomiasis, or African sleeping sickness, is caused by *Trypanosoma gambiense* (called after the Gambia river, in which district the fever is prevalent), and is carried by the tsetse fly, *Glossina palpalis*. The trypanosomes live in the blood, causing fever,

Fig. 10–4 Trypanosoma gambiense. x 1500

weakness, emaciation, and enlargement of the cervical and other lymph nodes. It is only later that they invade the central nervous system and cause true sleeping sickness with its characteristic lethargy and coma. Trypanosomes are easily demonstrated in the blood during attacks of fever and in the cerebrospinal fluid when symptoms of sleeping sickness have developed.

Toxoplasmosis. The protozoan *Toxoplasma gondii* is found throughout the world in many species of warm-blooded animals; members of the cat family appear to be the definitive host. The three forms of toxoplasma, the trophozoite, cyst, and oocyst, are variously responsible for the acute infection and the latent infection, but the oocyst exists only in the cat family (Fig. 10–5). When formed in cat intestine, the oocyst is excreted in the feces and matures in 1 to 21 days, after which it is infectious. This suggests that kitty litter boxes and human infants do not make a good match.

Toxoplasma is widespread in distribution, and results in lymphadenopathy in man. It causes congenitally acquired infection that is often characterized by cerebral calcifications and chorioretinitis in newborns (3,000 cases per year in the United States). In addition, toxoplasma often causes fatal encephalitis in the immunologically compromised host.

The disease is best diagnosed by serologic tests for specific toxoplasma antibodies. The trophozoite may be identified with Giemsa stains in tissues, and isolation by injection into mice is a useful procedure. A case can be made for serodiagnosis in all women before pregnancy, since acquisition of toxoplasma by the pregnant patient is a grave risk to the fetus. However, such testing is not yet routine in the United States.

An epidemic of toxoplasmosis occurred in patrons of a riding stable in Atlanta in 1976. Thirty-seven became ill with toxoplasmosis. The source was traced to 2 cats and 2 kittens; the incidence of disease was highest in the riders who came daily to the stable and spent most of their time at the end of the stable where cat feces were most abundant.

Leishmaniasis, or kala-azar, is simply referred to in passing as another worldwide protozoal disease.

NEMATODES OR ROUNDWORMS

Metazoal parasites are two cell layers thick and are unfortunately more complex structurally than protozoa; they include the worms, so far as this chapter is concerned, and we shall consider these parasites as follows: (1) nematodes or roundworms, (2) cestodes or tapeworms, and (3) trematodes or flukes. Such parasites can infest any compartment of the body and can navigate through the host during different parts of their life cycle. They have an awesome potential for travel through the intestinal tract across the gut barrier into the bloodstream to rest in the liver, or to migrate into the lung. From there, the egg or worm may be swallowed, or it may enter and obstruct the lymphatics, there to cause elephantiasis, or it may find its way into the eye or brain. Eosinophilia in the peripheral blood is often present. This is always suggestive of a helminth (parasitic worm) infection, being part of an allergic reaction to the foreign protein of the worm. In the case of the nematodes, which form the largest group, with a few exceptions, no intermediate host is required for completion of the life cycle.

Hookworm Disease (ankylostomiasis). This is one of the most prevalent diseases; it has been estimated that there are some 100,000,000 cases in the world. It is a disease of warm and tropical climates and used to be prevalent in the southern part of the United States. The worm, which is less than 3 cm in length, occurs in large numbers in the duodenum and jejunum. The mouth is armed with four teeth or hooklets that attach it to the wall of the duodenum and that give the worm its name (Greek *ankylos*, hooked, and *stoma*, mouth). The method by which the hookworm reaches the duodenum is one of the romances of medicine. The young embryo worm lives in warm, moist ground, bores through the skin of a person's bare feet, enters a vein, and is carried by the blood to the lung, where it is arrested. Here the worm escapes into the bronchi and starts to climb up the trachea. When it reaches the upper end, it descends the esophagus, passes through the stomach, and reaches the end of its long journey in the duodenum. Large numbers of hookworms arrive here and fasten themselves to the wall of the bowel. In time they produce marked anemia with profound lassitude and weakness. This is not remarkable, seeing that hundreds, sometimes thou-

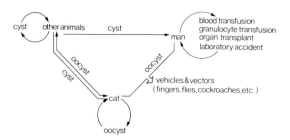

Fig. 10–5   This diagram illustrates the life cycle of the toxoplasma organism. The cat is a preferential host. The organism may be excreted in the feces of the cat and infest other animals, such as mice. The cyst in man may be transferred from man to man by blood transfusion, laboratory accident, or organ transplant. (From Krick, J.A., and Remington, J.S.: Toxoplasmosis in the adult—an overview. N. Engl. J. Med., 298:550, 1978.)

Fig. 10–6   This histologic section shows the method of attachment of the hookworm to the wall of the human intestine.

sands, of the little worms have been found hanging onto the wall of the intestine, sucking blood as a baby would suck milk (Fig. 10–6). No intermediate host is required for the development of the hookworm. As many as 10,000,000 eggs may be laid at one time. If these are deposited in warm, moist soil, they develop into active embryos, which await a passerby with bare feet, so that they may penetrate the skin and start on

Fig. 10–7   This photograph shows the Ascaris lumbricoides in the appendix. (Kindness of Dr. C.H. Lupton, Jr.; Boyd, W.: *Textbook of Pathology*. Philadelphia, Lea & Febiger, 1974.)

their odyssey to the duodenum, where they complete their life cycle.

Roundworm Disease (ascariasis). This worm resembles the earthworm in size and shape, and is a common inhabitant of the intestine, especially in children (Fig. 10–7). Infection is due to swallowing the eggs of the worm on uncooked vegetables.

This sounds simple, but the reality is far from simple. The capacity of the uterus has been estimated at about 27,000,000 eggs and the daily output for each female at 200,000, quite a difference from the human female. Indeed the ascaris seems to be bent on an "exploding population." But when the developing eggs hatch into larvae in the intestine, they are not content to develop there without following the strange example of the hookworm. So they penetrate the wall of the bowel, are carried to the heart and then the lungs, where they are filtered out, and pass up the trachea and down the esophagus into the intestine! With this voyage of discovery behind them, they are content to develop peacefully into adult worms. We can wonder how on earth such a method of development could have been evolved, but we are left without an answer.

Pinworm or Threadworm Disease (enterobiasis). *Enterobius vermicularis* is a common parasite in the intestine of children. The worms are only 8 mm long, and, when passed in the stools, they resemble a moving piece of white thread. They cause marked irritation and itching of the skin around the anus. Infection is due to swallowing contaminated vegetables and fruits. Masses of pinworms may be found in the vermiform appendix, but they are not responsible for acute appendicitis, as was once believed. An easy diagnostic procedure is to apply transparent adhesive (Scotch) tape to the perineal area of the person who has the irritation and itching. Pinworms may be readily identified when they stick to the tape, although they are not easily seen in the skin.

Trichinosis. Every parasitic worm seems to take pride in developing a special way of life, and trichinella, or trichina as it used to be called, is no exception. The disease trichinosis is caused by a tiny roundworm that passes its complete life cycle in the body of a single animal. However, unless the host is eaten by another animal, the embryos die, surely a curious arrangement to have been evolved by a worm, but apparently a satisfactory one. Owing to improvement in meat inspection and changes in the handling and distribution of meat, trichinosis has become comparatively rare (Fig. 10–8). Larvae in pork may be rendered noninfective by heating to 55°C (131°F) or by freezing at −15°C (5°F) for about 3 weeks.

The parasite infects a variety of animals, in particu-

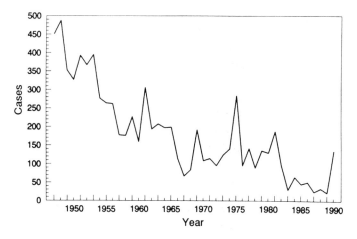

Fig. 10–8 Reported trichinosis cases—United States, 1947–1990. (Data for 1987–1990 are preliminary.) (From Centers for Disease Control, Morbidity and Mortality Weekly Report, 40(4):57, 1991.)

Fig. 10–9 This map of villages near Paris shows the outbreak of trichinosis at the dots. Source of this outbreak is believed to have been infected horse meat. (From Bourée, P., et al.: Outbreak of trichinosis near Paris. Br. Med. J., 1:1047, 1979.)

lar the rat, the bear, the pig, and man. The pig becomes infected by eating the rat, and man becomes infected by eating the pig, but the life cycle comes to an end with man because he is not eaten, normally. Epidemics occur, particularly in Germany, from eating imperfectly cooked pork in sausages. The embryos ingested in the infected pork develop in the intestine into tiny adult male and female worms, only 1 to 3 mm long. The resulting ova develop into embryos, which are discharged into the blood, are carried to all parts of the body, and invade various organs. However, the embryos can only develop in the voluntary muscles and die out elsewhere. Every muscle in the body may be infected, but full development of the embryo into an adult worm is not possible unless the parasite finds itself in the digestive canal of another animal. In man the embryos cause myositis, an acute inflammation of the muscles, which become hard, swollen, and often painful. Fever is a common symptom, and there is a marked and characteristic eosinophilia, of great diagnostic value. Diagnosis is made immunologically or by skin test, and only rarely today by biopsy.

The clinical pattern of trichinosis is fever (65%), headache (61%), muscle aches (59%), and periorbital edema (57%). An increased eosinophil count (97%) is the signal that alerts the clinician to the suspicion of trichinosis. Elevated muscle enzymes confirm this diagnosis and are present in 93% of patients. These figures are taken from an outbreak of trichinosis in the suburbs of Paris (Fig. 10–9).

Filariasis. In this infection by a nematode worm, the adult worm lives in the lymphatics while the larvae travel in the blood. It is a disease of tropical countries, because the culex mosquito is necessary for com-

pletion of the life cycle as well as for transmitting the infection.

The life history and habits of the filaria are remarkable even for an animal parasite. The adult worm, only 0.5 to 1 cm in length and extremely thin, lives in the lymphatics, especially in those of the groin and pelvis. The male and female live together, and the ova develop in the uterus of the female into active larvae, known as microfilariae, which are eel-like bodies so thin that they pass through the smallest capillaries. They are therefore found in the blood (Fig. 10–10),

Fig. 10–10 This microscopic view shows a microfilaria in blood. x 300.

but only at night, because it is at night that the culex makes its appearance, sucks the blood of the patient, and thus allows completion of the life cycle of the parasite. This beautiful piece of timing is made possible by a daily cyclical parturition by the females and by the rapid death of the microfilariae. Before midday, the turgid females are crammed with microfilariae, but after 2 P.M. the uterus is empty until the next day, for the larvae are in the blood awaiting the mosquito at sundown. The larvae do the patient no harm, and this nocturnal periodicity may go on for years. When the mosquito bites an infected person, the larvae pass with the blood into the insect's stomach. They penetrate the stomach wall and lodge in the thoracic muscles. Here they develop into young worms, which make their way to the base of the proboscis and await injection into man, where sexual development may be attained and reproduction takes place.

Although the larvae in the blood do no harm, the adult worms are apt to produce lymphatic obstruction, especially as they are present in masses. Elephantiasis may develop as a result of obstruction of the lymphatics. This is a condition in which the tissues become enormously thickened and indurated, the legs resemble those of a young elephant (hence the name), and the scrotum is huge. The diagnosis of filariasis is made by demonstrating the larvae in the blood at night, but it is elephantiasis caused by the adult worms that constitutes the real disease.

CESTODES OR TAPEWORMS

We now pass to a different type of worm. Tapeworms are of various kinds, but they all spend part of their life cycle in man and part in another animal. A tapeworm gets its name from its shape, for it is long and narrow, like a piece of tape (Fig. 10–11). The head is small and the body is long. There are four tapeworms of importance in human pathology. Three of these pass the sexual or adult stage in man and the asexual or cystic stage in an animal, hence the name cestode. The fourth passes the adult stage in an animal (dog) and the cystic stage in man. The easiest way to remember the names of tapeworms is by the name of the animal that acts as the second host. All of these worms are known by the generic term, taenia.

Beef Tapeworm (Taenia saginata, Taenia mediocanellata). This common tapeworm of the United States and Canada may be 10 meters long, but its head is only 2 mm in diameter. It lives in the intestine, and the body of the female is crowded with eggs that are discharged in the stools. If these eggs are swallowed by cattle, they are carried to the muscles, where they

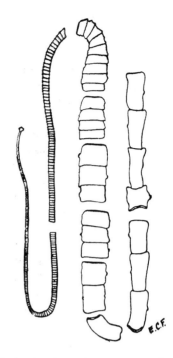

Fig. 10–11 This drawing shows the appearance of a tapeworm. Its head is in the small segment on the left. (From Faust: *Human Helminthology*. Philadelphia, Lea & Febiger.)

pass through a second phase of the life cycle and develop into cysts. If imperfectly cooked beef from an infected cow is eaten, human infection will result, and the cystic parasite will grow into the full-length adult in the intestine. The diagnosis is made by examining the stools for fragments of the worm (segments) that become broken off and discharged.

Pork Tapeworm (Taenia solium). This worm is similar to the beef tapeworm, but it is smaller, only three meters long. The second host is the pig, and human infection results from eating infected pork that contains the tiny cysts.

Fish Tapeworm (Diphyllobothrium latum). This very long worm passes the cystic stage in some of the larger freshwater fish, such as pike and perch. There is no danger in eating these fish provided they have been properly cooked, and the same is true of the beef and pork. Infestation used to be found chiefly among the fish-eating peoples in the Scandinavian countries, Russia, and parts of Asia, but more recently it has been imported into the United States and Canada, and is now indigenous in the districts around the Great Lakes and Lake Winnipeg. The eggs are discharged from the ripe segments at the rate of 1,000,000 a day, but the segments are empty and shriveled when shed, in this respect differing from the other two tapeworms. It follows that in stool examinations the presence of ripe segments indicates the beef or the pork tapeworm; the presence of eggs indicates the fish tapeworm.

Dog Tapeworm (Echinococcus granulosus). This disease is commonly called hydatid disease and is caused by 1 of 2 species (*Echinococcus granulosus,* or *E. multilocularis*) of tapeworm that live in the intestines of dogs and wolves. This worm is entirely different from the other three in the following respects: (1) It is small, 8 mm long. (2) It is the cystic stage that is passed in man; the adult stage occurs in the dog. (3) The cysts often cause serious symptoms in man and may prove fatal. Human infection is usually due to ingestion of unboiled vegetables soiled by the excreta of dogs. The dogs are infected by eating the flesh of infected sheep. The disease in man, which is most prevalent in Australia, South America, and other great sheep-raising countries where infected dogs and men come into close contact, is called **hydatid disease,** and the cysts are known as hydatid cysts. These cysts are formed principally in the liver, but may occur in any of the organs. They may attain a large size, and sometimes cause the death of the patient. The fluid of the cysts is clear and sterile, but it contains immature forms, which must not be allowed to escape during removal of the cysts. Intradermal injection of the fluid is said to give a specific skin reaction in cases of hydatid disease. Treatment is surgical removal of the hydatid cyst with appropriate precautions to prevent spillage of the infective agents. Hydrogen peroxide in dilute solution seems to be the agent of choice.

It seems that the history of echinococcal disease in the United States started early in this century. It was known in swineherds in the southeast, and by 1920 it had spread to the Mississippi Valley. Recently there have been serious outbreaks in western states, where the cycle involves sheep as intermediate hosts. Sheepranchers, Basque-Americans in California, Mormons in Utah, and the Navajo, Zuni, and Santo Domingan Indians in Arizona and New Mexico, are at risk wherever dogs are permitted to eat uncooked sheep offal.

Skin testing has shown a positive reaction in native populations of Alaska (22%), the Yukon (40%) and in Canadian Eskimos and Indians of British Columbia. To detect the presence of cysts, CT scans have become important and the Casoni test (intradermal injection of echinococcal antigen) is a useful diagnostic procedure.

TREMATODES OR FLUKES

These small, flat, leaf-shaped unsegmented worms include several varieties of flukes, infesting both animals and man in the Orient, of which the liver fluke in China and the lung fluke in China and Japan may

be mentioned. The life cycle of trematodes cannot continue without an intermediate host, which is a water snail.

Schistosomiasis. This is the most common disease caused by flukes. Again, there are several varieties responsible. The only one we shall mention is *Schistosoma haematobium,* generally referred to as bilharzia. This fluke causes widespread disease in Egypt and in other parts of northern Africa. The flukes live in the veins of the pelvis and bladder, and the ova, which are armed with a sharp spine, are laid in the wall of the bladder where they produce an intense inflammatory reaction with continual passage of blood in the urine and a marked predisposition to cancer of the bladder wall.

EXTERNAL PARASITES: ARTHROPODS

The parasitic arthropods, so called because they have joined legs, are numerous and cause many skin troubles, particularly in the tropics. Some are also carriers of disease. The most common skin parasites are lice, fleas, and acarus, the "itch insect," which causes scabies. The bites of arthropods always itch to some degree, the itching being due to the development of hypersensitivity to the saliva deposited at the site of the bite. The hypersensitivity may be so extreme that the itching becomes almost intolerable.

Acarus scabiei. The itch insect, which is the cause of scabies, is shaped like a turtle, but is only 0.5 mm long. The impregnated female bores a tunnel into the skin between the fingers, at the wrists, or in the axillas, laying her eggs at the end of the tunnel where the young are hatched. These in turn bore new tunnels, so that the irritation and itching may be intense. The male remains quietly on the surface and causes no trouble. This parasite can be transmitted easily from person to person. The disease is common among school-age children, and, as with other diseases, it may find a comfortable reservoir among the adults at the home of the child. Because of its benign nature (recurrent itching and a mild rash), it is often undiagnosed and unsuspected.

Pediculi. Various pediculi or lice may infest the skin. The head louse (*Pediculus capitis*) lives on the scalp, and causes some irritation. The "nits" we observe are ova, minute bodies attached to the hairs. The body louse (*Pediculus corporis*) lives on the surface of the skin and breeds in clothing. Not only does the body louse produce much greater irritation than the head louse, but it is responsible for carrying the infection of typhus fever, relapsing fever, and trench fever. It does this by biting first a sick and then a healthy person.

Fleas. The common flea is of little significance in relation to disease. The rat flea, on the other hand, is of great importance, because it conveys plague not only from one rat to another, but also from rat to man.

Arthropods as Disease Carriers

In the course of our study of infection, whether of bacteria, rickettsiae, viruses, or protozoa, we have seen that an arthropod vector or conveyer, usually an insect, is necessary in many instances for the continuation of the infection. A vector may be mechanical or biologic. The mechanical vector merely picks up the infecting agent from the body or excreta and deposits it on exposed food (house flies in relation to typhoid, or to bacillary and amebic dysentery) or conveys infection through contamination of the biting organ (flies and mosquitoes in relation to anthrax). The biologic vector plays an essential part in the completion of the life cycle of the pathogen rather than merely offering it a free ride. In many instances it is only the female that transmits disease, another illustration of the old saying that the female of the species is more deadly than the male.

SYNOPSIS

Parasitism is an evolutionary process.
Alternate hosts are necessary for many parasites.
Control of vectors in the life cycle of many parasites is the means of disease control.
Protozoa and metazoa are two great classes of animal parasites.
Parasites are causative agents of classic disease processes such as anemia, cirrhosis, and cancer.

Terms

Definitive host   *Cestode*   *Schistosomiasis*
Intermediate host   *Trematode*   *Trichinosis*
Malarial parasite   *Arthropod*   *Scabies*
Nematode   *Hydatid cyst*

FURTHER READING

Allason-Jones, E., et al.: Entamoeba histolytica as a commensal intestinal parasite in homosexual men. N. Engl. J. Med., 315:353, 1986.

Beisel, W.R.: Synergism and antagonism of parasitic disease and malnutrition. Rev. Infect. Dis., 4:746, 1982.

Bourée, P., et al.: Outbreak of trichinosis near Paris. Br. Med. J., 1:1047, 1979.

Cameron, T.W.M.: *Parasites and Parasitism.* London, Wiley, 1956.

Cheever, A.W.: Schistosomiasis and neoplasia. J. Natl. Canc. Inst., 61:13, 1978.

Craig, P.S., Deshan, L., and Zhaoxun, D.: Hydatid disease in China. Parasitology Today, 7:46, 1991.

Flegel, K.M.: Symptoms and signs of malaria. Can. Med. Assoc. J., 115:409, 1976.

Hagar, J.M., and Rahimtoola, S.H.: Chagas' heart disease in the United States. N. Engl. J. Med., 325:763, 1991.

Harries, J.: Amoebiasis: a review. J. Roy. Soc. Med., 75:190, 1982.

Hasleton, P.S. and Curry, A.: Pneumocystis carinii: the continuing enigma. Thorax, 37:481, 1982.

Hoffman, S.L., et al.: Immunity to malaria and naturally acquired antibodies to the circumsporozoite protein of Plasmodium falciparum. N. Engl. J. Med., 315:601, 1986.

Hopkins, D.R.: Eradication of Dracunculiasis: Update. Epidemiol. Rev., 13:316, 1991.

Katelaris, P.H., and Farthing, M.J.G.: Diarrhea and malabsorption in Giardiasis—a multifactorial process. Gut, 33:295, 1992.

Krick, J.A., and Remington, J.S.: Toxoplasmosis in the adult—an overview. N. Engl. J. Med., 298:550, 1978.

Lisker-Melman, M., and Martinez-Palomo, A.: Intestinal Amebiasis. In: *Gastrointestinal Infections in the Tropics.* Basel, Karger, 1990.

McLeod, R., Mack, D., and Brown, C.: *Toxoplasma gondii*—new advances in cellular and molecular biology. Exper. Parasitology, 72:109, 1991.

Mahmoud, A.A.F.: Schistosomiasis: clinical features and relevance to hematology. Semin. Hematol., 19:132, 1982.

Marcial-Rojas, R.A.: *Pathology of Protozoal Helminthic Diseases with Clinical Correlations.* Baltimore, Williams & Wilkins, 1971.

Marsden, P.D.: Leishmaniasis. N. Engl. J. Med., 300:350, 1979.

Meyer, E.A. and Jarroll, E.L.: Giardiasis. Am. J. Epidemiol., 3:1, 1980.

Miller, L.H.: Research in malaria vaccines. N. Engl. J. Med., 315:640, 1986.

Moser, R.H.: Trichinosis from Bismarck to polar bears. J.A.M.A., 228:735, 1974.

Mott, K.E., Desjeux, P., Moncayo, A., et al.: Parasitic diseases and urban development. Bull. W.H.O., 68:691, 1990.

Reed, S.L.: Amebiasis—an update. Clin. Infect. Dis., 14:385, 1992.

Rosenberg, I.H., and Bowman, B.B.: Intestinal physiology and parasitic disease. Rev. Infect. Dis., 4:763, 1982.

Schantz, P.M.: Echinococcosis in American Indians living in Arizona and New Mexico. Am. J. Epidemiol., 106:370, 1977.

Schantz, P.M., and Glickman, L.T.: Toxocaral visceral larva migrans. N. Engl. J. Med., 298:436, 1978.

Schmidt, G.D., and Roberts, L.S.: *Foundations of Parasitology,* St. Louis, C.V. Mosby Co., 1977.

Shou-Pai, M., and Bao-Ruo, S.: Schistosomiasis control in the People's Republic of China. Am. J. Trop. Med., 31:92, 1982.

Teutsch, S.M., et al.: Epidemic toxoplasmosis associated with infected cats. N. Engl. J. Med., 300:695, 1979.

11

NEOPLASIA

When you do not have any money the problem is food; when you have money it is sex;
when you have both it is health; and when everything is simply great then you are frightened of death.—J.P. DONLEAVY

Of all the disease processes we have to study in this book, none is more intriguing, more fascinating, and more perplexing than neoplasia. The term means new growth. There are, of course, various forms of new growth such as repair, the formation of granulation tissue, and compensatory hypertrophy of an organ. The term **neoplasm** is reserved for the formation of benign and, more particularly, malignant tumors or cancer. Tumor is a more general term signifying a swelling or lump, but there are many lumps that are not neoplasms, such as abscesses.

DISTURBANCES OF GROWTH

The normal organs and tissues of the body are made up of cells under the control of laws of growth. An organ such as the liver or bone increases in size, usually, not by an increase in cell size (the cells of a whale are the same size as the cells of a mouse), but by an increase in the number of cells. In youth, this multiplication is rapid, partly because of the abundance of growth hormone, and partly because of the genetic programming of the tissue. However, in adult life, cell replication is sufficient only to replace what is lost by continual turn-over or wear and tear. Occasionally, there is an increase in the number of cells in a tissue **(hyperplasia)** in the adult due to unknown or nonspecific causes. This increase happens most often in tissues such as the endocrine glands, which respond particularly to growth-promoting hormones. In many instances the hyperplasia seems autonomous.

Another phenomenon of growth is the adaptive response to work demand **(hypertrophy),** which may be best demonstrated by physical training in skeletal muscle; this also occurs in cardiac muscle and other tissues. An increase in the size of an organ is usually due to an increase in the size of individual cells. With specific work training, muscle cells increase the number of cytoplasmic myofilaments and thereby enlarge.

The converse of these adaptive responses is a loss of normal size or number of structural units, which results in **atrophy** of an organ or tissue. In muscle, this may be due to lack of use, to injury, to loss of innervation, or to interference with the normal blood. In other tissues it may be due to a loss of endocrine stimulus, as in pituitary hypofunction. A decrease in size of the tissue or organ may, on the other hand, have a congenital origin and may result from an abnormal blood supply or from a failure of development. The terms **agenesis, aplasia,** and **hypoplasia** have been applied to some of these conditions (Table 11–1).

A third general variation in the normal growth and structure of a tissue occurs frequently in response to different types of stimuli; some are irritative, some nutritional. These changes from normal are reflected in an unusual pattern of structure: the replacement of one type of epithelium by another, as occurs in the bronchi and trachea of long-term smokers. A change from the normal ciliated columnar epithelium of the

Table 11–1.   Disturbances of Growth

Agenesis	Complete absence of an organ or tissue.
Atrophy	Decrease in size of cells after they have achieved normal size.
Hypertrophy	Increase in size of cells, resulting in increase in size of organ.
Hypoplasia	Decreased number of cells in a tissue. Aplasia refers to absence of cells.
Hyperplasia	Increase in number of cells.
Metaplasia	A change in type of adult tissue to a type which is not found in that tissue.
Dysplasia	A change, usually found in proliferating cells, characterized by abnormal morphology affecting mostly the size and shape of nuclei.

tracheo-bronchial mucosa to squamous epithelium is called **squamous metaplasia**. The same change can also be observed in the endocrine which is normally columnar and can become squamous, usually as a result of chronic inflammation. A significantly different type of change warrants the use of the term dysplasia. As we shall discuss, this is interpreted as a warning sign that the normal controls over orderly growth and development of the tissue may be lacking.

We know that if one kidney is removed, the other kidney will increase in size, and we talk of this as a compensatory mechanism. What is the stimulus to this response? Equally, if a portion of the liver is removed, the liver will regenerate. Unfortunately, few tissues in man can react in this way. The stimuli to new growth are poorly understood and the factors that signal the end of the new growth are even less clear. However, we know that cells in a tissue are in direct contact with each other. When this contact is broken, as in a cut where cells are injured, the loss of contact may be the stimulus to new growth. When cells make contact with each other, there is cessation of movement. This process is comparable to the phenomenon of **contact inhibition** in cells growing in culture, which stop growing when they become confluent.

A neoplasm is a mass of new cells which proliferate without control and serve no useful function. This lack of control is particularly marked in malignant tumors (cancer). Cancer cells are the anarchists of the body, for they know few laws, pay no regard to the commonweal, serve no useful function, and cause disharmony and death in their surroundings. It used to be thought that cancer was a peculiarly human disease, but we now know that it occurs throughout the entire vertebrate animal kingdom. It seems to be a phenomenon of the extremes of age; most cancers seem to occur in the young and in the aged (Fig. 11–1 and Table 11–2). Babies and children are not spared, however. Cancer, including leukemia, is now a leading cause of nonaccidental death in children between the ages of 3 and 14 in industrialized countries. These cancers differ from those in adults in clinical features, sites of origin and types of tumor. Tumors of embryonic origin (embryonic tumors) are common in infants and young children, but correspondingly rare in adults. Four out of five of these tumors in children arise from the nervous system, the urinary system, or the lymphopoietic system, whereas in adults, four out of five cancers arise from the breast, alimentary, respiratory, or genital systems. Figure 11–2 shows cancer deaths by site and sex for all ages from 1921 to 1985.

Cancer has a fundamental characteristic that makes it life-threatening, and puts it in second place in the

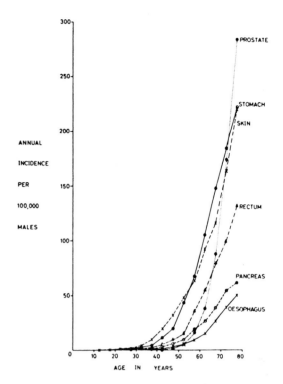

Fig. 11–1   The pattern of continued increase of incidence of cancer from adolescence to old age. (From Miller, D.G.: On the nature of susceptibility to cancer. Cancer, 46:1308, 1980.)

list of causes of death in North America, after cardiovascular diseases. Cancer kills because of invasion of tissue and by distant spread to vital organs, where it may compress, obstruct, or destroy vital functions by its metastases. In 1985 there were an estimated 480,000 deaths in the United States from cancer. The

Table 11–2.   The Increase in the Incidence* of Cancer with Age

TOTAL	<15	15–24	25–34	35–44	45–54	55–64	65–74
306.7	12.4	36.3	118.9	200.9	407.9	789.6	1344.0

All sites, total, and age specific.

* Crude rates, both sexes, per 100,000

(From Miller, D.G.: On the nature of susceptibility to cancer. Cancer, 46:1307, 1980.)

Table 11–3.   Sites of Cancer in Order of Frequency as Cause of Death in the United States (1989)

FEMALE	MALE
1. Lung	Lung
2. Breast	Colon/rectum
3. Colon/rectum	Prostate
4. Pancreas	Pancreas
5. Ovary	Leukemia

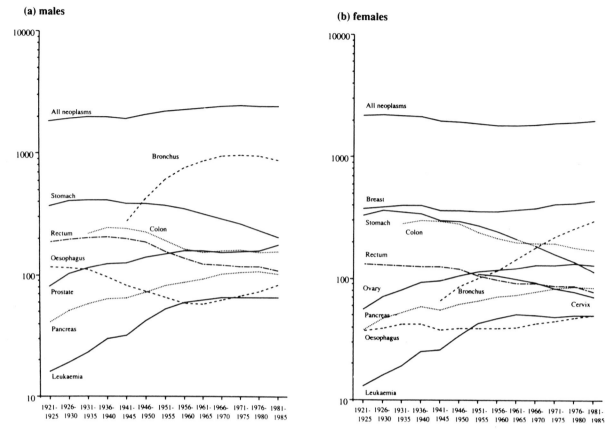

(a) males

(b) females

Fig. 11–2   Cancer deaths by site and sex, 1921 to 1985 (age-standardized death rate per million population). x axis = years and y axis = rate per million (log scale). (From Davis, D.L., Hoel, D., Fox, J., and Lopez, A.D.: International trends in cancer mortality in France, West Germany, Italy, Japan, England and Wales, and the United States. Ann. N.Y. Acad. Sci., 609:5, 1990.)

types of tumors that caused these deaths are shown in Table 11–3.

This pattern may change with earlier diagnosis and treatment, but it may also change with social and occupational exposures. For instance, breast cancer was the leading cause of cancer death among females until 1985, when lung cancer, which had been second, became first. Relative changes in mortality due to cancer and selected causes of death are shown in Figure 11–3.

NATURE OF NEOPLASIA

There is much talk about the mystery of cancer, as if it were the only mysterious process in the entire realm of disease. But inflammation is mysterious, and we have only partially solved the mystery by inventing such words as chemotaxis; diabetes is a mystery that has not been solved by the discovery of insulin; multiple sclerosis and schizophrenia remain mysteries without the suggestion of a solution. Most normal cells seem concerned more with function than with growth, but the cancer cell is concerned more with

growth, in the sense of reproduction of itself, than with function. The capacity for growth seems to have supplanted that for function. The nerve cells of the human brain represent the highest in specialization of function, but they have lost the power of reproduction. Most neoplasms of the brain consist not of nerve cells, but of neuroglia (supporting cells).

Cancer Cells

Cancer is a disorder of cell growth and differentiation, and the cancer cell appears to be a modified cell. An electron micrograph of a cancer cell is shown in Figure 11–4A and a drawing illustrating some of its features in Figure 11–4B. Another scheme (Fig. 11–5) shows the many differences between cancer and normal cells that have been identified in recent years, but not all these differences occur in all tumors, nor are any of them necessarily diagnostic. Unfortunately, we do not know all the mechanisms of normal growth and its regulation, so it is small wonder that we do not understand cancer. However, in recent years cell and molecular biologists have identified a number of

Fig. 11–3 Relative change in mortality (1950–1954 = 100) for selected causes of death in developed countries from 1950–1954 to 1986. (From Lopez, A.D.: Competing causes of death: A review of recent trends in mortality in industrialized countries with special reference to cancer. Ann. N.Y. Acad. Sci., 609:58, 1990.)

factors, among them growth factors, cytokines and interleukins, which are involved in the way cells regulate their growth. Consequently, those discoveries are being applied to the study of cancer cells and have begun to shed a new light on how they lose control of growth. The cancerous modification comprises loss of the more specialized functions, a process called dedifferentiation, in addition to the acquisition of increased growth function, changes accompanied by invasion of the surrounding tissue and the formation of the secondary growths at a distance known as **metastases.** The ability to form a metastasis is the ultimate criterion by which malignant tumors are distinguished from benign ones.

One of the fundamental questions related to the biology of a cancer cell is: assuming that there is one determinant change responsible for the transformation of a normal cell into a cancer cell, what is it? It is

fair to state that, at the present time, such a universal event has not been discovered that would present in all cancers. As will be apparent from the discussion below, cancer most often results from not a single but repeated assaults of different types of injury affecting the genome.

One concept is concerned with systems normally involved in regulating substances essential to cell division. Loss or disruption of such systems would make normal regulation of cell division impossible, with resulting unrestricted growth, that is to say, neoplasia. Carcinogens, or cancer-producing agents, whether chemicals or radiation, could be responsible for damage to such systems. The result would be unregulated cell proliferation.

Early steps on the path to cancer probably occur all the time in our bodies, but the path is most often aborted. This is due mainly to the different mechanisms: first, efficient systems can repair injured DNA. Secondly, transformed cells have not acquired the machinery for long-term multiplication. Thirdly, the immune system can eliminate certain types of transformed cells. Cancers that do establish themselves are the "successful ones," those most effective in growth, invasiveness, and metastasis. The "unsuccessful" tumor cells die spontaneously. There are a variety of strategies employed in the process of tumor cell progression. Tumor cells may well produce **proteases** (enzymes that digest proteins) that facilitate the crossing of barriers, such as basement membranes, into adjacent tissues. They also produce **angiogenesis** factors, which promote the growth of local circulatory vessels to feed the tumors. Furthermore, they might have modified or overexpressed receptor molecules which control the way they respond to growth factors.

A difference between the functions of cancer cells and that of normal cells may explain why a cancer, given sufficient time, kills its host unless treated promptly and efficiently. Of course, it may do this by blocking a natural passage such as the esophagus, or by causing ulceration of a mucus membrane with fatal hemorrhage. But apart from these complications, cancer causes loss of weight, wasting, emaciation, and finally, death. A large neoplasm acquires nitrogenous building blocks from the body stores to satisfy the continual demand for protein synthesis, but this supply is not unlimited. Cancer cells appear to exercise priority over the demands of normal tissues for amino acids, thus constituting a nitrogen trap. Small wonder that wasting and cachexia are a characteristic feature of the later stages of malignancy. A great part of this process is mediated by the immune system of the cancer patient which produces a protein called Tumor Necrosis Factor (TNF) that not only kills tumor cells

A

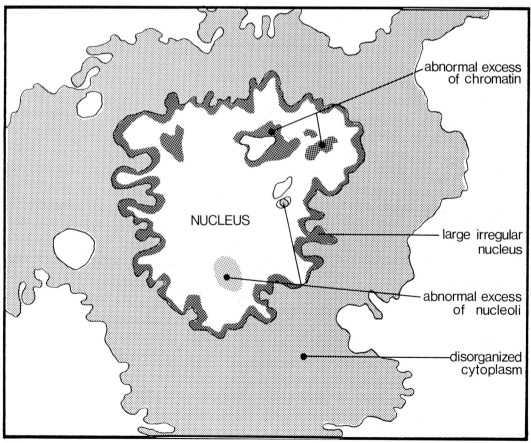

abnormal excess
of chromatin

NUCLEUS

large irregular
nucleus

abnormal excess
of nucleoli

disorganized
cytoplasm

B

impaired intercellular communication

increased lectin agglutinability

lost or modified glycolipids

nuclear modifications

CANCER CELL

altered surface enzymes

virus integration

altered permeability and transport

modified adhesion and contact inhibition

cytoplasmic alterations

lost or modified glycoproteins

new antigens & lost antigens

Fig. 11–5 This drawing shows peripheral and central abnormalities in the cancer cell, namely, impaired intercellular communications, increased cell surface substances, altered permeability and transport mechanisms, and modifications in the nucleus. (Adapted from Nicolson, G.L.: Transmembrane control of the receptors on normal and tumor cells. II. Surface changes associated with transformation and malignancy. Biochim. Biophys. Acta, 458:1, 1976.)

but also interferes with lipid metabolism and induces cachexia.

Much recent research has focused on the properties of cancer cells. There are experimental analogs of cancer cells cultivated in tissue culture, known as **transformed** cells, which exhibit comparable biochemical changes to cancer cells, and often cause tumors in vivo. Several conclusions can be drawn about the changes observed in transformed cells. Cell shape and cytoskeletal architecture are affected. The loss of "contact inhibition," whereby the growth of transformed cells is less inhibited by the contact with other cells, was mentioned above. The growth of transformed cells also depends less on attachment to the physical support of an underlying basement membrane. From this viewpoint an important test is this ability to grow freely in soft agar. This property correlates strongly with their ability to cause tumors in vivo. Normal cells placed in culture usually grow for a short time and then die; transformed cells are immortalized and will grow indefinitely. The ultimate test of transformation is the ability of transformed

cells to grow as a malignant tumor when transplanted to a special strain of mice called nude mice. Not only do these mice have no hair but, more important, they are immunodeficient and have lost the ability to reject transplants from other species.

Cancer cells display a different set of internal and surface proteins, or glycoproteins, from their cells of origin. Reappearance of embryonic marker proteins has been observed in a variety of cancers. Rather than suggesting a source of origin for tumor cells, these shared traits of embryonic and cancer cells may be those most conducive to their similar "lifestyles." Although there are profound differences, the two populations share steady growth, migration to new body sites, and a relatively undifferentiated state.

It is worth remembering that cancer is probably not a single disease with a predictable cause and a predictable program, but rather that it represents the visible manifestations of those multiple assaults or injuries resulting in errors in cell behavior that produce cells capable of uncontrolled division, invasiveness, and metastasis beyond the control of host regulation. The changes involved are stable and are passed on to the offspring of the tumor cells. Other changes might be added or deleted during this passage. One reasonable interpretation is that changes in the DNA are responsible for the inheritable alterations. That these structural DNA changes do occur has now been established in a number of cancers and they have been found to be quite diverse. For instance, DNA can be lost, a process called deletion, either through a loss of chromosome or of short segments of DNA. When we discuss later the concept of anti-oncogenes we will see that deletions can have a dramatic influence on the production of cancer. Another DNA change is a mutation whereby one or several of its nucleotides are exchanged for different ones. Sometimes the number or copies of a particular gene present in DNA can be increased, a process called gene amplification. Another possible change is named translocation, whereby a gene present on one chromosome is moved next to or within a different gene on another chromosome. All these and other DNA changes can potentially activate—or inactivate—genes exerting determinant roles in cell division or function associated with growth. Consequently, it may be the regulation of expression of DNA that is disarrayed in cancer. Perhaps genes can be altered in such a way that im-

Fig. 11–4 A, This electron microphotograph of a liposarcoma cell shows the irregular appearance of the cytoplasm and nucleus. The normal cell of this type is an adipose cell, which has a small and unremarkable nucleus, a large storage depot of triglyceride, and active but peripheral mitochondria. B, specifically illustrates the abnormalities in the electron microphotograph.

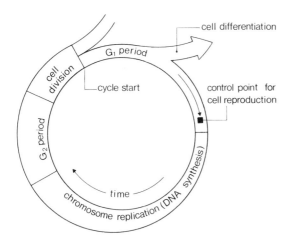

Fig. 11–6   This diagram of the cell cycle illustrates the point in the cycle at which alterations that may pervert the cell function are likely to take place. (From Thorn, G.W., et al. (Eds.): *Harrison's Principles of Internal Medicine*, 8th Ed. New York, McGraw-Hill, 1976.)

portant normal proteins are no longer produced, or else the cancer cell produces "cancer proteins"—modified proteins capable of inducing neoplastic transformation by altering the choice of active cell functions.

There is also evidence from an experimental system for an "epigenetic" change in gene expression, i.e., a change which does not imply a DNA modification. Such a model proposes a change in the specificity, timing, or stimulus requirements of existing regulatory factors with no irreversible change in the DNA. This is presumably the type of change that accompanies normal tissue differentiation. Cells from a mouse teratocarcinoma, a malignant tumor developed from an early embryo, have been mixed into a normal mouse embryo, and the fetus matured in a foster mother. Normal offspring developed even though many of their cells in many tissues derived from the teratocarcinoma cells. The conclusion is that in a nor-

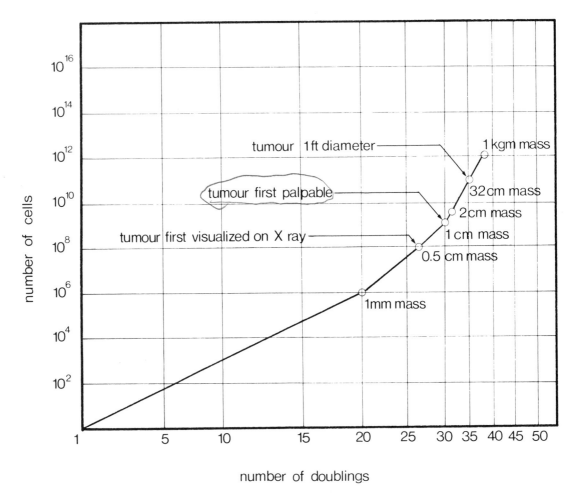

Fig. 11–7   This graph shows the number of cells, the number of doublings, and the size of the mass. It illustrates that a tumor may be first visible only after 25 or more doublings. The rapid growth from that point is indicated in the change in the slope of the curve. (From Thorn, G.W., et al. (Eds.): *Harrison's Principles of Internal Medicine*, 8th Ed. New York, McGraw-Hill, 1976.)

mal environment, the tumor cells are induced to reverse their phenotype and to behave and differentiate as normal cells. One interpretation is that the main teratocarcinoma DNA was unaffected in any irreversible fashion during transformation, but suffered an epigenetic alteration in its pattern of expression. The possibility of mutation is certainly not excluded, but these experiments suggest that a strictly epigenetic model of carcinogenesis may be relevant in some systems.

On the basis of what we know about the mechanisms by which a normal cell is transformed into a cancer cell, we can state that, in general terms, cancer is the result of changes in cell control mechanism. The regulator of cellular activity, the governor of the complex "micro-society" of a cell is DNA, and its ministers and secretaries of state are the RNA molecules transcribed from it. The intricate mechanism of chromosomes and genes with their nucleic acid, which controls cellular reproduction as well as metabolism, can be upset in various ways. Interference with the structure of genes or the regulation of their transcription into messenger RNA can induce changes that will permanently speed the rate of mitotic division, and the result will create the initial conditions for the induction of cancer. Just as the regulator of a watch may be moved to fast or slow, so may the mitotic rate be permanently accelerated by carcinogens or retarded by chemotherapy and radiation. The time at which cells are most susceptible to alterations in their growth controls is in the G1 period, shown in Figure 11–6. As one cell will produce 65,536 daughter cells after 16 divisions, it is apparent that even a slight increase in the rate and rhythm of cell division will soon produce a tumor. The rate of growth of a tumor is dramatically demonstrated in Figure 11–7, in which the number of doublings and the number of cells are related to the size of the mass of tumor.

CAUSES OF CANCER

The exact cause of cancer is not known. It is doubtful, indeed, whether there is any single, universal cause of all cancers, any more than we would expect to find any single, universal cause of all inflammations. Both inflammation and cancer are processes, not diseases, whereas inflammation of the appendix and cancer of the stomach are diseases in the ordinary sense of the term. Again, just as it would be absurd to expect to discover a single method of treatment that would cure all infections, so it is probably useless to hope for a single cure of all cancers. The alliterations "the cause of cancer" and "the cure of cancer" are unfortunate because they have become deeply im-

planted in the mind of the public. It is believed that there must be one cause and one cure, so that persons tend to reject the information that great advances have been made both in our knowledge of the causation and in the treatment of malignant disease. As a matter of fact, there are many chronic pathologic conditions, such as cirrhosis and emphysema, that are far less curable than cancer. Tumors form a group, just as do the infectious diseases, and each has to be considered by itself. We do know a good deal about certain factors that play a part in the production of cancer, just as we do know a good deal about treatment of the disease. Important factors in carcinogenesis are: (1) chemical carcinogens, (2) ionizing radiation, (3) viruses, (4) hormones, (5) heredity, (6) environment, and (7) chronic irritation. This does not mean that there may not be others, or that only one is responsible in a given case (Fig. 11–8). It will be noticed that some of the factors may be termed external, such as chemical carcinogens, others internal, such as heredity.

Chemical Carcinogens

The first observation on chemical carcinogenic agents was that of Sir Percival Pott in 1775, who made the association between the frequent appearance of cancer of the scrotum in chimney sweeps and the extraordinary amount of soot and coal tar in their clothing and on their bodies. This observation and recognition is widely quoted as the first instance of occupational cause of cancer.

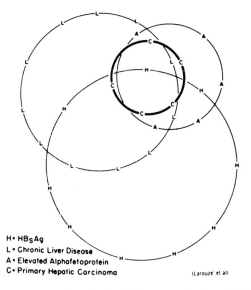

H = HBsAg
L = Chronic Liver Disease
A = Elevated Alphafetoprotein
C = Primary Hepatic Carcinoma   (Larouze' et al)

Fig. 11–8 An example of a Venn diagram employing clinical and biochemical data to define a subset of a population susceptible to cancer, in this case, cancer of the liver. (From Miller, D.G.: On the nature of susceptibility to cancer. Cancer, 46:1316, 1980.)

In 1915, 140 years after Pott's paper, Yamagiwa in Japan put this idea to the test by painting tar on a rabbit's ear every day for 6 months, and succeeded in producing cancer of the skin. This was an epoch-making discovery, because for the first time it was possible to produce a malignant tumor in an experimental animal. The carcinogens present in tar, including the tar of cigarettes, contain hydrocarbons which have polycyclic benzene rings as a common feature. It is perhaps significant that a slight change in the chemical structure of a substance may convert it from a noncarcinogen into a carcinogen. Any of these carcinogens can produce carcinoma (epithelial cancer) or sarcoma (connective tissue cancer) at the site of application. Some can even convert a tissue culture of fibroblasts into a culture of cancer cells.

The application of a chemical carcinogen to a tissue is not followed by the presence of a tumor in a matter of days. The time between the exposure to a carcinogen and the appearance of a tumor is called the latent period, which is variable, but may be as long as decades.

Berenblum and Shubik studied these phenomena and found that the development of such tumors could be enhanced by the application of a noncarcinogen, a mildly irritating substance such as croton oil. Thus they described two stages in experimental tumor production: **initiation,** in which the conversion to neoplastic potential is created by exposure to a carcinogen, and **promotion,** which may accelerate the rate at which the tissue has a chance to become malignant. This process is schematically illustrated in Figure 11–9.

Initiators are virtually always mutagens and as such they introduce sites of potential mistakes when DNA replication or transcription occur. Promoters are usually not mutagens. Promoters most often enhance cell division. This is often the result of a cascade of events during which various intracellular proteins are phosphorylated by enzymes called protein kinases. The eventual increase in cell proliferation mediated by promoters allows the initiation-induced mutations to be transmitted to daughter cells. It should be emphasized that neoplastic transformation through initiation and promotion is not a switch to a preprogrammed, well-defined "other state." Tumors undoubtedly evolve continuously. At each stage (primary growth, invasion, metastasis), few cells survive, and the result is the natural selection of the most "successful" neoplastic behavior. This is particularly true for the development of metastases. Indeed, experimental data suggest that cells in the primary cancer site undergo additional genetic changes when they acquire the ability to metastasize.

Some chemical compounds have a structure that suggests they might behave as initiators of carcinogenesis. Since initiators are mutagens, a screening test based on the induction of mutations in bacteria, called the Ames test, has been developed. Almost all known carcinogens have been found to be potent mutagens, although conversely all mutagens are not necessarily carcinogenic. A proportion of compounds found to be mutagenic with the Ames test have then been shown to be carcinogenic in animals. This is a powerful way of screening our environment for hazards and of testing new compounds before their use. It also has made clearer the relationship of mutation to carcinogenesis. Some compounds tested are found not be mutagenic in their pure state; however, after incubation with an extract of liver containing a sampling of metabolic en-

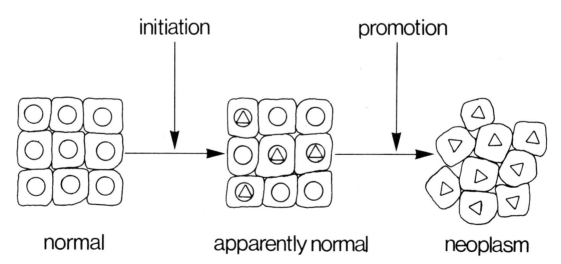

Fig. 11–9   Normal cells are shown at the left. Following initiation, some of these cells may have changes in their nucleic acids, as indicated by the presence of triangles within the nucleus. Following repeated exposure to agents, which is promotion, a tumor may appear.

zymes, they tested positive. Thus **some compounds are metabolized to carcinogens by our bodies**.

What we have learned from chemical carcinogenesis raises the challenging question whether malignant transformation is necessarily a unidirectional sequence of events. In experimental situations where this problem was investigated it was found that some chemical inducers of differentiation can exert antagonizing effects on tumor development; there is evidence in one neuroblastoma system that tumors can be induced to further differentiation along the normal pathway of their original cell type. Application of the appropriate hormone or inducer causes the cells to respond, to differentiate, and to lose their malignancy.

Ionizing Radiation

That ionizing radiations are important and powerful carcinogens became clear soon after Roentgen's discovery in 1895, when many early experimentalists developed skin tumors of their hands. Even today, lymphoma has a greater incidence than normal in radiologists (Table 11–4).

A single dose of 600 r is followed by benign and malignant tumors of the skin, connective tissue, and viscera in the experimental animal. The survivors of the first Hiroshima and Nagasaki atomic blasts show a 10-fold increase in leukemia in the heavily exposed group. The inducing effect of irradiation may be delayed for a long time. There is an increase in incidence of leukemia as new cases are diagnosed decades after exposure to radiation. The miners in Schneeberg and Joachimsthal, Germany, for centuries have suffered from a high incidence of carcinoma of the lung; this is now known to be due to radioactive uranium. Thyroid, breast and salivary gland cancer can also be induced by ionizing radiation. Ultraviolet light radiation is also carcinogenic, which explains the high incidence of cancer of the skin and lip among field workers in the white population of the tropics, Australia, and the southern United States. The increased risk is not restricted to these regions as epidemiologists have clearly documented that the overwhelming majority of skin cancers, including melanoma, are caused by excessive sun exposure. Skin cancer is rare in blacks, who are protected from ultraviolet light by a high pigment content of the skin.

Viruses

One of the most exciting modern discoveries relating to carcinogenesis is that of the role of viruses. As far back as 1911, Rous showed that a cell-free filtrate of a sarcoma of fowl could produce a new tumor when injected into another fowl of the same breed. This experiment was the breakthrough but it aroused no enthusiasm, for the only similar tumors were confined to birds. Then in 1932 a tumor due to a filter-passing viral agent was described in a wild rabbit by Richard Shope. A short time later, Bittner proved that cancer of the breast in mice can be transmitted to the newborn by an agent in the mother's milk. It should be noted at this point that in the human species there is no clear evidence for a viral involvement in the causation of breast cancer.

At present, the production of malignant tumors of a variety of types by cell-free filtrates in laboratory animals has become commonplace. It is even possible to induce cancer in cultures of human cells by the addition of the SV-40 virus.

Both DNA and RNA viruses can cause cancers in experimental animals. Among the DNA viruses, the polyoma, adenoviruses, and some herpesviruses are tumorigenic; among the RNA viruses mostly the retroviruses induce cancer. It should be recalled that the

Table 11–4. Neoplasms of Various Types and Sites in Irradiated Populations, Tentatively Quantified as in Excess or Not

NEOPLASM CATEGORY	ATOMIC BOMB SURVIVORS	OCCUPA-TIONALLY EXPOSED WORKERS	THERAPEUTICALLY IRRADIATED PATIENTS	
			ADULTS	CHILDREN
Bladder	−	−	+	−
Brain	−	−	−	+
Cervix uteri	+	−	+	−
Connective tissue	−	−	+	+
Cranial sinuses	−	+	+	−
Liver	−	−	+	−
Lymphoma	+	+	−	−
Multiple myeloma	+	+	−	−
Ovary	−	−	+	−
Pancreas	−	−	+	−
Pharynx	−	−	+	−
Rectum	−	−	+	−
Salivary glands	+	−	+	+
Skin	−	+	+	+
Vagina	−	−	+	−

Data from Albert and Omran (1968); Upton (1968); ICRP (1969); McIntyre and Pointon (1971); BEIR (1972); Pochin (1972); UN (1972); Nishiyama et al. (1973); Modan et al. (1974); Matanowski et al. (1975); Smith and Doll (1976).

(From Upton, A. C.: Radiation effects. In *Origins of Human Cancer, Book A.* Edited by H. H. Hiatt, et al. New York, Cold Spring Harbor Laboratory, 1977.)

latter form a DNA copy of their genome, which is then stably integrated into the host chromosome. It is probably their property of intimate and long-lasting association with host DNA that allows viruses to cause cancer.

In general, those viruses which are associated with the development of cancer are not lytic to the cell they infect. They induce or contribute to the transformation of a normal cell into a cancer cell by inserting genes which will drive the cell in a state of uncontrolled proliferation.

A major advance in our thinking on the subject of the viral origin of cancer is represented by Gross' concept of vertical transmission. A laboratory animal suffering from a bacterial or viral disease will readily spread the infection to its neighbors of the same generation. This spread may be termed "horizontal transmission." However, the same is not true of a neoplasm induced by a virus, such as leukemia or mammary carcinoma in the mouse. Leukemia in mice is an example of a latent virus infection that produces a neoplastic disease that develops in an inbred strain when the mice reach early adult life. Gross showed that the carcinogenic agent is transmitted vertically, that is to say, from one generation to another, through the germinal cells. In the case of mammary gland carcinoma in the mouse, the virus is transmitted through the mother's milk. The agent may remain latent throughout the life span of the host, which remains healthy, and yet carries and transmits the seeds for the subsequent development of breast cancer in the mouse offspring.

It will be recalled from the virology chapter that EBV (Epstein-Barr virus), a herpesvirus, causes mononucleosis in man, and that the EBV genome is thought to persist in a small population of lymphocytes in the host after the acute infection. EBV was also said to be closely associated with two human cancers, nasopharyngeal carcinoma and Burkitt's lymphoma. It is currently thought that these cancers are multicausal, with transformation by EBV as one of the steps, perhaps the first one. A number of additional events are implicated with Burkitt's lymphoma, including environmental factors such as endemic malaria, physiologic changes in the immune system, and molecular events, such as the characteristic chromosome translocation observed in the tissue of patients with Burkitt's lymphoma, as well as in some other types of lymphomas. In this case, then, EBV transformation is probably the initiator, and cancer follows after a long latency, if the appropriate promoters are supplied.

There is growing evidence that certain subtypes of papillomaviruses, which are sexually transmitted, can cause cancer of the cervix. Meisels remarked in the sixties that the cervix of women with different types of dysplasia have cytological changes consistent with an infection by a papillomavirus. This observation, made originally by a pathologist, was supported by the work of two molecular pathologists, Zur Hausen and Orth, who discovered that a high proportion of cases of cervical dysplasia are positive for specific subtypes of human papillomavirus. When one of the unfavorable outcomes of cervical dysplasia, cancer, is examined, 95% of affected women are positive for the virus. Interestingly, the male partners of these patients often have penile lesions harboring the same virus. This observation is in keeping with the concept that cancer of the cervix is a sexually transmitted disease. We now start to understand why human papillomavirus can cause cervical cancer. Its genome codes for a viral protein which inactivates a cellular protein, called p53, which normally regulates cell proliferation. This notion will be expanded when we discuss the concept of anti-oncogenes, since p53 is one of them.

There is recent evidence implicating another DNA virus in human cancer: hepatitis B virus (HBV) and primary hepatocellular carcinoma. The distribution of hepatocellular carcinoma coincides with that of chronic hepatitis virus infection. HBV causes acute infection which can be symptomatic or not. About 5% of cases progress silently to chronic hepatitis, which can be complicated by liver cirrhosis and finally cancer, called hepatocellular carcinoma. Overall, it should be noted that only a small fraction of patients with HBV-associated chronic hepatitis progress to cirrhosis and then cancer. Neonatal or infantile infection with HBV is common in such persons. In patients with primary hepatocellular carcinoma, evidence of HBV infection and expression has been reported in 70 to 95% of cases examined, and integrated HBV DNA has been detected in the hepatoma cell chromosomes. The factors involved in activating the chronic HBV or in promoting the change from hepatitis or cirrhosis to a hepatoma are as yet unknown. However, this correlation is new, and mass vaccinations in high endemic areas are in progress. If the incidence of hepatocellular carcinoma drops in a few years or decades, this will support the idea that HBV is either the cause or a determinant promoter of liver cancer in these areas. As in the case of cervical cancer, molecular biologists are investigating why a virus can cause liver cancer. Recently, Tiollais found that HBV integrates its genes in the hepatocyte within the gene of retinoic acid receptor. This receptor is involved in the maintenance of cell differentiation and it is hypothesized that viral gene integration into it contributes to cell transformation.

Finally, let us discuss the role of retroviruses and

cancer. Retroviruses have a genome made up of RNA, not DNA. A reverse (hence the prefix "retro") transcriptase makes a DNA copy from it, which is then integrated into the host cell genome. We owe a good deal of our understanding of the nature of neoplastic transformation in murine and avian systems to studies of leukemia-inducing and sarcoma-inducing retroviruses (Table 11–5). Their relevance to carcinogenesis in the wild is less certain. Endogenous retroviruses are inherited as stable genes in most species of mammals. We will focus this discussion on human disease and, specifically, the only clearly established prototype in which a retrovirus can cause cancer: adult T-cell leukemia/lymphoma (ATL). Epidemiological and molecular biology studies, done mostly by Gallo, have indicated that a retrovirus called HTLV-1 (human T-cell leukemia virus, type 1) is the cause of ATL. The disease is encountered mostly in Southern Japan and the West Indies. Some details of the mechanisms by which HTLV-1 causes ATL are already known. Indeed, a viral gene activates the production by the infected T cell of both interleukin-2 and interleukin-2 receptor. These two molecules are the driving force of the T cell, comparable to both its gasoline and its engine respectively. Once again, because the net effect is malignant transformation, one has to hypothesize that the activation of this driving force is not controllable any more. Although it appears to be an important step in the process of transformation leading to a leukemic T cell, it is likely that other mechanisms operate for the completion of the process.

Genetic Factors

In the experimental animal, of which pure strains can be bred with ease, the genetic constitution may be a factor of paramount importance. Thus we have high-cancer strains and low-cancer strains of mice for a particular tumor and organ. It is not possible to apply the results of breeding experiments in mice to men for obvious reasons, but a few human tumors show such a familial tendency so that up to half of the members of a family may die of the disease if they live long enough. Such tumors are neuroblastoma of the retina and malignant polyp of the large bowel in familial polyposis. An historic example of a familial tendency is that of Napoleon, who died at St. Helena of cancer of the stomach, although much has been made recently of possible death by arsenic poisoning. His father, his grandfather, his brother, and his three sisters all died of the same disease.

Several types of evidence make it clear that the genetic component of human cancer is relatively small. For instance, most cases of colonic polyps are not familial. Studies on identical twins show that their expe-

Table 11–5. Neoplasms of Viral Etiology

TYPE OF NEOPLASM	ANIMAL SPECIES	REFERENCES
Chicken leukoses	Fowl	Ellerman and Bang (1908)
Chicken sarcomas	Fowl	Rous (1911)
Chicken sarcomas	Fowl	Fujinami and Inamoto (1914)
Mill-Hill endothelioma	Fowl	Foulds (1934)
Chicken fibrosarcomas	Fowl	Duran-Reynals (1946)
Mammary cancer (adenocarcinoma)	Mice	Bittner (1936)
Maxillary gland tumors	Mice	Gross (1953)
Leukemia	Mice	Gross (1952)
Papillomatosis	Rabbit, cattle, horse	Shope (1932), Olson (1941)
Adenocarcinoma of kidney	Leopard, frog	Lucké (1934, 1938)
Papilloma (warts)	Humans	Green, et al. (1940) Strauss, et al. (1950)

(From Perez-Tamayo, R.: *Mechanisms of Disease.* Philadelphia, W. B. Saunders Co., 1961.)

riences with common types of cancer are no more similar than those of nonidentical twins. Most convincing are the studies on migrating populations in the context of worldwide epidemiology. The relative incidence of specific cancer varies greatly from country to country; this finding is consistent with the significance of environmental factors: diet, soil, water, air, industrial by-products. Japan has high levels of stomach cancer, but relatively lower levels of breast, large intestine, and prostate cancer as compared with the United States. When Japanese immigrants migrate to California, their cancer profile looks similar to that of native Californians within two generations. As breeding within the group remains prevalent, the dominant force here is environmental. Since the shift is not immediate, the environmental factors probably include elements, such as diet, that change slowly with cultural assimilation rather than automatic stimuli, such as air quality. Studies of other migrant populations illustrate the same point. Epidemiologists have attempted to define the environmental factors that correlate with the relative international frequencies of given cancers. For example, it appears that the increased incidence of cancer of the large intestine correlates well with high fat consumption in a society and with low fiber intake.

There are some situations, however, in which a genetic predisposition for a given cancer is apparently involved. Women whose sisters or mothers have suffered from breast cancer have a significantly greater likelihood of having breast cancer than do women in general. We used to separate in different disease categories those rare cancers, like retinoblastoma, which have a clearly defined and predictable, heritable transmission, from the more common types which have a so-called sporadic occurrence. Epidemiologists and geneticists are now telling us that there is a "grey zone" between those two categories in which genetics and environment combine in such a way that a member of a family which has more cases of cancers than the general population has himself or herself a higher likelihood of having cancer. This has now been clearly demonstrated in the case of breast and colon cancer.

A hereditary disorder known as xeroderma pigmentosum illustrates the role of inherited and somatic (not in the germ-line, but rather occurring independently in body cells) mutation (Table 11–6). Persons who inherit this mutation are more susceptible to DNA damage effected by environmental radiation, for example the ultraviolet irradiation of sunlight. Persons so affected have a significantly increased level of skin cancer. The basic molecular defect in these patients is that ultraviolet light-induced damage to the epidermal cell DNA remains unrepaired, in contrast with normal persons in whom the damaged segment of DNA is repaired by excision, and these accumulated mutations obviously exert a carcinogenic effect.

Oncogenes—Clues to the Molecular and Biologic Mechanisms of Tumorigenesis

The discovery of oncogenes by Bishop, Varmus and Weinberg represents one of the two most important recent advances in cancer research. Interestingly, the second one is the discovery of anti-oncogenes and will be discussed immediately after this section.

Table 11–6.   Genetic Abnormalities and Susceptibility to Cancer

I. Chromosome aberrations
  Trisomy 21 syndrome
  Klinefelter's syndrome (XXY)
  Female XY mosaicism
  13-q deletion syndrome
  The Philadelphia chromosome
II. Recessively inherited syndromes
  Bloom's syndrome
  Fanconi's anemia
  Ataxia telangiectasia
  Xeroderma pigmentosum
III. Dominantly inherited syndromes
  Retinoblastoma
  Gardner's syndrome
  Familial polyposis
  Basal cell nevus syndrome
  Neurofibromatosis
  Multiple endocrine adenomatosis syndromes

(From Miller, D.G.: On the nature of susceptibility to cancer. Cancer, 46:1307, 1980.)

Oncogenes were discovered from the study of retroviruses. There are two broad categories of retroviruses: "leukemogenic" or slow tumor viruses, and acute, or rapid tumor viruses. The former (such as Moloney leukemia virus or avian leukosis virus) contain only those functions required for viral growth and contain all the genetic machinery required for replication; the latter (for example, Harvey sarcoma virus, Abelson virus, Rous sarcoma virus) do not have the genes for replication but contain genes which confer oncogenicity, i.e., the ability to form a malignant tumor from the cells it infects. Such genes are now referred to as **viral oncogenes.** They encode membrane-associated, cytoplasmic or nuclear proteins which have the potential to induce malignant transformation, usually through a cascade of intracellular events. This potential can be measured by assaying in vitro and in vivo tumorigenesis. The main criterion of tumorigenesis is the ability of cells, transformed by an oncogene, to grow as a malignant tumor when transplanted into an immunosuppressed mouse. To date, at least 21 different viral oncogenes have been described, each of which confers the ability to rapidly induce tumors in specific tissue and cell types. Oncogenes are referred to by a 3-letter abbreviation that usually includes the name of the animal species or genus infected by the virus: src, abl, sis, erb, ras. Viruses containing oncogenes are usually replication defective, and their spread from cell to cell requires that they use the DNA replication machinery of the infected cell, or co-infection with a helper virus.

To summarize at this point, the genome of viruses capable of inducing malignant transformation are defective for cell replication but, almost as a "revenge," contain discrete gene sequences called oncogenes which will drive the cells they infect to replicate with them and, beyond that, to become malignant. This could be called the ultimate form of parasitism and this scenario could end here. However, molecular virologists asked the following question: Where do these viral oncogenes come from? The answer was extraordinary by its significance. It appears that viral oncogenes were acquired from the genome of **normal, non-infected cells.** Indeed, using techniques of nucleic acid hybridization, it was found that normal animal cells contain genes which are closely related, if not homologous, to the viral oncogenes. Such genes seem to be bona fide cellular genes, well conserved throughout evolution and expressed at particular stages of development. They are designated protooncogenes, or cellular oncogenes, and referred to as c-src, c-abl, c-ras, etc. The implication of these data is that we carry within ourselves the very instructions for cancer, which are latent or dormant, but that in the course of our lives, this potential for disease can be awakened. Our knowledge of the acute retroviruses implies that some viral infections may be one way of activating these genes. One can also postulate that other stimuli might equally well alter the expression of the cellular oncogenes with the result of provoking tumor formation. This disturbing thought has placed the study of oncogenes in cells and in the viruses that capture them at the very frontier of modern biology.

Now we come to the question of how the inclusion of the cellular oncogene in the virus changes it from a coordinated element of cellular information to an inducer of cancer. Acute retroviruses are the most rapid and surefire inducers of tumors known. A number of models have been proposed to explain this phenomenon. First, the viral signals for gene expression are very potent, and inclusion in the virus may increase the level of the oncogene's product far beyond the normal cellular level, past some "oncogenic" threshold. Second, the high level of expression mediated by the virus may occur in a cell or tissue type not normally expressing this protein, with consequences beyond the control of normal cellular regulation. Thirdly, the gene may undergo deletions, rearrangements or mutations during inclusion in the virus which qualitatively change the activity of the protein product, rendering it oncogenic. Experimental data suggest that all three of these models are operative in different circumstances. The third model is particularly common with many oncogenes. Although quantitative differences in gene expression are important, there is every indication that viral oncogenes always differ in some qualitative way from their cellular progenitors.

As we have suggested, oncogenes may well be activated by agents other than viruses. Mutagens (agents that introduce changes into DNA) have been shown to be carcinogenic in a majority of cases and may play a role in oncogene activation. Scientists are now actively examining the state of cellular oncogenes in animal and human tumors not associated with a known viral etiology. In some cases they found increased levels of expression of a particular oncogene; in several instances, this effect was accomplished by the actual physical amplification of the gene to yield a cell with numerous gene copies of the oncogene (for example, m-myc in human neuroblastoma). Of note is the observation that the degree of m-myc amplification is clinically significant: the more amplification there is present, the poorer the patient's prognosis. The same clinical observation is valid for another oncogene called neu in the prognosis of breast cancer patients.

Thirdly, there are some human cancers (Burkitt's lymphoma and chronic myelocytic leukemia) which have long been associated with characteristic chromosomal rearrangements. It has been shown recently that in these tumors, one of the break points of the translocation, i.e., the region of DNA moved to a new chromosomal environment, contains the sequences of a known cellular oncogene (c-myc in Burkitt's lymphoma, c-abl in CML). In the case of Burkitt's lymphoma, the c-myc oncogene located on chromosome 8 is translocated on chromosome 14 just downstream of genes coding for immunoglobulins. Since all this happens in B lymphocytes, cells that synthesize a large amount of immunoglobulin, the c-myc becomes highly transcribed in this very active neighborhood.

Although some types of cancer have oncogenes that are overexpressed but are not structurally different from normal oncogenes, it remains that in other tumors structural differences do exist. In one case, that of a human bladder carcinoma, the difference has been shown to be a point mutation which directs a change in one amino acid of the encoded ras oncogene protein. This mutated protein has a decisive effect on malignant transformation even though other events must also take place. Point mutations in the ras oncogene are frequently found in pancreas, colon and lung carcinomas. In the latter case, the presence of the mutation correlates with poor prognosis when compared with lung cancers that do not have it.

To recapitulate, chromosomal rearrangements, alteration of the local genetic environment by insertion of novel regulatory signals, or pinpoint mutations can activate an oncogene. Considering that many known carcinogens are DNA mutagens it is quite possible that they exert their action by affecting oncogenes.

What are the protein products encoded by the known oncogenes? Although not all are characterized, a picture is emerging of several categories of proteins. Many oncogenes code for proteins that activate protein kinases: i.e., these enzymes specifically phosphorylate other proteins. This modification is correlated with a change in activity in the affected substrates in ways that are not fully understood but which eventually increase DNA replication and transcription. Other oncogenes are nuclear proteins with presumed affinity for DNA probably at sites involved in the regulation of mitosis. Some oncogene products mimic naturally occurring growth factors although they might be slightly different from them in their structure. This is the case of the sis oncogene which has a high degree of homology with PDGF (platelet derived growth factor). Cells expressing the activated form of sis can have their own growth continuously stimulated by it when they happen to express the PDGF receptor. This type of unregulated self-stimulation is called autocrine.

Cancer is a complex phenomenon. The multi-step etiology and multi-step progression of tumors has long been discussed. No single molecular event seems likely to cause a fully developed tumor under natural conditions. Recent experiments, in which activated oncogenes are effectively implanted in a variety of cell types in culture, are addressing this question of the multiplicity of steps involved in cancer formation. Some activated oncogenes can transform primary embryo cells in culture, whereas others cannot and can only transform established cell lines. Some activated oncogenes enable the cells they transform to grow to self-limiting tumors in experimental animals, whereas combinations of oncogenes in the same cells may permit them to induce metastatic disease. There seems to be a hierarchy of cell stages between coordinately regulated growth and differentiation and the uncontrolled proliferation of cancer cells. These different stages involve a network of genes and protein products which direct growth and differentiation. The study of oncogenes brings together the diverse environmental insults and genetic factors implicated in causing cancer, and focuses our attention on the most likely target: a subset of important cellular genes. When these genes are properly expressed they program the complex steps of regulated cell growth and development, but when disturbed they can sabotage the very order they were designed to maintain. One could easily become dogmatic and state that cancer is a summation of insults characterized by the activation of several oncogenes in a cell resulting in the defeat of its various control mechanisms. Testing such an hypothesis is not an easy experimental task. Suffice it to say that this dogma has many fissures and if one wants to understand better the process of malignant transformation, one needs to introduce the important concept of anti-oncogenes.

Anti-Oncogenes

When the karyotype of cancer cells is examined by cytogeneticists, they usually see a large number of chromosome abnormalities and it is often difficult to detect a consistent pattern. There is, however, a special and rare type of eye tumor, called retinoblastoma, occurring in children, which has a consistent chromosomal change. This consists of the deletion of a specific segment of the long arm of chromosome 13, a region designated 13q14. The other chromosome 13 does not have such a gross 13q14 deletion but, in fact, it also carries a structural abnormality in the same region. What about the retinal cells around the retinoblastoma and all the somatic cells as well? The answer to this question depends on whether the child has a

familial or a sporadic form of retinoblastoma. In the familial form, one chromosome 13 is normal and the other is not, whereas in the sporadic form, both chromosomes 13 are normal. To summarize, children with the familial form of retinoblastoma are born with one mutation inactivating the gene, now called the Rb gene, and undergo a second inactivating mutation of Rb in their retinal cells. In the sporadic cases, both inactivating mutations occur after birth.

Those observations are derived from the recent pioneering studies of Knudson and Cavenee and have led to the fundamental concept of anti-oncogene, also called tumor suppressor gene. Basically this concept states that cancer arises from the loss of a normal function associated with cell growth, proliferation or differentiation. This challenging idea is supported by the observation that the Rb gene encodes a protein, the Rb protein, which binds to DNA.

One might wonder whether the concept of anti-oncogene applies to rare childhood tumors like the retinoblastoma, or whether it has a more general significance. When Bodmer and Vogelstein recently demonstrated that at least one anti-oncogene is involved in the much more common colorectal cancer, it became evident that the initial observation is not unique. Several genes are lost or inactivated in colorectal cancer and one of them called p53, which is located on chromosome 17, behaves as an anti-oncogene. This gene is inactivated through point mutations.

To conclude this section, we have to ask ourselves whether the concepts of oncogenes and anti-oncogenes are mutually exclusive in the causation and mechanisms of cancer. Although it looks a little bit premature to give a clear-cut answer one might propose the following scheme. Carcinogenic agents of different kinds, or spontaneous mutations, induce abnormalities in genes affecting the growth, proliferation or differentiation of cells. When activated, oncogenes produce proteins that activate and deregulate these normal processes. Inactivation of anti-oncogenes abolishes the normal down-regulation of cell proliferation. Thus it might well be that both activation of oncogenes and inactivation of anti-oncogenes are necessary for cancer to occur, whatever the chronology of these two events might be.

Environment

It is certainly the case that some forms of occupation bear a striking relation to cancer in particular sites. This is a subject of increasing importance in the industrial age in which we live, and in which the workmen's compensation claims a corresponding degree of attention. Mere mention need be made of workers with coal tar and petroleum distillates, aniline dyes, x-rays and radioactive material, and many other raw materials and products. Traditional and modern agriculture is not exempt from cancer risks as well. The truth is that throughout life we seem to swim in a sea of carcinogens, and it is more by good fortune than by good management that some of us escape to die from causes other than cancer. Chronic irritation used to be a favorite scapegoat, but it is seldom heard of now, although a few examples come to mind. For instance, cancer of the urinary bladder is common in persons chronically infected with *Schistosoma hematobium* which is very common in Egypt.

Environmental exposure to industrial hazards or simply to contaminants of the household has gained increasing attention as a possible etiologic factor in the rising tide of our ills (Table 11–7). It is now clear that asbestos offers real hazards to the industrial worker, whether a miner or a fitter engaged in using the material. It even appears that the worker's family is at increased risk, because when he returns home his clothing may carry sufficient asbestos particles to expose those who wait daily for the worker's return. The role of asbestos in producing cancer of the pleural surfaces is clearly recognized, although the latent period may be several decades.

Other recent connections between occupational exposure and cancer have been made. For example, in the plastics industry, exposure to vinyl chloride has been shown to produce a tumor of blood vessels in the liver. It has been known for decades that workers in the heavy metals industries (nickel, copper, cobalt) all may have significantly increased risks for different cancers, and it has even become clear that sawmill workers have an extraordinarily high risk of cancer of the nasal sinuses.

The incidence of different forms of cancer certainly varies greatly in different parts of the world (Table 11–8). We have already mentioned the high incidence of bladder cancer in Egypt, melanoma in Australia, and liver cancer in China and East Africa, which are associated with schistosomiasis, high ultraviolet light exposure, and hepatitis B, respectively.

Now that we have considered some of the contemporary ideas of how cancer is caused let us turn to a consideration of what tumors are, how they are identified, classified, and behave.

CHARACTERISTICS OF TUMORS

An operational and reasonable definition for all tumors is that of Willis: "A tumor is an abnormal mass of tissue, the growth of which exceeds and is uncoordinated with that of normal tissues, and persists in the same excessive manner after the cessation of the stimuli which evoked the change."

Tumors can be divided into two general classes: the one innocent or benign, the other malignant. Sometimes a benign tumor may develop into a malignant

Table 11–7. Occupational Cancers

AGENT	OCCUPATION	SITE OF CANCER
Ionizing radiations		
radon	certain underground miners (uranium, fluorspar, hematite)	bronchus
X-rays, radium	radiologists, radiographers	skin
radium	luminous dial painters	bone
Ultraviolet light	farmers, sailors	skin
Polycyclic hydrocarbons in soot, tar, oil	chimney sweeps	scrotum
	manufacturers of coal gas	skin
	many other groups of exposed industrial workers	bronchus
2-Naphthylamine; 1-naphthylamine	chemical workers; rubber workers; manufacturers of coal gas	bladder
Asbestos	asbestos workers; shipyard and insulation workers	bronchus pleura and peritoneum
Arsenic	sheep dip manufacturers; gold miners; some vineyard workers and ore smelters	skin and bronchus
Benzene	workers with glues, varnishes, etc.	marrow (leukemia)
Mustard gas	poison gas makers	bronchus; larynx; nasal sinuses
Vinyl chloride	PVC manufacturers	liver (angiosarcoma)
(Chrome ores)	chromate manufacturers	bronchus
(Nickel ore)	nickel refiners	bronchus; nasal sinuses
(Isopropyl oil)	isopropylene manufacturers	nasal sinuses
*	hardwood furniture makers	nasal sinuses
*	leather workers	nasal sinuses

* Specific agent not identified.

(From Doll, R.: Introduction. In *Origins of Human Cancer, Book A.* Edited by H.H. Hiatt, et al. New York, Cold Spring Harbor Laboratory, 1977.)

Table 11–8. Range of Variation in the Incidence of Common Cancers

TYPE OF CANCER	HIGH-INCIDENCE AREA	CUMULATIVE RISK[a] (%)	RANGE OF VARIATION[b]	LOW-INCIDENCE AREA
Skin	Australia, Queensland	>20	>200	India, Bombay
Esophagus	Iran, N.E.	20	300	Nigeria
Bronchus	England	11	35	Nigeria
Stomach	Japan	11	25	Uganda
Cervix uteria	Colombia	10	15	Israel, Jewish
Liver	Mozambique	8	70	Norway
Prostate	USA, black	7	30	Japan
Breast (♀)	USA, Connecticut	7	5	Uganda
Colon	USA, Connecticut	3	10	Nigeria
Buccal cavity	India, part	>2	>25	Denmark
Rectum	Denmark	2	20	Nigeria
Bladder	USA, Connecticut	2	4	Japan
Ovary	Denmark	2	8	Japan
Corpus uteri	USA, Connecticut	2	10	Japan
Nasopharynx	Singapore, Chinese	2	40	England
Pancreas	New Zealand, Maori	2	5	Uganda
Penis	Uganda, part	1	300	Israel, Jewish

[a] By 75 years of age in absence of other causes of death.
[b] At ages 35–64 years

(From Doll, R.: Introduction. In *Origins of Human Cancer, Book A.* Edited by H. H. Hiatt, et al. New York, Cold Spring Harbor Laboratory, 1977.)

one but this occurs very rarely. A malignant tumor differs from a benign one in the following particulars.

1. A malignant tumor, if untreated, will kill the patient wherever it occurs, even in the hand or foot because it spreads to distant organs. Usually a benign tumor may only cause death if it happens to grow in a vital organ such as the brain.
2. A malignant tumor infiltrates the surrounding tissue. It sends claws into it like a crab. The word cancer means a crab. A benign tumor grows by expansion, as a toy balloon does when blown up, and is usually separated from the surrounding tissue by a capsule so that it can be shelled out, or at least readily removed.
3. When a malignant tumor is excised, it may recur. This is because some of the outlying parts have not been completely removed; they are so minute that they cannot be seen by the surgeon, but they may soon grow to the size of the original tumor. When a benign tumor is removed, it usually does not recur.
4. Generally, a malignant tumor grows more rapidly than a benign one, although some cancers are remarkably slow in growth. It is important to note that the growth is not necessarily linear and that there might be phases of rapid expansion interspersed with slow growth. The rapid growth is because tumor cells divide rapidly. The presence of numerous mitotic figures, particularly abnormal mitotic figures, indicates to the pathologist that the tumor is almost certainly malignant.
5. A malignant tumor sets up secondary growths (metastases) in lymph nodes and in distant organs. This is because the cancer has invaded the lymph or blood vessels, and the tumor cells are carried to other parts of the body, where they settle down and form new tumors. This is the single most obvious criterion of malignancy: the presence of **metastases.**

There are microscopic differences of great importance to the pathologist in the task of determining whether the tumor removed by the surgeon is or is not cancer, but they need not be detailed here. Suffice it to say that a benign tumor has a different architecture compared to the organ it derives from. However, the morphology of the individual cells is quite normal. In a malignant tumor both the architecture and the cell morphology are abnormal. The cells of a malignant tumor show a lack of normal differentiation, a reversion to a more primitive and undifferentiated type, which is known as **anaplasia.** Both the histologic and cytologic changes may be so great that the pathologist can diagnose the case as one of cancer the moment he looks down the microscope. In other cases, a decision may be difficult, and different pathologists may disagree in their interpretations of the microscopic picture.

Carcinoma-in-situ. An important step in the fight against cancer is the recognition by the pathologist of

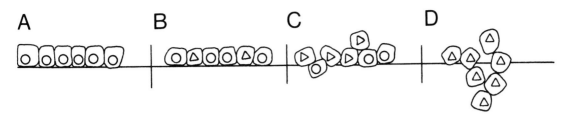

Fig. 11–10 *A,* illustrates normal cells, *B,* shows cells with some atypia that could be considered dysplastic. *C,* Microinvasive carcinoma is represented by breaching of the basement membrane, and *D,* invasive carcinoma with malignant cells penetrating deeply into the stroma, is shown. The triangles for nuclei rather than circles symbolize transformed cells, whatever the cause.

the earliest beginnings of the malignant process. When metastases have occurred, it is often too late. When invasion of the deeper tissues can be recognized it may be quite late, although this depends on the type of cancer. However, when the malignant change is still cytologic with no invasion beyond the normal anatomical barriers, such as the basement membrane, the disease is more easily curable. This is called *carcinoma-in-situ* or preinvasive carcinoma. In this lesion the cells do not mature normally and have a high rate of proliferation. The condition may be reversible, but in many cases, the *in-situ* state develops into a microinvasive and then an invasive one. In the case of carcinoma, this step is characterized by a breaching of the underlying basement membrane which normally separates the epithelium from stroma. It is in carcinoma of the cervix uteri that recognition of preinvasive carcinoma is of the greatest practical importance and has already saved the lives of countless women. A drawing to illustrate the concept is shown in Figure 11–10, in which *A* represents normal cells in a tissue, and *D* represents malignant cells invading the surrounding tissue.

Some of the principal distinguishing features between benign and malignant tumors are listed in Table 11–9. It must be understood that these are generalizations to which there are frequent exceptions.

Spread of Tumors

This subject has already been referred to. In contrast with a benign tumor a malignant one spreads locally and to distant parts. The local spread is due to the high motility of the tumor cells, their lack of adhesiveness, and, in the case of carcinomas, the secretion of proteolytic enzymes capable of digesting the underlying basement membrane. Once into the stroma, the tumor cells acquire the additional property of invading blood and lymphatic capillaries. Lymphatic invasion leads to migration of the tumor cells into local lymph nodes. Permeation of the lymphatics is particularly well seen in cancer of the breast. In the surgical treatment of cancer of the breast, the lymph nodes in the axilla, which receive the lymph from the breast, are removed together with the breast. This is done even though they are not enlarged, for they may contain cancer cells that have not yet had time to form a visible tumor.

Invasion of blood capillaries sets up the conditions for **tumor embolism,** the cancer cells forming emboli and being carried by the blood stream to distant parts in the same way as thrombi may become detached and converted into emboli. It should be pointed out that, fortunately, embolism of tumor cells in the blood circulation does not necessarily mean that the tumor will form metastases at distant sites. It appears that two conditions must be fulfilled: the distant site must process the proper soil for colonization, and the tumor must have gained new characteristics to be able to grow on a foreign ground.

In embolism through the blood stream, the tumor cells are carried to some other organ, where they are arrested in the capillaries and start secondary growths or metastases. In abdominal organs such as the stom-

Table 11–9.   Characteristics of Benign and Malignant Tumors

CHARACTERISTICS	BENIGN	MALIGNANT
1. Growth	Slow, expansive, often encapsulated	Rapid, invasive, nonencapsulated
2. Metastases	Absent	Frequent
3. Recurrence after removal	Absent	Frequent if incomplete removal
4. Histology	Relatively normal	Abnormal to a varying degree
5. Cytology	Normal	Varying degrees of anaplasia
6. Mitoses	Absent	Often numerous and abnormal
7. Constitutional effects	Rare, apart from endocrine adenomas	The rule

ach, metastases are usually in the liver, because the blood from the digestive tract is carried first to the liver. In the case of other organs, the metastases not uncommonly occur in the lungs, but any organ in the body may be involved.

Having reviewed some of the general aspects of tumor pathology, we may now briefly consider a few of the more important varieties of tumors. Many of these are described in more detail in connection with the organs in which they occur. It is difficult to give an interesting or even intelligible account of tumors without reference to the microscopic structure and the use of a large number of technical terms, but this is avoided as far as possible.

Benign Tumors

The general characteristics of a benign tumor have already been outlined, so they need not be repeated here. In describing benign tumors, and the same is true of malignant tumors, we name them after the tissue from which they arise, adding most often the suffix -oma, which indicates tumors, just as -itis indicates inflammation. Some of the principal tissues from which neoplasms are derived are as follows: (1) **epithelium,** which makes up the skin, the mucus membranes that line the mouth, stomach, intestine, and uterus, and most cells of others organs, such as the breast, liver, and urogenital organs; (2) **fibrous** or **connective tissue,** which forms a general framework of the body and therefore occurs in all organs; (3) **fat** or adipose tissue; (4) **bone** and cartilage; (5) **muscle;** (6) **blood vessels;** (7) **nervous tissue;** (8) **lymph nodes;** (9) **endocrine glands**. A brief description of the most common types of benign tumors follows.

Adenoma. This benign epithelial tumor is often glandular in structure; that is to say, the cells are arranged around secretory spaces. It occurs most commonly in organs that are themselves glandular, such as the gastrointestinal tract and thyroid gland.

Lipoma. A soft fatty tumor growing from fat (adipose tissue), lipoma may occur wherever fat is present, but is most common in the neck, shoulders, back, thigh and buttocks, and other places where fat is abundant.

Leiomyoma. This tumor is composed of smooth muscle which is normally found in the walls of the stomach and intestine, the blood vessels, and the uterus. Leiomyomas are common in the uterus, where they are frequently called "fibroids." Benign tumors derived from voluntary muscles are exceedingly rare.

Angioma. This tumor is composed of vessels, usually blood vessels, but sometimes lymphatic vessels.

It is therefore generally of a bright or dark red color, although a lymphangioma is colorless. A common site for hemangioma (angioma derived from blood vessels) is the skin, especially of the face or neck, where it forms a red patch known as a port-wine stain or birthmark. The latter term is used because the tumor is usually present at birth.

Nevus. A tumor of the skin, a nevus is composed of some epidermal cells filled with melanin pigment, called melanocytes, being usually dark in color and sometimes jet black. Also called moles, they are so common that nearly everyone has at least a tiny one, and many people have a large number of them. A nevus is a congenital condition, but it may not be apparent at birth. The common sites are the face, neck, and back. They are probably under hormonal influence for they tend to develop or increase in size at puberty. Less than 10% of the congenital nevi may become malignant. Some people have more and larger nevi than the rest of the population, and by the time they reach the age of 60 about half of them will have developed a melanoma. This is called the dysplastic nevus syndrome and has a tendency to be inherited as an autosomal dominant trait. The beginning of a malignant change in later life is indicated by an increase in size, inequality in shape, and heterogeneity of pigmentation, the presence of a pink halo due to congestion, and itching. The tumor has now become a **malignant melanoma.** The sites that have a poor prognosis are the palm, the sole of the foot, the fingers and toes, the genitals, and places exposed to continued trauma. The transformation is often slow and insidious and the tumor should be removed at once. A mole that shows no change need not be touched except for cosmetic reasons, but chronic irritation and trauma must be avoided at all costs.

Malignant Tumors

For almost every tissue of the body that can give rise to a benign tumor, a malignant tumor also may arise. In practice, however, nearly all malignant tumors can be divided into two great groups, **carcinoma** and **sarcoma,** both of which are included under the common term cancer. This simplification of nomenclature is possible because the epithelial tumors are called carcinoma, whereas the name sarcoma is applied not only to connective tissue tumors but also to tumors of bone, cartilage, fat and muscle, which are derived from or closely related to connective tissue.

Carcinoma. The commonest of malignant tumors spreads principally by the lymphatics, so that secondary involvement of the regional lymph nodes is common and has to be considered by the surgeon in every case. Spread by the blood stream is also common, and it sometimes happens that the first indication of cancer in an organ such as the lung is the development of a secondary tumor in the brain, the secondary tumor naturally being mistaken for the primary one until the original is discovered. It is evident that when tumors are present in two organs, it may be difficult to say which is primary and which secondary.

Carcinoma may arise either from the skin or from glandular organs (breast, thyroid), including the secreting glands in the mucus membrane of the stomach, intestine, and uterus. The microscopic structure differs in the two cases. In cancer derived from skin, cervix, and esophagus, there is some attempt at reproducing the normal arrangement of the epithelial cells in layers, so that this tumor is known as **squamous cell carcinoma** (resembling the squamous cells of the epidermis). Squamous cell carcinoma can also occur in the lung. In that case it is thought that the single columnar epithelium of the bronchi is first transformed into a metaplastic, multilayered squamous epithelium, and then into a squamous cell carcinoma. In glandular cancers, there is an attempt at arrangement of the cells around gland spaces, so that the tumor is known as **adenocarcinoma** (Greek *aden*, gland).

The degree to which carcinoma can resemble the normal squamous epithelium or glandular structure varies greatly. There may be absolutely no approximation to the normal arrangement of cells; such a tumor is said to be **undifferentiated** or **anaplastic**. These anaplastic tumors are usually highly malignant. Conversely, the tumor may reproduce the normal structure with a fair degree of success. It is then said to be **differentiated** and for most body sites has a better prognosis. It is evident from what has been said previously that, if a tumor is highly differentiated, the pathologist may have difficulty in distinguishing it from a benign epithelial tumor (adenoma, papilloma). The degree of differentiation is usually expressed in 4 grades, grade 1 being the most differentiated, grade 4 the most anaplastic.

The common sites of carcinoma are the breast, lung, colon and rectum, prostate, uterus, bladder, stomach, pancreas and skin. Skin cancers, whether they are basal or squamous cell carcinomas, are not widely invasive, with the noticeable exception of melanoma. Cancer of the other organs is described when the diseases of those organs are considered.

Sarcoma. This is a malignant tumor of connective (fibrous) tissue and of those structures such as vascular and intestinal smooth muscle, bone and cartilage that are derived from connective tissue. Sarcomas may occur in any part of the body, as connective tissue is present everywhere. These tumors are uncommon as compared with carcinoma. Distant spread of sarcomas is usually by the blood stream, and metastases are usually in the lungs.

Hodgkin's Disease and Lymphomas. These two disease entities refer to a malignant tumor of the lymph nodes. They are relatively common, accounting for the 5th most frequent cancer in both men and women. Its chief characteristics are its wide distribution and its sensitivity to radiation and chemotherapy. The response to these therapies is remarkable, large masses of tumor melting away in a few days or weeks. Some cases can be cured and many held in check for a long time by means of treatment.

Malignant Melanoma. This type of cancer was described above in the section on the nevus and its transformation. We need to reinforce that if this tumor is not diagnosed and treated by surgery, early and aggressively, it will disseminate rapidly to lymph nodes and distant organs. A remarkable new finding is that at least 10% of malignant melanomas respond to a new form of immunotherapy in which the patient's own lymphocytes are stimulated by interleukin-2 and injected intravenously. A significant proportion of kidney cancers also respond favorably to this exciting new therapy.

Glioma. This is a malignant tumor of the glia or neuroglia of the brain that separates the neurons from one another and acts as a kind of connective tissue. Except in children brain tumors are relatively uncommon, and such tumors practically never arise from neurons always from neuroglia. The gliomas vary greatly in malignancy, but even the least malignant ones show no attempt at encapsulation and merge with the surrounding brain tissue. Molecular biologists have documented that each rise in the grade of gliomas is characterized by, and may be due, to genetic changes in chromosome 17. This makes the task of the brain surgeon peculiarly difficult, because even when the tumor has been exposed, it is difficult to know how much of the surrounding brain to remove. Oddly, brain tumors do not metastasize outside the skull.

Symptoms of Cancer

The most important single fact about the clinical picture of cancer is that, in the early stages, the disease is often painless. If it were as painful as a toothache, far fewer people would die from the disease. The symptoms vary with the location of the tumor, but in most cases there are likely to be such general constitutional symptoms as weakness, loss of weight, anemia, and pain late in the disease. In a superficial part, such as the skin, subcutaneous tissue or breast, a lump may be felt. When the affected organ communicates with the surface, there may be a discharge or bleeding, as in cancer of the uterus.

Finally, it must be remembered that the symptoms may not be due to the primary tumor, which may remain latent, but to metastases. One of the best examples of this confusing occurrence is that of a silent carcinoma of the lung that metastasizes to the brain, so that the patient comes to the doctor with symptoms of a brain tumor, but no cough, shortness of breath, pain in the chest, or spitting of blood.

So far we have spoken of the clinical effects of cancer as those due to the local lesion and to metastases. But the most puzzling, indeed mysterious, effects are those known as systemic manifestations. These effects are too multiform to be enumerated, but they may be systemic with TNF-mediated cachexia; dermatologic; vascular, more particularly occlusion of veins by thrombi; hormonal disturbances involving many hormones; and neuromuscular symptoms suggesting lesions of the nerves and muscles. For some of these, the term **paraneoplastic syndrome** has been coined and its main significance is that it can signal an undiagnosed cancer.

TUMOR IMMUNITY

In the early animal carcinogenesis studies the experiments consisted of transplanting malignant tumors in animals into other animals. The recipient animal had to be of the same strain and species. The tumor would not grow in an animal of another species because the tumor tissue acted as a foreign antigen, which stimulated the formation of specific cytotoxic cells and antibodies that destroyed the antigenic tumor tissue. For this reason it was impossible to transplant successfully human cancer to laboratory animals. Resistance of heterotransplantation has now been overcome in three ways: (1) preliminary radiation of the animal, (2) administration of immunosuppressive drugs, and (3) grafting to special mice which are born without a thymus and are also hairless (nude mice). All three methods appear to depress immune response to heterologous antigens in the transplanted tumor, probably owing to a great reduction in the number of lymphocytes known to produce antibodies. The result of these procedures has been exciting, for it is now possible to transplant human cancer to other animals and to maintain the disease over successive generations allowing for the testing of new diagnostic and therapeutic protocols.

It has also been recognized that some malignant tumors are surrounded by lymphocytes and evoke a substantial inflammatory response. Now we know that patients with defective immune mechanisms are often visited by cancer. The commonest example of this phenomenon today is the person who has received steroids and radiation or drugs to depress the immune response after receiving an organ kidney transplant, for instance. There is a general concept that an immune system has a way to eliminate nonself cells, cells that have been phenotypically so modified that some lymphocytes recognize and eliminate them as foreign-body cells. This is called immune surveillance, and how powerful this system is in the recognition of early forms of human cancer remains to be fully documented. These observations have led to therapeutic attempts to stimulate the host defenses by using such nonspecific stimulants as attenuated tubercle bacilli (BCG). This method is effective in the treatment of one form of bladder cancer and has recently been approved for wide therapeutic use.

One of the most spectacular advances in medicine over the last four years has been the observation that it is now possible to induce the regression of certain types of cancer, some of which are known to behave aggressively. In 1985 Rosenberg, a surgeon, injected Interleukin-2 (IL-2), a hormone-like substance normally produced by lymphocytes, into mice having widespread melanoma with metastases to the lung. The tumor, which carries a dreadful prognosis in mice as it does in humans, was found to regress markedly with the disappearance of a large number of metastases. Rosenberg concluded that the mice could not by themselves generate killer cells but that with the help of injected interleukin cells these cells could be activated and acquire the capability of killing the melanoma cells in the animal.

Subsequently, Rosenberg and his group found that this mode of treatment would be even more effective if the killer cells, which belong to a subgroup of lymphocytes and are now called LAK (for Lymphokine Activated Killer cells), were generated in vitro by incubating inactive lymphocytes with IL-2 before the LAK, thus generated, were reinfused in the patient. The activity of the LAK cells was then maintained in the cancer-bearing animal by repeated injections of IL-2. Cures were obtained. A more recent variant of this form of immunotherapy consists of harvesting and stimulating tumor infiltrating lymphocytes (TIL).

How could this important observation on mice be applied to patients? The first clinical results were reported in 1986. This and subsequent trials were performed mostly on patients with widely metastatic tumors for whom no alternate therapy was available. What was found, using strict clinical and radiological criteria, was that in some patients with melanomas and kidney cancer, tumor growth was arrested, and furthermore, in more than 10% of these patients regression was observed to the point where no tumor metastases could be demonstrated. For any health professional who has attended cancer patients with disseminated disease, this remarkable effect of IL-2 stimulated lymphocytes on metastatic tumors represents an effect far beyond the natural history of cancer, especially disseminated melanoma.

Although spontaneous regression can occur, this outcome is exceedingly rare and, therefore, cancer diagnosis has to be followed by appropriate, and sometimes aggressive, therapy.

SYNOPSIS

Cancer is a process in which multiple factors play a role.

Chemical carcinogenesis has been interpreted in terms of initiation, promotion, and a variable latent period.

Viral carcinogenesis has been identified mostly in animals so far. In humans, cancer of the cervix is thought to be associated with the papilloma virus.

Hormonal dependence of some tumors has been shown and is used therapeutically in some human cancers.

Hereditary factors predisposing cancer are now being identified in larger numbers and with greater accuracy thanks to the application of molecular biology techniques.

The causation and progression of cancer involve both activation of oncogenes and inactivation of anti-oncogenes.

Environmental carcinogens may be difficult to incriminate because of a long latent period (decades).

The distinctions between benign and malignant tumors are clear on theoretical, histologic, and cytologic grounds in most cases.

The recognition that immune mechanisms play a role in resistance to tumors offers new modes of therapy.

Some serologic tests for cancer are valuable, but cytologic and biopsy methods form the backbone of diagnosis.

Cancer may produce systemic signs such as fever, weight loss, hormonal signs, and nonspecific signs.

Terms

Neoplasia	Adenoma	Paraneoplastic syndrome
Contact inhibition	Nevus	Oncogene
Metastases	Melanoma	Anti-oncogene
Cachexia	Carcinoma	Platelet derived growth factor
Carcinogen	Sarcoma	Chromosomal rearrangement
Human papilloma virus	Lymphoma	Gene amplification
Burkitt's lymphoma	Leukemia	
Anaplasia	Exfoliative cytology	
Dysplasia	Biopsy	
Carcinoma-in-situ	Carcinoembryonic antigen	

FURTHER READING

Baldwin, R.W.: Mechanisms of immunity in cancer. Pathobiol. Ann., 11:155, 1981.

Becker, F.F.: Recent concepts of initiation and promotion in carcinogenesis. Am. J. Pathol., 105:3, 1981.

Berenblum, I.: Cancer prevention as a realizable goal. Cancer, 47:2346, 1981.

Bishop, J.M.: Molecular themes in oncogenesis. Cell, 64:235, 1991.

Bishop, J.M.: Retroviruses and oncogenes II. Bioscience Reports, 10:473, 1989.

Bittner, J.J.: Milk factor in mammary mouse cancer. Science, 84:162, 1936.

Bodel, P.: Tumors and fever. Ann. N.Y. Acad. Sci., 230:6, 1974.

Burkitt, D., and Hutt, M.S.R.: Geographic pathology in developing countries. Int. Pathol., 7:1, 1966.

Burton, A.C.: Why do human cancer death rates increase with age? A new method of analysis of the biology of cancer. Perspect. Biol. Med., 20:327, 1977.

Busch, H.: The final common pathway of cancer: Presidential address. Canc. Res., 50:4830, 1990.

Cairns, J., and Logan, J.: News and views: step by step into carcinogenesis. Nature, 304:582, 1983.

Catalona, W.J., Smith, D.S., Ratliff, T.L., et al: Measurement of prostate-specific antigen in serum as a screening test for prostate cancer. N. Engl. J. Med., 324:1156, 1991.

Cavanee, W.K.: Recessive mutations in the causation of human cancer. Cancer, 10:2431, 1991.

Cross, M., and Dexter, T.M.: Growth factors in development, transformation and tumorigenesis. Cell, 64:271, 1991.

Doll, R.: The epidemiology of cancer. Cancer, 45:2475, 1980.

Effron, M., et al.: Nature and rate of neoplasia found in captive wild mammals, birds and reptiles at necropsy. J. Natl. Cancer Inst., 59:185, 1977.

Fidler, I.J., and Hart, I.R.: Biological diversity in metastatic neoplasms: origins and implications. Science, 217:998, 1982.

Folkman, J., and Haudenschild, C.: Induction of capillary growth in vitro. In Cellular Interactions. Edited by Dingle and Gordon. New York, Elsevier North-Holland Biomedical Press, 1981.

Fraumeni, J.F., Jr.: High-rate cancers among low-risk populations. J.N.C.I., 65:1187, 1980.

Friedman, H., and Southam, C.: International conference on immunobiology of cancer. Ann. N.Y. Acad. Sci., 276, 1976.

Gold, P.: Biological markers of human tumors. In Gastrointestinal Cancer. Edited by J.R. Stroehlein and M.M. Romsdal. New York, Raven Press, 1981.

Goldenberg, D.M.: Immunobiology and biochemical markers of gastrointestinal cancer. In Gastrointestinal Cancer. Edited by J.R. Stroehlein and M.M. Romsdal. New York, Raven Press, 1981.

Goldsmith, H.S.: Unanswered mysteries in the death of Franklin D. Roosevelt. Surg. Gynecol. Obstet., 149:899, 1979.

Hall, E.J.: From chimney sweeps to oncogenes: The quest for the causes of cancer. Radiology, 179:297, 1991.

Henderson, B.E.: Observations on cancer etiology in China. Natl. Cancer Inst. Monogr., 53:59, 1978.

Henle, W., Henle, G., and Lennette, E.H.: The Epstein-Barr virus. Sci. Am., 241:48, 1979.

Hollingsworth, R.E., and Lee, W.H.: Tumor suppressor genes: New prospects for cancer research. J.N.C.I., 83:82, 1991.

Hunter, T.: Cooperation between oncogenes. Cell, 64:249, 1991.

Kohn, J.I., and Fry, R.J.M.: Radiation carcinogenesis. N. Engl. J. Med., 310:504, 1984.

Krontiris, T.G.: The emerging genetics of human cancer. N. Engl. J. Med., 309:404, 1983.

Linos, A., et al.: Low dose radiation and leukemia. N. Engl. J. Med., 302:1101, 1980.

Liotta, L., et al.: Cancer metastasis and angiogenesis. Cell, 64:327, 1991.

Markert, C.L.: Cancer: the survival of the fittest. In Cell Differentiation and Neoplasia. Edited by G.F. Saunders. New York, Raven Press, 1978.

Marshall, C.J.: Tumor suppressor genes. Cell, 64:313, 1991.

Meyskens, Jr., F.L.: Coming of age—the chemoprevention of cancer. N. Engl. J. Med., 323:825, 1990.

Miller, D.G.: On the nature of susceptibility to cancer. Cancer, 46:1318, 1980.

Miller, R.W.: Cancer epidemics in the People's Republic of China. J. Natl. Cancer Inst., 60:1195, 1978.

Møller Jensen, O.M., Estève, J., Møller, H., and Renard, H.: Cancer in the European Community and its member states. Eur. J. Cancer, Vol. 26, 1990.

Pitot, H.C.: The natural history of neoplastic development: the relation of experimental models to human cancer. Cancer, 49:1206, 1982.

Roizman, B.: The structure and isomerization of herpes simplex virus genomes. Cell, 16:481, 1979.

Rosenberg, S.: Adoptive immunotherapy for cancer. Sci. Am., 262:62, 1990.

Rous, P.: Transmission of a malignant new growth by means of a cell-free filtrate. J.A.M.A., 56:198, 1911.

Shope, R.E.: A filterable virus causing a tumor-like condition in rabbits and its relationship to virus myxomatosum. J. Exp. Med., 56:803, 1932.

Shopland, D.R., Eyre, H.J., and Pechacek, T.F.: Smoking-attributable cancer mortality in 1991: is lung cancer now the leading cause of death among smokers in the United States? J. Natl. Cancer Inst., 83:1142, 1991.

Shubik, P.: Vascularization of tumors: a review. J. Cancer Res. Clin. Oncol., 103:211, 1982.

Solzhenitsyn, A.I.: Cancer Ward. New York, Dial Press, 1968.

Stanbridge, E.J., and Nowell, P.C.: Origins of human cancer revisited. Cell, 63:867, 1990.

Stewart, S.E., et al.: Viral production of cancer. Virology, 3:380, 1957.

Travali, S., Koniecki, J., Petralia, S., and Baserga, R.: Oncogenes in growth and development. FASEB J., 4:3209, 1990.

Stevenson, F.K.: Tumor vaccines. FASEB J., 5:2250, 1991.

Tisdale, M.J., and Beck. S.A.: Cancer cachexia. Intl. J. Pancreatology, 141, 1990.

Wagner, H.N., Jr., and Conti, P.S.: Advances in medical imaging for cancer diagnosis and treatment. Cancer, 67:1121, 1991.

Wagoner, J.K.: Occupational carcinogenesis: the two hundred years since Percival Pott. Ann. N.Y. Acad. Sci., 271:1, 1976.

Warren, S.: Radiation carcinogenesis. Ann. N.Y. Acad. Sci., 46:133, 1970.

Weinberg, R.A.: Finding the anti-oncogene. Sci. Am., 259:44, 1988.

Wiklund, K., Holm, L.-E., and Eklund, G.: Cancer risks in Swedish Lapps who breed reindeer. Am. J. Epidemiol., 132:1078, 1990.

APPENDIX

Diagnosis of Cancer

The final diagnosis of cancer, that is to say, whether a lump is a neoplasm, and whether that neoplasm is innocent or malignant, must be made in the laboratory. The clinician can be suspicious, but not certain. Unless there are exceptional circumstances, no patient should be treated for cancer unless a tissue diagnosis of the tumor has been firmly established by a pathologist. A number of techniques can be employed in this diagnosis.

Exfoliative Cytology. Cancer cells tend to lose the adhesiveness characteristic of normal cells, so that they may be cast off or exfoliated from the surface early in the disease, even in the preinvasive stage. These cells are found in exudates, secretions, washings, and scrapings. This diagnostic method, called diagnostic cytology or cytopathology, has opened up new vistas in the early diagnosis of cancer. Its greatest value at present is in cancer of the cervix, bronchus and bladder, where it is easy to obtain fresh cells that have not yet autolyzed. By this means it is possible to detect early cancers. In advanced cancer the test may be negative, because the cells have become necrotic and therefore unrecognizable. The test was first described by Papanicolaou, hence the widely used name of "Pap smear" given to the cytological diagnosis of cervical cancer.

Fine-Needle Aspiration Cytology. More recently, a new technique has been introduced allowing physicians to obtain cells, which do not normally enfoliate, from deeply located organs such as the thyroid gland, lymph nodes, breast, or pancreas. Small cell clumps are aspirated through a long needle attached to a syringe. The main advantage of this technique is that not only can cells be obtained from organs which do not desquamate, but the procedure can also be performed outside of the operating room. As discussed in the urogenital section, there is now evidence that the serological assay of PSA (Prostate Specific Antigen) can be an important adjunct to digital rectal examination in the diagnosis of cancer.

Biopsy. When a tumor is removed by a surgeon in the operating room, it is sent to the pathology laboratory where it is fixed, sectioned, and stained. It is on the microscopic examination of these sections that the final diagnosis is made by the pathologist as to whether or not the lesion is malignant. Under some circumstances, particularly in the case of lumps of the breast, it may be desirable for the surgeon to have a report on the nature of the lesion during the course of the operation, so that he may determine the extent of the subsequent procedure which could be as extensive as a mastectomy. For this purpose, a frozen section is cut and stained enabling a "rush diagnosis" to be made in the course of a few minutes. This is a reliable way to establish a diagnosis although, in a few cases, the pathologist defers her/his decision until regular histological sections are obtained.

Chemical Tests. Enormous amounts of time and money have been spent on the search for a chemical test of the blood or of the secretions that would indicate that neoplasia was in progress. The liver synthesizes many different proteins, but it has been discovered that, early in its development, it synthesizes alpha-fetoprotein (AFP) that is no longer made in the adult life unless there is an hepatocellular carcinoma or embryonal carcinoma of the testis. By contrast, other tumor markers are important not in diagnosis, but in the progress of cancer. This is the case with carcinoembryonic antigen (CEA) which is a marker for several types of carcinomas, mostly colorectal carcinoma. The main use for the serological assay of CEA is the detection of recurrence following surgery for colorectal cancer. Scientists have developed a number of monoclonal antibodies to CEA and other tumor markers and they label them with radioactive isotopes or drugs in an attempt to use these modified molecules in radioimaging or immunotherapy targeted at cancer cells.

For the few tumors known to secrete hormones (parathyroid, adrenal) it is possible to determine their site of origin by serum assays.

Molecular probes. In this and other chapters we mention several times the impact of molecular biology on the knowledge of disease mechanisms. Beyond this fundamental aspect there is now the beginning of a new story: the contribution of molecular biology to the **diagnosis** of cancer. You recall that one of the basic characteristics of cancer is some structural change of critical genes. A typical example is lymphoma. Like any cancer, this malignancy first involves a very small portion of the affected organ, in this case, the lymph node. Consequently, histological examination might easily miss this early focus of lymphoma. It happens, however, that lymphomas are characterized, from their very beginning, by a rearrangement of the T-cell receptor or immunoglobulin genes. This rearrangement can be detected using short DNA probes that do not bind the same way to intact and rearranged genes. This technique is very sensitive and can detect 1% of the rearranged DNA from lymphoma cells amongst 99% of unchanged DNA from the non-tumoral lymph node. Molecular probe technology is the newest development in the practice of pathology, is already being used extensively in the diagnosis of various inherited diseases, and will probably be applied to the diagnosis of an increasing number of cancers.

Staging of Tumors

The treatment and prognosis of cancer has been modified by new insights into the variability of different types of cancer and by their response to different protocols or types of therapy. One important factor in treating cancer has been to determine its extent in a given patient before beginning treatment. This is called staging of cancer. By staging we mean defining the extent of the cancer in a patient, that is, whether the tumor involves only a small part of an organ or whether it is widespread and involves regional lymph nodes and other organs at anatomically remote sites. The implications of this widespread distribution are that the tumor not only is great in total mass, and therefore both burdens the body metabolically and is likely to involve critical sites, but that it is likely as well to continue to metastasize because of multiple foci that have become sites for tumor growth. The staging procedure has allowed comparisons to be made among groups of patients treated at widely different centers and groups of patients treated by radically different methods for the same cancer (surgery, chemotherapy, radiotherapy, immunotherapy, or any combination thereof). The system most widely used for staging has been called the TNM system, after the abbreviations for *t*umor, lymph *n*odes, and *m*etastases. The tumor is considered in terms of its size and extent at the primary site, it is appraised in terms of the presence and extent of lymph nodes involved, and it is judged by the presence of metastases.

The classification is based on involvement of different anatomic sites and is shown in the accompanying Table A11–1. The oldest staging procedure is Duke's classification of cancer of the bowel shown in Table A11–2.

Table A11–1.   The TNM System

T:	PRIMARY TUMOR
N:	REGIONAL LYMPH NODES
M:	DISTANT METASTASES

TUMOR	
T_0	No evidence of primary tumor
T_{is}	*Carcinoma-in-situ*
T_1, T_2, T_3, T_4	Ascending degrees of increase in tumor size and involvement

NODES	
N_0	Regional nodes not demonstrable
N_{1a}, N_{2a}	Demonstrable regional lymph nodes; metastases not suspected
N_{1b}, N_{2b}, N_3	Demonstrable regional lymph nodes; metastases suspected
N_x	Regional lymph nodes cannot be assessed clinically

METASTASES	
M_0	No evidence of distant metastases
M_1, M_2, M_3	Ascending degrees of metastatic involvement of the host including distant nodes

(From Thorn, G.W., et al. (Eds.): *Harrison's Principles of Internal Medicine*, 8th Ed. New York, McGraw-Hill, 1977.)

Table A11–2.   Duke's Classification of Colorectal Cancer

Type A.	Growth confined to the rectum. No extra-rectal spread, no lymphatic metastases.
Type B.	Spread by direct extension into extrarectal tissues; no lymphatic metastases.
Type C.	Lymphatic metastases present.

Table A11–3. Radiosensitivity of Human Tumors

GROUP I	GROUP II	GROUP III
(Sensitive tumors: disappearance of tumors with doses less than 2500 r; normal tissues unaffected)	(Intermediate tumors: regression with doses of 2500 to 5000 r)·	(Resistant tumors: more than 5000 r with irreversible changes in normal tissues)
Lymphosarcoma	Basal cell carcinoma	Carcinoma of the breast
Lymphoepithelioma	Some epidermoid carcinomas of the skin and uterine cervix	Carcinoma of the stomach
Ewing's sarcoma		Osteogenic sarcoma
Chronic leukemia	Carcinoma of the thyroid	Chondrosarcoma
Some parotid tumors		Malignant melanoma

(From Perez-Tamayo, R.: *Mechanisms of Disease.* Philadelphia, W.B. Saunders Co., 1961.)

A second and important aspect in understanding the biologic behavior of cancer, both treated and untreated, is called grading. This can be done by the histologic appearance of a tumor. Tumors are graded according to the degree of anaplasia or undifferentiation and the number of mitotic figures, which reflects the rate of growth. Tumors are usually graded 1 to 4, with the lower numbers implying a lesser degree of malignancy. Unfortunately, one tumor may differ histologically in different parts of the body, so such attempts to predict the biologic behavior of a given cancer have not always been valuable.

Cancer Therapy

At the present time, cancer can be treated effectively by surgical removal, by radiotherapy, by chemotherapy and by immunotherapy. The ideal therapeutic agent would be one with a selective action on malignant cells that leaves normal cells untouched, just as antibiotics lead to the destruction of bacteria, but do not interfere significantly with the metabolism of normal tissues (Fig. A11–1).

Benign tumors are treated with complete success by local removal, that is to say, only the tumor itself needs to be removed and none of the surrounding tissue. With malignant tumors, the reverse is the case. Not only the tumor, but as much of the surrounding tissue as is feasible, must be excised, for it may harbor cancer cells that cannot be detected by the eye or hand, but only by the microscope. Depending on the part of the body affected, the regional lymph nodes also may have to be removed, but cancer of each organ must be considered as a separate entity, and

what is true of one is not necessarily true of another. The presence of distant metastases implies that surgical treatment alone offers small hope of cure.

It should be emphasized that we believe every cancer is curable in the early stage before it has begun to spread. How do we measure cure or the effect of a given treatment? The most common figure is 5- or 10-year survival. Another measure is the disease-free interval, that is, the time between treatment and the first recurrence. Other studies mention the percentage of patients with complete or incomplete remission at a specific time following completion of the treatment.

The concept we put forward is that cancer has a single focus in which the neoplastic cells originate, and that if that focus is removed soon enough, the cancer will not disseminate. However, there is abundant evidence that some tumors (skin cancer in those exposed to sunlight for many years, carcinoma of the bowel in families with polyposis, alveolar cell carcinoma of the lung, to name a few) occur in multiple foci and are called multicentric in origin. Thus the

Table A11–4. Choice of Treatment in Localized and Regional Tumors and Hematologic Malignancies

DIAGNOSIS	SURGERY	TREATMENT RADIO-THERAPY	CHEMO-THERAPY
Carcinomas			
Breast	P	Alt/adj	T
Uterine cervix	P	P	T
Choriocarcinoma	Alt	—	P
Lung	P	Alt	T
Stomach	P	—	T
Pancreas	P	—	T
Leukemias and Lymphomas			
Leukemia			
Acute myeloblastic	—	—	P
Hodgkin's disease	Alt	P	T

P   —Primary method of treatment
Alt —Alternative method of treatment, or one useful in special situations
Adj—Used as adjunctive therapy
T   —Currently under clinical investigation as adjunctive treatment
— —No data available on this form of treatment

(From Thorn, G. W., et al. (Eds.): *Harrison's Principles of Internal Medicine,* 8th Ed. New York, McGraw-Hill, 1977.)

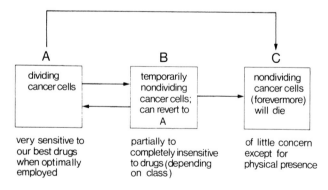

Fig. A11–1 This drawing shows when cells may be susceptible to chemotherapy. (From Thorn, G.W., et al. (Eds.): *Harrison's Principles of Internal Medicine,* 8th Ed. New York, McGraw-Hill, 1976.)

paradigm of a single site of origin may be a fiction of our way of looking at some cancers and this is an important consideration in their follow-up.

Radiation is a well-tried and valuable method of treating certain forms of cancer. This treatment is made possible because radiations have a greater destructive action on rapidly growing cells than on normal cells. They, therefore, have a selective action on cancer cells compared with that on the surrounding tissue. It is possible, however, to kill all the tissue by radiation, and this danger has constantly to be borne in mind by the radiotherapist. His/her aim is to use the maximum amount of radiation on the cancer, but to stop just short of damaging the normal tissue.

Radium and certain other radioactive atoms give off radiations (gamma rays) that are similar in nature to x-rays and that have a similar action on tumor tissue. Both may be used for attacking some tumors, but, in most cases, one or the other is preferable.

Tumors vary tremendously in their response to radiation (Table A11–3). Some, such as lymphoma, are highly radiosensitive; others, such as malignant melanoma, are as highly radioresistant. An intimate knowledge of tumor pathology is therefore necessary before treatment of cancer by radiation can be attempted. Speaking generally, external irradiation is used for the treatment of widely diffused tumors such as lymphoma, as well as for deep-seated tumors such as cancer of the lung. Irradiation from internally implanted radioactive sources is used for advanced cancer of the cervix of the uterus. Frequently, the various forms of treatment are combined, e.g., surgery and radiation (Table A11–4). An increasing number of cancers and leukemias combine multiple therapeutic approaches for which there are well-defined protocols designed by national or international panels of experts including biostatisticians. Informed consents are requested from patients who are then randomized between various "arms" of these therapeutic protocols. When physicians and biostatisticians observe a statistically significant benefit from one therapeutic arm, this becomes the new standard of treatment with which future studies will be compared.

An example of such therapeutic approaches would contrast in breast cancer patients: surgery vs. surgery plus chemotherapy vs. surgery plus irradiation. These types of multi-center studies are very powerful and help in increasing significantly the therapeutic response in various forms of cancer.

12

INHERITED DISEASE

Heredity is nothing but stored environment.—BURBANK

It has been suspected for centuries that some diseases are transmitted from parent to child. The earliest understanding of inheritance appears in the ancient Hebrew writings which decreed that if two boys in a family died from bleeding following circumcision, then later sons of the same mother or her sisters should not be circumcised. Thus it was recognized that disease could be transmitted from unaffected related females to their sons.

It was not until the 1800s that the laws governing inheritance began to be elucidated. Mendel's laws of inheritance were first published in 1866, although the significance of his work was not recognized until much later. Archibald Garrod pioneered the study of inherited disease; he noticed that some diseases occur in clusters of a single family, and although the parents of an affected child did not show any stigma of the disorder, they were discovered to be cousins or closely related. He identified not only the mode of inheritance for some disorders, but also the biochemical abnormalities responsible for the disease (alkaptonuria, albinism, cystinuria and pentosuria). He summarized his theories and observations in the classic work *Inborn Errors of Metabolism* published in 1909, although the significance of this work was also not recognized for some 35 years.

Since Garrod's time the field of human genetics has expanded tremendously. Today we have detailed knowledge of how traits are inherited, how genetic information is "decoded" and expressed during development, how defects in a gene can lead to disease, and we are working on treatment for these disorders.

Genetics has become one of the most important aspects of medicine. In our search for causes of disease we increasingly point the accusing finger not at a bacterium or virus but at our own genetic blueprints. We recognize that given a sinful life-style some of us are "predisposed" to succumb to myocardial infarcts, some to lung disease, and others to thrive.

Modern genetic engineering has enabled us to identify specific genes and to move them from one cell to another, providing much for the imaginations of science fiction writers, spawning a number of political, social and ethical problems since this is tampering with "creation" itself. Yet this technique has given us a way of producing insulin and interferon from bacteria. We may be able to insert normal genes into genetically defective human cells to cure genetic disease.

INHERITED DISEASE

In discussing hereditary disease, we should define some terms that are often used congruently and casually. Congenital disease refers to those diseases that are recognized as a result of occurrences during development and are present at birth, but do not necessarily have a hereditary (genetic) cause. The best examples of congenital disease are the deafness and the cardiovascular lesions that occur in the infant born to a mother who was infected with rubella virus during her first trimester of pregnancy. It is estimated that more than two-thirds of mothers so exposed to rubella have children with severe defects. This information has made strong arguments for abortion in the first trimester.

It is necessary, nonetheless, to recognize that it is not always possible to be certain about the origin of a given defect that is apparent at birth. Since some abnormalities are associated with genetic factors, it is appropriate to discuss briefly some frequent and important structural defects that appear at birth and are generally called congenital malformations. They are listed in Table 12–1 with their approximate frequency and sex ratio.

At this time, it is difficult to distinguish between congenital and genetically determined disease, and it is probably wise to use the purest definition: **congeni-**

Table 12–1. Approximate Frequency and Sex Ratio of Common Congenital and Genetic Malformations

MALFORMATION	FREQUENCY/ 1000 BIRTHS	M:F
Congenital heart disease	2.5	1:1
Talipes equinovarus (club foot)	2.0	2:1
Myelomeningocele	1.5 (0.5–4.4)	1:1
Anencephaly	2.0	1:2
Down's syndrome (mongolism)	1.6	1:1
Cleft lip ± cleft palate	1.0	2:1
Klinefelter's syndrome	1.0	1:0

(From Bearn, A.G.: Congenital malformations. In *Cecil Textbook of Medicine*, 15th Ed. Edited by P.B. Beeson, W. McDermott, and J.B. Wyngaarden. Philadelphia, W.B. Saunders Co., 1979.)

tal disease is considered to be one in which there is no recognized genetic determinant.

The conventional approach to classifying genetic disorders is to group them into three subsets:

1. Chromosomal disorders. This category includes diseases shown to be due to abnormalities in the structure or number of chromosomes.
2. Monogenic disorders. These are diseases in which there is clear-cut evidence of genetic disorder but no change in the chromosome is visible. They result most likely from mutations in single genes, and follow specific, straightforward patterns of inheritance. The subset includes the inborn errors of metabolism and a number of diseases whose precise genetic defect is not known, but whose inheritance pattern suggests a monogenic disorder.
3. Multifactorial disease. These disorders are relatively common and result from the interaction of several genes with multiple environmental factors. They are said to "run in families," but inheritance is complex.

CHROMOSOMAL ABERRATIONS

Chromosomal anomalies fall into two general categories: changes in number of chromosomes and changes in the structure of individual chromosomes. The incidence of such anomalies is generally estimated at about 6.5 per 1,000 live births; however, this is thought to represent only the tip of the iceberg of aberrant conceptions (Table 12–2). For instance, most embryos with chromosomal aberrations are aborted spontaneously.

Abnormalities in Chromosome Number. Some of the most common aberrations result from the presence of an extra chromosome, for example XXY instead of the normal XY, or three autosomes instead of two. The extra chromosome, which is in every cell of the body, owes its existence to a meiotic error in the development of the egg or sperm. The most frequent error of meiosis is called **nondisjunction,** which occurs when a pair of homologous chromosomes fail to separate as the cell divides. This produces gametes (either ova or sperm) with two copies of one chromosome where there should only be one. When the abnormal gamete meets its partner in fertilization, the unfortunate zygote will be endowed with three copies or 47 chromosomes in all (Fig. 12–1). This condition is referred to as **trisomy. Monosomy,** which also results from nondisjunction, is the condition in which only one chromosome of the normal pair exists in the zygote. Both of these are rare, but monosomy appears to be particularly incompatible with life—almost all are spontaneously aborted.

Trisomy 21, also known as Down's syndrome, is that condition in which autosome number 21 is in triplicate. It is quite common with a prevalence of 1 in 700 births. The newborn child has slanted eyes, hyperextensibility of the joints, short stature, and, as becomes apparent only too soon, mental retardation. Abnormalities of the cardiovascular system, intestines and kidneys are also common.

Table 12–2. Frequency of Selected Chromosome Aberrations

	A SPONTANEOUS ABORTIONS	B LIVE-BORN
Sex chromosome abnormalities:		
Turner's syndrome (all types)	1/18	1/3,500 "females"
Klinefelter's syndrome (all types)	Probably same as in live-born	1/500 "males"
Extra X chromosomes (females mainly XXX)	Probably same as in live-born	1/1,360 "females"
Autosomal abnormalities:		
Trisomy G	1/40	1/600
Trisomy 18	1/200	1/4,500
Trisomy D	1/33	1/14,500
Trisomy 16	1/33	Almost 0
Triploidy	1/22	Almost 0

(From Wintrobe, M., et al. (Eds.): *Harrison's Principles of Internal Medicine*, 7th Ed. New York, McGraw-Hill, 1974.)

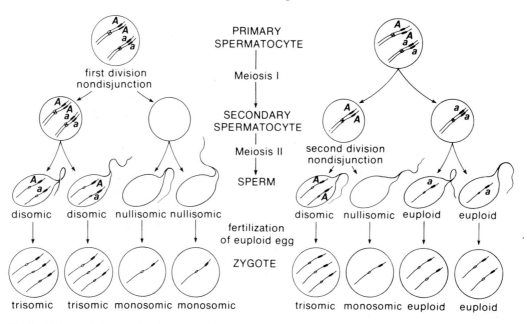

Fig. 12–1 Results of meiotic nondisjunction involving a single pair of chromosomes with a heterozygous gene. Assume that all other chromosome pairs segregate normally. *Left:* When nondisjunction occurs in the first division, the eventual gametes are two disomic, two nullisomic, and no euploid. *Right:* When nondisjunction occurs in the second division (in just one of the two secondary spermatocytes) the gametes are one disomic, one nullisomic, and two euploid. (From *Genetics: Human Aspects,* by Arthur P. Mange and Elaine J. Mange. Copyright 1980 by Saunders College/ Holt, Rinehart and Winston. Reprinted by permission of Holt, Rinehart and Winston, CBS College Publishing.)

The incidence of Down's syndrome rises with maternal age (Fig. 12–2). This may be related to the fact that all the ova of a female are present at birth, arrested in prophase of meiosis I. Thus a woman at age 40 is ovulating ova which are also 40 years old. We must keep in mind, however, that an older woman still has a 97% chance of delivering a normal baby, that half the cases of the disorder are born to women under the age of 35 (they have a lower risk but they produce far more babies), and that in 20% of cases the extra chromosome comes from the father. Patients with Down's syndrome can live beyond the age of 30. Besides the consequences of cardiac malformation, their lifespan is also limited by an increased susceptibility to infections, by the development of acute leukemia, and of brain lesions resembling those usually observed in Alzheimer's disease.

The common sex chromosome anomalies are Klinefelter's syndrome (XXY) and Turner's syndrome (a single X). The diagnosis of these disorders is made with the use of sex chromatin, a darkly staining mass in the nucleus of all normal female cells which never appears in normal male cells. It usually lies against the inner surface of the nuclear membrane (Table 12–3). The method used to find sex chromatin is the **buccal smear**—cells are scraped from the inside of the mouth and examined under the microscope.

Sex chromatin has been shown to consist of one

Fig. 12–2 This graph shows the relative frequency of Down's syndrome with increasing maternal age. (Adapted from Thorn, G.W., et al. (Eds.): *Harrison's Principles of Internal Medicine,* 8th Ed. New York, McGraw-Hill, 1976.)

Table 12–3.   Correlations of Phenotype, Sex Chromatin, and Sex Chromosomes

	SEX PHENOTYPE	BARR BODIES (MAXIMUM NUMBER PER CELL)	SEX-CHROMOSOME CONSTITUTION
Normal male	Male		XY
Testicular feminization syndrome	Females (with testes)		XY
Double Y (or XYY) male	Male		XYY
Turner's syndrome	Female		XO
Normal female	Female		XX
Klinefelter's syndrome	Male		XXY
Klinefelter's syndrome	Male		XXYY
Triple X syndrome	Female		XXX
Triple X-Y syndrome	Male		XXY
Tetra X syndrome	Female		XXXX
Tetra X-Y syndrome	Male		XXXXY
Penta X syndrome	Female		XXXXX

(From Wintrobe, M., et al. (Eds.): *Harrison's Principles of Internal Medicine.* New York, McGraw-Hill, 1974.)

tightly condensed X chromosome which is genetically inactive. At the start of development in the female, both X chromosomes are active, but at some stage still early on, one becomes inactive, a process now known as **lyonization** (after Mary Lyon who did the original studies). The end result is that although females have twice as many X chromosomes as males, they have the same number of active X genes, and in the case of extra X chromosomes there will be extra sex chromatin.

Klinefelter's syndrome is the most common of the sex chromosomal anomalies (Fig. 12–3). As we have indicated, it is caused by the chromosome complex XXY. An individual with Klinefelter's syndrome has small testes with infertility, the breasts may be slightly enlarged, and the presence of sex chromatin in the buccal smear confirms the clinical diagnosis. Decreased mental capacity may be noted in some Klinefelter males. The extra chromosome is thought to arise

almost entirely through nondisjunction which occurs about 60% of the time in the mother and about 40% of the time in the father.

Turner's syndrome (Fig. 12–4) is one in which a single X (written XO) occurs (about 1 in every 3,000 births). In some cases only a part of the second X chromosome is missing. The rarity of Turner's syndrome is due to the high spontaneous abortion rate for all monosomies; an estimated 98% of all XO embryos are lost in early pregnancy. It is not known why only 2% survive, particularly given the relative mildness of the deformity.

The syndrome includes short stature and lack of secondary sexual characteristics; ovaries do not develop accounting for primary amenorrhea, and sterility ensues. Coarctation of the thoracic aorta is common and causes hypertension. Most patients are of normal intelligence. Nondisjunction is again the cause.

Fig. 12–3   This photograph shows the phenotypic appearance of a Klinefelter patient. Note the long extremities, narrow shoulders, and relatively wide hips. (By permission of the Upjohn Company, Kalamazoo, Michigan, monograph on cytology.)

In contrast with Turner's syndrome there is a commonly occurring syndrome called multi-X female, in which there is an excessive number of X chromosomes. The patients are phenotypically normal females but present with a number of menstrual irregularities. Interestingly they may display mental retardation and this is somewhat proportional to the number of excessive chromosomes.

Males, who are usually of tall stature, can have a chromosomal abnormality characterized by an additional Y chromosome. There is a controversy as to the significance of this genetic change as some reports found it is associated with aggressive behavior.

Screening of subjects with mental retardation not associated with Down's syndrome has demonstrated a large number of cases with a chromosomal change named fragile X syndrome. It is seen as an unstained region of the long arm of chromosome X which tends to break easily, hence the name. Two-thirds of patients are male, and characteristically they have enlarged testes.

It must be remembered that the anomalies associated with changes in chromosome numbers result from chromosomal imbalance not gene mutation; most likely the gene products are qualitatively normal

Fig. 12–4   This photograph shows the phenotypic appearance of Turner's syndrome. The chest is relatively wide and the neck is short. (By permission of the Upjohn Company, Kalamazoo, Michigan, monograph on cytology.)

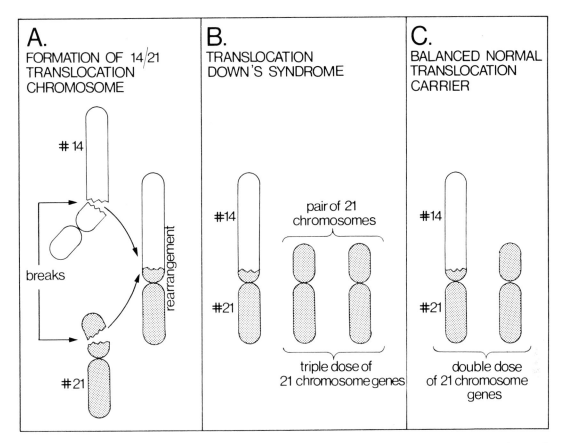

A.
FORMATION OF 14/21 TRANSLOCATION CHROMOSOME

#14

breaks

rearrangement

#21

B.
TRANSLOCATION DOWN'S SYNDROME

#14

#21

pair of 21 chromosomes

triple dose of 21 chromosome genes

C.
BALANCED NORMAL TRANSLOCATION CARRIER

#14

#21

double dose of 21 chromosome genes

Fig. 12–5 These drawings show the mechanism of translocation *(A)* resulting in Down's syndrome at *B,* and in a balanced, normal translocation at *C.* (From Thorn, G.W., et al. (Eds.): *Harrison's Principles of Internal Medicine,* 8th Ed. New York, McGraw-Hill, 1976.)

but too much or too little is present. The fact that so many systems of the body tend to be affected suggests that normal metabolism and development are critically dependent upon the concentration of the gene product as well as its structure.

Abnormalities in Chromosome Structure. Occasionally parts of chromosomes break off, are lost, or reattach themselves to other chromosomes. The loss of a piece is called a **deletion,** which can result in partial monosomy if the loss is sufficiently large. Deletions of more than a few genes (this includes monosomies) tend to be lethal. In a **translocation** pieces of chromosome ends break off and exchange positions. About 4% of children with Down's syndrome have only 46 chromosomes, one of which is abnormally long and results from a translocation involving chromosomes 14 and 21 (Fig. 12–5). This type of Down's syndrome is inherited from a normal parent who carries the translocation; he or she is normal because the abnormally long chromosome is balanced by an abnormally short one. Meiosis and late fertilization yield monosomies which miscarry, trisomy and normal zygotes among the various possibilities. The translocation

may be transmitted to more than one child in the family.

Translocations are not restricted to congenital diseases. They can occur after birth and this is a feature of several types of leukemias and lymphomas as discussed in Chapter 23.

MONOGENIC DISORDERS

Monogenic disorders are those caused by a mutation in a single gene. This produces an abnormality in a single protein. It may seem trivial at first glance, but many proteins are essential molecules; they are crucial constituents of cell membranes, and they play vital roles in the transport of many substances. As enzymes they catalyze or regulate all the reactions of metabolism. The structure of a protein is usually vital to its function, and each protein owes its unique structural features to its primary amino acid sequence, which in turn depends upon the base sequence of the gene.

The best known monogenic diseases have been classified into three groups: enzyme deficiencies, transport protein deficiencies, and receptor protein malfunctions. Enzyme defects have been the most extensively studied; the events which accompany such defects are outlined in Figure 12–6. The three major events, each of which may be harmful in and of itself are accumulation of substrate, overuse of alternate metabolic routes for the substrate and product deficiency.

Monogenic disorders show one of three simple (Mendelian) patterns of inheritance: autosomal dominant, autosomal recessive, and X-linked inheritance (Table 12–4). A dominant disorder is one which will be manifest when the individual has only a single dose of the mutant gene (i.e., is heterozygous for it). Recessive diseases do not become clinically evident unless the individual is homozygous for the mutant gene. Persons who are heterozygous for a recessively inherited mutation are referred to as carriers; they themselves do not have the disease, unlike the dominant case in which possession of the gene is always accompanied by expression of the disease. In spite of the fact that they are not clinically affected, carriers often have biochemical abnormalities which show up on laboratory examination. X-linked disorders are those caused by mutations in genes located on the X chromosomes. These are far more commonly expressed in males than in females because males have only one X chromosome and so will show the disease whether it behaves in a dominant or recessive fashion.

Dominant Inheritance. This is the easiest type of inherited disease to recognize because each affected individual has an affected parent and grandparent (unless the mutation is new). The character can be transmitted by a parent of either sex to a child of either sex. The affected individual possesses one mutant allele and one normal allele, each of which will go to separate gametes at meiosis so that half the gametes will receive the mutant allele and the other half the normal gene. Thus there is a one in two chance that offspring inherit the disease (Fig. 12–7). If the mutation is new, the parents of the patient will, of course, be unaffected, but his offspring and their descendants will inherit the disease as described.

Dominance may not always be as pure as we have suggested here. It is not necessarily a matter of all or nothing. The degree of dominance, the grade of potency, is expressed by the term **penetrance.** When a dominant gene fails to manifest itself in the individual carrying it, there is said to be partial penetrance. A dominant gene with 80% penetrance will express itself only in 80% of cases; in the remaining 20% the disease will skip a generation.

Dominantly inherited disorders include various diseases listed in Table 12–4. Some of these are covered in the chapters that are relevant to the affected organ systems.

Recessive Inheritance. Autosomal recessive mutations are more difficult to identify. Such mutations often lie dormant for many generations, the carrier going happily through life unaware that genetically he possesses a program that may be devastating for his offspring. Only when two unsuspecting carriers have children is the disorder finally expressed. Before this begins to sound like the tale of the unlucky few,

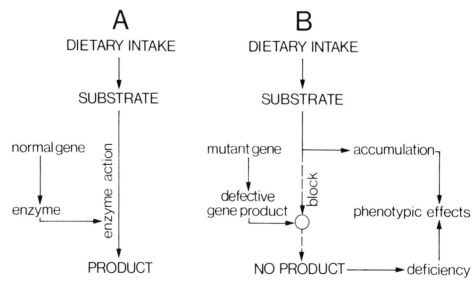

Fig. 12–6 This figure shows the effect on the accumulation of substrate in a person with a mutant gene, which results in the defective gene product. The treatment of this problem is to remove the accumulation of material, or to substitute a normal gene for a defective one. (From Whaley, L.F.: *Understanding Inherited Disorders.* St. Louis, C. V. Mosby Co., 1974.)

Table 12–4.   Some Relatively Common Mendelian Disorders

AUTOSOMAL DOMINANT	AUTOSOMAL RECESSIVE	X-LINKED
Familial monogenic hypercholesterolemia	Cystic fibrosis	Hemophilia A
Marfan's syndrome	Deaf mutism	Classic agammaglobulinemia (Bruton)
Adult polycystic disease	Phenylketonuria and other heredity aminoacidurias	Pseudohypertrophic muscular dystrophy
Huntington's chorea	Wilson's disease	Testicular feminization
Neurofibromatosis	Homocystinuria	Vitamin D-resistant rickets
Osteogenesis imperfecta	Albinism	
Von Willebrand's disease	Emphysema (due to alpha-1 antitrypsin deficiency)	
Achondroplastic dwarfism	Friedreich's ataxia	

(From Bearn, A.G.: Pedigree analysis in inherited disease. In *Cecil Textbook of Medicine*, 15th Ed. Edited by P.B. Beeson, W. McDermott, and J.B. Wyngaarden. Philadelphia, W.B. Saunders Co., 1979.)

we should note that a large number of us carry a certain load of genes or groups of genes which, when homozygous, would be harmful or lethal in our offspring. However, most of these are so rare that they would only be revealed in matings between individuals with very similar genes, such as members of the same family. Studies of inbreeding show that infant and child mortality is slightly higher in first cousin marriages than in unrelated parents.

The pattern of recessive inheritance is illustrated in Figure 12–8. The most common case is that of two carrier parents who are normal, whose offspring have a 1 chance in 4 to have the disease, 1 chance in 4 to be completely normal, and 1 chance in 2 to be phenotypically normal but to carry the trait.

X-Linked Inheritance. X-linked, or sex-linked, inherited disease is much less frequent than the other types we have discussed. The mutations involved are located on the X chromosome. As we reviewed briefly before, females have two X chromosomes and males have one X and one Y. Both sex chromosomes carry additional nonsexual genes known as sex-linked genes. As the female has two X chromosomes, she will most likely be heterozygous and therefore a carrier for a mutant gene in a single X chromosome, whereas the male with a single X chromosome will be homozygous for the mutant gene, so that the trait will become apparent. The gene in question may be passed from father to daughter, from mother to son and never from father to son, but if it is recessive it is only in the male in which it is unmasked, that it be-

Fig. 12–7 This diagram shows the proportions of affected children in dominant inheritance.

Fig. 12–8 This diagram shows the proportions of affected persons and of carriers in recessive inheritance.

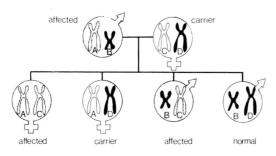

Fig. 12–9 This figure shows the effect of sex-linked inheritance on the numbers and carriers of the offspring.

comes apparent (Fig. 12–9). In the female the abnormal gene is masked by the normal dominant gene on the other chromosome.

The inherited diseases that are relatively common are discussed in the Appendix, p. 284.

MULTIFACTORIAL DISORDERS

As the name suggests, a multifactorial disease is one which develops from the interaction of many factors, specifically, hereditary and environmental factors. This category includes some of the common diseases of adults (such as hypertension, heart disease, diabetes mellitus, duodenal ulcer) as well as some of the common birth defects (such as cleft lip and palate and congenital heart disease). Many normal traits, such as height, may be considered multifactorial—to be tall one must have genes for tallness, whatever they are (hence tall parents usually have tall children),

and the right nutritional and other environmental conditions.

Multifactorial traits and diseases have long been known to "run in families," but the exact nature of the hereditary component still eludes us. However, such diseases are best explained not in terms of a single-gene effect (and no chromosomal abnormality has been identified), but on the basis of multiple gene dosage. In fact, the whole idea of health and disease can be reviewed with this concept of multiple genic factors in mind. This may explain why some family groups seem singularly successful, live to ripe old age, and are relatively free of mortal disorders, whereas other families seem fated to a short and ailing life. René Dubos, in *The Mirage of Health*, has interesting and important things to say in this respect.

Diseases with a multiple gene component are described as **polygenic.** The genes concerned can be thought of as "risk genes." In certain families, large numbers of risk genes may be present, and when these reach a certain concentration in one unfortunate individual the likelihood of developing the disease becomes very great. This is termed the "threshold effect" (Fig. 12–10). It is thought that at the genetic threshold, environmental factors come into play, determining whether and to what extent the individual will be clinically affected. A good example of a threshold trait is cleft palate. The palate, which forms the roof of the mouth and the floor of the nose, develops from two pieces of tissue that initially hang down on either side of the tongue. These processes must shift

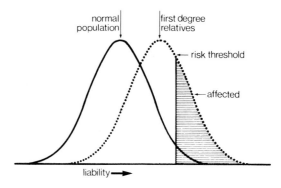

Fig. 12–10 This graph shows the effect on the appearance of disease of multiple factors. The normal population is shown in the curve at the left. Persons with a hereditary risk, which depends on several genes being present and working together to make a particular disease evident, move the curve to the right. Not all persons with a particular complement of genes will necessarily show the disease, as the manifestation of disease may depend in addition on some environmental factors. Thus those who show the disease are represented on the right-hand part of the right curve. (From Bearn, A.G.: Polygenic and multifactorial inheritance. In *Cecil Textbook of Medicine*, 15th Ed. Edited by P.B. Beeson, W. McDermott, and J.B. Wyngaarden. Philadelphia, W.B. Saunders Co., 1979.)

upward so that they come to lie horizontally above the tongue, and fuse to form the palate. If, for some reason, this shift occurs late in development, the growth of the head may have moved the palatine processes so far apart that when they shift they will be unable to fuse, resulting in a cleft palate. Many genetic and environmental factors influence the stage at which the shift occurs, but certainly genes which code for late timing of the shift would confer an increased risk of developing the defect. According to this theory, late timing genes represent the genetic threshold; families with such genes sit closer to the threshold and are more prone to cleft palates. For these families, any event which further delays the shift, or interferes in some other small way, can move the fetus into the danger zone. However, we should note that the risk of this event is far lower than if the defect were inherited in an autosomal recessive fashion; no more than 5 to 10% of first degree relatives will be affected.

Gout is another example of a multifactorial disease. It is associated with an elevated serum uric acid (hyperuricemia), which in turn may develop in a variety of different ways. Secondary gout may arise as a consequence of another disorder, such as leukemia or the X-linked recessive disorder Lesch-Nyhan syndrome. Primary gout refers to those cases in which hyperuricemia is the central manifestation of the disease and for which no cause of mendelian mode of inheritance can be demonstrated. This form of gout has a complex mode of inheritance and appears to be influenced by

multiple environmental factors, as with all multifactorial diseases.

In theory, an elevated serum uric acid level can be produced in 1 of at least 3 ways: (1) by an increased production of uric acid, (2) by an increased absorption of precursors, (3) by a decreased excretion or decreased breakdown of uric acid. Recent evidence points to increased uric acid production and reduced excretion by the kidneys as the principal causes of elevated serum levels.

What is gout and what does this serum uric acid level have to do with the exquisitely painful big toe, or other joint?

Gout is a most intriguing disease that may involve any joint and many other areas of connective tissue (Fig. 12–11). An attack of acute gouty arthritis is usually unheralded, and the patient is often awakened in the middle of the night by a severe pain, often in the great toe (Fig. 12–12). The pain is attributed to the presence of crystals of sodium urate in the tissue of this afflicted part. One proposed mechanism of onset of this disease is a cycle of crystallization of urate from supersaturated body fluids that evoke an inflammatory response (Fig. 12–13).

Chronic gout is due to the formation of masses of crystals in connective tissues of the joint and other sites, where they appear as chalky white deposits, rather like drops of paint, an appearance from which the name gout is derived (Latin, *gutta*, a drop). These crystal deposits may have a destructive effect on the

Fig. 12–11   Marked formation of gouty tophi in the hands of a man who was supposed for years to have rheumatoid arthritis, and was treated as such. (Boyd, W.: *Pathology for the Physician*).

Fig. 12–12 Perhaps the most famous imaginative portrayal of a disease is James Gillray's interpretation of Gout: it does manage to suggest the "feel" of the malady in an expressive way. It could also serve as the perfect illustration of the four cardinal signs of inflammation as enumerated by the great Roman physician, Celsus: *Calor, Dolor, Rubor, Tumor* (fever, pain, redness, swelling). The Romans were acquainted with gout, and the poet Ovid, speaks of it as *podagra nodosa*, the adjective nodosa being used in the sense of tying up in knots. The disease has long been associated with rich living; and it is one of the maladies, along with apoplexy, epilepsy, stone, and quartan agues, which doctors of old frankly said they could not cure. The death of Gillray in 1815 was caused, it is said, by intemperance. It is quite possible, therefore, that his vivid rendering of the pains of gout was based upon actual experience. (From Philadelphia Museum of Art: Smith Kline Collection.)

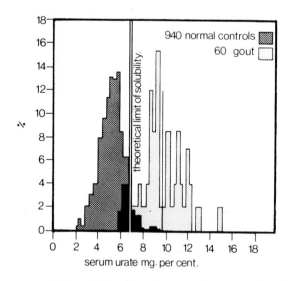

Fig. 12–13 This graph illustrates the range of serum urate levels in 940 normal persons and in 60 persons with gout. The limit of solubility of uric acid ranges around 6.5 mg%. Thus those who have higher levels of uric acid precipitate crystals. (From Seegmiller, J.E.: Diseases of purine and pyrimidine metabolism. In *Duncan's Diseases of Metabolism*, 7th Ed. Edited by P.K. Bondy, and L.E. Rosenberg. Philadelphia, W.B. Saunders Co., 1974.)

cartilage of the joint and cause an arthritis similar to osteoarthritis. The kidneys may accumulate deposits in the collecting system, and urate crystals here may lead to serious and chronic renal dysfunction. The occurrence of kidney stones should always suggest gout as a possible cause in men over 40 years of age. Renal failure is a serious and sometimes fatal complication of gout.

The familial and hereditary nature of gout has been known since earliest times, and many pedigrees have been analyzed to determine the mode of inheritance. It is reasonable on the basis of all the current data to suggest that the serum uric acid level is controlled by multiple genes, any one of which may appear dominant in any selected population. This theory implies that whereas multiple metabolic defects may be responsible for hyperuricemia, a single defect may be characteristic of a particular family. This important concept is relevant to other diseases that can be considered multifactorial and/or polygenic.

As alluded to earlier, in some disorders of the hematopoietic system such as leukemia and lymphoma, there may be an accelerated turnover of nucleic acid, which may lead to overproduction of uric acid, which in turn may become chemically apparent with urate deposits. Most other instances of secondary gout are traced to decreased excretion of uric acid, as in chronic renal diseases (polycystic kidney, chronic glomerulonephritis, and pyelonephritis). There are also specific interferences with renal tubular function which may result in uric acid accumulation (e.g., lead poisoning, use of therapeutic drugs, e.g., chlorothiazide). However, the important thing to recognize is that although the expression of the disorders may be the same (arthritis, tophi), these vastly differing causes can be elucidated and the patient successfully treated by the use of drugs to aid in the excretion of the uric acid and remission of its symptoms.

CANCER AND HEREDITY

A number of cancers are directly or indirectly caused by inherited or acquired genetic changes. These include the cases of colon cancer developing in patients with familial adenomatous polyposis, retinoblastoma, and certain forms of leukemia. These conditions are discussed in Chapters 17, 11, and 23, respectively. The genetic changes consist of mutations, translocations, gene loss, and can effect oncogenes as well as anti-oncogenes, as discussed in Chapter 11.

BEHAVIORAL GENETICS

Before we conclude with treatment for genetic diseases we might mention here a new area of study, a territory that is still relatively unexplored, i.e., the field of behavioral genetics, in which early results indicate that the dualism of environment and heredity is just as important as in the more obvious areas of nutrition and disease. Gene effects for aggressive behavior, maze-learning, and avoidance learning performances have all been described in animals. Some genes are known to affect behavior in humans. The first genetic disorder identified with a definite behavioral component was Lesch-Nyhan syndrome, an X-linked recessive disorder characterized by the absence of an important enzyme involved in the metabolism of two of the DNA bases. Behavioral features of this disorder include self-mutilation, aggressive behavior and mental retardation (although poor IQ scores may be due in part to difficulties in communication). Afflicted individuals chew off their finger-tips and bite their lips all the time crying out for assistance, and pinch and spit at others while at the same time apologizing for this behavior.

GENETIC SCREENING

Screening is the process of looking through a population for individuals at risk for inherited disease either in themselves or in their children. There are two basic purposes. First, to detect genetic disease before it is fully expressed so as to institute treatment to prevent symptoms from developing. Screening for phenylketonuria is a good example. Screening programs for this disease exist in most States and Canada, in which all newborns are examined with a simple blood test. For those shown to have the disease, early dietary restrictions can prevent the devastating mental retardation which otherwise ensues. Such a program is costly, particularly in light of the fact that the disease appears about once in every 10,000 births (in Caucasian populations); however, the cost of caring for untreated individuals over their entire lifetimes is often far greater, to say nothing of the suffering of affected families.

The second use of screening is detection of heterozygotes for recessive diseases to provide reproductive counseling to couples in which both parents are found to be carriers (Table 12–5). Screening for Tay-Sachs and sickle cell trait carriers provides examples of this method. Sickle cell screening has been fraught with problems, particularly confusion of the trait with the disease (remember carriers of the trait are heterozygous and phenotypically normal); difficult reproductive choices for carrier couples who run a 25% risk of having an affected child with each pregnancy (Table 12–6). Their options are to take the risk or not to have children at all—a tough choice, but a frequent dilemma in genetic disease, which more often than not confronts parents who were not screened but whose carrier status was revealed by the birth of an affected child.

Prenatal diagnosis has improved the picture considerably for a few diseases; where the carrier status of the parents is known, each pregnancy can be tested and abortion is offered as an option in the event that the fetus is actually affected. Prenatal diagnosis can be achieved using a variety of methods. Ultrasound and fetoscopy can be used to actually look at the fetus, though many defects will not be picked up unless they are specifically looked for. Amniocentesis is a widely used technique for examining fetal cells; a sample of amniotic fluid (the fluid surrounding the fetus) is withdrawn from the womb using a needle, and the cells in it are cultured and examined. Chromosomal abnormalities may be detected, and the sex of the child is easily seen, which is important information for mothers who carry X-linked disorders and who may decide to abort all male offspring. Enzyme stud-

Table 12–5.   Genetic Diseases-Carrier Detection* Advisable for Reproductive Decisions

DISORDER	MODE OF INHERITANCE	METHOD OF CARRIER DIAGNOSIS	PREVENTIVE MEASURES IN CARRIERS	POPULATION AFFECTED
Duchenne muscular dystrophy	X-linked	CPK level	Amniocentesis for male sex	All
Hemophilia	X-linked	AHG level and AHG cross-reactive material	Amniocentesis for male sex	All
Lesch-Nyhan syndrome	X-linked	HGPRT assay	Amniocentesis—HGPRT assay	All
Translocation Down's syndrome	Empirical recurrence risks apply	Chromosomal tests for balanced carrier	Amniocentesis—chromosomal study	All
Sickle cell anemia	Autosomal recessive	Hemoglobin electrophoresis	Genetic counseling	Blacks
β-Thalassemia major	Autosomal recessive	Red cell abnormalities Hb A_2 increased	Genetic counseling	Mediterranean and tropical population
Tay-Sachs disease	Autosomal recessive	Hexosaminidase A assay	Amniocentesis— hexosaminidase assay	Ashkenazic Jews

* Limited to translocation Down's syndrome, X-linked, and *frequent* autosomal recessive diseases. Detection of carriers for many rare inborn errors associated with enzyme deficiency is possible, but the risk for normal sibs of affected patients to have affected offspring is small, because the frequency of the carrier state for such inborn errors is low in the population.

(From Motulsky, A.G.: Genetic counseling. In *Cecil Textbook of Medicine*, 15th Ed. Edited by P.B. Beeson, W. McDermott, and J.B. Wyngaarden. Philadelphia, W.B. Saunders Co., 1979.)

ies may be done on fetal cells to detect inborn errors of metabolism like Tay-Sachs disease. Another technique involves looking for fetal proteins in the mother's blood, which has the great advantage of not invading the uterus. Two abnormalities of the central nervous system, anencephaly (absence of brain) and spina bifida (a deformity of the spine and spinal cord) can be diagnosed by observing higher than normal levels of the fetal protein, alpha fetoprotein, in the

amniotic fluid and in the maternal blood. Again, abortion is the solution offered.

The technique of Restriction Fragment Length Polymorphism (RFLP) has already been alluded to in this section. This test is being applied to the detection of an increasingly large number of genetically determined diseases such as thalassemia, sickle cell anemia, cystic fibrosis, Duchenne muscular dystrophy, polycystic kidney disease and Lesch-Nyhan syn-

Table 12–6.   Risks for Rare Mendelian Disorders in Families

MODE OF INHERITANCE	FIRST DEGREE RELATIVES AT RISK	RISK	OTHER RELATIVES AT RISK	RISK
Autosomal dominant	Sibs, parents, children (both sexes)	50%	Uncles, aunts, nephews, nieces	26%
			First cousins	12.5%
Autosomal recessive	Sibs (both sexes)	25%	Uncles, aunts, nephews, nieces, cousins	Negligible
	Children	Negligible*		
X-linked recessive	Brothers	50%**	Maternal uncle	50%**
	Sisters (carriers)	25%**	Maternal aunt (carrier)	50%**
			Maternal male cousin	25%**
			Maternal female cousin (carrier)	25%**

* Risks for children of patients affected with common autosomal recessive diseases depend on gene frequency (highest risk [2%] for sickle cell anemia [0.08 × 0.25]).

** Risks are negligible when the disease in an affected patient is caused by a new mutation. Recent work suggests that the proportion of new mutations may be much less than the expected 33% in X-linked lethal diseases.

(From Motulsky, A.G.: Genetic counseling. In *Cecil Textbook of Medicine*, 15th Ed. Edited by P.B. Beeson, W. McDermott, and J.B. Wyngaarden. Philadelphia, W.B. Saunders Co., 1979.)

drome. It also happens in quite a large number of inherited diseases that the exact location of the gene is not known. If, however, the defective gene is located near a noncoding sequence which differs between individuals, RFLP can be used to identify the disease not only in affected individuals but also in fetuses and children at risk.

The RFLP technique can be performed on a very small amount of material such as 0.1 g. It can also be performed even if the material available is smaller than that, such as a drop of blood, a small fragment of chorionic villi, dried semen, or even a single hair. In these cases, the tiny amount of DNA can be amplified a million times or more using the technique of polymerase chain reaction (PCR). The target gene of interest is copied using a special DNA polymerase, and each copy in turn is copied further. The enormous amplification provided by PCR produces a detectable amount of the gene sequence which is then tested by RFLP or another technique based on visualization with specific probes. PCR is also used in the diagnosis of a number of infectious diseases.

Another direct approach used in modern diagnostic technology consists of synthesizing short oligonucleotide probes that hybridize specifically to the normal or the mutated gene. This is used, for instance, in the demonstration of mutations of the ras oncogene in certain cancers (Chapter 11), and the identification of carriers with alpha$_1$-antitrypsin deficiency who are at risk to develop lung emphysema (Chapter 15).

The ethical issues surrounding prenatal diagnosis are many and complex, not the least of which is the treatment for a defective child. No family should suffer the agony of helplessly watching their blind, retarded toddler with Tay-Sachs disease slowly deteriorate, or of rearing a retarded child, who may live to the age of 50 without ever learning to tie his or her shoes. But in remedying the situation some have adopted the principle that defective children should not be born. Exactly where this principle might lead us is neither clear nor pleasant to contemplate. One example of its widespread use may be found in John Wyndham's *The Chrysalids*, a science fiction tale of intolerance toward genetic malformations in an imaginary post-nuclear war society.

TREATMENT

In order to be effective, the treatment of genetic disorders requires a clear knowledge of the nature of the defect. Despite rapid growth in our knowledge of many disorders we are not yet able to modify many inborn errors of metabolism, although for a few (phenylketonuria, cystinuria) there are impressive statistics to show a change in prognosis. Reverting for a moment to conceptual expression, we may list several approaches to genetic diseases.

Dietary restrictions. The accumulation of toxic abnormal products is prevented by limiting the amount of precursor in the diet. For example, the treatment for phenylketonuria consists largely of eliminating phenylalanine from the diet.

Product replacement. Diabetes mellitus, hemophilia and congenital hypothyroidism may be effectively managed by supplying the deficient protein.

Surgery. Cleft lip, cleft palate and congenital dislocated hip can be corrected surgically.

Bone marrow transplantation. This approach is being used with significant success in severe combined immune deficiency, an inherited disorder characterized by a severe deficit of both humoral and cellular immunity.

Gene replacement. This is an experimental, still controversial form of treatment, involving genetic engineering, or the fabrication of designer genes. To replace a gene, such as a defective beta globin gene in sickle cell anemia or thalassemia, the normal gene must be identified, isolated, purified and attached to a "carrier" molecule of DNA. The carrier and gene, collectively referred to as a **recombinant DNA,** must then be introduced into precisely the right cells (bone marrow cells in the case of the beta globin gene). This is best done by removing a few such cells from the patient beforehand and reinjecting them after they take up the new DNA. Each of these steps is now technically feasible, but there remain the following serious questions. First, how can we make sure that the gene enters only the right cells and stays there? Second, how will the new gene be regulated? Its product should be made in sufficient but not harmful amounts and it is not yet certain what mechanism will control this. Third, will the new gene be harmful to the present or future generations of cells? A few successful genetic therapy experiments have been attempted with animals and at least one unsuccessful and controversial experiment has been tried with humans.

Gene replacement is far from the only medical application of genetic engineering. Various mammalian genes have been transferred into bacteria so that they can produce insulin, growth hormone or interferon. Through such developments genetics is fast becoming a big business, and at the same time promises to play a role of ever increasing importance in modern medicine.

SYNOPSIS

Genetic controls of subcellular, cellular, tissue, organ, and integrated mechanisms may often be abnormal. Mutations may affect either the structure or the amount of a cellular product.

Genetic diseases may be inherited as dominant, recessive, X-linked, or with differing degrees of penetrance. They may be classified anatomically, in relation to their importance, or as diseases of chromosomal aberration, due to mutations, or of polygenic etiology.

Klinefelter's, Turner's, and Down's syndrome are examples of chromosomal disorders. Hemoglobinopathies and familial polyposis are examples of mutation. Gout is an example of a disease process of both multifactorial and polygenic etiology.

Genetic disorders can be treated by supplying the missing product, by limiting the abnormal precursor, by administering an inhibitor, by depleting the body of the abnormal stores, and by using family counseling.

Terms

Gene	*Turner's syndrome*	*Trisomy*
Chromosome	*Recessive*	*Down's syndrome*
Mutation	*Dominant*	*Gout*
Sickle cell disease	*Sex-linked*	*Polymorphism*
Klinefelter's syndrome		

FURTHER READING

Antonarakis, S.E.: Diagnosis of genetic disorders at the DNA level. N. Engl. J. Med., 320:153, 1989.

Ash, P., Vennart, J., and Carter, C.O.: The incidence of hereditary disease in man. J. Med. Genet., 14:305, 1977.

Bell, J.A.: The epidemiology of Down's syndrome. Med. J. Australia, 155:115, 1991.

Bishop, D.T., and Burt, R.W.: Genetic epidemiology and molecular genetics of colorectal adenomas and cancer. Frontiers in Gastrointestinal Research, 18:99, 1991.

Brown, M.S., and Goldstein, J.L.: A receptor-mediated pathway for cholesterol homeostasis. Science, 232:34, 1986.

Byers, P.: Genetic disorders of mineralized tissues. Conn. Tiss. Res., 27:169, 1992.

Connor, J.M., and Riggs, A.D.: *Essential Medical Genetics.* Oxford, Blackwell Scientific, 1987.

De Braekeleer, M.: Hereditary disorders in Saguenay-Lac-St-Jean (Quebec, Canada). Hum. Hered., 41:141, 1991.

Defries, J.C., and Plomin, R.: Behavioral genetics. Annu. Rev. Psychol., 29:473, 1978.

Dubos, R.: *Mirage of Health: Utopias, Progress, and Biological Change.* New York, Harper & Row, 1979.

Fraser, F.C., and Nora, J.J.: *Genetics of Man.* Philadelphia, Lea & Febiger, 1986.

Goodenough, U., and Levine, R.P.: *Genetics.* New York, Holt Rinehart and Winston, 1979.

Hirschhorn, R.: Therapy of genetic disorders. N. Engl. J. Med., 316:623, 1987.

Holmes, L.B.: Congenital malformations. N. Engl. J. Med., 295:204, 1970.

King, M.-C.: Genetic analysis of cancer in families. Cancer Surveys, 9:417, 1990.

Levitan, I.B.: The basic defect in cystic fibrosis. Science, 244:1423, 1989.

McKusick, V.A.: *Mendelian Inheritance in Man.* Baltimore, Johns Hopkins University Press, 1987.

McKusick, V.A.: Mapping and sequencing the human genome. N. Engl. J. Med., 320:910, 1989.

Mudd, S.H., et al.: A study of cardiovascular risk in heterozygotes for homocystinuria. Am. J. Hum. Genet., 33:883, 1981.

Narod, S.: Counselling under genetic heterogeneity: a practical approach. Clin. Genetics, 39:125, 1991.

Rakic, M.T., et al.: Observations on the natural history of hyperuricemia and gout. Am. J. Med., 37:862, 1964.

Rossiter, B.J.F., and Caskey, C.T.: Molecular studies of human genetic disease. FASEB J., 5:21, 1991.

Schull, W.J., Otake, M., and Neel, J.V.: Genetic effects of the atomic bombs: a reappraisal. Science, 213:1220, 1981.

Scriver, C.R.: Garrod's legacy to the nations of mice and men. In *Mammalian Genetics and Cancer.* The Jackson Laboratory Fiftieth Anniversary Symposium. New York, Alan R. Liss, 1981, p. 169.

Scriver, C.R.: Window panes of eternity. Health, disease, and inherited risk. Yale J. Biol. Med., 55:487, 1982.

Spaeth, G.L., and Barber, G.W.: Homocystinuria and the passing of the one gene-one enzyme concept of disease. J. Med. Philos., 5:8, 1980.

Spielman, R.S., Baker, L., and Zmijewski, C.M.: HLA and the genetics of disease susceptibility. In *HLA in Endocrine and Metabolic Disorders.* New York, Academic Press, Inc., 1981.

Stanbury, J.B., Wyngaarden, J.B., and Fredrickson, D.S.: *The Metabolic Basis of Inherited Disease,* 4th Ed. New York, McGraw-Hill Book Co., 1983.

Suzuki, D.T., et al.: *An Introduction to Genetic Analysis.* New York, W.H. Freeman & Co., 1989.

Weatherhall, D.J.: *The New Genetics and Clinical Practice.* Oxford, Oxford University Press, 1990.

Wilson, E.O.: *On Human Nature.* Cambridge, Harvard University Press, 1978.

Young, F.E.: DNA probes. Fruits of the new biotechnology. J.A.M.A., 258:2404, 1987.

APPENDIX

Genetic Information

Chromosomes

All hereditary information is contained in molecules of deoxyribonucleic acid (DNA) which reside in the nucleus of each cell (except for less than 1% which is in the mitochondria). During interphase (when the cell is not dividing but going about the routine of daily life) DNA is dispersed and not visible as a discrete structure under a light microscope. In preparation for mitosis DNA replicates, and then in prophase each DNA strand begins to coil upon itself. Gradually the strands become compacted into **chromosomes.** At metaphase the chromosomes are at their shortest, thickest, and most easily visible. They can be photographed at this time and arranged in order of size; such a picture is called a karyotype (Fig. A12–1). Here chromosomes consist of two chromatids, one chromatid being the original DNA and the other its copy, joined together at the centromere. This conformation resembles a small cross, with short and long "arms." Special dyes have been used to examine chromosomes more closely. These dyes bind preferentially to regions of the chromosome producing a banded pattern (Fig. A12–2).

Each species of animal has its own specific karyotype and its own specific number of chromosomes. Humans have 46; 44 autosomes, and 2 chromosomes. Both autosomes and sex chromosomes are arranged in pairs, one member of each pair being maternal and the other paternal in origin. Each of the 44 autosomes contributed by a male gamete is homologous with a corresponding chromosome contributed by a female gamete. The sex chromosomes, which determine the sex of the individual are known as the **X and Y chromo-**

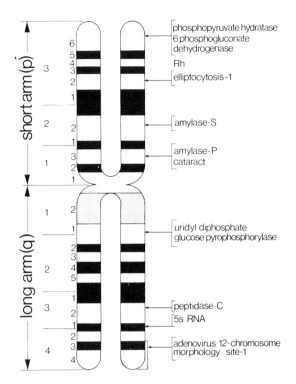

Fig. A12–2 This drawing of a chromosome shows the banding that is now visible with modern staining techniques. The arrows show the loci for the location of a variety of enzymes on a human chromosome. (From Thorn, G.W., et al. (Eds.): *Harrison's Principles of Internal Medicine,* 8th Ed. New York, McGraw-Hill, 1976.)

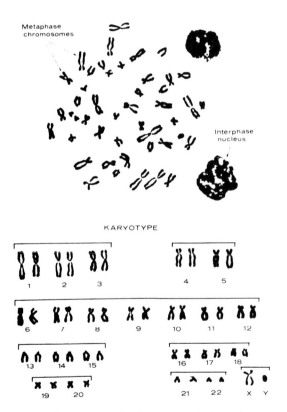

Fig. A12–1 Photomicrograph of human metaphase chromosomes from a stained culture of leukocytes. In the lower half of the figure is a human karyotype constructed by cutting out the chromosomes from photographs like that above and arranging them in several groups according to their size and sites of attachment of spindle fibers (primary constrictions). There are 22 pairs of autosomes and an X and Y chromosome. (Photomicrograph courtesy of L. Lisco and H. Lisco. From Bloom, W., and Fawcett, D.W.: *The Textbook of Histology,* 10th Ed. Philadelphia, W. B. Saunders Co., 1975.)

somes. In female somatic cells there are two homologous X chromosomes, whereas in the male the arrangement is heterologous, with one X and one Y chromosome. The Y chromosome is as small as the smallest autosome and carries few genes.

In **meiosis** (the reduction division) pairs of homologous chromosomes separate; each goes to a separate gamete. First, the chromosome replicates itself, and forms the familiar cross shape seen in the karyotype. Then the cell divides, whereupon the paternally derived chromosome and its duplicate go to one daughter cell and the maternally derived chromosome with its duplicate goes to the other. Daughter cells then divide, this time separating the original chromosome (chromatid) from the duplicate and sending each to a different gamete. Thus four gametes are formed, each with 23 chromosomes. Amazingly enough, most of the time these complicated travel plans are followed without a hitch.

Sex chromosomes undergo the same process, resulting in two types of spermatozoa, a set with one X chromosome, which on fertilization will result in a female offspring, the other with one Y chromosome, which results in a male. The father passes on the Y chromosomes received from his father to all his sons, and the X chromosomes received from his mother to all his daughters.

It seems that a chromosome is made of a single, extremely long strand of DNA, coiled upon itself many times. The structure and function of DNA has been covered in Chapter 1, but a few essentials are worth reviewing here. DNA molecules are composed of two complementary strands which interact with each other to form a double helical structure.

Each strand contains a sequence of bases (adenine, guanine cytosine and thymine) which pair up with bases in the complementary strand (always A with T and G with C). The entire structure resembles a twisted rope ladder, the base pairs forming the rungs.

Genes

Genes are encoded in specific sequences of DNA bases. Segments of the sequence can be "read" by messenger RNA (transcription, Fig. A12–3) which carries the message out of the nucleus to the ribosomes where the code is translated (Fig. A12–4), resulting in the manufacture of polypeptides. A **gene** is defined as a segment of DNA which codes for the amino acid sequence of a single polypeptide. It is the gene, not the chromosome, which is the unit of heredity. Genes are located on chromosomes and have specific, normally fixed addresses or "loci" where they can be found. Gene mapping is now a frontier in human biology and medicine. The details of how the genetic machinery operates in the cell are outlined in Chapter 1.

Alleles

Alleles are different forms of one gene. A given gene X which codes for polypeptide X does not always have exactly

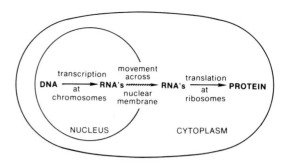

Fig. A12–4 The scheme for decoding a gene. Overall, a particular sequence of nucleotides in DNA causes a cell to assemble a particular sequence of amino acids into a protein. It is a two step process in which RNA molecules are intermediaries, carrying copies of genetic information across the nuclear membrane. The first step (DNA → RNA) is called **transcription,** and the second step (RNA → protein) is called **translation.** Some genes are transcribed into RNA but not translated. (From *Genetics: Human Aspects,* by Arthur P. Mange and Elaine J. Mange. Copyright 1980 by Saunders College/Holt, Rinehart and Winston. Reprinted by permission of Holt, Rinehart and Winston, CBS College Publishing.)

the same base sequence in all individuals. These variations in a gene are called alleles. This can mean that some individuals produce a form of polypeptide X which is different from that in other individuals; there can be slight variations in structure and/or function. An example is the variant of hemoglobin. Hemoglobin is the molecule which carries oxygen around the body, and gives the blood its familiar color. It is composed of 4 amino acid chains; 2 alpha and 2 beta chains of globin. The beta globin chains are translated and transcribed from the beta globin gene, of which we have two copies, one from each parent. A number of different forms or alleles of the beta globin gene are known to exist, all of which produce some form of beta chain. However, some alleles of the beta gene have base sequences that produce beta chains which are structurally unstable, such as the one which causes red blood cells to sickle.

If an individual possesses two identical beta globin alleles, he is said to be **homozygous** for the beta globin gene. He could be homozygous normal or homozygous for the sickle cell gene. If the two alleles are different, then the individual is **heterozygous**; he has inherited a different form of the beta globin gene from each parent. We are all homozygous for about 80% of our genes.

Before we move on, one last point requires definition; that is the matter of genotypes and phenotypes. The entire collection of genes of an individual forms his **genotype.** The outward expression of the genotype is called the **phenotype.** The way you look is your phenotype; the real you is your genotype! Environmental factors can alter both genotype and phenotype.

Mutation

A mutation is a change in a gene or genes which is transmitted to the next generation of cells. Such alterations can take the form of loss or addition of one or more bases, or substitution of one base for another. The effects of a mutation depend upon the importance of the new amino acid

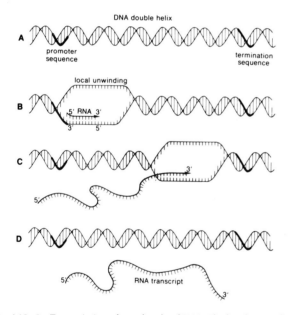

Fig. A12–3 Transcription of a molecule of RNA. The local unwinding of the DNA helix *(B)* is brought about by the attachment of the enzyme RNA polymerase at the promoter sequence on one of the two strands. Transcription into RNA proceeds along *this* strand of DNA *(B, C)* in the same direction as in DNA replication: the other strand of DNA is not "read" (at least not in this region). The complementary RNA transcript does not remain bound to the DNA template but peels off as the molecule is formed. In this way, the same stretch of DNA can be transcribed repeatedly, many RNA molecules being started successively before the preceding ones complete their transit to the termination site. The bubble formed by the separation of the DNA double helix travels along with the formation of the RNA transcript. (From *Genetics: Human Aspects,* by Arthur P. Mange and Elaine J. Mange. Copyright 1980 by Saunders College/Holt, Rineholt and Winston. Reprinted by permission of Holt, Rinehart and Winston, CBS College Publishing.)

arrangement to the polypeptide or protein, and the importance of the polypeptide or protein to the body machinery.

All biochemical processes in the body are under the direct or indirect control of genes. Each biochemical reaction can be resolved into different steps, each step controlled by a different gene coding for a specific enzyme. Therefore a mutation in a single gene will most likely affect only one step of a reaction. The structure or the amount of the product of the reaction may be affected, and if the reaction is blocked, precursors may accumulate which may also be harmful. Some mutations are harmful, although the effect can range from a minor clinical manifestation to death.

Mutations can arise spontaneously, i.e., irrespective of environmental conditions. Occasionally, during DNA replication, bases are mispaired, left out or rearranged. Usually these are repaired but, if not, the defect is passed on. This may occur in somatic cells or in germinal cells. If it occurs very early in development before germ cells have differentiated, both somatic and germinal cells may be affected.

Mutations may also be induced by environmental agents. We know that x-rays damage DNA indirectly by producing free radicals in the vicinity of DNA, perhaps by creating peroxides, such as H_2O_2 from H_2O. Ultraviolet light, the most common cause of skin cancer, acts directly on DNA by causing breaks in chain continuity due to alterations in base pairing. Indeed, most carcinogens act by causing mutations.

Most of the time we regard mutations as dreadful and dangerous events. But they are also the key to much of our individuality. Genetically, no two people are the same, just as no two people look exactly alike, unless they are genetically identical, i.e., monozygotic twins. Genetic individuality yields biochemical individuality: there are normal variations in protein composition, in the constituents of tissues and body fluids, in needs for specific nutrients and in pharmacologic responses to drugs. This last variation forms the basis of the field of pharmacogenetics. It has been estimated that in each of us, more than 20% of our proteins exist in a form that differs from the one present in the majority of the population. Such variability is due largely to mutation giving rise to many different alleles and is called **polymorphism** (literally "many forms"). This means that each of us is adapted to the environment in a different way, and among us there is considerable variability in ability to handle every kind of environmental challenge, including those that cause disease. In fact, we can even redefine disease in these terms: disease can be considered to represent an incompatibility between an individual's genetic make-up and his environment. Of course, in some disorders, the genetic component is so overwhelming that the term genetic disease is used.

Recently, new technologies have been introduced to identify the genes involved in the differences between individuals. The main approach is called restriction fragment length polymorphism (RFLP) because it uses special enzymes that cut DNA at discrete locations, producing fragment lengths that are specific to a given individual. In fact, forensic pathologists, the police, paleopathologists, and population geneticists, among others, are using this approach to identify people, living or dead, from a tiny piece of tissue, blood, semen or hair.

Mutation is also the mechanism by which each species evolves into a more efficient form. Helpful mutations are inherited just as are harmful ones. The story of sickle cell hemoglobin gene provides us with a good example of the work of evolution in this regard. Indeed, a significant number of Africans are heterozygous for sickle cell anemia, and they are found in areas with a high incidence of malaria. When sickling occurs, it creates an environment which is hostile for the malaria parasite which normally inhabits red blood cells. Therefore, the parasite is forced to escape the cell and this results in a milder form of malaria as compared to people who are not carriers of the sickle cell trait. As a result, carriers of sickle cell disease are better protected against the lethal effects of malaria and are therefore relatively more numerous in geographic areas where malaria has been endemic for many centuries.

When an allele is harmful in the homozygous state, but advantageous when heterozygous, it is said to possess **heterozygote advantage**. Overall this genetic phenomenon is rare.

Relatively Common Inherited Disorders

Dominant Inheritance

Familial monogenic hypercholesterolemia is the most common mendelian disorder of the human species. As the name implies, it is characterized by a high level of circulating cholesterol. This sets up an important condition for the causation of atherosclerosis and its complications, myocardial infarction and strokes, as discussed in Chapter 13. The autosomal dominant genetic defect is a mutation in the gene coding for the receptor of low-density lipoprotein (LDL), the main carrier of cholesterol. In fact, this gene is very long and can be affected by one of several possible mutations.

Marfan's syndrome can best be remembered by looking at a portrait of President Abraham Lincoln. His morphological features included a tall stature, long fingers, prominence of the forehead. The significance of this otherwise uncommon condition is the development of a dilatation of the thoracic aorta, with a significant risk of lethal dissection rupture. It is possible that more than one type of mutation accounts for Marfan's syndrome. Based on the recent discovery of the genetic defect, museum authorities have recently allowed scientists to extract DNA from a few hair follicles sampled from Lincoln's scalp and investigate whether he had the disease.

Huntington's chorea is a neurological disorder, mapped to a gene located on chromosome 4, which becomes evident after the second decade of life with choreiform, i.e., jerky movements and dementia.

Neurofibromatosis is relatively common and is characterized by multiple skin tumors composed of cells present in peripheral nerves (Fig. A12–5). The same tumors can also be associated with acoustic nerve. In addition, the patients have several large, light brown skin lesions, called "café au lait" spots. This autosomal dominant disease has a 100% penetrance and its gene has now been located on chromosome 17.

Adenomatous polyposis and **adult polycystic kidney disease**, two relatively common and severe autosomal dominant disorders, are discussed in Chapters 17 and 20, respectively.

Recessive Inheritance

The most striking example of recessive inheritance is **Tay-Sachs** disease. A moving account of this condition will be found in H.G. Wells' short story *The Valley of the Blind*, written many years ago. The parents are always normal, although both must carry the recessive gene. No affected per-

Fig. A12–5 This photograph, taken at the turn of the century, shows a number of warty protrusions all over the body, characteristic of **neurofibromas**. It has been remarked that "if you need to examine more than one of these growths, you do not know what it is". Multiple neurofibromas, described by von Recklinghausen, are benign tumors. (The Evans Collection, Osler Library, McGill University.)

son ever grows up to be a parent, as the disease is fatal in early life.

Tay-Sachs disease is an autosomal recessive disorder in the catabolism of gangliosides. A ganglioside is a type of lipid found in high concentrations in "ganglion" cells or neurons of the brain. It forms part of the nerve cell membrane. Gangliosides, like all membrane components, are continually broken down and replaced, so as to ensure that the membrane remains in good working order. The breakdown process occurs in several steps, each step catalyzed by a different enzyme. Powerful enzymes are sequestered inside lysosomes. The lysosome completely contains the catalytic process, allowing only small products of degradation to diffuse out.

In Tay-Sachs disease, one catalytic enzyme, hexosaminidase A, is deficient. Breakdown beyond this step is blocked

leading to an accumulation of the partially degraded ganglioside inside the lysosome. Lysosomes themselves accumulate inside the nerve cells, the nucleus is pushed aside, and the cytoplasm bulges. Eventually the nerve axons degenerate and, as the structure of the brain is destroyed, so is its function.

Although this process begins long before birth, for the first 3 to 6 months of life the infant looks and behaves normally. Then, at the time when he should be growing strong enough to sit unsupported, the child in fact becomes weaker and appears apathetic. Mental and motor deterioration progress rapidly after one year, with eventual paralysis, deafness, blindness and seizures. The child usually dies from pneumonia by the age of 3 or 4.

Tay-Sachs disease is rare except in Jewish populations of Eastern European origin where the carrier state is estimated at about 1 in 30. Today, carriers can be identified because they have a reduced serum level of hexosaminidase A. In addition, the homozygous state is detectable in utero through the use of amniocentesis. We will have more to say on this subject later.

Tay-Sachs disease is the prototype of conditions associated with the deleterious storage of unprocessed metabolic products. There are, however, other types of storage diseases, and some of them, like Niemann-Pick disease, Gaucher's disease, and mucopolysaccharidosis are transmitted as autosomal recessive traits.

Another example of recessive inheritance is **albinism**, a startling defect in pigmentation that leaves the skin, hair, and eyes a varying degree of white. An albino will usually marry someone who does not carry that particular and unusual gene; all the children will be heterozygotes. If an albino marries someone who is a heterozygote, half the children will be albinos and half unaffected heterozygotes. If two albinos marry, all the children will be albinos.

Other recessively inherited mutations include **cystic fibrosis** and **alpha₁-antitrypsin deficiency** (Chapter 15), **sickle cell anemia** and **thalassemia** (Chapter 23), and **hemochromatosis** (Chapter 18).

X-linked Inheritance

Hemophilia, the "bleeding disease," is the most famous example of a sex-linked inherited disease.

The most famous example of hemophilia arose in the royal families of Europe. The mutant gene, located on the X chromosome, should normally code for clotting factor VIII, without which the blood will not clot. The mutation originally occurred in Queen Victoria who had one hemophiliac son and two carrier daughters (see Fig. 4–10). Between them, Victoria's offspring spread the mutation among the ruling houses of Prussia, Russia, and Spain. A striking account of the effects of this disease on the patient, his family, and the course of modern history can be read in *Nicholas and Alexandra*, by Robert Massie.

Fabry's disease is a form of storage disorder which, unlike the other members of this disease category, is X-linked. Recognized first as hemangiomas of the skin, its significance derives from the widespread intra-cellular accumulation of a complex lipid. This material accumulates predominantly in the kidney and most patients die of renal failure.

Other X-linked disorders include the hemolytic anemia associated with **glucose-6-phosphate dehydrogenase deficiency** (Chapter 23), immunodeficiency caused by **agammaglobulinemia** (Chapter 6), and **Duchenne's muscular dystrophy** Chapter 25).

2

The Organs and Their Diseases

13

THE HEART

The physics of a man's circulation are the physics of the waterworks of the town in which he lives, but once out of gear you cannot apply the same rules for the repair of one as of the other.—Sɪʀ Wɪʟʟɪᴀᴍ Oꜱʟᴇʀ

From the earliest of times, our ancestors have realized the importance of the heart to life itself. Our language testifies to this, particularly the language of the poets. We say that a man is brokenhearted, or wounded to the heart, or that he wears his heart on his sleeve, or that it is in his throat, or in his boots. Our knowledge of the anatomy and physiology of the heart has advanced incredibly in recent years. We pass catheters into its cavities, measure the electrical changes in its muscle, record pressures and gradients, estimate the degree of injury by enzyme assays, and probe it by sound waves (echocardiography) and by computer-assisted radiology. We also cool it for operations and shock it to make it beat again. We still do not understand how it is that one person may have extensive myocardial scarring without suffering unduly, whereas another dies of sudden heart failure without adequate explanation.

Structure. The average weight of the human heart is 300 grams in the male, 250 grams in the female, about the size of a person's fist, but the heart is considerably larger in a big, muscular laborer, or smaller in a tiny, fragile, aged, woman. It is composed of muscle and valves (Fig. 13–1). Viewed with routine x-rays, the important structures of the cardiovascular system are shown in posterior/anterior and lateral views in Figure 13–2. The valves consist of a thin and delicate membrane, the endocardium, which also lines the cavity. Although so thin as to be translucent, the valves prevent a single drop of blood from leaking through when closed. On the right side of the heart, the tricuspid valve divides the chamber into an atrium or auricle, which receives the venous blood from the body, and a ventricle, which sends blood to the lungs by the pulmonary artery, whose mouth is guarded by the pulmonary valve. The left side of the heart is divided by the mitral valve into an atrium, which receives blood from the lungs, and a ventricle, which sends this blood out into the great artery, the aorta, whose opening is controlled by the aortic valve. The function of the valves is to prevent backflow of blood between the beats.

Just as the interior of the heart is lined by the endocardium, so its outer surface is covered by another delicate membrane, the epicardium. The part of the chest in which the heart is situated is lined by a second layer of pericardium, so that between the two layers there exists a space, the pericardial cavity, in which the heart can contract and expand. This cavity normally contains a small amount of serous fluid (20 ml), which lubricates the sliding surfaces. After injury or infection in the pericardium, fibrin can accumulate and can roughen these pericardial surfaces, even causing a noise similar to that of sandpapering (friction rub).

The heart muscle or myocardium has an abundant blood supply, which is much more important than in other muscles, because, unlike them, the heart does not rest for long. This blood supply is provided by two arteries, the right and left coronary arteries, which arise from the aorta immediately above the aortic valve and carry blood to every part of the heart muscle; the maximum flow is during the filling phase or diastole.

These arteries are different from others of the same size in the body, having an extra layer of longitudinal smooth muscle, perhaps because they are subject to intermittent stretching that takes place with each contraction of the heart.

Coronary sinus catheterization now enables us to look into the physiology of the myocardium and cardiac metabolism in a way never before possible. Physiologists have explored the electrical activity of single heart muscle cells by inserting a microelectrode into the interior of a cell to map the function of heart muscle during open heart surgery.

Function of the heart is reviewed in the Appendix, p. 315.

ATRIAL NATRIURETIC PEPTIDE

During the last 10 years, abundant evidence has accumulated to show that the atria of the mammalian heart not only act as passive chambers and the repository of the conduction bundles, but have an endocrine function as well. Many years ago, atrial cells were shown by electron microscopy to contain granules similar in appearance to some endocrine organs, but their function was not identified until recently.

Extracts of atrial cells are now known to increase the excretion of salt by renal tubules. Atrial peptide

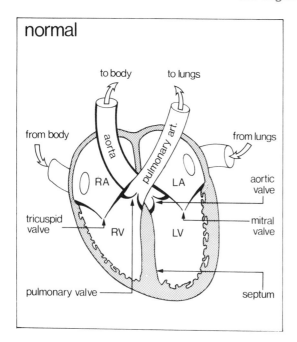

Fig. 13–1 This diagram of the normal heart shows the relative proportions of the sizes of the ventricles and the atria, RV, LV, RA, LA, that is, right and left ventricles and right and left atria. It also illustrates the relative wall thicknesses of the aorta and pulmonary artery, and the placement of the respective atrial ventricular valves, the tricuspid on the right and the mitral on the left, the pulmonary valve, and the aortic valve. IVC is the inferior vena cava.

seems to be twice as concentrated in the right atrium as the left. There are, in fact, specific receptors for these atrial peptides in kidney tubule cells. Endothelial and arteriolar cells also have receptors for this hormone, as do cells of the adrenal cortex. It is now clear that a coordinated physiological response to atrial peptide includes renal excretion of salt, a decrease in diastolic pressure (vasodilation), and an inhibition of secretion of aldosterone. All of these responses can best be viewed as homeostatic attempts to restore the circulation to a normal volume. The primary stimulus to the secretion of atrial peptide by cardiac myocyte appears to be distention of the atria, arising principally from volume overload. Recent studies on patients in congestive failure confirm this by demonstrating a linear increase in peptide concentrate concomitant with increased right atrial pressure. Thus a newly described hormone acts to coordinate the regulation of plasma volume and blood pressure by regulating salt secretion, renal function, and vascular resistance.

Clinical symptoms of heart disease may be caused by lesions in any of the anatomic subdivisions of the heart. We have **endocardial** diseases (which include valvular diseases), **myocardial** diseases, and **pericardial** diseases. The patient's medical history and the

A

B

Fig. 13–2 A, This figure shows a normal chest x-ray in PA (posteroanterior, or back to front) projection. The cardiac silhouette is seen in the center of the chest, with left ventricle (LV), right ventricle (RV), left atrium (LA), right atrium (RA), aortic knob (AO), left and right pulmonary artery (LPA and RPA), azygous vein (AZ). The trachea is shown at T, and the remainder of the chest film is unremarkable. IVC is inferior vena cava and the arrows outline the mainstem bronchi which contain air. B, In the lateral projection, the left pulmonary artery is seen at LPA, the right pulmonary artery at RPA, and the main stem bronchus to the right upper lobe at RUL.

physical examination should give much insight into the possible reasons for a particular patient's heart failure.

Laboratory Investigations. The myocardium is rich in enzymes, the most important of which, from the clinical standpoint, is an enzyme specific for muscle, creatine phosphokinase (CPK). Another enzyme found in heart muscle is glutamic oxaloacetic transaminase, called GOT or SGOT (S for "serum") for convenience. The normal serum level is low, from 4 to 40 units, but in myocardial infarction a large amount is released into the blood, so that the serum level is a sensitive and valuable index of recent necrosis of the myocardium (Fig. 13–3).

Chest x-rays and specific techniques for outlining the chambers of the heart, as with the use of barium in the esophagus, may demonstrate ventricular enlargement. Angiography (contrast media injected into veins or arteries) and cardiac catheterization are special techniques done in diagnostic centers. Modern use of isotopes allows us to visualize areas of heart muscle that do not function (Fig. 13–4). At least two different techniques are used for imaging of infarcts with modern methods. Some isotopes are taken up

by the normal myocardium, so that an infarct of any age or an area of hypoperfusion is shown as an area of absent or reduced activity (cold spot). Other isotopes are taken up by the damaged tissue, so that an acute infarct is shown as a positive image (hot spot). The mechanisms by which isotopes are taken up are debated but they may be related to the deposition of calcium in or near mitochondria of damaged cells. The optimal time for these scans is between 24 and 48 hours after the beginning of the infarct, scanning 1 to 2 hours after injection of the isotope, and viewing in 3 projections. A positive result with a technetium scan, for example, may be obtained up to 6 days after the infarct. The use of such scans is being developed day by day, and as we learn more about the value of such methods, they may be put to greater use. At the present time, most scans are not reliable for assessing the size of an infarct, because the uptake or radioactivity depends greatly on the blood flow and may not be proportional to the volume of the infarct itself. These methods are currently used to confirm the presence of infarcts rather than to establish the original diagnosis. Routine electrocardiography is helpful, particularly when tracings can be compared with earlier records. Precordial leads detect the sequential passage of electrical impulses and help to show which parts of the ventricular muscle are not functioning (Fig. 13–5). Echocardiography allows direct estimate of ventricular wall thickness and competence of valves (Fig. 13–6).

Heart disease heads the causes of death. As we stated earlier, in the developed world of about 1.2 billion people (25% of the total world population) there are an estimated 11 million deaths each year. Of these, 2.4 million are attributed directly to ischemic heart disease and another 1.5 million to stroke, which is usually due to atherosclerosis of cerebral vessels or hypertension, or both. The incidence has been steadily rising over the last hundred years until the late 1960s partly, at least, because of the increased number of older people. Arbitrary classifications of subsets of heart disease show some changes with time of the incidence of different diseases. These changes can be credited both to changes in life-styles (different eating and exercise habits) and to changes in medical treatment (open heart surgery), as well as to artificial differences because of new diagnostic methods and different diagnostic classifications (Fig. 13–7).

The principal categories of heart disease that we consider in this chapter are: (1) coronary artery disease, (2) hypertensive heart disease, (3) congenital heart disease, (4) valvular heart disease, (5) heart disease due to infections, and (6) rheumatic heart disease. Of these, by far the most common are hypertensive heart disease and coronary artery disease, then

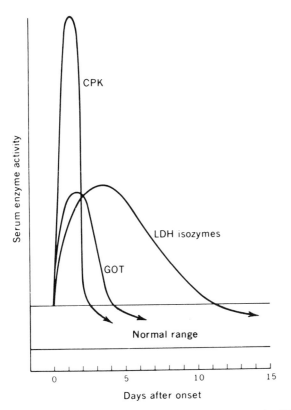

Fig. 13–3 This graph shows the time relationships between the CPK, LDH (lactic dehydrogenase) and GOT enzymes following myocardial infarction. (From Wintrobe, M., et al. (Eds.): *Harrison's Principles of Internal Medicine*, 7th Ed. New York, McGraw-Hill, 1974.)

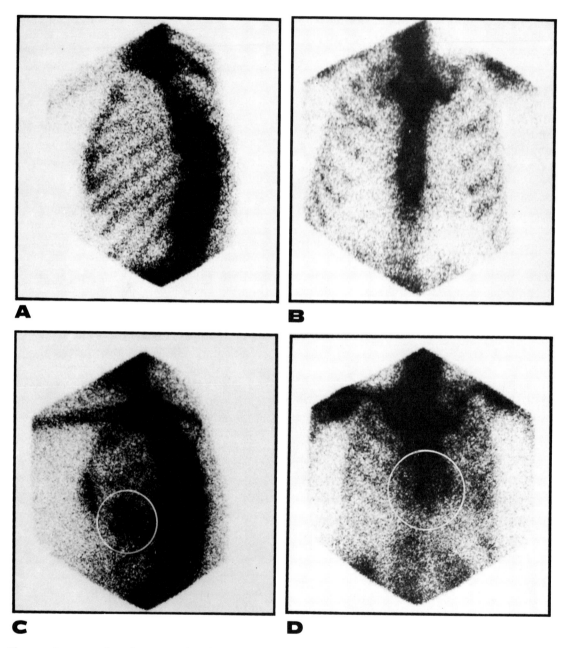

Fig. 13—4 These nuclear scans show the pattern of uptake of TC99mPP, a calcium-seeking agent in the normal person (A & B) and in a patient with a myocardial infarct (C & D). A, lateral view of the heart and chest, B, frontal view of the heart and chest. C and D show an area of increased uptake in the area of the infarction, which is shown within the circle. The resolving power of this new method allows one to see areas that are comparatively large; a very small lesion (1 centimeter square) will not be visible. However, one can identify the presence of the isotopes that are concentrated in the necrotic area.

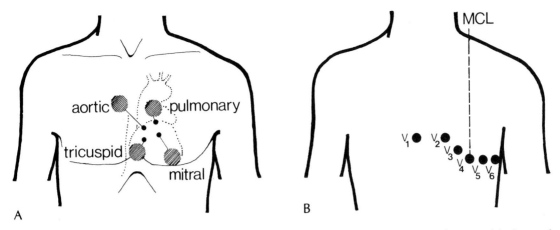

Fig. 13–5 *A* shows the location of the heart sounds. The small black dots in the center are the anatomic location of the heart values; the larger shaded areas are the points to which the valve sounds are usually referred. *B* illustrates the electrode positions of the precordial leads for an electrocardiogram: V₁ and V₂ are placed at the fourth intercostal space on either side of the sternum; V₃ halfway between V₂ and V₄; V₄ at the midclavicular line (MCL) and fifth intercostal space; V₅ and V₆ directly lateral to V₄. (Adapted from Andreoli, K. G., et al.: *Comprehensive Cardiac Care*, 4th Ed. St. Louis, C. V. Mosby Co., 1979.)

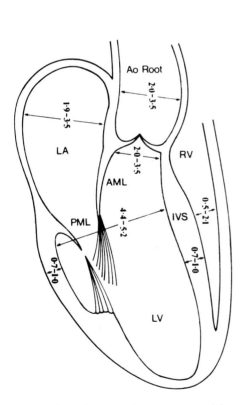

Fig. 13–6 This scheme illustrates the appearance of the chambers and wall thicknesses of a heart as determined by **echocardiography.** This should be compared with Figure 13–1 to show the dimensions of the chambers and their walls. The **echocardiogram** is used as a direct measurement of wall thickness and chamber size. LA is left atrium, LV left ventricle, PML posterior mitral leaflet, AML anterior mitral leaflet and IVS interventricular septum.

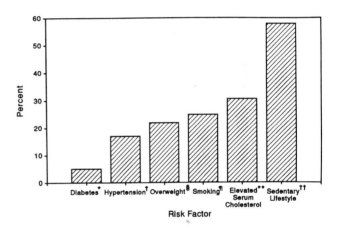

Fig. 13–7 Prevalences of modifiable risk factors for coronary heart disease—Behavioral Risk Factor Surveillance System, 1988, and Second National Health and Nutrition Evaluation Survey (NHANES II), 1976–1980. (From Centers for Disease Control, Morbidity and Mortality Weekly Report, 39(32):542, 1990.)

Table 13–1. Age-Adjusted Death Rates by Cause in the United States, 1968 and 1973

	RATES PER 100,000 POPULATION		
CAUSE OF DEATH	1968	1973	PERCENTAGE OF CHANGE
All deaths	743.8	692.9	− 6.8
All cardiovascular diseases	372.1	336.6	− 9.5
Ischemic heart disease	241.6	218.9	− 9.4
Cerebrovascular disease	71.3	63.7	− 10.7
Hypertensive disease	9.5	6.3	− 33.7
Rheumatic heart disease	7.2	5.4	− 25.0
Congenital heart disease	3.7	3.4	− 8.1
Other cardiovascular disease	38.9	38.9	0.0
All other diseases	371.7	356.3	− 4.1

(Source: The National Heart and Lung Institute, Bethesda, MD, from unpublished data from the National Center for Health Science.)

295

rheumatic heart disease; much less common are bacterial endocarditis and congenital heart disease. Table 13–1 shows the relative frequency of different types of heart disease in the population, but it is important to remember that regardless of the overall rarity or abundance of any particular disease, to the person afflicted there is no more important type of disease than the one from which he suffers.

CORONARY ARTERY DISEASE

In a previous chapter, we studied the effect of cutting off the arterial blood supply to an organ not provided with good collateral circulation, and we found that the effect usually depended on whether the closure of the artery was slow or sudden. Gradual closure due to narrowing of the lumen of the artery by atherosclerosis led to atrophy and death of the specialized cells of the part (e.g., heart muscle) and their replacement by scar tissue. Sudden closure by embolism or by thrombosis caused the formation of an infarct, an area in which all the tissue was killed by the sudden ischemia.

Unfortunately, the coronary arteries are frequently affected by atherosclerosis. This process narrows the lumen of the vessels and predisposes a person to thrombosis and occlusion. Coronary artery narrowing seems to accompany old age, but it is more severe in men than in women at earlier ages. Many factors predispose a person to atherosclerosis in general, and we think of coronary artery disease as having multifactorial etiology. Physical activity, heredity, obesity, metabolic disease such as diabetes mellitus, hypertension, abnormalities of lipid metabolism, and personal and social factors such as smoking and stress all play a role.

Traditionally, whenever there is pain in the chest, we jump to the conclusion that there is an impending "heart attack." Ischemia (lack of oxygen) of the myocardium is heralded by such pain; the most common cause of ischemia is arterial narrowing or occlusion. Narrowing of the coronary vessels by atheromatous plaques (which may be only segmental) and the occurrence of thrombi with or without plaques are the most common findings at autopsy in cases of acute myocardial infarction. We know that thrombi are constantly forming and being broken down by fibrinolysins; an additional etiologic factor, then, may be changes in our fibrinolytic mechanisms. In some instances, no anatomic lesion of the coronary artery can be found, but the monitor in the intensive care unit clearly records acute ischemia. In such cases we speak of "spasms" of the vessels, but are no better able to explain their etiology than in those rare cases of "sympa-

thetic" death, when sudden death occurs on hearing bad news or following bereavement.

To recapitulate, although the public speaks of a "coronary" (at best an inaccurate and slangy term), from the standpoint of the patient the essential feature is the presence or absence of a myocardial infarct. An infarct may occur without thrombosis, the lumen of the coronary artery being greatly narrowed by atherosclerotic thickening of the inner coat (intima), and the final obstruction produced occasionally by rupture of the soft atheromatous material into the lumen. Or thrombosis may occur without the production of an infarct, because the area of cardiac muscle is supplied with blood from one of the other coronary arteries (collateral circulation). It is the ischemia of the heart muscle, not the thrombosis of the coronary artery, that produces the symptoms and distress from which the patient suffers. The infarct is a soft, yellow area of dead muscle in the wall of the left ventricle, varying greatly in size (Fig. 13–8). The softness of the dead tissue makes it a weak spot in the wall of the ventricle which may rupture during the first week.

In myocardial infarction, enzymes are liberated from the dying cells and pass into the blood. Both the CPK and SGOT levels may rise from 2 to 20 times the normal within 24 hours of an infarction, not returning to normal for 3 to 6 days. The level of CPK is more specific for muscle damage—there are specific muscle isozymes that can be tested for—and rises more rap-

Fig. 13–8 This photograph of the inside of a left ventricle of a recently infarcted heart shows a dilated chamber with a massive infarction. The variegated appearance of the venticular myocardium at the arrows on the left shows the hemorrhage and necrosis. The arrow at the right shows mural thrombus material. (McGill University, Department of Pathology Museum.)

idly than transaminase; CPK levels also fall more quickly. In response to necrosis, the white blood cell count will rise (leukocytosis) as will the body temperature (fever), and we may be able to detect changes in the cellular function of the muscle by changes in the wave of repolarization (ECG). Today, radioisotope scans may be used to show the infarct in a questionable case as we have discussed. Ancillary methods to support the diagnosis are determinations of the central venous pressure and the pulmonary wedge pressure by catheters that demonstrate the loss of functional capability of the ventricular muscle.

The prognosis in coronary artery occlusion varies greatly, depending on the functional importance of the artery that is blocked, the extent of the damage to the heart muscle, and the availability of collateral circulation. The annual mortality rate of patients with disease of 1 coronary artery is 2.2%; with 2-vessel disease it is 6.8%; and with 3-vessel disease it is 11.4% per year. Patients with left main artery disease have the same life expectancy as those with 3-vessel disease. The patient may die instantaneously; this, indeed, is the most classic cause of sudden death. However, if the heart survives the shock, as is frequently the case, a collateral circulation is established in time. When this occurs, the patient may make a reasonably

satisfactory recovery. The recent development of cardiopulmonary resuscitation methodology, which is being taught at every level, and the availability of emergency mobile resuscitation equipment, all leading to intensive care units, is changing the pattern of survival from acute infarctions (Fig. 13–9). The immediate mortality of coronary artery thrombosis is believed to be around 10%.

Considerable emphasis is placed today on early support and treatment of the patient with acute myocardial infarction. If he can be taken to an intensive care unit alive within the first hour, his chances of survival are greatly improved over 15 years ago, because of modern pharmacotherapy with drugs such as propranolol and lidocaine. If the patient survives the attack, the infarcted area needs about 6 weeks to become strengthened by scar tissue. The patient should therefore be protected from unusual physical efforts for this period. Once the infarct has healed, the patient may live for 15 to 20 or more years in good health.

Recently, it has become possible to identify as the principal cause of death two major, different types of pathophysiology. Ventricular fibrillation is the first and most common. This process has been managed increasingly successfully with electrical shock and

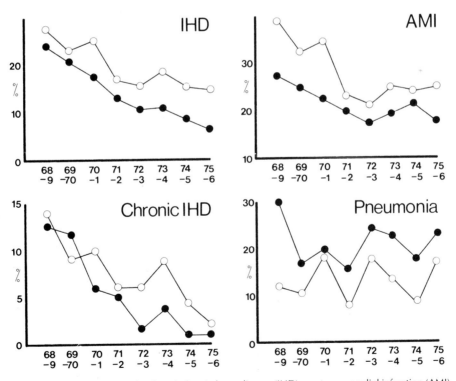

Fig. 13–9   These graphs show the decreasing mortality from ischemic heart disease (IHD), acute myocardial infarction (AMI), and chronic ischemic heart disease, as compared with pneumonia. Clearly, there has been a remarkable decline in mortality from ischemic heart disease and from chronic ischemic heart disease. The dark dots represent the female population and the light circles, the male. (From Craig, I. H., et al.: Changing mortality from ischemic heart disease and acute myocardial infarction. Med. J. Aust., 2:463, 1978.)

drugs such as lidocaine, which decrease the irritability of the ischemic muscle. In-hospital deaths from acute fibrillation used to account for 30% of cardiovascular deaths; this figure has been halved by recognizing that arrhythmias occur most commonly soon after symptoms are present. The greatest success in managing heart disease is the salvage of 65% of male patients who used to die within the first hour of symptoms. Today, up to 85% of first-attack patients seen within the first 30 minutes leave the hospital alive (Fig. 13–10). The second type of pathophysiology is represented by patients with significant pump failure. These persons are managed better now with diuretics, vasodilator agents, calcium channel blockers, inotropic drugs, and pacemakers.

Attempts have been made to categorize and to classify heart failure in order to assess the effectiveness of different management protocols, as shown in Table 13–2.

In angina pectoris, which refers to pain in the chest due to relative ischemia, the patient should be advised to live within his exercise tolerance, i.e., he should do no more activity than can be performed without production of anginal pain. The use of nitroglycerin may give relief of the anginal pain at the time of its occurrence.

More attention should be paid to decreasing the risk factors in coronary artery disease. In addition, diabetes mellitus, obesity, smoking, a sedentary life, high serum lipids, and hypertension all materially in-

Table 13–2. Classes of Heart Failure

		HOSPITAL MORTALITY
Class I.	No pulmonary edema	0.5%
Class II.	Moderate failure: rales, S3 gallop, tachypnea, right heart failure, jugular venous distention	10 to 20%
Class III.	Severe pulmonary edema	35 to 45%
Class IV.	Shock with systolic pressure less than 90 mm, peripheral constriction, cyanosis, mental confusion, decreased urine output	85 to 95%

crease a person's predisposition to coronary artery thrombosis.

Apart from "sudden death," the complications of an infarct include chronic heart failure, about which more will be said later. During the time when the necrotic muscle is weakest, a rupture may occur. Frequently, this is accompanied by hemorrhage into the pericardial space (tamponade), which interferes with cardiac filling and causes death. Sometimes the necrotic area is replaced by scar that does not contract, and a bulge or aneurysm of the ventricle is formed. In this area, or in any area where the endocardium has been injured, thrombus material may accumulate. This thrombus on the wall of a ventricle (mural thrombus) may then break off and embolize to remote organs such as brain, kidney, or extremities, resulting in loss of function. But the most common complication of these is heart failure, which has been increasingly well managed with new drugs. Finally, of course, one infarction may be followed by another, the risk of which is always enhanced in someone who has experienced a first infarction. Table 13–3 and Figure 13–11 show the classic complications of infarction, and Table 13–4 lists the classic anatomic and histologic changes found at intervals after the acute event has taken place. These patterns seem to be changing today as newer ways of managing infarcts are used (vasodilators, *beta* blocking drugs, and pacemakers).

To summarize, the **complications of an infarct include arrhythmia, shock, rupture, tamponade, aneurysm, thrombus, embolism, and chronic heart failure.**

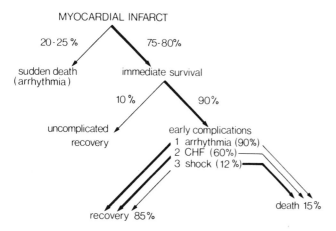

Fig. 13–10 This scheme illustrates the outcome, at the present time, following a myocardial infarct. The rate of recovery of 85% of afflicted persons as a result of early and effective treatment, which is based largely on the widespread use of cardiopulmonary resuscitation and on rapid hospital support, represents a radical change from 10 years ago, when as many as 60% of the patients with an infarct died before reaching a hospital. (From Robbins, S., and Angell, M.: *Basic Pathology.* Philadelphia, W.B. Saunders Co., 1976.

Table 13–3. Classic Complications of Myocardial Infarct

Arrhythmias	Mural thrombus	Aneurysm
Rupture	Embolism	Intractable failure

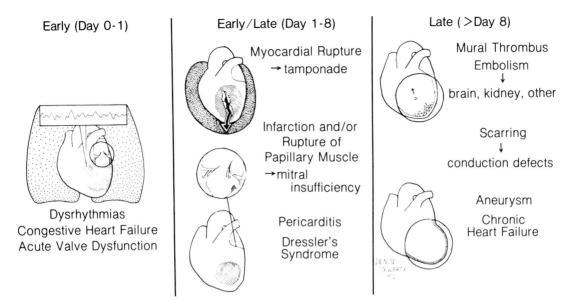

Fig. 13–11 Complications of myocardial infarction. (Courtesy Dr. D. Skwarok.)

Table 13–4. Sequence of Changes in Myocardial Infarction

TIME	GROSS CHANGES	LIGHT MICROSCOPE	HISTOCHEMISTRY	ELECTRON MICROSCOPE
0 to 2 hours	None	Waviness of fibers at border; Contraction bands and wavy lines	↓ Glutaminase I and β-hydroxybutyrate dehydrogenase; ↓ K^+ and ↑ Na^+ and Ca^{++}	Mitochondrial swelling and granules; distortion of cristae
4 to 12 hours	Swollen area	Beginning coagulation; edema; hemorrhage; marginal neutrophils	Succinic dehydrogenase negative	Relaxation of myofibrils (prominent I-bands); aggregation and margination of nuclear chromatin
18 to 24 hours	Pallor	Continuing coagulation (pyknosis of nuclei; shrunken eosinophilic cytoplasm)	Succinic dehydrogenase negative	
24 to 48 hours	Pallor, sometimes hyperemia	Total coagulative necrosis with loss of nuclei and striations; heavy interstitial infiltrate of neutrophils and mononuclear leukocytes	Succinic dehydrogenase negative	
2 to 4 days	Hyperemic border; central yellow-brown softening; pericarditis (11%)	Beginning fatty change		
10 days	Maximally yellow and soft; beginning scarring at margins	Beginning fibrosis		
Seventh week	Scarring complete	Collagenization		

(From Robbins, S.L., and Angell, M.: *Basic Pathology*, 2nd Ed. Philadelphia, W.B. Saunders Co., 1976.)

HYPERTENSIVE HEART DISEASE

If the heart has to work for years against a greatly increased resistance in the form of high blood pressure, it will gradually become exhausted and fail. The strain falls principally on the left ventricle, and in a while, the wall of this ventricle becomes thicker, or hypertrophied (Fig. 13–12), so as to be able to overcome the increased resistance. When the heart is grasped at post mortem examination, it feels like a closed fist. Finally, however, its power is lost, the heart fails, the ventricle becomes dilated, and the end

Fig. 13–12 This photograph shows, on the right, marked concentric left ventricular hypertrophy compared with a normal left ventricle on the left. (McGill University, Department of Pathology Museum.)

picture is much like that of other forms of heart failure. The symptoms are similar to those of heart failure from other causes, such as valvular disease and coronary artery disease. It must be pointed out, however, that many persons with hypertension live vigorous lives for decades without developing signs of heart failure. In the opinion of some, such persons would be happier if they were ignorant of their high blood pressure. There is good evidence, however, that treatment of hypertension is changing the pattern of this disease.

It should be stated here that there is an important difference between hypertension with a slightly elevated systolic pressure and a diastolic of 95 mm Hg and a diastolic pressure of over 120 mm Hg which represents a medical emergency. All hypertension is not the same.

The principal causes and varieties of hypertension are discussed in the next chapter. In the most common form, known as essential hypertension, small arteries throughout the body are narrowed; and this leads to increased peripheral resistance to the blood

flow, so that the diastolic pressure is elevated. A patient with hypertension may not die of heart failure, but rather as the result of rupture of a blood vessel in the brain (cerebral hemorrhage). Narrowing of the small arteries in the kidneys may lead to dysfunction of these organs, and the patient may die of renal failure. Thus death in hypertension may be due to disease of the heart, the brain, or the kidneys.

CONGENITAL HEART DISEASE

Heart disease may be congenital rather than acquired. A child is born with cardiac defects due to failure in the process of development. One important predisposing cause is rubella (German measles) in the mother during the first 3 months of pregnancy. This circumstance assumes practical importance, because surgical operations are available for the treatment of several of these defects. Many congenital abnormalities of the heart may occur, some rare, others incompatible with life. Table 13–5 shows the relative frequency of each of the more important congenital anomalies. Those amenable to current surgical treatment will be described.

The key to most of the defects lies in variations in the formation of the septum, which divides the heart into a right and a left side. The most important feature of congenital heart disease is the possibility of a mixing of the blood in the systemic and pulmonary circulations as the result of a shunt. Three common causes of shunts are (1) atrial septal defect (Fig. 13–13), (2) ventricular septal defect (Fig. 13–14A,B), and (3) patent ductus arteriosus (Fig. 13–15). In all of these defects, the lungs become overloaded with blood. Another distinction may be made between cases with cyanosis and those without cyanosis. Cyanosis (a bluish color due to inadequate oxygen saturation of arterial blood) is caused by a right to left venous-atrial shunt, because poorly oxygenated venous blood then enters the systemic circulation.

Table 13–5. Common Congenital Heart Diseases

ANOMALY	MALE TO FEMALE RATIO	DEFINITION	% OF INCIDENCE OF CHD IN INFANTS	DISORDERS ASSOCIATED WITH INCREASED INCIDENCE
Ventricular septal defect	1:1	Abnormal opening between the ventricles	28.3	Down's syndrome
Patent ductus arteriosus	1:3	Persistence of the fetal connection between the aorta and pulmonary artery	12.5	Rubella syndrome
Atrial septal defect	1:3	Abnormal opening between the atria	9.7	Down's syndrome
Coarctation of the aorta	4:1	Stricture in the thoracic aorta	8.8	Turner's syndrome
Tetralogy of Fallot	1:1	Ventricular septal defect, pulmonic stenosis with right ventricular hypertrophy and aorta overriding the ventricular septum	7.0	Thalidomide ingestion

(Adapted from Whaley, L.F.: *Understanding Inherited Disorders*. St. Louis, C.V. Mosby Co., 1974.)

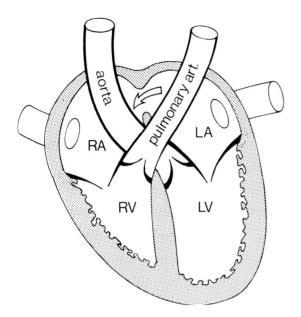

Fig. 13–13 This diagram shows an **atrial septal defect.** Since pressure in the left atrium is higher than in the right, blood is shunted into the right atrium. This creates extra work for the right side of the heart, resulting in right atrial and ventricular hypertrophy.

Congenital defects also commonly predispose a patient to endocardial infections with bacteria for reasons that remain obscure. Sometimes the patient with congenital heart disease dies of bacterial endocarditis.

At least 90% of the patients with congenital disease of the heart and great vessels fall into 1 of 4 groups. These are, in their order of frequency, although not in their order of discussion: (1) septal defects, (2) coarctation of the aorta, (3) patent ductus arteriosus, and (4) the tetralogy of Fallot. All of these are treatable by surgery.

Septal Defects. Atrial septal defects may be trivial or serious. Patency of the foramen ovale, the opening in the septum between the two atria that is normally present at birth, is the most common and the least important of congenital cardiac anomalies. As the opening is small and oblique, little blood usually passes from one side to the other. A true septal defect due to failure of development is another matter. The opening may be large, and blood passes readily from the left to the right side where the pressure is lower, so that both the right atrium and the right ventricle become greatly dilated and hypertrophied. There is no cyanosis until cardiac failure sets in; the patient may live from 30 to 50 years.

Ventricular septal defects may be uncomplicated by other cardiac anomalies. The opening is usually small, situated in the membranous part of the septum, and causes little disturbance. Here again cyanosis will be absent except as a terminal phenomenon. Bacterial endocarditis, however, occurs at the margin of the opening in many cases, so that surgical closure of the

A   **B**

Fig. 13–14 A, This figure shows a **defect in the ventricular septum.** Blood is shunted into the right ventricle, which results in right ventricular hypertrophy and in increased pulmonary blood flow. Life expectancy depends on the size of the defect. B, This arteriogram shows a remarkably enlarged pulmonary artery with all of its branches dilated.

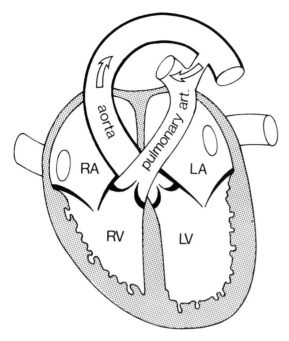

Fig. 13–15 Patent ductus arteriosus. Shunting of blood from the aorta into the pulmonary artery results in right ventricular hypertrophy and in increased blood flow and pressure in the pulmonary arterial system.

defect is appropriate. When the defect is small, the characteristic physical sign is a loud systolic murmur. Defects smaller than 5 mm are of little physiologic significance.

Tetralogy of Fallot. This is a most important congenital lesion of the heart, and the most common of the lesions causing cyanosis, for reasons that will soon become obvious. The most significant physiologic part of this condition is pulmonic valve stenosis. The pulmonary valve is narrowed, so that the blood is unable to pass in sufficient quantity from the right ventricle to the lungs. Fallot described three other changes in addition to the pulmonic valvular stenosis. (1) The aorta, which normally receives blood only from the left ventricle, overrides the right ventricle. (2) There is incomplete closure of the interventricular septum (a high septal defect exists). (3) As a result of the increased resistance to outflow, the right ventricle becomes hypertrophied. So the four defects that constitute the tetralogy are: pulmonic stenosis, ventricular septal defect, overriding aorta, and right ventricular hypertrophy (Fig. 13–16). The tetralogy of Fallot is the most common cause of the condition known as the "blue baby," a name given because of the extreme degree of cyanosis, the blue color being most marked on the lips, ears, cheeks, and hands. The principle of the corrective operation is to bypass the obstruction

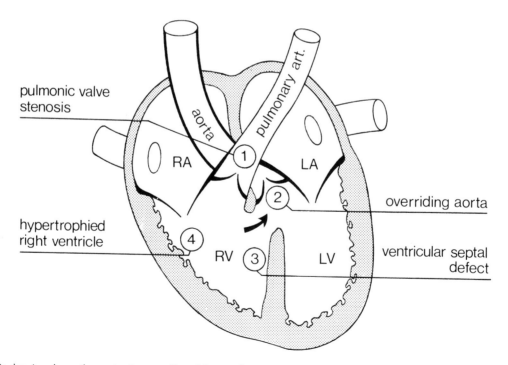

Fig. 13–16 This drawing shows the anatomic anomalies of the **tetralogy of Fallot.** They are pulmonary valvular stenosis, which leads to right ventricular hypertrophy, a ventricular septal defect, and an overriding aorta. The principal physiologic problem is the failure of blood to flow though the lungs for oxygenation, which leads to the classic "blue baby."

at the opening of the pulmonary artery. This is done by anastomosing (connecting) the left subclavian artery, a branch of the aorta, to the pulmonary artery beyond the obstruction, so that the blood now reaches the lungs, although from the left ventricle instead of from the right. Reference to Figure 13–16 may make the matter clearer, although the branches of the aorta are not shown in the diagram. The improvement in the child's condition is immediate and dramatic, the cyanosis and shortness of breath often being improved by the time the patient is returned to bed from the operating room.

Patent Ductus Arteriosus. The ductus arteriosus is a short vessel that passes from the pulmonary artery to the aorta. During intrauterine life, the blood from the right side of the heart passes along this channel into the aorta without passing through the lungs, as these organs are not used for respiration while the child is still in utero. The ductus should become closed a few weeks after birth. It may, however, remain open or patent. Thus the blood continues to flow from the aorta into the pulmonary artery because the pressure is higher in the former than in the latter. Blood therefore receives sufficient oxygen from the lungs, and there is no cyanosis except in cases complicated by other congenital defects. Although the condition is compatible with a long and active life, in most cases life expectancy is considerably shortened. This is because the increased flow and increased pressure in the pulmonary arterial system eventually cause a thickening of the walls of the pulmonary arterioles and raise the pulmonary arterial pressure. In turn, the right ventricle must do more work, and, as the resistance increases, the right ventricle may fail. Another danger is the development of bacterial endocarditis at either end of the ductus. The treatment is surgical division of the ductus, a relatively simple operation.

Coarctation of the Aorta. This condition is a narrowing of the aorta (Latin *coarctare*, to press together)

in the region where it is joined by the ductus. It is usually beyond the origin of the large arteries to the head and arms, so that there is an abundant flow of blood to these parts and the blood pressure in the arm is high. Little blood passes through the narrowed aorta to the abdomen and legs, where the blood pressure is low, and the pulse can hardly be felt. Usually enough blood manages to bypass the obstruction through abundant collateral vessels that open up. Recognition of this collateral circulation by means of radiography greatly assists the physician in making a correct diagnosis. The surgical treatment consists of clamping the aorta above and below the obstruction, excising the narrowed segment, and sewing the divided ends of the aorta together. This dramatic operation is usually attended with complete success.

VALVULAR DISEASE

Although this form of heart disease used to be a sentence of limited life, since the early 1950s, with the development of intrathoracic surgery and techniques for intracardiac operative procedures, the valvular heart diseases have been operated on with increasing success. Nowhere is the illustration clearer that progress in medicine depends on technical developments as much as on the particular skill of a single physician. Extracorporeal circulation machines, cardioplegic drugs (which bring the heart to a standstill) and the evolution of new valvular prostheses have effected a revolution in the management of these disorders. We have already seen that there are four valves in the heart, 2 on the left side and 2 on the right. We shall confine our attention to the valves on the left side, namely the mitral and the aortic. Either of these may be too narrow (stenosed) or too wide (insufficient or incompetent) (Fig. 13–17). There are thus four possibilities.

Mitral Stenosis. Most, if not all, cases of mitral stenosis are rheumatic in origin. The condition is much

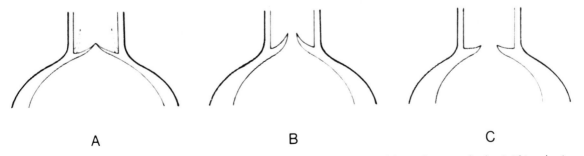

| A | B | C |

Fig. 13–17 A, This drawing shows the appearance of a normal valve, which may open widely or close completely. B, This valve is unable to open completely, and is considered stenotic. C, This value is unable to close and is considered insufficient.

more common in women than in men. The valve opening may be a mere buttonhole, which will hardly admit the tip of the little finger (Fig. 13–18), whereas the normal opening should admit two fingers with ease. The valve looks like a deep funnel, the walls of which are formed by the fused cusps. The blood rushing through this rigid funnel on its way from the left atrium to the ventricle causes a vibration of its walls, which is responsible for the characteristic diastolic murmur heard and the thrill felt. If the reader will pause to think of the anatomy of the heart and of the direction of the blood flow, he will not need to be told that, owing to the obstruction, the left atrium and eventually, the right side of the heart become greatly dilated (Fig. 13–19). A thrombus may form in the dilated left atrium, and this may become detached and give rise to cerebral embolism. The general effects of mitral stenosis are those of chronic venous congestion.

The stenosis can now be treated surgically by valvotomy and reconstruction of the valve or by replacement with an artificial valve. Figure 13–20 shows two x-ray studies of the chest of a patient whose diseased mitral valve has been replaced by a Starr-Edwards ball-in-cage prosthesis. The ball is a Silastic, long-lasting structure kept in an open or shut position by three metal struts, as shown in the accompanying photograph. The two x-ray studies show the ball's position in systole and diastole. In assessing the value or desirability of the operation, it must be remembered that the condition is not necessarily progressive, and that well over 50% of the patients survive without operation for 20 years or more, many showing little change in their clinical condition.

Mitral Insufficiency. This is the least well defined of the four principal valvular lesions. Incompetence is

Fig. 13–19 This posteroanterior film of the chest shows the typical configuration of the heart in mitral valvular disease, in which there is both stenosis and insufficiency of the mitral valve. The prominent finding at the white line is the presence of an enlarged left atrium. The cardiac silhouette is of a globular shape, reflecting the hypertrophy of the right heart which may have a ventricular wall as thick as the normal left ventricle.

Fig. 13–18 This photograph shows the mitral valve as seen from above the tricuspid valve at T, the aortic valve at A, and the mitral valve at M. The arrow shows the free margin of this fish-mouth stenotic valve, which is unable to open adequately. (McGill University, Department of Pathology Museum.)

caused by sclerosis and contraction of the cusps or by dilatation of the valve ring. One common cause is rheumatic endocarditis, but bacterial endocarditis may also cause incompetence. Although it is convenient and appropriate to speak of stenosis or incompetence as if they were discrete and specific entities, and whereas it is important to learn the signs and symptoms of these particular forms of valvular disease, it is also true that even if the physiologic lesion is predominantly stenotic, there is usually a measure of incompetence, and if the physiologic abnormality is predominantly insufficiency, there is some measure of stenosis.

Aortic Stenosis. Pure aortic stenosis usually occurs in men over 50 years of age, whereas mitral valve stenosis is commoner in women at an earlier age. The stenosis is of the calcified nodular type, best called calcific aortic stenosis. The cusps adhere together to form a kind of diaphragm as in mitral stenosis, but the most striking feature is the presence of warty calcified masses, which may cover the cusps (Fig. 13–21). The entire valve is incredibly hard and rigid. This stenosis has three accepted causes: it may be rheumatic in ori-

Fig. 13–20 *A*, These two chest x-rays show an artificial (Starr-Edwards) ball-in-cage mitral valve. The x-ray on the left shows the ball of the valve closing the orifice in left ventricular systole. On the right, the ball or poppet is in the cage and the left ventricle is filling. *B*, A Starr-Edwards prosthetic mitral valve.

Fig. 13–21 These drawings show the appearance of the aortic valve, normal in the left area, a severely stenotic valve with only two cusps on the middle, and an even more severely stenotic atherosclerotic valve in the right view.

Fig. 13–22 *A*, **Aortic stenosis** and resulting left ventricular hypertrophy. *B*, This posteroanterior chest film shows a prominent, straight left cardiac silhouette, which is usually seen in left ventricular hypertrophy.

gin, it may occur on congenital bicuspid valves, or it may be an expression of atherosclerosis without known contributing factors. Calcific aortic stenosis is certainly being encountered more frequently than it was formerly. The heart shows a perfect example of pure or concentric hypertrophy of the left ventricle (Fig. 13–22*A*,*B*). The most characteristic physical sign is a rough rasping systolic murmur and thrill at the aortic area. Cardiac surgery offers relief with a reasonable degree of safety. The radiologic demonstration of calcification in the area of the aortic valve may serve to confirm the diagnosis. It must be noted that calcific aortic stenosis is often well tolerated into old age, even after evidence of severe obstruction to the aortic outflow has been noted, but once heart failure occurs, the prognosis is poor.

Aortic Insufficiency. Insufficiency or incompetence of the aortic valve may be due to endocarditis of the valve cusps or to dilatation of the aorta and the aortic ring. The former may be caused by rheumatic endocarditis or by bacterial endocarditis. The latter used to be a common result of syphilitic aortitis before the days of modern treatment of syphilis. It was the syphilitic form that used to give the classic picture of the disease, which was well known to French poets, but this is now becoming rare.

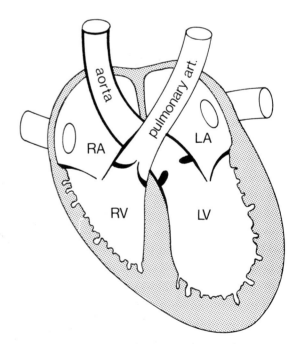

Fig. 13–23 **Aortic insufficiency.** The aortic valve is incompetent. Blood flows back into the left ventricle in time and causes it to dilate and to become hypertrophied.

In this condition, the heart is all left ventricle, which is greatly hypertrophied as well as dilated, on account of the regurgitant flow of blood from the aorta into the ventricle through the incompetent valve during systole (from the dilated ventricle), and of too little blood during diastole (owing to the backward flow) (Fig. 13–23). This process accounts for the "water-hammer pulse" of leaping character felt at the wrist. The loud diastolic murmur, which is the most characteristic physical sign, is due to the rush of blood back into the ventricle during diastole.

RHEUMATIC HEART DISEASE

This disease is not nearly so common today as it used to be. The simple reason may be that its origin as a reaction to the antigens of a streptococcal sore throat has been modified by the frequent and extraordinary use of antibiotics. Rheumatic heart disease is attributed to an inflammatory process with an immunologic etiology, as demonstrated by a rise in titer of antistreptolysin antibodies (antibodies to group A hemolytic streptococci) that occurs about three weeks after a streptococcal sore throat. At this time, all parts of the heart may be inflamed in a pancarditis.

As a result, the valves (commonly the mitral) become inflamed, and from the blood flowing over them, blood platelets and fibrin are deposited on them. These deposits form little nodules called vegetations, each about the size of a pin's head, which form a row along the margin of the cusps. The inflamed cusps, normally almost as thin as gossamer, become markedly thickened and tend to adhere to one another, just as do inflamed loops of bowel when brought in contact. As the inflammation subsides, fibrous tissue takes the place of the inflammatory exudate, and this slowly contracts, causing retraction of the cusps. This process takes months or years.

The effect of all this on the function and use of the valve may be 1 of 2 kinds, although often both result. Owing to the adhesions between the thickened cusps, they are unable to open properly when the blood flows through the valvular opening, so that this opening becomes permanently narrowed (stenosis). This narrowing may become so extreme that finally the opening is no larger than a buttonhole, whereas normally it should admit two fingers. The mitral valve is the common site of rheumatic endocarditis, and mitral stenosis is one of the most serious forms of heart disease, for not enough blood can flow from the left atrium into the left ventricle, and so is dammed back first in the lungs, then in the right side of the heart, and finally in the veins of the body (Fig. 13–24A,B). The left atrium may become greatly dilated behind the obstruction (Fig. 13–25). Mitral stenosis is three times more common than all other rheumatic heart lesions. The second result is incompetence of the valve. Here the retraction of the cusps is much more marked than their self-adhesion. The result is that the cusps are unable to meet when the valve tries to close, and the blood escapes back from the ventricle into the atrium in the case of the mitral valve, and from the aorta into the ventricle in the case of the aortic valve.

It is important to realize that a person with chronic valvular disease of the heart is not necessarily an invalid, nor should such a person be encouraged to consider himself as one. The evidence of a valvular lesion is a murmur heard by the stethoscope over the heart, but a person with a cardiac murmur may lead a full and vigorous life. If the heart muscle is healthy, it is able to compensate for the valvular lesion, unless the latter is marked and progressive. Today, thoracic surgery offers valve replacements with ingenious plastic and metal devices that function as well as normal valves, and hundreds of patients have their symptoms relieved by surgical intervention.

In addition to causing inflammation of the valves, rheumatic fever also damages the heart muscle and pericardium. Small areas of inflammation and destruction, known as Aschoff bodies or nodules, are scattered through the muscle, and later these become converted into scar tissue. Such a scarred myocardium cannot fail to be weakened. On account of the damage to the wall of the atrium, the peculiar condition known as atrial fibrillation is apt to develop, especially in mitral stenosis. Normally the atria beat at the same rate as the ventricles; this is natural, because normally the wave of muscular contraction starts in the atria and passes on to the ventricles; it is the beat of the ventricles that produces the pulse. In atrial fibrillation, the atria no longer contract in a regular manner; they seem to be trembling instead of contracting. The result is that the ventricles contract in a rapid and irregular manner, this irregularity being reflected in marked irregularity of the pulse. The ventricles tend to become exhausted, with resulting heart failure, the symptoms of which are palpitation and dyspnea. The administration of drugs prevents the irregular impulses from the atria from reaching the ventricles, which then commence to beat in a much slower and more regular manner, with immediate relief to the patient.

The pericardium also becomes inflamed (pericarditis (Fig. 13–26), and the two inflamed layers of pericardium may stick together and form adhesions that may seriously hinder the heart's action. The truth of the remark made in the general discussion of rheumatic fever will now be evident, that it is a disease that licks

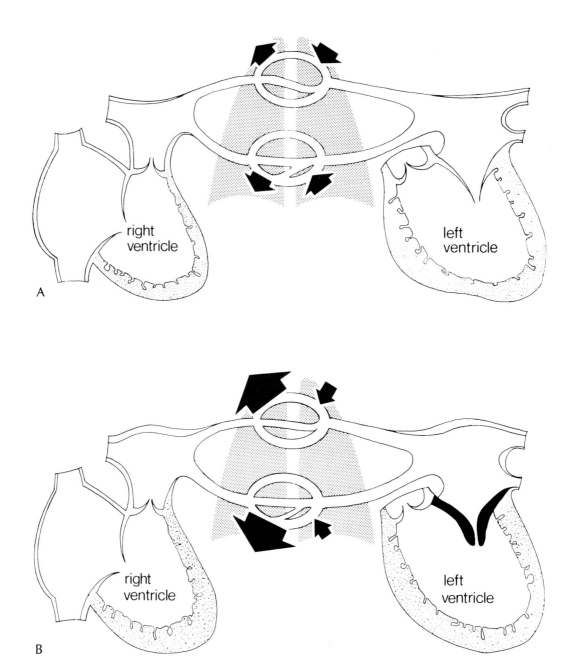

Fig. 13-24 *A* illustrates schematically the appearance of a normal right ventricle, pulmonary vascular bed, left ventricle, and mitral valve. The arrows indicate the traditional balance in the Starling hypothesis. *B* shows the effect of mitral valve stenosis on the pulmonary vascular bed; the large black arrows represent the extravasation of fluid into the interstitial space, which is greater because of the increased hydrostatic pressure owing to the failure to empty the left atrium. This pulmonary edema then causes the patient to feel short of breath. The right ventricle is shown as hypertrophied in this drawing; it is a compensatory hypertrophy. (From Edwards, J.: Pathology of chronic pulmonary hypertension. Pathol. Annu., 9:1, 1974.)

Fig. 13–25 This photograph of the left atrium, mitral valve, and left ventricle shows the remarkable dilatation and hypertrophy of the left atrium in a representative case of prolonged mitral stenosis. The thickened, shortened chordae tendinea so typical of rheumatic heart disease are shown at the arrow. (McGill University, Department of Pathology Museum.)

the joints but bites the heart, for the patient is left with permanent lesions that may cripple his heart to the day of his death, although the day may be far removed.

INFECTIOUS ENDOCARDITIS

In the continually changing picture of disease, it would be difficult to name a condition that has altered its appearance more completely in recent years than infectious endocarditis. It used to be a malady in which the heart beat a muffled march to the grave, in quick time in the acute form, with a slower but just as deadly rhythm in the subacute variety. Now, thanks to antibiotics, it has become a curable disease when treated early. This, indeed, is one of the great triumphs of antibiotic chemotherapy and cardiovascular surgery. A sharp distinction has been drawn in the past between the acute and subacute forms of infectious endocarditis. The importance of this distinction has faded, and more emphasis is laid on the infecting agent and on whether the patient can have the infected valve replaced by a prosthesis. It is, however, still convenient to speak of acute and subacute varieties.

Subacute Bacterial Endocarditis. This form of endocarditis is much less common than the rheumatic form, but it used to be much more fatal. Until the

Fig. 13–26 This photograph of the epicardial surface of the heart shows the ragged fibrinous adhesions, which have been described as bread and butter, that may be seen in chronic uremic disease, in persistent rheumatic injury, or even in a purulent pericarditis. (McGill University, Department of Pathology Museum.)

Fig. 13–27 This photograph shows large vegetations attached to the mitral valve at the arrow. These are present in endocarditis. (McGill University, Department of Pathology Museum.)

introduction of antibiotic therapy, the mortality was practically 100%. The disease used to run its course in a number of months, sometimes a year. It is commonly caused by a variety of nonhemolytic streptococcus (*Streptococcus viridans*). One peculiarity is that the disease is usually superimposed on an old rheumatic endocarditis, healthy valves being seldom affected. The bacterial colonies are called vegetations and are large and extremely friable (Fig. 13–27). The cusps of the valve are sometimes destroyed. The vegetations are teeming with streptococci, and these are discharged into the blood stream where they can be detected by blood culture. This procedure is of great value in the diagnosis of difficult or suspected cases.

The most striking feature of the disease is the formation of large numbers of emboli due to the breaking off of fragments of the friable vegetations. These sail off into the blood stream and come to rest in various organs, where the emboli give rise to characteristic symptoms of the disease. Some of the emboli are large, and if these lodge in the blood vessels of the brain, they may cause paralysis or abscesses, whereas in the kidney they may cause blood to appear in the urine. Sometimes they are minute, but if these tiny

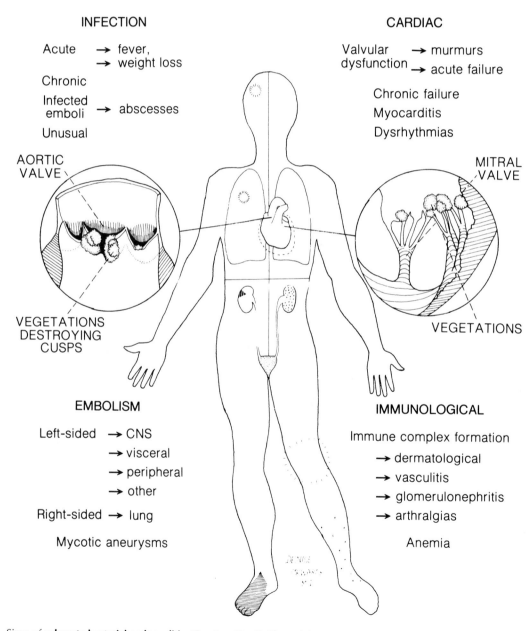

Fig. 13–28 Signs of **subacute bacterial endocarditis**. (Courtesy Dr. D. Skwarok.)

Fig. 13–29 This is a photograph of destructive bacterial endocarditis, destroying the noncoronary cusp of the aortic valve. This leads to aortic valve insufficiency and left ventricular failure. (McGill University, Department of Pathology Museum.)

emboli should lodge in the smallest vessels of the skin, they will cause these vessels to rupture, with the formation of multiple pinpoint hemorrhages known as petechiae. Petechiae in the skin, blood in the urine, and streptococci in the blood culture, together with enlargement of the spleen and long-continued fever, are principal clinical features that point to the correct diagnosis. The low-grade fever combined with any known valvular heart lesion or heart murmurs should clinch the diagnosis (Fig. 13–28).

Acute Infectious Endocarditis. This is a much rarer form of endocarditis caused by enormous numbers of pyogenic bacteria such as *Staphylococcus aureus* and *Streptococcus hemolyticus*. The cusps of the valves are rapidly destroyed (hence the term acute) (Fig. 13–29), and the patient used to die in less than 6 weeks without antibiotic therapy. Today, early surgical removal of the infected valve, together with antibiotic therapy, has improved the life expectancy of such patients.

Five types of disease of the heart have been outlined, together with the four principal valvular lesions. Practically nothing has been said about diseases of the myocardium, apart from the effect of coronary artery occlusion, nor about the pericardium, which may be involved in various forms of inflammation in addition to rheumatic pericarditis. Such discussions would be out of place in this *Introduction*. It may be mentioned, in addition, that tumors of the heart, both benign and malignant, do occur, but fortunately are rare.

CLINICAL PATTERNS OF HEART DISEASE

The chief symptoms of heart disease are pain, palpitation, and dyspnea or shortness of breath. Pain has already been discussed in connection with coronary artery occlusion. Palpitation, a condition in which the

patient becomes aware of the forcible beating of the heart, may be a symptom either of valvular or myocardial disease. Frequently, however, it does not indicate any organic heart disease, but rather is caused by anxiety, too much stress (often associated with too much tea or coffee), or perhaps by such a disorder as hyperthyroidism. Disorders of rhythm may take the form of increased rate (tachycardia) or irregularity of rhythm, occasional beats being missed. Murmurs, which may be heard with the stethoscope, are caused by the blood leaking back through an incompetent valve or forcing its way through a stenosed one. Heart block is a condition in which the pulse rate drops to about one-half the normal, and is caused by scars or inflammation often due to coronary artery disease interfering with the "conduction bundle," which carries the electric impulse necessary for muscular contraction from one part of the heart to the other.

Dyspnea is the most common symptom of heart failure. The shortness of breath is caused by the inability of the failing heart to move blood through the lungs. Fainting attacks (syncope) may occur in aortic valvular incompetence because part of the blood, instead of going to the brain, escapes back into the left ventricle. This causes cerebral ischemia, which is the primary cause of most fainting attacks. Congestive heart failure is a picture presented by patients, the right side of whose heart is becoming exhausted, and is particularly well seen in mitral stenosis. There is damming back of the blood in the veins that empty into the right atrium, so that the veins in the neck stand out prominently; the liver is enlarged and tender because the blood accumulates in its substance (Fig. 13–30). The lips, ears, and fingers are cyanosed or blue because of insufficient oxygenation of the blood flowing through them, for it is the presence of oxygen that imparts to the blood in the arteries its bright red color.

Edema generally is evidence of congestive heart failure, although it may also be caused by other conditions, such as kidney disease. In heart disease, it occurs because the hydrostatic pressure of the venous end of the capillary circulation is raised, and interstitial fluid gradually increases in volume and collects in the tissues; it is most marked in the feet and legs, where it causes a swelling in which a depression can be made by steady pressure of the finger (pitting on pressure). The reason for this transudation of fluid from the blood vessels is partly the increased pressure in the microcirculation caused by the back pressure from the heart, and partly damage to the vessel walls with an increase of their permeability owing to an insufficient supply of the oxygen that is necessary for their own health.

NORMAL

HEART FAILURE

RIGHT HEART FAILURE

INCREASED VENOUS PRESSURE
    SYSTEMIC CIRCULATION

STASIS OF CIRCULATION

ANOXEMIA OF VISCERA

DECREASED LIVER FUNCTION

HEPATOMEGALY

ASCITES

PEDAL EDEMA

LEFT HEART FAILURE

INCREASED VENOUS PRESSURE—
    PULMONARY CIRCULATION

PULMONARY EDEMA

DECREASED KIDNEY PERFUSION

SODIUM RETENTION

WATER RETENTION

INCREASED BLOOD VOLUME

hepatomegaly

ascites

H$_2$O

H$_2$O

edema

Fig. 13–30   This diagram illustrates end-stage **congestive heart failure** and many of its complications. The primary lesion is in the heart, whose ability to pump blood forward becomes severely compromised. This leads to venous congestion and to reduced arterial blood flow. The inset shows the *normal balanced circulation.*

Congenital heart disease has its own special signs and symptoms. Cyanosis is the most characteristic of these signs, sometimes being present from the moment the blue baby makes its appearance in the world, but usually developing later. Dyspnea on exertion is equally common, but may range from the slightest to the most severe. Polycythemia (increased number of red blood cells), which is compensatory in nature, serves for a time to offset the deficiency in oxygen. Clubbing of the fingers, one of the most striking of the physical signs, is due to a disturbance of nutrition of the tissues that affects both the terminal phalanges and the nails, the latter becoming thickened and curved. Cerebral symptoms such as faintness, dizziness, and even syncope are frequent owing to the anoxia.

Perhaps the most important fact to remember is that the majority of people with structural heart disease are able to lead useful lives. The discovery that a cardiac murmur is present does not mean that the patient's whole mode of life has to be changed. Someone with valvular disease of the heart may live comfortably for many years due to the compensatory ability of the heart muscle.

Sometimes one can do little about the underlying heart disease, but the edema can be treated in most cases. The most important part of the treatment is the use of a diet that is low in salt. In heart failure, salt tends to be retained. This results in the retention of water and in edema. Salt and water can be eliminated from the body by the use of diuretics. After an episode of heart failure, the patient may again be able to resume activity, but may be instructed to limit exertion until he has acquired a tolerance for physical activity. This may be done with a supervised rehabilitation program. Education of the patient with heart disease as to the mode of life best suited to him is a most important item in the treatment. Too great solicitude can be as unfortunate as too great recklessness.

Finally, it must be remembered that no organ is influenced to so marked a degree by nervous stimuli and the emotions. The simple everyday words of our language testify to the truth of this statement. We say that the person is heavyhearted, hardhearted, heartless, good-hearted, that his heart aches with loneliness, flutters with alarm, or stops with fear. It is evi-

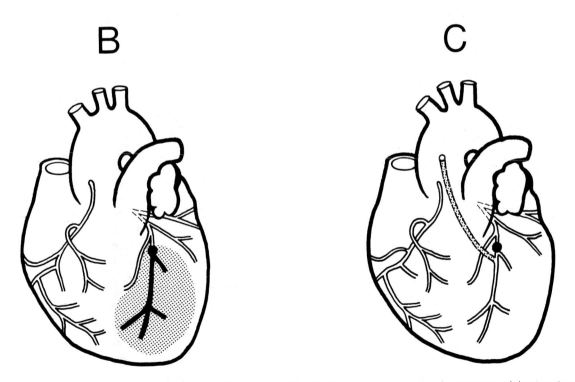

Fig. 13–31 *A* shows the normal coronary circulation, which supplies blood to the heart. (Reprinted with permission of the American Heart Association.) In *B*, an infarct has occluded the anterior descending branch of the left coronary artery. This has cut off the blood supply to that portion of the left ventricle that is supplied by this vessel. The infarct results in tissue damage or death. *C* illustrates an aortocoronary bypass. A vein graft (usually from the patient's leg), is attached to the aorta at one end and to the coronary artery at the other, beyond the occlusion.

dent that many cardiac symptoms may have an emotional rather than an organic basis, and to confuse one with the other is a serious matter for both the physician and the patient.

HEART TRANSPLANTATION

The general subject of tissue transplantation has already been discussed. Transplantation of the heart or mechanical replacement has naturally aroused keener interest and greater excitement than in the case of any other organ. The principal problem is rejection of the transplanted heart, a problem that has not yet been completely solved, in spite of the use of many immunosuppressive drugs. Indeed the heart sometimes seems more vulnerable to rejection than the kidney. This may be because we have vastly more experience with kidney transplants than with heart transplants. Kidney transplantation has been successful now for nearly 50 years. The rejection of the heart may be early, in 1 to 4 weeks, or later, in weeks or months, with occlusion of the coronary arteries. It is evident that immunosuppressive therapy must become more efficient and cyclosporine has achieved this. One patient has survived 20 years with a heart transplant.

Over 2,000 heart transplants will have been carried out in the 20 years since the first. The cost effectiveness of this procedure will always be debated; it is currently three times as expensive as routine valve replacement or as aortocoronary bypass procedures. Lack of suitable donors remains a major obstacle; one-third of patients accepted into a program die before a donor heart becomes available. In the best hands, however, there is nearly a 70% 1-year survival rate, and nearly a 60% 5-year survival rate (Shumway). The

considered opinion today, however, is that heart transplantation offers therapy for only a few carefully selected patients with end-stage heart disease who would surely die without it. It is a last resort, if you will, rather than a panacea for most pains in the chest.

AORTOCORONARY BYPASS SURGERY

The surgical approach to the treatment of vascular disease of the coronary arteries has now developed to the point where it is being demanded by almost every anxious man over 40 with pain in the chest. The existence of the technical feasibility does not obscure our ignorance of its real value in prolonging life. As this is written, it is not clear that this expensive procedure ($35,000), which now has an acceptable operative mortality (0.5 to 3%) does improve prognosis. It does seem to alleviate the disabling angina in most cases (80%), and exercise testing shows that more than half the patients who have the procedure gain benefit. In this domain, however, psychogenic factors have been recognized as playing a major role for at least three decades. A comparative study of the effects of medical versus surgical management of coronary artery disease has demonstrated though, for one class of patient, the A-C bypass (Fig. 13–31) offers better results than more conservative medical treatment. The present indications for surgery are stable angina pectoris, which is disabling, unstable angina which is medically uncontrolled, or symptomatic patients with angiographic evidence of left main coronary artery stenosis. It is felt by most conservative and thoughtful physicians that each case must be decided on its own merits, and the decision for operation should be made on factors other than prolongation of life.

SYNOPSIS

Heart muscle supplies blood for two circulations: the systemic and pulmonary.

Preload, afterload, contractility, and heart rate are the principal determinants of cardiac output.

Heart function can be assessed by measuring pressure, flow, size, sounds, electrical activity, and the presence of muscle enzymes in the serum.

The heart has a limited adaptability to work, but its effectiveness can be improved by training.

Heart diseases may be classified by several different methods, e.g., endocardial, myocardial, pericardial or congenital, vascular, metabolic, infectious, inflammatory, iatrogenic, idiopathic, or on some other taxonomic basis.

Complications of ischemic heart disease are: failure, arrhythmias, rupture, thrombus, embolism, and aneurysm.

Complications of congenital heart disease include: failure, shunts, compensatory hypertrophy, pulmonary hypertension, polycythemia, and endocarditis.

Complications of valvular heart disease depend on the valve or combinations of valves involved and include: failure, arrhythmias, dilatation, hypertrophy, sudden death, thrombosis, embolism and endocarditis.

Terms

Myocardium

Endocardium

Pericardium

Systole

Diastole

Tamponade

Essential hypertension

Septal defect

Coarctation

Valvular stenosis

Valvular insufficiency

Pancarditis

Endocarditis

Syncope

Angina pectoris

Aortocoronary bypass

FURTHER READING

Editorial: Images of the heart. Br. Med., J., 285:527, 1982.

Abrams, J.L.: Coronary arteriography: pathologic and prognostic implications. AJR, 139:1, 1982.

Baum, D., Bernstein, D., Starnes, V.A., et al.: Pediatric heart transplantation at Stanford: Results of a 15-year experience. Pediatrics, 88:203, 1991.

Braunwald, E.: Regulation of the circulation. N. Engl. J. Med., 290:1124, 1974.

Braunwald, E., Ross, J., Jr., and Sonnenblick, E.H.: *Mechanisms of Contraction of the Normal and Failing Heart.* Boston, Little, Brown and Co., 1968.

Burke, M.: Viral myocarditis. Histopathology, 17:193, 1990.

Connolly, J.E.: The history of coronary artery surgery. J. Thorac. Cardiovasc. Surg., 76:733, 1978.

Copeland, J.G., Emay, R.W., et al.: Selection of patients for cardiac transplantation. Circulation, 75:2, 1987.

DeBold, A.J.: Atrial naturietic factor. Science, 230:767, 1985.

DeFeudis, F.V.: Coronary atherosclerosis: Current therapeutic approaches and future trends. Life Sciences, 49:689, 1991.

E.P.S.I.M. Research Group: A controlled comparison of aspirin and oral anticoagulants in prevention of death after myocardial infarction. N. Engl. J. Med., 307:701, 1982.

Fuster, V., et al.: Mechanisms of disease: the pathogenesis of coronary artery disease and the acute coronary syndromes (First of Two Parts). N. Engl. J. Med., 326:242, 1992.

Gomez-Marin, O., et al.: Improvement in long-term survival among patients hospitalized with acute myocardial infarction, 1970 to 1980: The Minnesota Heart Survey. N. Engl. J. Med., 316:1353, 1987.

Gould, S.E.: *Pathology of the Heart*, 3rd Ed. Springfield, Charles C Thomas, 1968.

Griffith, B.P., Hardesty, R.L., et al.: Heart-lung transplantation: lessons learned and future hopes. Ann. Thor. Surg., 43:6, 1987.

Grobbee, D.E., et al.: Coffee, caffeine and cardiovascular disease in man. N. Engl. J. Med., 323:1026, 1990.

Gruentzig, A.R., et al.: Long-term follow-up after percutaneous transluminal coronary angioplasty: The early Zurich experience. N. Engl. J. Med., 316:1127, 1987.

Hager, W.D., and Kats, A.M.: Management of shock in acute myocardial infarction: Changing concepts; past, present, and future. Cardiol., 74:286, 1987.

Hillis, L.D., and Braunwald, E.: Coronary-artery spasm. N. Engl. J. Med., 299:695, 1978.

I.S.A.M. Study Group: A Prospective trial of intravenous streptokinase in acute myocardial infarction (I.S.A.M.): Mortality, morbidity, and infarct size at 21 days. N. Engl. J. Med., 314:1465, 1987.

Isom, O.W., et al.: Does coronary bypass increase longevity? J. Thorac. Cardiovasc. Surg., 75:28, 1978.

Jude, J.R., Kouwenhoven, W.B., and Knickerbocker, G.G.: Cardiac arrest: report of application of external cardiac massage of 118 patients. J.A.M.A., 178:1063, 1961.

Kieller, L.H., and Perper, J.A.: Sudden-death and the decline in coronary heart disease mortality. J. Clin. Dis., 39:1001, 1986.

Leaf, A., and Weber, P.C.: Cardiovascular effects of n-3 fatty acids. N. Engl. J. Med., 318:549, 1988.

Little, R.C., and Little, W.C.: Cardiac preload, afterload, and heart failure. Arch. Intern. Med., 142:819, 1982.

Luchi, R.J., et al.: Comparison of medical and surgical treatment for unstable angina pectoris: results of a veterans administration cooperative study. N. Engl. J. Med., 316:977, 1987.

McCaffrey, F.M., Braden, D.S., and Strong, W.B.: Sudden cardiac death in young athletes. Sports Med., 145:177, 1991.

Muller, J.E., et al.: Myocardial infarct extension: Occurrence, outcome, and risk factors in the multicenter investigation of limitation of infarct size. Ann. Intern. Med., 108:1, 1988.

Murphy, J.G., Gersh, B.J., McGoon, M.D., et al.: Long-term outcome after surgical repair of isolated atrial septal defect— follow-up at 27 to 32 years. N. Engl. J. Med., 323:1645, 1990.

Paffenbarger, R.S., Jr., and Hale, W.E.: Work activity and coronary heart mortality. N. Engl. J. Med., 292:545, 1975.

Parisi, A.F., Folland, E.D., and Hartigan, P.: A comparison of angioplasty with medical therapy in the treatment of single-vessel coronary artery disease. N. Engl. J. Med., 326:10, 1992.

Ragland, D.R., and Brand, R.J.: Type A behavior and mortality from coronary heart disease. N. Engl. J. Med., 318:65, 1988.

Relman, A.S.: Artificial hearts—permanent and temporary. N. Engl. J. Med., 314:644, 1986.

Shumway, N.E., and Stinson, E.B.: Two decades of experimental and clinical orthotopic homotransplantation of the heart. Perspect. Biol. Med., 22:S81, 1979.

Smith, M., and Little, W.C.: Potential precipitating factors of the onset of myocardial infarction. Am. J. Med. Sci., 303:141, 1992.

Stary, H.C.: Regression of atherosclerosis in primates. Virchows Arch. Path. Anat., 383:117, 1979.

Sytkowski, P.A., Kannel, W.B., and D'Agostino, R.B.: Changes in risk factors and the decline in mortality from cardiovascular disease. N. Engl. J. Med., 322:1635, 1990.

Taussig, H.B.: *Congenital Malformations of the Heart*, 2nd Ed. Cambridge, New York Commonwealth Fund, 1960.

Tosteson, A.N.A., et al.: Long term impact of smoking cessation on the incidence of coronary heart disease. Am. J. Publ. Health, 80:1481, 1990.

Weinblatt, E., et al.: Relation of education to sudden death after myocardial infarction. N. Engl. J. Med., 299:60, 1978.

APPENDIX

Function of the Heart

The heart is a hollow muscular pump whose function is to circulate the blood through the body. It is a common misconception to think that the heart is the master of the

Fig. A13–1 This diagram illustrates interactions between components that regulate cardiac activity. (From Braunwald, E.: Regulation of the circulation. N. Engl. J. Med., 290:1124, 1974.)

body; the reverse is more reasonable—that the heart is the servant of the body and is subject to many forces, as shown in Figure A13–1. It sends venous blood to the lungs, where oxygen is taken up and carbon dioxide given off, and then pumps oxygenated blood to the tissues, where the oxygen is used.

The heart can be trained or will adapt to training. With regular exercise, the amount of blood that is expelled with each contraction can be increased, and the rate of the heart will be lowered. An Olympic athlete may have a heart rate as low as 40 beats per minute, half the resting rate of a sedentary office worker.

We do not know actually what makes the heart beat, although we know a lot about what regulates its rate. What we call the beat is a contraction, similar to that of other muscles, but, unlike other muscles, the beat can go on after the nerves that supply the heart are cut, and even after the animal (or person) is dead. The contraction of the myocardium, which drives the blood out of the ventricles into the arteries, is known as systole. The succeeding relaxation during which the cavities become refilled with blood from the veins is called diastole (Fig. A13–2). In health, valves prevent a backflow of blood from the arteries into the right and left ventricles, and from the ventricles into the atria. The sinoatrial (auricular) node, a small area of specialized tissue in the upper part of the right atrium close to the entry of the superior vena cava, is called the pacemaker. A current of electricity passes through the myocardium from the sinoatrial node each time the heart beats. Impulses pass out in all directions, reaching the ventricle, where they are carried by a specialized branch of muscular and nervous tissue called the atrioventricular bundle of His. If this bundle is interfered with by disease, the result is known as heart block, which is characterized by a much slower rate of con-

traction, because the impulses are generated separately in atria and ventricles.

There are many ways in which medical treatment can influence the pacemaker, some old, such as digitalis, originally an infusion or brew made from the leaves of the purple foxglove, *Digitalis purpurea* or ladies' fingers, and some new, such as the electric pacemaker. When the heart is diseased, a quivering of the atria in place of a regular beat often sets in, known as atrial or auricular fibrillation. Impulses now pass into the bundle of His so rapidly that the ventricles respond irregularly and ineffectively.

The electric pacemaker has been used in those serious cases of heart block known as Adams-Stokes disease (also called Stokes-Adams disease) with a slow pulse rate, which may be associated with severe congestive heart failure. The condition may be a later after-effect of myocardial infarction involving the bundle of His. A tiny transistorized pacemaker driven by a long-life battery may be placed under the skin of the abdominal wall and connected to electrodes implanted in the heart muscle. Heart block is now overcome and a new rate is established. The cardiac output may be best at induced rates different from that of the natural sinoatrial pacemaker.

An electric current is normally generated in the contracting myocardium. When this is recorded it is an electrocardiogram. This shows a series of waves, known by the letters Q, R, and S, due to contraction of the ventricles (Fig. A13–3). The accompanying diagram relates the electrical activity system to the other functions of the heart (Fig. A13–4). In heart disease, these waves may show a change in shape and position, which may help the physician to arrive at an explanation for the alterations in function (Table A13–1).

When the normal heart is listened to with the assistance

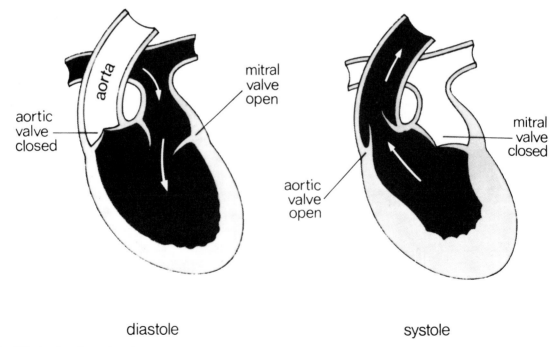

diastole   systole

Fig. A13–2   This drawing shows the relative sizes and positions of the mitral valve, left ventricle, aortic valve, and aorta in diastole and systole, illustrating that the pump depends not only on contractions but on the integrity of the valves.

of a stethoscope applied to the chest wall, two heart sounds are heard. The first sound is longer, softer, and of deeper pitch than the second sound. The first sound, which is caused partly by contraction of the heart muscle and partly by closure of the valves (mitral and tricuspid) between the atria and ventricles, is likened to "lubb;" the second sound, short, hard and of a higher pitch, is represented by "dup." A change in the quality of these sounds may indicate disease of the valves.

The rate of the heartbeat, i.e., the pulse, varies. The normal rhythm of the heart depends on the balance of two sets of nervous impulses, one tending to slow, the other to accelerate the heart's action. Both nerves belong to the involuntary or autonomic nervous system. The vagus nerve is responsible for the retarding impulses; acetylcholine is liberated at the nerve endings of the vagus and acts on the heart muscle. The accelerating impulses pass along the sym-

pathetic nerve fibers, and another substance is liberated at their nerve endings. In the resting heart the influence of the slowing vagal impulses is greater. If all nervous input to the heart were removed, the heart would beat at approximately 100/min. The quickening of the heartbeat that results from emotion, the feeling that your heart is in your mouth or in your boots, is due to a disequilibrium in the exquisite balance that normally exists between these sets of influences.

Heart rate also depends on the demand of the tissues for oxygen. The runner's heart beats faster and he breathes more quickly in response to an increase in this demand. Muscular work is an expenditure of energy, and energy is obtained from the oxidation of food. As food cannot normally be burned without oxygen, the heartbeat is quickened and breathing becomes deeper and faster to supply this need.

The condition of the blood vessels must also be taken into

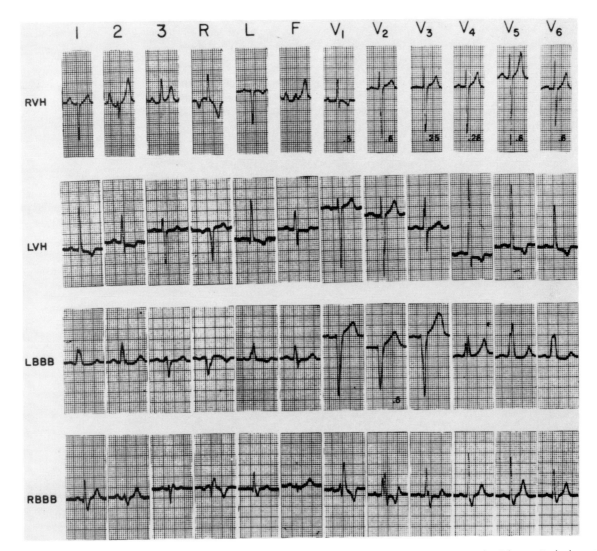

Fig. A13–3   Shown here is the typical appearance of electrocardiograms in a variety of abnormal conditions, namely, right ventricular hypertrophy (RVH), left ventricular hypertrophy (LVH), left bundle branch block (LBBB), and right bundle branch block (RBBB). The numbers at the top of the illustration are the numbers of the electrocardiographic leads. Compare the direction and amplitude of the QRS complex in lead 1 in RVH and LVH. Their opposite direction results from the different ventricular mass; hypertrophy of the right ventricle in one instance, the left in the other. (From Wintrobe, M., et al. (Eds.): *Harrison's Principles of Internal Medicine*, 7th Ed. New York, McGraw-Hill, 1974.)

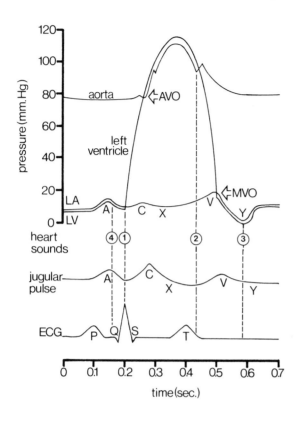

Fig. A13–4 Simultaneous ECG, pressures obtained from the left atrium, left ventricle, and aorta, and the jugular pulse during one cardiac cycle. For simplification, right heart pressures have been omitted. Normal right atrial pressure closely parallels that of the left atrium, and right ventricular and pulmonary artery pressures correspond closely to their left heart counterparts, except that the former are reduced in magnitude. The normal mitral and aortic valve closures precede tricuspid and pulmonic closures, respectively, whereas valve opening reverses this order. The jugular venous pulse lags behind the right atrial pressure.

During the course of one cardiac cycle, the electrical events (ECG) initiate and therefore precede the mechanical (pressure) events, and the latter precede the auscultatory events (heart sounds) that the mechanical events themselves produce. Shortly after the P wave, the atria contract to produce A wave; a fourth heart sound may succeed the latter. The QRS complex initiates ventricular systole, followed shortly by left ventricular contraction and by the rapid build-up or left ventricular (LV) pressure. Almost immediately, LV pressure exceeds left atrial (LA) pressure. This imbalance closes the mitral valve and produces the first heart sound. When LV pressure exceeds aortic pressure, the aortic valve opens (AVO), and when aortic pressure is once again greater than LV pressure, the aortic valve closes, which produces the second heart sound and terminates ventricular ejection. The decreasing LV pressure drops below LA pressure to open the mitral valve (MVO), and a period of rapid ventricular filling commences. During this time, a third heart sound may be heard. (From Andreoli, K. G., et al.: *Comprehensive Cardiac Care*, 4th Ed. St. Louis, C. V. Mosby Co., 1979; modified with permission from Hurst, J. W., et al.: *The Heart, Arteries, and Veins*, 3rd Ed. New York, McGraw-Hill, 1974.)

account in any consideration of the heart's action. When the heart pumps blood into the arteries, it does so against a certain amount of resistance (peripheral resistance). This resistance may become too high or too low in pathologic conditions; in hypertension, narrowing of the arterioles increases the peripheral resistance, whereas in shock, there may be little or no peripheral resistance. No organ works continually at its maximum capacity; the heart has a large amount of reserve in order to cope with emergencies. When hypertension develops, the heart adapts to the increased workload by hypertrophy or increase in the muscle mass. We call this compensatory hypertrophy. In the course of

Table A13–1.   Elements of Electrocardiography

	PATHOLOGY/ABNORMALITIES
P Wave Represents spread of electrical impulse from atria (activation or depolarization of atria)	Increase in amplitude usually indicates atrial hypertrophy in atrioventricular valve disease, hypertension, cor pulmonale congenital heart disease
PR Interval Measures time taken by impulse to travel all the way from SA node to ventricular muscle fibers	PR interval may be increased in congenital disease, rheumatic heart disease, or from drugs (digitalis) as well as in heart block (ischemic)
QRS Complex Represents spread of impulse from ventricular muscle (activation or depolarization of ventricles)	(1) an increase in duration indicates abnormal intraventricular conduction, usually meaning block of 1 of the bundle branches (2) if the amplitude is too low, it may indicate cardiac failure, widespread myocardial damage
T Wave Represents recovery period of ventricles when they recruit their spent electrical forces (repolarization)	Unusually tall T waves suggest myocardial infarct of K^+ intoxication, or myocardial ischemia without infarction. Low T wave indicates low K^+
QT Duration From beginning of QRS to end of T represents total duration of ventricular systole	(1) Prolonged QT occurs in congestive heart failure, myocardial infarction, hypocalcemia (2) QT can be shortened by digitalis, Ca excess, K^+ intoxication

HEART RATE

AFTER LOAD
diastolic pressure

CARDIAC
OUTPUT

PRELOAD
stretching of
ventricular muscle

CONTRACTILITY
OF HEART MUSCLE

MUSCLE CONDITION

Fig. A13–5 This diagram illustrates the relationship between cardiac output and several different factors. Cardiac output depends on the interrelationship of all the factors shown. If the heart rate falls below 40/min or exceeds 180/min, the cardiac output cannot support normal metabolic requirements. If the ventricular muscle is not slightly stretched, the ventricle will not contract with sufficient force to provide an adequate systolic pressure to maintain the circulation. If the myocardial muscle is deprived of oxygen or if it is subject to either an excess or a deficiency of potassium, the muscle will not be able to contract, regardless of the rate per minute or of the stretch of the muscle. Thus all the factors shown are important in the maintenance of cardiac output.

time or because of disease of the heart muscle, this power may fail and decompensation sets in.

The amount of blood that the heart puts out is determined by several factors (Fig. A13–5). We can organize them under four headings. Many years ago, the English physiologist Starling observed that the heart responded as any other muscle to stretch. He stated that the strength of contraction was proportional to the filling of the heart. This concept, that stretching the ventricular musculature results in increased cardiac output, is referred to as **preload.**

Clearly, the effectiveness of each contraction of heart muscle depends on the state of health of the muscle, which in turn depends on its nutritional supply, e.g., the correct amount of intracellular potassium and calcium. The well-being of cardiac muscle governs the strength of contraction and is a determinant of cardiac output. This state is called the **contractility** of heart muscle.

Within the hydraulics of the vascular system, the pressure for continuous perfusion of the capillaries (diastolic pressure) and the size of the left ventricle, which dictates the pressure that is developed by the muscle fibers (wall tension), are factors that govern how much blood can be delivered with each systole into the aorta. This notion is called **afterload** in contemporary nomenclature.

Finally, the **rate** at which the heart beats naturally affects the circulatory efficiency, so that heart rate is important in a consideration of the mechanics of the circulation.

14

BLOOD VESSELS

A man is as old as his arteries.—SYDENHAM

This chapter should be regarded as a direct extension of the preceding, just as the arterial tree and vascular system are in continuity with the heart, and cannot be separated from it, speaking from a functional point of view. In this section we discuss the arterial tree (Figs. 14–1 and 14–2) and its diseases, review the relationship of atherosclerosis to hypertension, and then go on to discuss disorders of the venous circulation. In earlier chapters, we considered such disorders of the circulation as thrombosis, embolism, edema, and shock; there is no need to include them here.

ARTERIES

A sound heart is greatly to be desired, since it has to pump from 9 to 10 tons of blood every day, but if it must do so into a diseased arterial tree, it will have its work greatly increased. The aorta acts not just as a tube, such as a garden hose or a piece of plumbing, but as an elastic reservoir, which receives a cupful of blood from each heartbeat by distending in an elastic way so as to cushion the body from this jolting shock. The effect of each heartbeat can be visualized by crossing one leg over the other knee and watching the movement made with each heartbeat by the foot that hangs as a pendulum. As the arteries lose their elasticity with age or disease, or if the aortic valve loses its competence, the shock of each heartbeat becomes more abrupt, until the whole head will shake with the force of each beat. The value of the elastic recoil of the aorta is to provide a reservoir of energy that permits continuous flow through the capillary bed during the intervals between each beat, much as one builds up pressure in a better grade garden sprayer, which permits the vapor to continue to cover foliage between pumping actions. To achieve this important facility of continuous perfusion, we have evolved blood vessels that consist of three layers, an inner coat (intima), which includes the nonwettable lining cells, the endothelium; a middle coat composed mainly of muscle (media), which includes elastic tissue in the arteries and arterioles; and an outer coat of connective tissue, the adventitia (Figs. 14–3 and 14–4).

We must not forget, however, that the 100,000-km network of the blood vessels of the body is composed largely of capillaries (Figs. 14–5 and 14–6), which form connecting links between the arteries and veins and which allow all the exchange to take place within a tissue. These links are about 10 microns (μ) in diameter, and their walls are only 1 μ thick, an ideal structure for the passage of substrates and oxygen between the circulating blood and the tissues.

The principal site of resistance or cause of work for the heart is the arteriolar bed, the small precapillary muscular arterioles, which respond to pressor agents, such as angiotensin, and to the increase of salt and water that occurs in heart and kidney failure (Fig. 14–7).

Diseases of the arteries are among the most common causes of morbidity and mortality in people of middle age and later life. These diseases belong to two groups: those that are sometimes called degenerative and are represented principally by arteriosclerosis, and those that are inflammatory and are often grouped under the heading of arteritis. Numerically, instances of arteritis are uncommon, whereas arteriosclerosis is so universal in the western world that we usually consider it to be a concomitant of aging. In fact, we exclaim when an elderly person is found to exhibit only a little arteriosclerosis at autopsy.

Arteriosclerosis

Before describing arteriosclerosis (Fig. 14–8), it may be well to mention that the arteries can be divided into three main groups: (1) the larger or elastic arteries, such as the aorta and its main branches; (2) the

Fig. 14—1 This drawing from Vesalius shows the distribution of the arterial tree of the whole human body. Wood engraving from Andreas Vesalius, *De Humani Corporis Fabrica*.

form of arteriosclerosis that commonly predisposes a person to thrombosis, which lends to atherosclerosis a sinister significance.

This patchy or nodular thickening of the intima of the artery, with accumulations of lipid, often results in narrowing of the lumen (Fig. 14–9). The blood supply may be cut down to the danger point, and a thrombus is apt to form on the diseased wall and to obstruct the narrowed lumen. It is worth recognizing, however, that an artery may be lined with atheromas or plaques and still be functional. The normal perfusion does not fall off until more than two-thirds of the diameter of any vessel lumen is occluded. If obstruction has been gradual, as sometimes occurs in the femoral artery, even complete occlusion may not cause symptoms, because a collateral circulation has had time to develop. This presupposes that the demand for arterial oxygen remains relatively constant and that a collateral circulation is available to compensate for the obstruction. Unfortunately, in some situations (some hearts) collateral circulation is not available, and sometimes the demands are unusual and excessive (as in snow shovelling), and the narrowing due to atheromatous plaques is sufficient to result in serious or fatal ischemia. This is the mechanism of production of coronary thrombosis, cerebral thrombosis, and thrombosis in the arteries of the leg. Atherosclerosis is an extremely common condition and is the chief cause of ischemia of the heart muscle, the brain, and the extremities.

At different times, emphasis has been placed on different aspects of the anatomic lesions: on the abundance of lipid, on the presence of fibrous tissue, on the smooth muscle hyperplasia, on the intimal injury, and on the deposition of platelets and thrombus material. The significance of atherosclerosis lies in its potential to (1) obstruct, (2) weaken the wall of the vessel, and (3) predispose a person to thrombus formation and all its complications.

Etiology. It is remarkable that, in spite of the frequency of atherosclerosis and the enormous amount of time and money expended in its investigation, we know as little about its real cause as about the cause of cancer. That is to say, we know a great deal, but the pieces of the puzzle are not yet in place to reveal the total pattern. This lack of comprehension has proved to be an obstacle to devising some method of preventing this crippling and often fatal condition, which is the curse of the declining years of life. It is perhaps better to speak of the pathogenesis of atherosclerosis, rather than of its etiology, which implies a causal agent. The large amount of experimental work has brought forth several lines of thought, but unfortunately the natural condition is almost exclusively a

medium-sized distributing or muscular arteries, which carry the blood from the main trunks to the various organs and tissues; (3) the small arteries and arterioles, which extend from the ends of the distributing arteries to the capillary beds. Arteriosclerosis is a general term that really signifies hardening of the arteries; arteriolosclerosis is a medial and intimal hyperplasia of arterioles.

Atherosclerosis is a term best reserved for the local lesion in the wall of the artery. It is a focal process—composed of fat-laden cells, smooth muscle cells, collagen, and fibrin and platelets—that affects principally the large arteries, especially the aorta and its main branches, but also the small arteries, particularly the coronary and cerebral arteries. This is the

Fig. 14-2 This graph illustrates the mean radius of the branchings of the aorta and its major vessels. (From Fry, Griggs, Jr., and Greenfield, Jr.: In vivo studies of pulsatile blood flow. In *Pulsatile Blood Flow*. Edited by Attinger. New York, McGraw-Hill, 1963.)

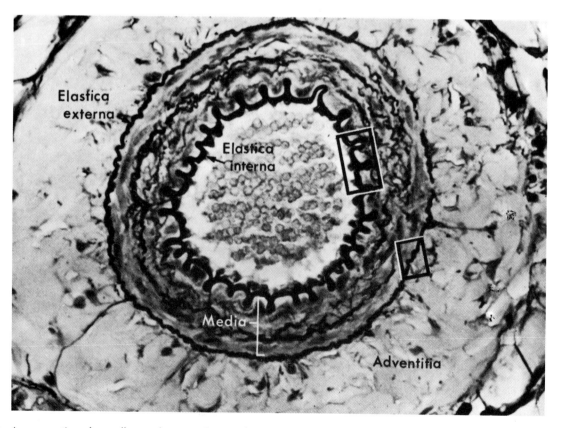

Fig. 14-3 A cross section of a small muscular artery showing the internal and external elastic lamellae, and the relative thickness of the wall. (From Bloom, W., and Fawcett, D. W.: *A Textbook of Histology*, 10th Ed. Philadelphia, W. B. Saunders Co., 1975.)

322

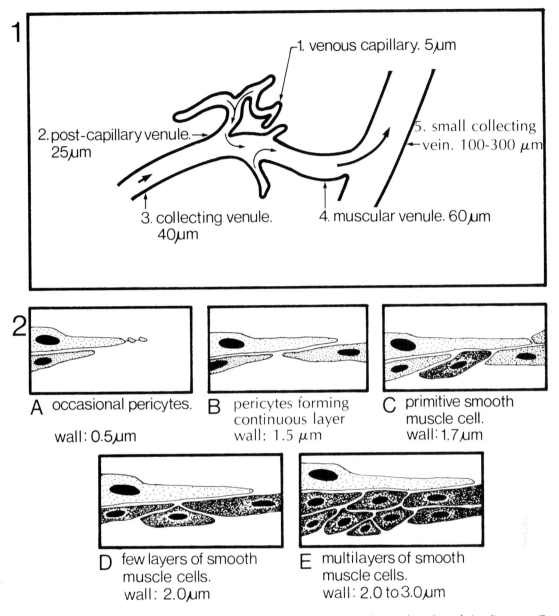

Fig. 14–4   These drawings show the relationship of the capillary bed and its cell walls to the venule and its relative diameters. (From Rhodin, J. A. G.: Ultrastructure of mammalian venous capillaries, venules and small collecting veins. *J. Ultrastruct. Res.*, 25:452, 1968.)

human disease, and does not occur spontaneously in the laboratory animal.

There have been many attempts to create a unifying hypothesis to explain all the observations, but before we enter the realm of hypotheses, it is better to record some of the observations themselves.

1. Atherosclerosis increases with age. It is significantly more noticeable in those who live to 60, but there are exceptions and some octogenarians die with arteries a 30-year-old would be proud of.

2. It apparently progresses more rapidly in women after the menopause and seems to be more severe in men than in women under the age of 40.

3. There are worldwide differences in the severity of atherosclerosis, and many studies testify to the changing prevalence of the disease in homogeneous genetic pools as people move, for example, from Japan to Hawaii, or from Asia to North America. The disease has been characterized as being of affluent societies.

4. The disease is more severe in those with hypertension. Other risk factors of significance are

Fig. 14–5 This whole-mount preparation of the retinal vessels shows an artery (art), the adjoining capillary bed (cap), and a venule (ven), to illustrate the relative proportions of the microcirculation. (Courtesy of T. Kuwabara.)

obesity, cigarette smoking, high fat intake, an intense "achiever" personality, and coincidental disease such as diabetes mellitus.

In 1974, for the first time in two decades, the United States statistics showed a decline in the deaths attributed to coronary artery disease, atherosclerosis, and its complications.

5. A factor, the significance of which is undetermined but that may be extremely relevant to our understanding of atherosclerosis, is exercise. A sedentary occupation is clearly one of the major risk factors, and the rise in participation in physical work/exercise may be partly responsible for the leveling off in premature deaths attributable to atherosclerosis.

There is also the observation that populations that reside in areas where the water is "soft" have a higher incidence of ischemic heart disease attributable to coronary artery atherosclerosis than populations that drink "hard" water. An imbalance with respect to zinc and copper in the diet has been shown to play a role in the experimental production of atherosclerosis. Table 14–1 shows some of these relationships.

The final point is to note that atheromas are reversible. Baboons shown to have atherosclerosis from an atherogenic diet lose their plaques when placed back on a normal diet, and recent studies in man have confirmed this observation. This holds out hope for the millions of people who may regard atherosclerosis as a necessary consequence of living beyond their 20s.

These, then, are the principal observations: epidemiologic, clinical, and experimental. How do they relate to the diseased blood vessel?

The classic theories have been (1) the lipid theory, (2) the encrustation theory, and (3) the insudation theory.

The lipid theory, based principally on the presence of lipid in the wall of the aorta, and on the identification of the similarity of such lipids with those that occur in the serum, has received wide attention. It has been suggested that these lipids, which are stored or possibly synthesized by cells in the aorta, interfere partly through sheer bulk and partly because of the

Fig. 14—6 These photographs of the microcirculation of the retina show *A*, the normal capillary cells and *B*, the presence of microaneurysms in a diabetic patient. (Courtesy of Dr. S. Brownstein.)

CARDIAC OUTPUT

stroke
volume

BP
120
60

autonomic
nervous
system

BLOOD
VOLUME

PERIPHERAL
RESISTANCE

renin
NaCl
aldosterone

Fig. 14–7 This figure shows the major factors that affect the blood pressure.

inflammation that they may elicit with the normal elastic nature of the aorta. The inflammatory cells secrete enzymes that destroy the elastica; the lipid merely makes it inelastic.

Other suggestions have been that the lipid accumu-

lates (a) because of a caloric overload, and (b) because cells in the vessel wall are injured by some other unidentified process, implying that atheroma is a symptom but not the agent of the arterial change.

The second classic theory is based on (a) the observations that atheroma forms most commonly at sites of turbulence in the blood stream, where arteries divide, or at parts where smaller subdivisions arise, (b) the fact that the intima is the target for much of the injury, and (c) the similarities between the organization of a thrombus and atheromatous plaques, a fact that proposes that arteriosclerosis is the result of surface injury in which platelets and fibrin are laid down. It supposes that the lipids are the result of degradation processes that digest and deposit the materials in macrophages or in pools of cholesterol crystals.

The third most popular hypothesis has a little of both of the other two theses and states that the materials of the bloodstream enter the wall of the aorta by insudation, and that they enter the wall more rapidly under increased pressure (hypertension). The serum proteins and lipids are sequestered there, if they cannot be metabolized by the resident cells, and thereby lead to the fibrin or lipid-containing plaques that we recognize.

A fourth theory suggests that atherosclerosis really

Fig. 14–8 These whole preparations of the coronary arteries and aorta illustrate the relative amounts of atherosclerosis, ranging from 1 to 7. Seven is severe and involves thrombosis and ulceration.

Fig. 14–9   This set of photographs from experimentally induced atheromas of the carotid arteries and aortas of rats shows: *A*, some thickening in a carotid artery that has been injured; *B*, a more marked degree of atheroma in a cholesterol-fed animal; *C*, the thoracic aorta of the control animal; and *D*, the foam cells from the addition of cholesterol to the diet of a rat. (From Clowes, A.W., et al.: Regression of myointimal thickening following carotid endothelial injury and development of aortic foam cell lesions in long term hypercholesterolemic rats. Lab. Invest., 36:73, 1977. Copyright 1977 by the U.S./Cdn. Div. of the International Academy of Pathology.)

is the product of a clone of new smooth muscle cells, akin to a tumor. The new smooth muscle cells proliferate and have an abnormal metabolism, which preferentially synthesizes lipids or secretes fibrin.

All these theories have one thing in common: none explains all of the observations, and each is partly valid.

To summarize, we must acknowledge that we do not have any single explanation for this widespread disorder of blood vessels. The recognition that many factors may contribute to its development has been the greatest contribution of the last two decades (Fig. 14–10).

Arteriolosclerosis. The smaller arteries of the visceral organs such as the kidney have been designated the "intimate vasculature," or, more recently, the

microcirculation. These vessels may participate in changes similar to the changes of the aorta, with thickening of the wall and narrowing of the lumen. However, lipid deposits are seldom seen and the changes are not so dramatic. Intimal hyperplasia and medial hypertrophy, even with accumulations of fibrin, are common reactions to hypertension and are designated as arteriolosclerosis (Fig. 14–11). In cases of accelerated hypertension, there may be necrosis of these arteries, and the entity then goes by the name of *arteriolonecrosis*.

Vascular Disease and Hypertension

We might review hypertension and underscore its relationship to vascular disease at this point. Earlier,

Table 14–1. Epidemiology of Ischemic Heart Disease (IHD)

ENVIRONMENTAL CHARACTERISTICS	IHD RISK*	POSSIBLE EXPLANATION
Diets low in fat and sucrose and high in vegetable fiber	<	Have low Zn/Cu; or contain phytate, a protective chelate
Nursing of infants	<	Human milk has low Zn/Cu
Cirrhosis of the liver	<	Increased loss of Zn
Exercise	<	Zn/Cu of sweat = 16; or synthesis of muscle and bone traps Zn
Chronic kidney disease	>	Bone loss releases Zn; or Zn infused during treatment
Availability of hard water	<	Decreased absorption of Zn

*< decreased; > increased

(From Klevay, L.M.: Elements of ischemic heart disease. Perspect. Bio. Med., 20:186, 1977.)

Fig. 14–11 This photomicrograph shows the arterioles entering a glomerulus that had been subject to hypertension for many years. The lumen of the arteriole is narrowed and the wall is hyalinized. This is **arteriolosclerosis.** (McGill University, Department of Pathology Museum.)

we defined hypertension as having two components, systolic (elevations over 150 mm Hg) and diastolic (elevations over 90 mm Hg), and recognized that blood pressure readings are variable in the same person, depending on such different factors as the patient's anxiety, whether the patient is supine or standing, or whether the blood pressure cuff is appropriate to the task. For practical purposes, because the diagnosis of "hypertension" carries with it such a dread implication, it is wise to determine the blood pressure

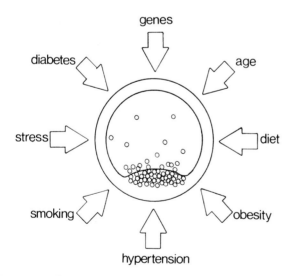

Fig. 14–10 There are no clear-cut "causes" of arteriosclerosis, but several factors are known to increase the risk of this disease. Those shown here increase the concentration of lipid in the blood as well as in the artery wall. Many of these factors are interrelated; for example, high-fat diets lead to obesity, obesity and smoking raise blood pressure. The coexistence of more than one factor increases a person's risk of arteriosclerosis and of myocardial infarction.

on three separate occasions (days) and to check the results both sitting and lying, because the anxiety of the visit to the doctor's office alone may cause a falsely high reading. After all, what one is trying to determine is the measurable level of work that the heart is called on to do during the daily life of the individual patient in question. It is important to recognize that a constant pathologic elevation of the blood pressure carries with it a considerable risk for stroke, accelerated atherosclerosis, and heart failure (Fig. 14–12).

The diagnosis of essential hypertension, as we have stated earlier, is a diagnosis of exclusion. Of all causes of hypertension, only about 6% are surgically curable (4% being due to renovascular disease, 1% to coarctation of the aorta, 1.5% to aldosterone-secreting tumors, 0.2% to Cushing's syndrome, and 0.2% to pheochromocytoma). The remainder are considered "essential."

Hypertension, however, must be put in a perspective of general occurrence. It is important to recognize that the incidence of hypertension increases with age, is higher in relatives of people with hypertension, is lower in people with active jobs (as opposed to sedentary), and is higher in people who are obese or have severe atherosclerosis.

In one primitive society in the Solomon Islands, for instance, there are two populations; one cooks its vegetable diet in sea water, the other lives nearby, a few kilometers from the sea, and uses stream water for cooking. Those with the diet enriched with salt have significantly higher blood pressures. Similarly, a group of Kenyans with low blood pressure left their

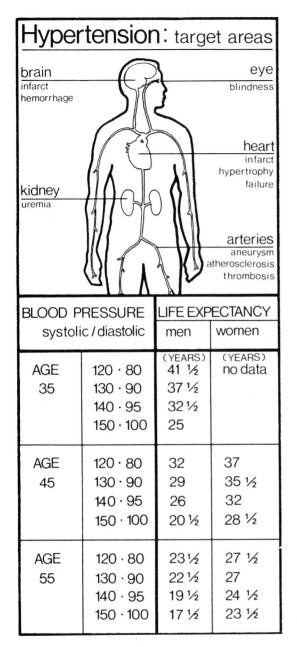

Hypertension: target areas

brain
infarct
hemorrhage

eye
blindness

heart
infarct
hypertrophy
failure

kidney
uremia

arteries
aneurysm
atherosclerosis
thrombosis

BLOOD PRESSURE		LIFE EXPECTANCY	
systolic / diastolic		men	women
AGE 35	120 · 80	(YEARS) 41 ½	(YEARS) no data
	130 · 90	37 ½	
	140 · 95	32 ½	
	150 · 100	25	
AGE 45	120 · 80	32	37
	130 · 90	29	35 ½
	140 · 95	26	32
	150 · 100	20 ½	28 ½
AGE 55	120 · 80	23 ½	27 ½
	130 · 90	22 ½	27
	140 · 95	19 ½	24 ½
	150 · 100	17 ½	23 ½

Fig. 14–12 This diagram illustrates the changes in life expectancy with elevations in blood pressure and shows the sites of complications of hypertension. (From Metropolitan Life Insurance Co.)

farms and entered the army, where they ate a diet containing as much as 18 g of salt per day. They all developed hypertension; this took about a year to occur. This effect of salt on blood pressure is probably one of the most important environmental factors in producing hypertension, and our diets are routinely rich in salt. It seems clear from studies on rats that not all individuals in any population are susceptible to such a factor as increased salt in the diet.

Hypertension is clearly known to accelerate the

process of arteriosclerosis in the aorta and the arteries. How it does so, whether by enhancing the permeability of the cells of the wall, by loosening junctions, by the effect of direct pressure (pressure necrosis), which may lead to cell death in the intima or media, or by increasing the likelihood of thrombus formation by increasing the mechanical interaction between platelets and endothelium, is not known. However, a rapid rise in blood pressure alone may cause injury to the arterioles and create a sequence of lesions in these vessels that is called **malignant hypertension.** This disease of unknown etiology is best remembered because of the clinical pattern. Usually a person so afflicted may complain of headaches and visual difficulties. Examination shows that, in addition to the elevated systolic and diastolic pressures (200/140), there is an abnormal protrusion of the optic nerve (papilledema), and microscopic hemorrhages and exudation can be seen in the retina with the ophthalmoscope. These same changes are probably occurring in the microvascular bed throughout the body. They have particularly damaging effects in the kidney (leading to renal failure) and brain (causing intracerebral hemorrhages and coma, eventually).

Perhaps nowhere is the relationship of arteriosclerosis and hypertension better illustrated than in the blood vessels of the pulmonary circulation. Usually this system, a low pressure (20/10 mm Hg), low-resistance circulation, shows no atheromas even in persons who have high serum lipids and who develop severe atherosclerosis in their aorta and systemic vessels. Even in obese, sedentary smokers (provided they have not developed severe lung disease), atheromas of the pulmonary circulation are rare. When, however, owing to a shunt or some other cause, pulmonary hypertension occurs, then one can expect to see and usually finds atheromas and arteriosclerosis in the pulmonary arteries, just as they appear in the systemic circulation.

Although multiple factors that contribute to atherosclerosis have been enumerated, it is not clear yet how each of them is related to the etiology of this ubiquitous disorder. However, the role of hypertension in promoting atherosclerosis cannot be doubted.

Arteritis

So far we have been considering the conditions to which the arteries and arterioles are liable. We may now turn to the much less common inflammatory lesions. A number of these appear to be manifestations of allergy or of hypersensitivity, although little or nothing is known about the substances to which the person is allergic.

Polyarteritis Nodosa. This is one of the diffuse collagen diseases (the collective phrase "collagen diseases" or "collagen vascular diseases" represents an attempt to group diseases of unknown etiology that manifest morphologic changes in the histologic appearance of connective tissue) and is also known as periarteritis nodosa, by reason of the periarterial inflammatory exudate that is often a prominent microscopic feature. It is an acute inflammation that involves the small arteries of the viscera. The cause is unknown, but strong evidence suggests that this disease represents a type of hypersensitivity. The disease often runs an acute course with fever, ending fatally in a few weeks or months. Symptoms vary widely, depending on which arteries are involved. The principal vessels affected are those of the gastrointestinal tract, the kidney, and the heart. There may be acute abdominal symptoms due to involvement of the mesenteric arteries, acute cardiac symptoms from coronary artery involvement, or neuritic pains due to lesions of the arteries supplying the peripheral nerves.

Disseminated Lupus Erythematosus. In this confusing name, the word "lupus" originally signified wolf, but is now taken to denote the distribution of the facial rash mentioned below. This is another of the collagen diseases, similar in many ways to polyarteritis nodosa, for it involves the small vessels of the viscera. The heart, kidneys, skin, and serous membranes are also involved. A butterfly-like red rash over the bridge of the nose and both cheeks is a common and striking feature. A peculiar occurrence is the finding of what are known as LE (lupus erythematosus) cells. These are polymorphonuclear leukocytes containing a large homogeneous inclusion mass. The inclusion has been shown to be altered DNA and the presumed antigen is believed to be the patient's own DNA. The LE cells were first found in the bone marrow of patients suffering from the disease, but it is now known that the phenomenon depends on the presence of some factor in the patient's blood serum that acts on the cells. When a test is made for the LE phenomenon, the patient's blood serum is mixed with his white blood cells, and a smear is made and searched for the development of LE cells. It must be realized that the test is in vitro, not in vivo. Today, the outlook for patients with SLE (systemic lupus erythematosus) is greatly improved because of new ways of using immunosuppressive and anti-inflammatory drugs.

Thromboangiitis Obliterans. A thrombotic occlusion (obliteration) of the vessels of the legs in relatively young men, this disease results in gangrene of the toes and then the feet. Buerger, in 1908, brought this condition to the attention of the medical profession, so that it is commonly referred to as Buerger's disease. The sex incidence is striking, for the disease is practically confined to men. The cause is unknown, but it is believed that there is a condition of allergic hypersensitivity in the arterial wall, as a result of which an acute inflammatory reaction develops. Patients seem to be especially hypersensitive to tobacco, and the sufferer is often found to be a heavy cigarette smoker. In the treatment of the disease, one of the most important points is to give up tobacco. Buerger called the lesion angiitis, meaning an inflammation of vessels, both arteries and veins, but at the present time thrombosis is coming to be regarded as the dominant feature of the disease.

Syphilis. This disease attacks two important sets of vessels: (1) the thoracic aorta, including the coronary artery ostia, more especially the ascending portion, and (2) the cerebral arteries.

Syphilitic Aortitis. Formerly one of the most common and most important of the lesions of syphilis, modern antibiotic therapy has made this condition a rarity until the last few years. The destruction caused by the *Treponema pallidum* in the wall of the aorta may produce aortic valvular insufficiency or aneurysm. Aortic insufficiency or incompetence is caused by destruction of the aortic ring to which the cusps of the aortic valve are attached. This destruction occurs by ischemic injury to the elastic tissue that forms a chief constituent of the wall, so that gradual stretching and dilatation occur and the valve becomes incompetent. The three cusps of the valve are shrunken and show a characteristic cord-like thickening, becoming separated from one another, and thus further adding to the incompetence. The smooth intimal surface of the aorta becomes pitted, scarred, and wrinkled like the bark of a tree. An aneurysm is a localized or diffuse dilatation of the wall of the thoracic aorta caused by damage to the elastic tissue of the wall. Syphilitic aneurysm is considered in the next section, together with other varieties of aneurysm. The common mechanism of injury was said to be occlusion of the vasa vasorum or the small vessels that supply the aortic wall itself. However, the spirochete itself may have initiated some of the injury. It is important to recognize that only one-third of all people with primary syphilis ever suffered this type of cardiovascular syphilis (see Chapter 7).

Aneurysms

This localized dilatation of an artery may be saccular, an outpouching of the vessel at a single point (Fig. 14–13), or fusiform, a uniform dilatation of an entire segment of the artery. Every aneurysm is due to weakening of the arterial wall. As a rule, it is the media that is damaged. Syphilis used to be the most

Fig. 14–13 This photograph shows the arch of the aorta in a patient who had syphilis several decades ago. The bulging protruding mass at the top of the picture is an **aneurysm** that is lined with thrombus material. This aneurysm has ruptured, causing the death of the patient. (McGill University, Department of Pathology Museum.)

Fig. 14–14 This aortogram shows multiple small aneurysms, seen at the arrows, in a case of periarteritis nodosa, a rare disease of arteries.

important cause of aneurysm of the aorta and its main branches. With the modern control of syphilis and with the increasing age of the population, atherosclerosis has come to replace it. Polyarteritis nodosa may weaken the artery and lead to the formation of multiple small aneurysms (Fig. 14–14). Finally, congenital weakness of the media in the arteries at the base of the brain has been suggested as a cause of so-called congenital aneurysms in this region. We shall confine our attention here to aneurysms of the aorta.

Aortic Aneurysm. Aneurysm due to atherosclerosis occurs at a later age than the syphilitic form; it generally affects the abdominal aorta, and it usually causes diffuse dilatation of the vessel (Fig. 14–15). Recent studies have shown a hereditary/familial incidence in aneurysms, and further studies may show the significance of the presence of aneurysms of the aorta in kindreds. The site of the involvement is the lower part of the aorta below the origin of the renal arteries. This is singularly fortunate, because it makes possible the replacement of the aneurysm by an aortic homograft or a plastic tube that may be a lifesaving procedure. Unfortunately, the aneurysm may press on the lower dorsal and lumbar vertebrae, with disastrous results. A syphilitic aneurysm usually involves the ascending aorta or the arch, is usually saccular, and presses on the surrounding structures, causing pain in the back, dyspnea, and difficulty in swallowing. It may rupture on the surface or internally, killing the patient at once.

Dissecting aneurysm is not a true aneurysm, as the

vessel is not dilated. A hemorrhage occurs in the media of the aorta at a point of weakness, and spreads along the vessel, dissecting the media into two layers (Fig. 14–16). The usual pattern may be a sudden sharp or excruciating pain in the chest or the abdomen, accompanied by prostration. The patient often experiences what he describes as a tearing sensation. The pain passes, but in a typical case death occurs some days later from the rupture of the aneurysm into the

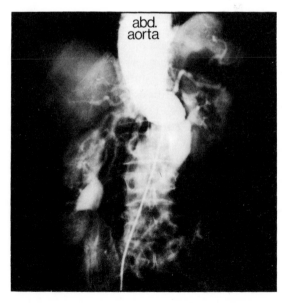

Fig. 14–15 This arteriogram shows a markedly dilated atherosclerotic aorta, in which the dilatation extends from the diaphragm to the level of the internal iliac arteries.

Fig. 14–16 *A,1,2,3,* The drawings show different routes for the accumulation of blood within the wall of the aorta in different types of dissecting aneurysms. (From Slater, E. E., and DeSanctis, R. W.: Dissection of the aorta. Med. Clin. North Am., 63:146, 1979.) *B,* This cross section of a carotid artery shows the effect of hemorrhage in the wall of the aorta. It narrows the lumen and thus obstructs blood flow. (McGill University, Department of Pathology Museum.)

chest or the abdominal cavity. This clinical pattern is not the only one, since the dissection may take a number of routes. It may separate the walls of the aorta and narrow the renal arteries; it may close off the mesenteric supply to the bowel; or it may dissect retrograde to narrow the coronary arteries. The aneurysm may also rupture into the pericardium, thereby preventing normal ventricular filling and killing the patient because of the effect of what is called tamponade. Studies of collected cases show that 3% of patients with a dissecting aneurysm die immediately; 20% die within a day; 60% die within two weeks; and 90% die within three months. In a few lucky cases, the person may survive many years. It is important to make the diagnosis as distinct from a myocardial infarction with which it is usually confused, because there is some hope from an early surgical approach to the aneurysm. Hypotensive agents certainly seem to have increased the short-term outlook for patients with dissecting aneurysms.

VEINS

The pathology of veins is entirely different from that of the arteries. Veins differ from arteries in two respects, both of which have a bearing on the development of disease. (1) They have valves (Fig. 14–17). Failure of the valves is one of the important features of varicose veins. (2) They have lymphatics, which explains why malignant growths invade veins with the greatest ease, but seldom invade the walls of arteries, which are lacking in lymphatics. Bacteria from without can also readily penetrate the vein wall by way of the lymphatics.

Phlebitis or inflammation of the veins used to be of great importance, but antisepsis and chemotherapy have changed the picture completely. The danger of phlebitis used to be an associated thrombosis, often septic in character. This has disappeared, but venous thrombosis unassociated with phlebitis still remains a threat and an unsolved problem. Two conditions that

Fig. 14–17 This illustration from William Harvey's *De motu cordis* (1628) shows how Harvey demonstrated valves in the venous system and the direction of the blood flow in veins by applying pressure from below.

affect veins in which thrombosis is common and sometimes serious, namely varicose veins and hemorrhoids, will be considered here. The two really belong to the same group, for hemorrhoids are merely varicose veins at the lower end of the intestinal canal.

Varicose Veins. These are veins that are dilated and tortuous. The dilatation may be extreme, so that the valves that normally guard veins and prevent a back-flow because of gravity become incompetent and cease to function. As a result of this failure, the stagnation and accumulation of blood in the vein greatly increase. The common site of varicose veins is in the superficial veins of the leg, just under the skin. Bluish knuckles of veins can be seen pushing the skin in front of them. These nodules are liable to injury, with resulting hemorrhage into the surrounding tissue. Thrombosis may occur due partly to the slow blood flow in the dilated vessels, partly to the frequency of injury to the vessel wall. The circulation in varicose veins is interfered with, the legs become swollen, and varicose ulcers are formed in the lower part of the leg. These ulcers used to be chronic and difficult to treat, but the outlook has been changed by modern methods of treating the varicose veins by surgical removal.

The causes of varicose veins are obscure. Heredity undoubtedly plays a part, and the condition may run in a family. The active factor is increase of pressure in the vein. This may be due to prolonged standing, intermittent, increased venous pressure (in the case of hemorrhoids), or the pressure of a tumor in the pelvis, a pregnant uterus, or even a continually loaded rectum.

The treatment of varicose veins is directed at the relief of the congestion, the accumulation of stagnant blood, in the dilated vessels. This may be accomplished by the application of a uniform support to the leg in the form of an elastic bandage or stocking which should extend to the groin rather than to the knee, as is more often the case. If this method fails to relieve the condition, the veins may be removed. The varicosity only affects the superficial veins, and as these communicate with the deep veins of the leg by small collateral channels, the circulation is reestablished through the leg veins. For the same reason there is no danger of emboli passing from the superficial veins into the general circulation.

Hemorrhoids. The condition in which the veins at the lower end of the rectum become varicose and enlarged is known as hemorrhoids. Internal hemorrhoids are those covered by the mucus membrane of the lower end of the rectum; they may "come down" through the anal opening and appear on the surface, although they can be replaced by pressure. External hemorrhoids are covered by the skin in the neighborhood of the anus.

The causes are those of varicose veins, i.e., heredity and increased pressure in the venous system. This is also true of the presence of hemorrhoids in patients with cirrhosis of the liver, in which the rise in portal pressure makes the collateral circulation of the esophagus and rectum anatomically important but susceptible to rupture.

The possible effects that may render the condition serious are hemorrhage, phlebitis, and thrombosis. Hemorrhage when the bowels are moved is usually small in amount, but may be continued over a long period, so that anemia may be produced without the patient's suspecting its cause. Phlebitis or inflammation of the dilated veins together with inflammation of the surrounding tissue is commonly referred to as an "attack of the piles." Its danger is that it may lead to the formation of an infected thrombus, which readily becomes converted into an embolus.

The treatment of hemorrhoids is partly indirect, partly direct. By indirect treatment we mean keeping the bowels loose by means of bland laxatives and suitable food. Direct treatment is aimed at the dilated veins. These veins may be closed by the injection of sclerosing solutions, and no more may need to be done. In more severe cases, operative removal of the hemorrhoids may be necessary.

SYNOPSIS

Arteriosclerosis is common in persons over 50 years of age.
Arteriosclerosis is likely of multifactorial etiology.
Arteriosclerosis is reversible.

The pathogenesis of arteriosclerosis is debated, but hypertension, platelet aggregation, turbulent flow, intimal injury, hyperlipidemia, and damage to smooth muscle cells have been implicated.

Arteriolosclerosis may both result from and contribute to hypertension.

The presence of arteriosclerosis contributes to systolic hypertension, arteriolosclerosis to diastolic hypertension.

Collagen vascular diseases are a group of diseases that share clinical features of fever, connective tissue and serosal involvement, pathologic features of uncertain etiology, and aspects of hypersensitivity reaction.

Terms

Arteriosclerosis
Arteriolosclerosis
Arteriolonecrosis

Atherosclerosis
Arteritis
Collagen vascular disease

Aortitis
Aneurysm
Phlebitis

FURTHER READING

Editorial: New evidence linking salt and hypertension. Br. Med. J., 282:1983, 1981.

Bailie, M.D., and Mattioli, L.F.: Hypertension: relationships between pathophysiology and therapy. J. Pediatr., 96:789, 1980.

Brown, J.J., Fisher, L.D., Schaefer, S.M., et al.: Regression of coronary artery disease as a result of intensive lipid-lowering therapy in men with high levels of Apolipoprotein B. N. Engl. J. Med., 323:1289, 1990.

Crawford, E.S., and Cohen, E.S.: Aortic aneurysm: a multifocal disease. Arch. Surg., 117:1393, 1982.

DeSanctis, R.W., et al.: Aortic dissection. N. Engl. J. Med., 317:1060, 1987.

Dobrin, P.B.: Mechanical properties of arteries. Physiol. Rev., 58:397, 1978.

Fauci, A.S. (Moderator): The spectrum of vasculitis. Clinical, pathologic, immunologic, and therapeutic considerations. Ann. Intern. Med., 89:660, 1978.

Glagov, S., et al.: Compensatory enlargement of human atherosclerotic coronary arteries. N. Engl. J. Med., 316:1371, 1987.

Golditz, G.A., et al.: Menopause and the risk of coronary heart disease in women. N. Engl. J. Med., 316:1105, 1987.

Goldstein, J.L., and Brown, M.S.: The LDL receptor defect in familial hypercholesterolemia. Med. Clin. North Am., 66:335, 1982.

Goldstein, J.L., and Brown, M.S.: Lipoprotein receptors: genetic defense against atherosclerosis. Clin. Res., 30:417, 1982.

Grobbee, D.E., Rimm, E.B., Giovannucci, E., et al.: Coffee, caffeine, and cardiovascular disease in men. N. Engl. J. Med., 323:1026, 1990.

Hansen, O., and Johansson, B.W.: Epidemiologic aspects of coronary heart disease in Malmö, Sweden, 1935–1988. Am. J. Epidemiol., 133:721, 1991.

Hartung, G.H., et al.: Relation of diet to high-density lipoprotein cholesterol in middle-aged marathon runners, joggers, and inactive men. N. Engl. J. Med., 302:357, 1980.

Heptinstall, R.H.: Malignant hypertension: a study of fifty-one cases. J. Pathol. Bacteriol., 65:423, 1953.

Karnovsky, M.J.: Endothelial-vascular smooth muscle cell interactions. Am. J. Pathol., 105:200, 1981.

Keith, N.M., Wagener, H.P., and Kernohan, J.W.: The syndrome of malignant hypertension. Arch. Intern. Med., 41:141, 1928.

Knapp, H.R., et al.: In vivo indexes of platelet and vascular function during fish-oil administration in patients with atherosclerosis. N. Engl. J. Med., 314:937, 1986.

LeQuesne, L.P.: Relationship between deep vein thrombus and pulmonary embolism in surgical patients. N. Engl. J. Med., 291:1292, 1974.

Liddell, M.J., et al.: The role of stress hormones in the catabolic metabolism of shock. Surg. Gyn. Obstetr., 149:822, 1979.

Majumder, P.P., St. Jean, P.L., Ferrell, R.E., et al.: On the inheritance of abdominal aortic aneurysm. Am. J. Hum. Genet., 48:164, 1991.

Mann, G.V.: Diet-heart: End of an era. N. Engl. J. Med., 297:644, 1977.

Murdoch, J.C., et al.: Down's syndrome: an atheroma-free model? Br. Med. J., 2:226, 1977.

Parks, J.S., and Rudel, L.L.: Effect of fish oil on atherosclerosis and lipoprotein metabolism. Atherosclerosis, 84:83, 1990.

O'Neil, W., et al.: A prospective randomized clinical trial of intracoronary streptokinase versus infarction. N. Engl. J. Med., 314:812, 1986.

Ordovas, J.M., et al.: Apolipoprotein A-I gene polymorphism associated with premature coronary artery disease and familial hypoalphalipoproteinemia. N. Engl. J. Med., 314:671, 1986.

Reid, L., and Meyrick, B.: Microcirculation: definition and organization at tissue level. Ann. N.Y. Acad. Sci., 384:3, 1982.

Sniderman, A.D., et al.: Association of hyperapobetalipoproteinemia with endogenous hypertriglyceridemia and atherosclerosis. Ann. Intern. Med., 97:833, 1982.

Sprafka, J.M., et al.: Continued decline in cardiovascular disease risk factors: Results of the Minnesota Heart Survey, 1980–82 and 1985–87. Am. J. Epidemiol., 132:489, 1990.

Stampfer, M.J., Sacks, F.M., Salvini, S., et al.: A prospective study of cholesterol, apolipoproteins, and the risk of myocardial infarction. N. Engl. J. Med., 325:373, 1991.

Stehbens, W.E.: Reduction of serum cholesterol levels and regression of atherosclerosis. Pathology, 23:45, 1991.

Sytkowski, P.A., Kannel, W.B., and D'Agostino, R.B.: Changes in risk factors and the decline in mortality from cardiovascular disease: the Framingham heart study. N. Engl. J. Med., 322:1635, 1990.

Taylor, A.E.: Capillary fluid filtration. Starling forces and lymph flow. Circ. Res., 49:557, 1981.

Tsevat, J., Weinstein, M.C., Williams, L.W., et al.: Expected gains in life expectancy from various coronary heart disease risk factor modifications. Circulation, 83:1194, 1991.

Walker, W.J.: Diet-heart era: Premature obituary. N. Engl. J. Med., 298, 1978.

Waters, D., and Lespérance, J.: Regression of coronary atherosclerosis—an achievable goal—review of results from recent clinical trials. Am. J. Med., 91 (Suppl.1B):S10, 1991.

Webster, M.W., et al.: Ultrasound screening of first-degree relatives of patients with an abdominal aortic aneurysm. J. Vasc. Surg., 13:9, 1991.

Wissler, R.W.: Update on the pathogenesis of atherosclerosis. Am. J. Med., 91 (Suppl.1B):S3, 1991.

Yamamoto, A.: Regression of atherosclerosis in humans by lowering serum cholesterol. Atherosclerosis, 89:1, 1991.

Young, S.G.: Recent progress in understanding Apolipoprotein B. Circulation 82:1574, 1990.

Zilversmit, D.B.: Atherogenesis: a postprandial phenomenon. Circulation, 60:473, 1979.

15

THE RESPIRATORY TRACT

Almost all the fallacies of medicine, perpetuated in popular belief, were once scientifically accepted theories.—W. LOFFLER

STRUCTURE AND FUNCTION

The principal function of the lungs is oxygenation of the blood, a business in which the heart and lungs are partners. Blood laden with the waste products of the body in the form of carbon dioxide is brought to the lungs, where carbon dioxide is given off and fresh oxygen is taken up. Respiration is essential to life; when it ceases, so does life. Oxygenated blood returns directly to the heart and is then sent through the arteries to supply the needs of the body. The lungs constitute the greatest mixing place of air and blood. Each lung is a honeycomb, with air in place of honey in the cells of the comb, and an infinite number of capillaries in their walls. These walls are virtually only two plasma membranes; gases (carbon dioxide and oxygen) readily pass through in either direction (Fig. 15–1). During inspiration, air is carried to the alveoli by the bronchi and their terminations, the bronchioles, which subdivide and ramify throughout the entire lung. The partial pressures of oxygen in the different compartments dictate the availability of this essential fuel. Under conditions of respiration at sea level (standard temperature and pressure) in a normal lung, hemoglobin will approach maximal saturation. With decreased ventilation, or at high altitudes, or with disease in the lung, there will be a departure from normal values as shown in Figure 15–2. A synoptic section reviewing lung structure and function appears in the Appendix, p. 358.

TECHNIQUES FOR STUDYING LUNG DISEASE

In medicine, the examination of the chest is one of the most challenging clinical adventures. By viewing the respiratory excursions, the use of accessory muscles, the rate and rhythm of breathing, one can adduce much about the effectiveness of the physiology of ventilation. Indirect examination of the anatomy of the lungs is now a changing art, as percussion and auscultation of the chest give way to newer radiographic methods (scans) (Fig. 15–3) and to the measurement of blood gases. It used to be that the diagnosis of pneumonia or abscess was made by hearing dullness to percussion or tubular breath sounds, or by hearing a change in voice sounds over an abscess cavity. This clinical observation was confirmed by the chest x-rays and culture.

Today, we depend on tomograms, technetium scans, and serial studies to make the diagnosis as well as transtracheal biopsies for culture, fiberoptic scopes for intrabronchial biopsy, and vast experience in nearly four decades of exfoliative cytology. The first diagnosis has always been anatomic, and in this chapter we attempt to show both the radiographic and morbid anatomic representations of most of the lesions we discuss.

INFECTIOUS DISEASES

The limits on this book make it impossible to consider all diseases of the nose, throat, larynx, and trachea, which form the upper part of the respiratory tract, but brief mention must be made of the universal ailment, the common cold.

Although this is the most common of all infectious diseases, it is only during the last few years that we have become certain of its cause. The causal agent is a **filterable virus**, which can be grown in tissue of human and monkey embryo kidney, in which it produces recognizable degenerative changes. The virus is spread with extreme readiness from one person to another, so that epidemics of colds are frequent. Unlike most other filterable viruses, it fails to confer any immunity on the infected person, so that he may suffer from several attacks in the course of a winter. Several groups of viruses may be involved in different epidemics. It is little wonder, then, that a first attack

A

Fig. 15–1   *A*, This cast of the lung shows the extensive branching of the airways that starts at the junction of the left and right main stem bronchus and continues for as many as fourteen divisions before the alveoli are reached. (From West, J.B.: *Respiratory Physiology*. Baltimore, Williams & Wilkins, 1974.) *B*, This drawing of the microscopic appearance of the lung shows the terminations of the respiratory bronchioles in the alveolar ducts and spaces. Note the communication (pore) between alveoli. Both air and inflammation can use these portals for transalveolar spread. (From Sorokin, S.: In *Histology*, 2nd Ed. Edited by R.O. Greep. New York, McGraw-Hill, 1966.)

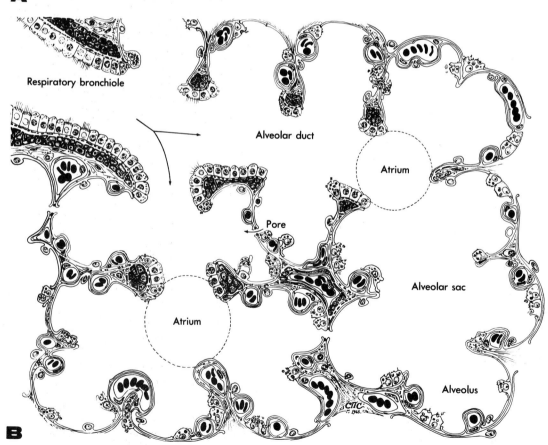

Respiratory bronchiole

Alveolar duct

Atrium

Pore

Atrium

Alveolar sac

Alveolus

B

Fig. 15–2 This scheme illustrates the function of the lung by showing the gradient of oxygen from the atmosphere to the intracellular sink (mitochondria) where oxygen is used. (From West, J.B.: *Respiratory Physiology.* Baltimore, Williams & Wilkins, 1974.)

does not immunize a person against a second. Predisposing or contributing factors probably play an important part, such as the chilling of the body as a result of sitting in a draft, wet feet, and the like.

This viral infection is acute, and, like other acute infections, it may clear up in the course of a few days. Too often, however, secondary invaders follow the primary infection and convert the acute into a chronic disease, which may drag on for many weary weeks. The most common of the secondary bacterial invaders are pneumococci, staphylococci, and streptococci.

The virus of the common cold and the secondary invaders attack first the nose and throat. Later they may spread down to the larynx, trachea, and bronchi, and up into the sinuses that open into the nose. For the first day or so, the mucus membrane lining the nose and throat is swollen, red, and dry, giving the well-known "stuffed-up" feeling, but soon a watery fluid is poured out that runs from the nose continually. If the secondary invaders gain a hold, the inflammation becomes suppurative in type, and the watery secretion is replaced by a purulent one, which may continue to be discharged for many weeks.

Bacterial Pneumonias

Pneumonia denotes an inflammatory condition of the lung caused by infection; a better name, therefore, would be pneumonitis. However, the term "pneumonia" is hallowed by tradition and will continue to be used and continue to have to be explained. Since the lung is an organ in the body that is in direct contact with the outside air, it is natural that bacterial infection is frequent. The most important causes of acute bacterial pneumonias are *Streptococcus pneumoniae,*

Streptococcus hemolyticus, Staphylococcus aureus, and *Friedlander's bacillus.* The diffuse or lobar form of pneumonia is nearly always caused by the pneumococcus, whereas the patchy or bronchopneumonic form is likely to be due to one of the other organisms just enumerated.

Pneumococcal Pneumonia (Lobar). The normal habitat of the pneumococcus is the mucus membrane of the upper respiratory tract (nose and throat), from which it may pass down into the lungs. About 40% of healthy people carry pneumococci in their throat and nose. Infection is acquired from another person, usually someone who harbors pathogenic pneumococci in the throat (a carrier) rather than someone suffering from the acute disease. As in the case of other infections, predisposing causes are of great importance. Anything that lowers the resistance may act as a predisposing cause, but some of the most important are alcohol, malnutrition, congestive heart failure, and exposure or fatigue.

When a person with pathogenic pneumococci in the throat is exposed to a predisposing cause, the pneumococci pass down the trachea and bronchi and gain access to the alveoli, where they cause acute inflammation. As the thin-walled blood vessels in the walls of the lung are in such intimate relation with the alveoli, an abundant, acute inflammatory exudate pours from the vessels into the air spaces. This exudate consists of the various elements that have already been described in the chapter on **inflammation,** but the predominating elements are polymorphonuclear leukocytes and serum, with formation of abundant fibrin from the latter. It is in essence a **fibrinopurulent exudate.**

The result of all this is replacement of the air in the alveoli by the exudate, so that the affected part of the lung is no longer air-containing, but is solid. This part of the lung is now said to be **consolidated.**

The inflammation spreads throughout a lobe, and may involve the entire lung. Often, however, the consolidation is confined to 1 or 2 lobes, hence the term lobar pneumonia (Fig. 15–4). Such a consolidated lung is about as different from the normal spongy structure as it is possible to imagine and can be seen on chest film (Fig. 15–5). The infection reaches the pleura, and the beautifully smooth surface is now covered with a shaggy, fibrinous or fibrinopurulent exudate. This exudate may be detected because the two surfaces are now roughened as sandpaper and a noise similar to the rubbing together of the palms of your hand is audible with each breath. This is called a **pleural friction rub** and is a sign of fibrinous pleurisy indicating underlying inflammation in the lung.

Lobar pneumonia usually runs its course in about

A

B

A

Fig. 15–4 *A,* Gross specimen of a lung shows the difference in color and consistency between the upper and lower lobe. The lower lobe contains no air due to replacement of the air space by pus. We call this pneumonia and refer to it as **lobar pneumonia,** when a whole lobe is involved. (McGill University, Department of Pathology Museum.) *B,* Microscopically the alveoli are filled with white blood cells.

a week. By the end of that time, provided the patient survives (which he usually does), the pneumococci are dead; the exudate dissolves and is finally removed by being coughed up in the sputum. The removal, which is called **resolution,** is extraordinarily complete, and in a few weeks, the lung is restored to its normal spongy condition, the alveoli being filled with air instead of with pus.

The foregoing description applies to the classic case of lobar pneumonia before the days of antibiotics. Naturally, if the infection is nipped in the bud by the administration of antibiotics, the lesions will not have time to develop, nor will the case come to autopsy.

Bronchopneumonia. This disease is usually caused by staphylococci, streptococci, or pneumococci. It is primarily a bronchitis, an inflammation of the bronchi, and is widespread throughout one or both lungs. Here and there the infection penetrates into the al-

veoli and produces a small patch of inflammatory consolidation. These patches may be seen throughout the lung, but they are separated by an abundance of air-containing lung tissue. Such a lung is not usually consolidated.

Bronchopneumonia is much more common than lobar pneumonia. It occurs at the extremes of age, being most frequent in young children and in the aged or the chronically ill or immunocompromised individual. It often accompanies the infectious fevers of childhood, and is so commonly found at postmortem examination as a terminal condition that it hardly attracts the attention of a pathologist unless it is unusually marked. Nevertheless, the disease must often serve as some ministering angel to snuff out the flickering flame when life is ebbing away.

In these days of prevalent staphylococcal hospital infections, bronchopneumonia has assumed a new

←

Fig. 15–3 *A,* Normal lung **perfusion scan** using technetium 99m macroaggregates of albumin, which demonstrates areas of vascular perfusion. All areas that are dense are receiving blood. *B,* Normal lung **ventilation scan** using xenon 133, a radioactive gas, which fills all ventilated air spaces. Poor ventilation may be due to air space disease, chronic obstructive pulmonary disease, or obstructing lesions. Compare with the previous figure; if the airways are blocked, there will be no dark areas with xenon; if the blood vessels are blocked, there will be no dark areas from technetium.

Fig. 15–5   This x-ray shows air space consolidation in the right upper lobe, consistent with lobar pneumonia. The dense material (inflammatory exudate) absorbs radiation, whereas normal alveoli do not.

twofold significance. (1) When admitted to hospital, persons suffering from some pre-existing lung disease readily become infected with the antibiotic-resistant staphylococci residing in the hospital, and the resulting bronchopneumonia may prove fatal. (2) Such staphylococcal lesions, especially if they develop into lung abscesses (Fig. 15–6), may act as an important reservoir and source of infection, which can be widely disseminated by the coughing of the patient.

Viral Pneumonias

It is now recognized that viral pneumonias outnumber all other pneumonias, especially during epidemics. In addition to the pneumonitis complicating such viral infections as influenza and measles, there are many cases of primary lung infection caused by a variety of different viruses.

Influenzal Pneumonia. Influenza is an acute inflammatory disease of the upper respiratory tract (throat, trachea, and bronchi), associated with marked general debility. The special peculiarity of influenza is that usually it is the mildest of infections, lightly referred to as "a touch of the flu." At long intervals, it assumes a virulent form, and like "a blast from the stars," as an old writer said, great epidemics sweep across the world and kill millions of people. At such times, as in the pandemic of 1918 and 1919, it seems, as John Bright remarked in another connection, that "the Angel of Death is abroad in the land; you can

Fig. 15–6   This photograph of a lung shows (at arrow) abscess cavities with a thin wall. Frequently, such an abscess is the result of aspiration. (McGill University, Department of Pathology Museum.)

almost hear the beating of his wings." In the pandemic of 1918 and 1919, there were some 500,000,000 cases throughout the world, of whom 15,000,000 died. By comparison, a more recent pandemic of Asian influenza was comparatively mild. It is in these virulent outbreaks that pulmonary complications in the form of influenzal pneumonia acquire a fearful significance. These epidemics may spread with extraordinary rapidity. In a United States Army camp in

1918 there were 3 cases on one day and 3,000 on the next!

The cause of influenza is a filterable virus of various strains or groups. This virus is inhaled and sets up an acute inflammation in the nose and throat that may spread upward into the sinuses and downward into the trachea and bronchi, causing the feeling of rawness so familiar to everyone. The virus causes not only a characteristic feeling of profound weakness and lassitude, but in some cases lowers the resistance of the respiratory tract, so that other bacteria, secondary invaders, like the 7 devils of Holy Writ, pass down into the lungs and produce pneumonia. This is much more likely to happen during the great epidemics, thus explaining the high mortality on these occasions. Influenzal pneumonia differs from the lobar variety in that both lungs are always involved, and, in place of being consolidated and dry as a result of containing a more or less coagulated exudate, they are wet and waterlogged. When the lung is examined at autopsy, it is found to be intensely congested with blood, so that it is a bluish-purple color. Under the microscope, the appearance of viral pneumonia differs from that of bacterial lobar pneumonia in that the interstitium is the principal site of inflammation, not the alveoli. The septa of the alveoli are thickened by the congestion and inflammation which increase the diffusing distance and may cause respiratory embarrassment.

Among the symptoms the dry, hacking **cough,** which is so common, is caused by acute irritation of the trachea and large bronchi. The profound **prostration** is due to a general toxemia. In influenzal pneumonia there may be marked **cyanosis** (blueness of lips and face) and **dyspnea. Fever** is present as in all acute infections. The most important complication of viral pneumonia is the frequent superinfection by bacteria. Viral infections typically cause cell death, and when the living cells of the bronchi are killed, the primary defense barrier to bacterial infection is broken, predisposing the patient to bacterial pneumonias. It is important to recognize that viral infections do not respond to conventional antibiotic therapy, and the diagnosis may be missed during the early phase of the disease (Fig. 15–7).

Primary Atypical Pneumonia. This relatively new arrival among the pneumonias appears to be a group rather than an entity, so designated because it is not caused by bacteria or fungi. The disease may appear

Fig. 15–7 Pneumonia and influenza (P&I) deaths reported from 121 cities in the United States, as a percentage of total deaths—October 1985-February 11, 1989. P&I deaths include all deaths for which pneumonia is listed as a primary or underlying cause or for which influenza is listed on the death certificate. The predominant virus type is shown above the peak of mortality for each epidemic season. The epidemic threshold for each influenza season was estimated at 1.645 standard deviations above the values projected on the basis of a periodic regression model applied to observed P&I deaths for the previous 5-year period but excluding the observations during influenza outbreaks. (From Centers for Disease Control, Morbidity and Mortality Weekly Report, 38(6):115, 1989.)

in small epidemics, usually in schools and army camps where young people are congregated. One of the most common causes of this disease is an organism called *Mycoplasma pneumoniae* (sometimes referred to as PPLO—pleuropneumonia-like organisms, or the Eaton agent). These organisms are smaller than bacteria and larger than viruses. There is an acute inflammation of the upper respiratory tract, only involving the lungs to a minor degree, so that, although the morbidity is high, the mortality is low. Even when pneumonia does develop, the physical signs are largely absent, a characteristic feature, but there is x-ray evidence of a patchy, ill-defined consolidation seldom involving more than a part of a lobe. The course is usually mild, with recovery occurring in 2 or 3 weeks.

Clinical Pattern. Lobar pneumonia will be taken as an example. Most of the symptoms can be explained by the pathologic lesions. The face is flushed, the breathing rapid, shallow, and painful; there is cough with blood-streaked sputum; fever and leukocytosis are present; and examination of the chest reveals changes in the lung. The dyspnea and rapid breathing are caused by interference with the free interchange of gases between the blood and air, owing to the exudate in the alveoli. The cough is due to irritation of the bronchi. The sputum is sticky, so that it can be pulled out in strings and is characteristically red or rust-colored. The stickiness is caused by the fibrin and mucus and the color by the red blood corpuscles in the exudate. The sputum consists largely of polymorphonuclear leukocytes (pus cells) and contains large numbers of pneumococci. The pain on breathing is an indication of pleurisy, the rough and inflamed surfaces of the pleura being rubbed together each time the patient takes a breath. Fever is caused by the toxins produced by the pneumococci. Leukocytosis is the natural result of the demand for enormous numbers of leukocytes to be poured into the alveoli of the lung. When the healthy chest is percussed, a resonant, drumlike note is heard, but when the lung is consolidated, there is dullness on percussion, owing to replacement of the air by exudate.

Abscess

In lobar pneumonia there is no true destruction; the walls of the alveoli are not destroyed. This phenomenon makes the complete structural recovery of the lung possible. Sometimes, however, especially when accessory factors are present that weaken resistance, the lung tissue is destroyed, and abscesses are formed. This complication is more likely to happen in bronchopneumonia, and, as we have already seen, staphylococcal infection is often responsible.

Abscess of the lung can be divided into three groups, depending on the method of causation. These are the aspiration, the embolic, and the pneumonic types.

Aspiration is the largest and most important cause today. Lung abscess is a constant threat in operations on the mouth, nose, and throat, especially tonsillectomy and extraction of teeth. Infected material passes down the trachea and bronchi. Abscess is more frequent in the right lung, which has a more vertical bronchus, and in the lower lobe. Stomach contents may be vomited during general anesthesia and inhaled into the lungs. Foreign bodies, especially peanuts and coins, may pass from the mouths of children down the trachea and cause lung abscess.

The embolic type of abscess is due to a septic thrombus' being carried by the venous blood to the right side of the heart, and then through the pulmonary artery to the lung. Two sources of an infected embolus may be mentioned: those from the veins of the female pelvis, and the lateral venous sinus of the skull which becomes infected in infections of the middle ear and mastoid.

Another type of abscess represents a complication of pneumonia, usually streptococcal or influenzal in type; abscess formation is rare in lobar pneumonia.

The clinical pattern is fever, cough, copious expectoration of pus, foul breath, and foul sputum. An important complication of lung abscess is the development of abscess of the brain, owing to infected materials being carried by the blood from the lung to the left side of the heart and thence to the brain. This process may also occur in bronchiectasis.

Pulmonary Tuberculosis

The general pattern of tuberculous infection has already been discussed, together with the observation of the decrease in the incidence of the disease from 700 deaths per 100,000 population in 1910 to 5 deaths per 100,000 today. As the infection is acquired in most cases by inhalation, it is natural that the lung should be by far the most common site of the disease. We have seen that tuberculosis is a struggle between attack and defense, usually on fairly even terms, but with the odds considerably in favor of the defense. When infection is established there are three possible courses: (1) **healing with scarring;** (2) **fibrocaseous tuberculosis;** (3) **acute tuberculous pneumonia.** The result depends on the size and frequency of the dose of tubercle bacilli on the one hand and on the natural powers of defense on the other. It is important to distinguish between primary infection and reinfection, often called secondary infection.

Primary Infection. The first infection usually occurs

in childhood, but now, as the result of public health measures, it may be delayed until adult life. The primary lesion is a small caseous focus, seldom more than 1 cm in diameter, usually situated at the periphery of the lung. A consequence of this infection is the drainage of macrophages that contain the tubercle bacillus to a centrally located lymph node. In the lymph node, further reaction takes place and leads to cellular hypersensitivity, but often the lymph node also shows a caseous lesion. This combination of the peripheral lesion (where the tubercle bacteria first gain their foothold) and the central lymph node lesion is called the **Ghon complex,** after its discoverer (Fig. 15–8).

In the Ghon complex, the primary infection contrasts sharply with the secondary lesion, which nearly always makes its first appearance at the apex of the lung. Infection spreads by the lymphatics, so that the regional lymph nodes become enlarged and caseous,

again in contrast to what is found in secondary infection. The patient with primary infection either recovers or dies; the disease does not become chronic, nor is there any cavity formation. Recovery is marked by disappearance of the pulmonary and lymph node lesions, or by their conversion into fibrous tissue with calcification. However, the patient is rendered hypersensitive or allergic to a subsequent infection, as shown by the tuberculin test. If healing fails to occur, there may be generalized septicemia with rapidly fatal bronchopneumonia.

Reinfection. The reaction of the now-allergic tissues to reinfection is different from that of the primary infection. The right lung is attacked more often than the left, and the lesion is usually just below the apex. There are now four possibilities: (1) healing with fibrosis, (2) chronic fibrocaseous tuberculosis, (3) acute tuberculous caseous pneumonia, and (4) acute miliary tuberculosis. The result will depend both on the size

Fig. 15–8   This photograph shows the peripheral lesion (round white mass) and the central lymph node with caseous necrosis (arrow) of the **Ghon complex,** the primary response to tuberculosis. (McGill University, Department of Pathology Museum.)

and frequency of the dose of tubercle bacilli and on the patient's own resistance to disease. This may be expressed by the formula

$$D = \frac{V \times N \times H}{Rn + a}$$

in which D is expression of the disease, V is virulence of organism, N is number of organisms, H is hypersensitivity of host, and R is resistance, both native (n) and acquired (a).

Healing with Scarring. This course, fortunately, is by far the most common for the infection to run, as shown by the frequent presence of old tuberculous scars at the apex of one or both lungs in persons who come to autopsy. The reason why tuberculosis localizes at the apex of the lungs is unknown. Two physiologic factors may play a role. First, the concentration of oxygen per unit volume of tissue at the apex is greater than elsewhere in the lung, and second, the venous and lymphatic pressures are less. Perhaps the tubercle bacillus thrives there because of the better environment and the potential difficulties of mobilizing adequate defenses. There is a limited amount of destruction of tissue, but if the bacterial dose is not large and if the person is in good health, the healing process asserts itself, the bacilli are overcome, fibrous tissue surrounds and invades the area, and finally only a scar is left, in which calcium salts are often deposited. Even during the active stage, the patient shows no symptoms, and is unaware that he has acquired tuberculosis, but the positive tuberculin test of the skin will show that this is the case.

Fibrocaseous Tuberculosis. This is the usual form in the person who shows active signs of tuberculosis. The name indicates that both main processes of the disease are at work. There is fibrosis, indicating healing, and caseation, indicating destruction. The basic lesion, as usual, is the tubercle. The tubercles coalesce to form caseous or cheese-like masses. The caseous material becomes softened, liquified, discharged into a bronchus, and finally expectorated as tuberculous sputum filled with tubercle bacilli. A **cavity** is formed in the place formerly occupied by the caseous material (Fig. 15–9). This cavity may be small, or it may be so large as to involve the greater part of a lobe. Sometimes an artery is left traversing a cavity. Should this vessel rupture, profuse hemorrhage may occur. In time, numerous cavities are formed. The intervening parts of the lung show tuberculous consolidation, the alveoli being filled with inflammatory cells and caseous material. If the progress of the disease is slow, fibrosis may be marked, especially around the cavities, but true healing does not occur. The disease spreads from the apex downward, so that the oldest

Fig. 15–9 This x-ray demonstrates a cavity lesion in the left upper lobe, in this case due to a cavitated tuberculous abscess.

and most advanced lesions are at the top. In a case with extensive lesions, there may be cavities in the upper part of the lung, consolidation in the middle, and separate tubercles at the base. Pleurisy is always present, and adhesions are formed between the two layers of the pleura.

Acute Tuberculous Pneumonia. Here the infection overwhelms the resistance, and runs through the lung like a forest fire, giving rise to the clinical picture of galloping consumption. There are no discrete tubercles, but in their place there is a diffuse pneumonic process. There is no fibrosis, no attempt at limitation of the infection. The disease may prove fatal in a few months or even weeks without therapy.

Acute Miliary Tuberculosis. This is a fourth type of tuberculosis, which may be regarded as a complication of any of the previous three. The tuberculous process may penetrate the wall of a blood vessel or a lymphatic, which may effectively do the same thing—discharge large numbers of bacilli into the blood stream. These bacilli are carried throughout the body, where they cause an infinite number of miliary tubercles in all the organs. The lungs are no exception so that, in addition to a small lesion at the apex of one lung, both lungs may be peppered with fine tubercles. The term miliary is derived from the similarity of the tubercles seen with the unaided eye to millet seeds, small white grains. Miliary tuberculosis can be present in any or all organs, such as the liver, spleen, and kidney (Fig. 15–10).

Clinical Pattern. The cause of general symptoms, such as fever, loss of weight, and weakness, is uncertain. They become more marked when secondary infection with pyogenic bacteria is added to the pure tuberculous infection. **Cough** is due to irritation of the larger bronchi. **Pain in the side** is due to tuberculous pleurisy. The character of the **sputum** depends on the nature of the lesions. In acute miliary tuberculosis, there may be no sputum. Until cavities have formed, it is scanty and may contain no bacilli. After cavity formation, it is copious and purulent, often owing to secondary infection, and contains large numbers of bacilli. The more rapid the disease, the more bacilli will there be; the more stationary the disease, the fewer are their numbers.

Hemoptysis, the coughing up of blood, is due to erosion of a blood vessel. It has been said that hemoptysis marks the end of the beginning or the beginning of the end of the disease. At first, there may be erosion of a small vessel in the early process of softening, and the sputum becomes blood-streaked. In the advanced stage, a large artery or vein crossing a chronic cavity may give way and cause a severe and possibly fatal hemorrhage.

It must not be forgotten that the patient with pulmonary tuberculosis is a potential source of danger to

Fig. 15–10   This photograph shows lesions with the appearance of small white millet seeds scattered throughout the lung, typical of **miliary tuberculosis.** Similar lesions can appear in the kidney, spleen, liver, and other organs. (McGill University, Department of Pathology Museum.)

those with whom he comes in contact. This danger may remain potential and not become acute if he is educated in the principles of hygiene. The two sources of danger are sputum and droplet contagion from coughing at close quarters. If sputum is safely disposed of and the danger of coughing infected droplets in the direction of another person is recognized, the tuberculous patient need not be a source of infection to those with whom he lives. But the danger is always present, and precautions must not for a moment be relaxed. This is the reason that tuberculosis is so common in crowded living conditions of poor neighborhoods.

In 1992 there is a re-emergence of tuberculosis as a public health problem due to two reasons. New strains of drug-resistant organisms have been identified in 17 states. One-third of all patients are resistant to one drug, one-fifth to two drugs, and many patients resistant to all drugs. One reason for resistance is the failure of patients to complete the full course of treatment. A second reason is the simultaneous appearance of tuberculosis in patients with AIDS who have few immune mechanisms. The number of new cases of tuberculosis in New York City alone rose from 1,300 in 1978 to more than 3,000 in 1991.

Bronchitis

Bronchitis may be acute or chronic. The acute form usually involves the trachea as well as the larger bronchi.

Acute Tracheobronchitis. The irritant responsible for the acute inflammation may be bacterial, mechanical (various dusts), or toxic (poisonous gases). The mucus membrane is red and swollen, and the lumen is filled with pus. When the irritant is removed, the inflammation is likely to subside.

Chronic Bronchitis. The definition of chronic bronchitis is "the presence of a productive cough for at least three months of the year over at least two consecutive years without other cause."

The inflammatory disease of the lung, characterized by cough and increased sputum production, is a common and serious disease in the middle-aged and older person. The disease occurs particularly in industrial areas and in heavy cigarette smokers. It has been identified in Great Britain as the most common chronic respiratory ailment, exceeded only by the common cold. The prevalence and seriousness of the disease was an incentive to clean up the endemic air pollution in the late 1960s in London. Although attempts to culture organisms have been made frequently, it is now accepted that environmental pollution, whether from the waste of factories or from the carbon and tars of smoke (household or tobacco), is the principal etiologic agent that leads to the hyper-

Fig. 15–11 This photomicrograph shows an area of lung in which a mucous plug obstructs a bronchiole (arrow).

plasia of the mucus glands, the hypertrophy of the smooth muscle, and the increased thickening of the bronchial wall. The excess secretion of mucus as a response to irritants leads to plugging of the small airways (Fig. 15–11) and a loss of local ventilation. The residual lung volume becomes increased, the vital capacity reduced, and the patient complains of wheezing and shortness of breath (Fig. 15–12). Because some areas of the lung are well ventilated and perfused, the level of arterial oxygen may remain within normal limits for many years. When the obstruction becomes more widespread, CO_2 is retained, arterial hypoxemia results, and, because of reflex vasoconstriction in the arteriolar bed of the lung, the resistance of this circulation is increased. This change then leads to increased demands on the right heart and eventually to hypertrophy and failure (cor pulmonale).

In patients with chronic bronchitis, the plugging of bronchioles sets the scene for bacterial infections, and frequently in winter they may have bronchopneumonia, which is naturally much more serious than in a person with normal lungs. The outstanding feature of this disease is the obstructive element that leads to the general designation of **chronic obstructive pulmonary disease** for chronic bronchitis.

EMPHYSEMA

This extraordinarily common disease of the lung is also classified under the umbrella of chronic obstructive pulmonary disease (COPD), but is anatomically different from chronic bronchitis, although both processes often, or usually, exist in a patient at the same time. There is much discussion as to the possible relationships between them. Emphysema is characterized by an increase in the volume of the lung (Figs. 15–13 and 15–14), which is attributed to the overdistension and destructive changes that can be seen distal to the terminal respiratory bronchioles. In Figure 15–15, the

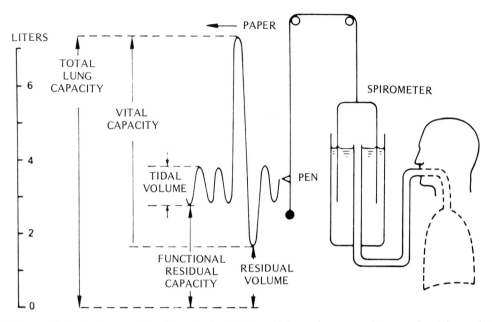

Fig. 15–12 This diagram illustrates the respective elements of ventilation which may be measured in normal and diseased states. Different lung diseases may affect different components of ventilatory function, as mentioned in the text. (From West, J.B.: *Respiratory Physiology*. Baltimore, Williams & Wilkins, 1974.)

Fig. 15–13 *A* and *B*, These x-rays show the changes of chronic obstructive pulmonary disease. The lungs are overinflated, larger, and appear much less dense than normal because there is more empty space and less tissue. Note the increased diameter of the chest and the flattened diaphragm.

Fig. 15–14   These sections of whole lung should be compared: *A*, a normal lung, and *B*, a lung with extensive emphysema. Note the coarser texture of *B*, which is the result of destruction of the small airways and coalescence into large empty pockets. (Courtesy of Dr. J. Hogg, Department of Pathology, McGill University.)

normal bronchial tree is contrasted with the dilated bronchial tree, and a dilatation, like a rotten apple on the branch of a tree, is seen at high magnification in Figure 15–15C. The alveolar spaces that are normally delicate and uniform have been destroyed, and they coalesce in emphysema to create a large saccule. Typically, the injury may be limited to the center of a secondary lung lobule. The destruction frequently occurs together with chronic bronchitis. This type of emphysema is referred to as **central lobular**. Large balloons of lung may occur less commonly, and these are called **bullae**. Another type of change has been recognized, in which the injury involves more than just the central portion of the lung lobule, and this is referred to as **panacinar** emphysema. Typically, as may be seen in Figure 15–14, emphysema is more extreme in the upper lobes of the lung and in the apical segment of the lower lobe.

It should be remembered that, although the disease is primarily one of the small airways and is associated with injury (pollution) and inflammation (bronchitis), and its association with injury and inflammation is well accepted, another association to explain the disease process has been made.

There is a rare hereditary form of emphysema in which a deficiency in a serum enzyme inhibitor (alpha-antitrypsin) has been found in members of a family who develop emphysema and chronic obstructive lung disease. It is suggested that the integrity of the lung depends on the presence of such an enzyme inhibitor. The lung destruction is explained in part by enzymatic damage to lung tissue. It has been suggested that the lack of antitrypsin may allow the trypsin, believed to come from bacteria and inflammatory cells, to digest the lung parenchyma and to cause the enlarged air spaces.

Emphysema is a crippling disease, feared because the patient does not die quickly, but drags out a miserable existence for many years, a trial and tribulation to himself, his family, and his physician. He has difficulty with every breath taken and breathes some 20,000 times every 24 hours. It has been said that perhaps the most compelling of human appetites is the need for air, and probably no distress is so agonizing as that which results from the inability to breathe adequately.

The effects of emphysema may be serious and far-reaching. The chest becomes barrel-shaped (see Fig.

Fig. 15–15 These preparations demonstrate a normal bronchial tree, *A*, and a bronchial tree that is dilated saccular and distinctly pathologic, *B*. A higher magnification of an area of emphysema is shown in C. (Courtesy of Dr. J. Hogg, Department of Pathology, McGill University.)

15–13), respiratory movements are diminished, and expiration is difficult and prolonged. Owing to the widespread atrophy and destruction of the alveolar walls, the small blood vessels that run in the septa are obliterated, with resulting obstruction to the pulmonary circulation.

CARCINOMA OF THE LUNG

At the present time, cancer of the lung is perhaps the most interesting and challenging of all malignant tumors. It is interesting because of the problems it presents with respect to: (1) **increased incidence,** (2) **possible relation to external carcinogens.** It is challenging because, of all the malignant tumors of internal organs, it is often readily seen by means of the bronchoscope, and yet the prognosis is among the worst.

During the past 80 years, bronchogenic carcinoma has become the commonest of the killing cancers, especially in the male. One in three men with cancer has carcinoma of the lung. There can be little doubt that there has been a real increase (Fig. 15–16), but it is equally true that we know what we see. It was not until the beginning of the present century that coronary thrombosis and myocardial infarction were recognized. No one suggests that the disease started then, yet the lesions, which any medical student can

now tell at a glance, were not appreciated by such masters as Virchow and Rokitansky, who may have given them different names.

If there were differences of opinion as to the question of an increased incidence of cancer of the lung, these differences are multiplied many times when we come to the matter of **causation.** The trouble is that there are so many possible carcinogens. The exhaust gases and soot from automobiles, especially when idling at stop lights in the city, are rich in carcinogenic agents. The same is true of such new events as radiation fallout, although that modern hazard can hardly be blamed for the development of cancer 50 or more years ago.

Cigarette smoking is the etiologic agent that has aroused the greatest interest and the most heated debates. Statistical evidence certainly supports the idea that excessive smoking is a factor of importance. If you do not smoke, the incidence of carcinoma of the lung is 3.4 per 100,000 population; if you smoke less than 1 pack per day, it is 59 per 100,000, and if you smoke more than 1 pack per day, it is 217 per 100,000. It is clear that cigarette smokers have a greater risk of dying of lung cancer than nonsmokers, and that the risk increases with the number of cigarettes smoked.

It is important to recognize that there are several distinct tumors of the lung that can collectively be called carcinoma, but at least three different subsets

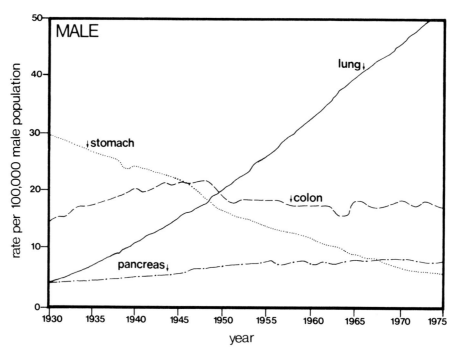

Fig. 15–16 This graph shows the remarkable increase in the rate of lung cancer during the years 1930 to 1975. Compare with the rate for stomach (falling), and colon (relatively constant). (From Gilbert, E.F., and Huntington, R.W.: *An Introduction to Pathology.* New York, Oxford University Press, 1978.)

are distinguished by microscopic examination, by their behavior, and by their prognosis and response to therapy. They probably are also different in that their cause may differ. Thus, we recognize one type of lung carcinoma as having a small cell pattern, arising in or around central bronchi and metastasizing early in the typical 50-year-old male patient. This type is called an "oat cell carcinoma" by popular designation, or, more correctly, **small cell carcinoma.** These cells have been shown to arise from cells other than those normally lining the respiratory tract. Instead, they are interstitial cells that stain with silver stains and contain secretory granules. These tumors sometimes are associated with syndromes of excess ACTH (adrenocorticotropic hormone) or ADH (antidiuretic hormone) production, and are responsible for the paraneoplastic syndrome, because of the ectopic hormones that these cells can secrete. It is important to recognize that this type of tumor (oat cell) accounts for only about 15% of all lung cancers (Fig. 15–17).

The most common type is **squamous carcinoma** (40%), which arises in the metaplastic epithelium of the major bronchi. The tumor grows into and surrounds one of the major bronchi, gradually narrowing the lumen until it becomes partially blocked (Fig. 15–18). Two results follow from this blockage. (1) In the first place, the part of the lung supplied by the

Fig. 15–18 The right lung is shown with a large area of **bronchogenic carcinoma** rising in the bronchus, which is narrowed (arrows). (McGill University, Department of Pathology Museum.)

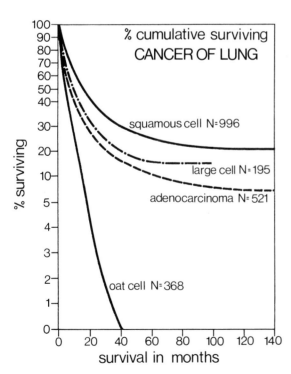

Fig. 15–17 This graph illustrates the survival rates for different histologic types of cancer of the lung. (From Mountain, C.F., et al.: A system for the clinical staging of lung cancer. A.J.R., 120:130, 1974.)

bronchus is cut off from a fresh supply of air, the air in this part of the lung is gradually absorbed into the blood, and finally the affected area of the lung undergoes collapse (atelectasis). This collapse can readily be recognized in the chest x-ray even though the tumor itself may be invisible, and by this means the correct diagnosis can be inferred. (2) The second possible outcome is recurrent infection beyond the obstruction, that is, an abscess or pneumonia that does not resolve. This is because the secretions in the blocked part of the bronchus cannot escape and therefore stagnate and contribute a suitable medium for infection. Cancer cells from the surface of the tumor that projects into the lumen of the bronchus are shed and coughed up in the sputum. Examination of the sputum for these cells, either by making smears or by coagulating the sputum into a block and cutting microscopic sections, is an extremely valuable means of making early diagnosis, especially in cases in which the tumor cannot be seen by the bronchoscope.

Other types of lung carcinomas are often thought of as subsets of this "bronchogenic" carcinoma. They may appear as large anaplastic cells (30%) or more poorly differentiated carcinomas. Another group that seems different comprises those carcinomas that show a glandular pattern (adenocarcinoma) (10%) and that arise in the periphery of the lung rather than in the larger central bronchi. Finally, there is another rare type (alveolar cell) (3%), which appears in many sites at once and resembles a disease in sheep attributed to a virus infection. Despite these morphologic differences, most lung cancers appear in persons who can give a history of heavy smoking for many decades; yet there are smokers who do not develop cancer, too!

One of the chief features of all carcinomas of the lung is the formation of metastases. Most frequently, carcinoma of the lung metastasizes to regional lymph nodes (80% at the hilum of the lung); then it is seen in the liver (40%), brain (15%), bone marrow (15%), and adrenal (15%). Even when the tumor in the bronchus is comparatively small, the cancer cells may spread by lymphatics to the lymph nodes in the chest, where they form a large tumor mass, or by the blood stream to distant organs such as the liver, brain, and bones. The first indication that the patient has cancer of the lung may be increase in girth due to metastases in the liver, severe headache due to a brain tumor, or a fracture caused by weakening of a bone from the presence of a secondary tumor. The adrenal and kidney are often involved. In addition to distant metastases, the tumor may spread widely throughout the lung and involve the pleura.

Clinical Pattern. The symptoms are due to metastases and obstruction. The **persistent cough** is due to irritation of the bronchus by a growth. When a patient in the cancer-prone age, particularly a man, has suffered from a cough and expectoration without obvious cause for more than a few weeks, it is always wise to suspect carcinoma and to examine the sputum for cancer cells or to pass a bronchoscope and inspect the lining of the bronchi. *Bloody sputum* is caused by the opening of a tumor in the bronchus into a blood vessel. **Dyspnea** may be due to the cutting off of air from the lung, to pressure by the enlarged glands, or to interference with the heart's action. **Pain** in the chest and back is caused by pressure on the nerves. Pleural effusion is common, and is due to irritation of the pleura by spread of the tumor. Other symptoms may be due to metastases in the brain and elsewhere.

Certain round, circumscribed benign tumors cannot be distinguished radiologically from inflammatory lesions (Fig. 15–19). These tumors are called **hamartomas** because they are attributed to a developmental defect, and the problem of the cause of this "coin lesion" is best solved by surgical removal and histologic examination.

It is important, however, to realize that not all tumors that can be identified in the lung have arisen there. The lung is a favorite site for metastasis of

Fig. 15–19 This x-ray demonstrates a calcified "coin lesion" in the right upper lung, so-called because of its size and shape. The cause in this case was histoplasmosis.

tumor from other organs, particularly tumors of the breast, kidney, or colon. Often these tumors appear as solitary lesions, but sometimes they are multiple, as shown in Figure 15–20. By the time such tumors are identified in the lung, it is usually too late to do much about them.

PNEUMOCONIOSIS

The long-continued irritation of certain substances may cause a chronic interstitial inflammation known as pneumoconiosis (Greek *konis*, dust). These dusts are often encountered as the result of industrial processes. The most common dangerous element in the dust is silica.

Silicosis is the most widespread, the most serious, and the oldest of all occupational diseases. It provides a serious hazard in the gold-mining industry in certain districts such as the South African Rand and northern Ontario. If, in coal mining, hard rock has to be drilled through, coal miners may also suffer. Other occupations in which there is danger are tin mining, stoneworking, metal grinding, and sandblasting. In all these cases, dust containing fine particles of silica may be inhaled over long periods of time.

The silica dust is carried by phagocytes from the bronchioles into the septa of the alveoli. There the dust acts as a stimulant to the formation of large amounts of connective tissue. This fibrosis goes hand in hand with destruction of the lung structure. At first

Fig. 15-20 *A*, The cloudy patches on this chest film are called "cannonball" lesions, and are consistent with multiple metastases to the lungs. *B*, The gross appearance of similar lesions throughout both lung fields, typical of metastatic tumor to the lungs from the kidney or bowel. (McGill University, Department of Pathology Museum.)

there are discrete nodules of fibrous tissue, but in time these coalesce to form large fibrous areas, which are useless from the point of view of respiratory function. These fibrous areas give a characteristic x-ray picture, by means of which an accurate diagnosis can be made.

We have spoken as if the silica particles explained everything. Another concept, an immunologic theory, has come into fashion. Silica, instead of having a simple toxic effect on the tissue, is now believed to combine with body protein to form antigen, so that there may be some element of an antigen-antibody reaction in the production of fibrosis.

The condition is progressive, and the patient continues to worsen even after he or she has been removed from the source of dust for a number of years. Many silicotics die of tuberculosis, because the presence of silica in tissues favors the growth of tubercle bacilli to an astonishing degree. There is gradually increasing shortness of breath, with developing heart failure owing to the difficulty the right ventricle has in pumping blood through the densely fibrosed lungs. This is one of the few conditions for which there is no treatment (except lung transplant) and it is evident that in this case prevention is all-important.

This can be done by adequately ventilating factories and by providing miners with masks that filter out the dust. Silicosis remains a serious occupational hazard.

Anthracosis, sometimes called "black lung," is the name given to the lung filled with coal dust. All city dwellers have a degree of anthracosis, as they inhale heavily soot-laden air and filter out the soot that stains their tissues. If the coal is hard coal, damage will result because the rock from which the coal was mined contains silica. **Asbestosis** is an important disease caused by the inhalation of asbestos dust. The disease may be acquired either during the crushing of asbestos rock, in the process of the manufacture of asbestos, or from handling building materials or insulation that is composed of asbestos. The simple act of sawing asbestos insulating board creates a fine dust that, when inhaled, can cause chronic injury to the lung. As the great bulk of asbestos comes from the province of Quebec, it is natural that many cases should be found in that locality. The lung shows the same airless and fibrous condition that is so characteristic of silicosis. Both in asbestosis and in silicosis there is a marked tendency to the development of pulmonary tuberculosis.

The most important aspect of asbestosis is not fibrosis, but rather the relation certain asbestos has to cancer of the lung and its covering, the pleura. We now recognize that the relatively rare tumor of the pleura, mesothelioma, is unequivocally associated with asbestosis but the latent period between exposure and tumors is extremely long. It now seems clear that occupational exposure to asbestos carries a risk for gastrointestinal cancers as well.

VASCULAR DISEASES OF THE LUNG

The most common pathologic state of the respiratory tract that causes serious symptoms, apart from the common cold, is **pulmonary edema.** This state arises when there is heart failure or, less commonly, when some other cause such as high altitude upsets the equilibrium in the capillary bed of the lung. By far the most common cause of pulmonary edema, which causes marked **dyspnea,** is heart failure from any cause. The mechanism by which the edema occurs is simply an elevation in the pressure at the venous end of the capillary bed. Other mechanisms, such as valvular heart disease (aortic stenosis, mitral stenosis), which raise the left atrial pressure, result in pulmonary edema that can be recognized in the patient by the moist, bubbling sounds heard through a stethoscope. These sounds are called rales. The same rules, in general, govern the occurrence of pulmonary edema as dictate the presence of edema in other places in the body.

Emboli to the lung from leg veins or from areas of thrombophlebitis, or even from the right heart, are frequently life-threatening, if not fatal. The occurrence of pulmonary emboli is often overlooked clinically, particularly if they are small. One of the classic presentations is the occurrence of a sudden pain in the chest accompanied by blood-tinged sputum. This presentation is relatively easy to recognize, but in many instances there may be no hemoptysis, and the embolus may elicit no inflammatory reaction (Fig. 15–21). Therefore the patient may be unaware that it has occurred. Because the lung has a dual blood supply (bronchial vessels arising from the aorta and pulmonary vessels from the right heart), unlike other organs such as the kidney that have an endarterial supply, **infarction** does not inevitably accompany every embolus. It is only when the systemic circulation (bronchial arteries) is compromised and sluggish, as in cases of chronic heart failure, that occlusion of a branch of the pulmonary artery causes an infarct. These infarcts classically are wedge-shaped, reflecting the distribution of the smaller vessels, and reach to the pleural space. A fresh infarct in the lung is often visible radiologically, and, if you should examine it grossly, it will appear hemorrhagic.

Large pulmonary emboli often arrest at the bifurcation of the pulmonary arteries and are a cause of sudden death, presumably on a reflex basis. The most common predisposing cause of pulmonary emboli, big or small, are areas of thrombosis in the deep veins of the leg or pelvis. Prolonged bed rest, surgical oper-

Fig. 15–21 These figures are lung scans. *A* shows multiple defects of perfusion due to pulmonary thromboembolism. Normal perfusion can be seen in *B*.

ations, and immobilization following orthopedic procedures are all significant predisposing causes of this serious vascular catastrophe.

A third but relatively rare disease of the pulmonary vasculature is prolonged and persistent hypertension. The pulmonary, as contrasted with the systemic, circulation is a low-pressure system in which the right ventricular pressure and main pulmonary artery pressure seldom exceed 30 mm Hg, about a quarter of the systolic pressure in the systemic circulation (120 mm Hg). It is a low-resistance, distensible system that receives the same volume of blood as the aorta, and even with exercise or after pneumonectomy there is only a slight increase in pressure. However, when there is narrowing of the pulmonary arteries due to chronic lung disease, or recurrent pulmonary emboli, or a reflex (vasomotor) constriction due to anoxemia or acidosis, then the pulmonary artery pressure will rise and approach systemic values.

Increased resistance may be caused by increased flow, whatever the cause (congenital defects of the heart or great vessels), by increased pressure in the left atrium (mitral stenosis, left heart failure), or by reflex vasoconstriction (chronic lung disease). Many conditions may lead to a rise in pulmonary arterial pressure and may eventually result in right heart failure **(cor pulmonale),** but they are beyond the scope of this chapter.

An even rarer disease is **primary pulmonary hypertension,** which is also referred to as idiopathic. This simply means that all of the recognized causes of pulmonary hypertension, such as recurrent pulmonary emboli, have been excluded as contributing to the disease, and this particular case has no known explanation for the hypertension and failure.

ASTHMA

This difficult and distressing disease is well named, for it is derived from the Greek word for panting. Literally, the term means difficult breathing and has been traced in English as far back as 1540. It is a disease of uncertain etiology, characterized by an increased responsiveness of the trachea and bronchi to various stimuli, many of which have been identified as allergens. The chief symptoms are marked wheezing and difficulty with expiration. The patient with asthma is subject to acute episodes of extreme **dyspnea,** principally due to prolonged and difficult exhalation of air. The smaller bronchi and bronchioles are narrowed and often occluded with excessive, tenacious mucus. The asthmatic patient has little difficulty with inspiration but the narrowing and valve-like constriction causes a sensation of tightness that may be frightening, and a wheezing that is loud and can be heard by others. This attack may subside within a few minutes or may continue sometimes for hours or may lead to death. The chest may become distended by nature of the air-trapping, and the patient may become cyanotic and be desperately anxious. Immediate relief is usually obtained with the administration of epinephrine or aminophylline.

The cause of asthma is not clear. There is often a family history of allergy and an individual history of hypersensitivity. In addition, there is abundant evidence that psychologic factors play a role in some cases, and that asthmatic attacks can be precipitated by emotional factors.

ATELECTASIS

This word means collapse of the lung. The lung is a sponge filled with air. When compressed, it collapses. Before birth there is, of course, no air in the lungs, and they are therefore completely collapsed, a condition of **congenital atelectasis.** As soon as the newborn breathes after birth, the lungs become expanded with air. In medicolegal work, the absence of atelectasis is proof that the child has lived after birth.

Apart from the congenital form, collapse of the lung may be produced in two entirely different ways: by compression of the lung or by obstruction of a bronchus. Compression of the lung may be caused by pleural effusion, by empyema, or by the presence of air under pressure in the pleural cavity (pneumothorax). Obstruction of a bronchus may be caused in a variety of ways. A foreign body such as a peanut, coin, or tooth may pass down the trachea and become lodged in a bronchus. No air can now enter that part of the lung supplied by the blocked bronchus; the air already there is absorbed into the blood, and the lung collapses. In debilitated children suffering from bronchitis, mucus may collect in the bronchi in such a large amount that obstruction and atelectasis result; owing to the debility, the mucus is not expelled by vigorous coughing. For the same reason, areas of collapse may develop after an abdominal operation, because mucus collects in the bronchi owing to the irritation of the anesthetic, and coughing is interfered with by the abdominal wound.

Pneumothorax

Pneumothorax is air in the pleural cavity. The air may come from the lung, usually as the result of rupture of an emphysematous bulla, occasionally of a tuberculous cavity on the surface. More rarely it may come from the outside, as in a perforating wound of

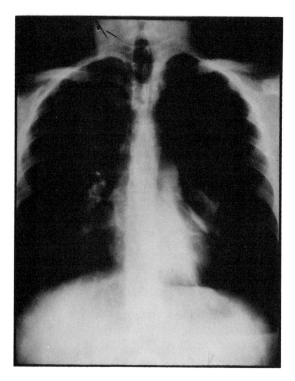

Fig. 15–22 This x-ray demonstrates a left-sided pneumothorax. The lung is completely collapsed on the left side and lies against the heart. Compare this with the right side, which is normal.

the chest or a fracture of a rib. Whatever the cause of the pneumothorax, the air accumulates in the pleural cavity and compresses the lung, causing collapse in the same way as an accumulation of fluid may lead to collapse. The presence of air can easily be detected by the physician by the physical signs it produces and by the appearance in the chest x-ray (Fig. 15–22). Pneumothorax may be an emergency and requires rapid diagnosis and treatment, or suffocation will result.

ADULT RESPIRATORY DISTRESS SYNDROME

This is the name given to acute respiratory failure characterized by hypoxia with radiologic evidence of an extensive, bilateral infiltrate with an alveolar pattern. This life-threatening disorder has been found in many medical and surgical disorders, ranging from burns and aspiration of gastric contents to overdose of drugs and viral infections. It is seen most commonly in shock syndromes and has in fact been called "shock lung." The reason for the massive leakage of erythrocytes into the interstitial and alveolar spaces is unclear, but injury to the alveolar capillary tissue seems to be a common denominator. It does not seem to matter whether the injury is anoxemia, a chemical or toxic insult, or a physical injury such as high tem-

perature, as in fire, the effect is the same, a marked respiratory impairment in the ability to oxygenate blood and to expand and ventilate the lung because of its increased turgor or stiffness. The hypoxemia may be fatal, and the treatment of this disorder remains uncertain.

BRONCHIECTASIS

Bronchiectasis is a condition of dilatation of one or more of the smaller bronchi. It is similar to aneurysm of an artery, and, like an aneurysm, it is caused by weakening of the wall of the bronchus. This weakening has traditionally been attributed to infection. A single agent is seldom sufficient to produce the condition. It is most common in children after such viral infections as whooping cough or measles, in both of which the bronchial walls are inflamed, but it often occurs in young adults, and may persist into middle life. The most significant lesion is the destruction of the musculature and elastic tissue, for it is these that weaken the wall of the bronchus and allow the dilatation to occur. The bronchus dilates and forms a sac in which infection can occur. In time, a regular cesspool is formed, the wall of the bronchus is destroyed, and an abscess results.

The chief symptom of bronchiectasis is the coughing up at intervals of great quantities of purulent material that may be foul-smelling. In abscess, also, large quantities of pus are brought up and the breath may be foul. The disease may be confined to one or more segments, a point of great importance when it comes to a question of surgical removal of the lesion. (A segment is a section of lung parenchyma more or less completely separated from neighboring segments and supplied by a separate bronchus.)

RESPIRATORY FAILURE

The inability of the respiratory system to maintain normal arterial gas tensions of either oxygen or carbon dioxide, or both, may be caused by many or most of the pathologic processes outlined in this chapter. Today, the diagnosis of respiratory failure depends on laboratory examination of blood gases to determine the partial pressures of oxygen and carbon dioxide. Beyond the arbitrarily defined limits of arterial PO_2 of less than 60 mm Hg or PCO_2 of greater than 50 mm Hg while breathing room air, the situation is interpreted as respiratory failure that may be either acute or chronic.

The principal cause of the fall in arterial oxygen or the rise in arterial CO_2 is interference with the normal mechanisms of oxygen transfer or alveolar ventilation. This interference may be caused by inappropriately matched gas exchange and circulatory perfusion (ventilation-perfusion inequality) (Fig. 15–21). For example, when an alveolus is full of inflammatory exudate and air cannot fill the alveolus (as in acute bacterial pneumonia), the pulmonary capillary blood will return to the heart with a decreased capacity for carrying oxygen. In this instance, the alveolar oxygen tension is reduced, and this is reflected in the arterial oxygen level. Elevations in arterial carbon dioxide occur when the alveoli are poorly ventilated.

The physiologic effects of these disorders of oxygen and CO_2 transport are important, since hypoxia seriously interferes with the metabolism of all tissue, particularly that of the brain. The nature of the association between hemoglobin and oxygen dictates that, so long as the arterial oxygen level remains above 65 mm Hg, hemoglobin transportation will be effective. When the level falls below 60 mm Hg, there is a large decrease in the oxygen available to tissues. On the other hand, elevations of CO_2 are not so dangerous to tissues themselves, but rather have a decided effect on the central nervous system that results in a progressive loss of higher faculties, so that with CO_2 retention a person loses the ability to react or to think, and finally lapses into coma. This phenomenon is known as CO_2 narcosis and is well described, for example, by Charles Dickens in his account of the fat boy in the *Pickwick Papers*. The behavior of the fat boy was considered strange, perhaps drunken, because he was always falling asleep, even while eating. In his instance, CO_2 narcosis could be postulated because his obesity prevented his diaphragm from moving normally, and this impairment of a person's normal ventilatory excursions insidiously leads to carbon dioxide retention. Therefore the condition has been called the "Pickwickian syndrome."

A third effect of any disorder in gas exchange may be the change in arterial pH. Since blood has a limited buffering capacity, or a limited capacity, particularly with respect to carbonic acid, any increase in PCO_2 will rapidly lead to acidosis. The most important obvious effects of such an acidosis are increased irritability of cardiac muscle, which may in turn lead to cardiac arrhythmias, or, on the other hand, to such changes as increased resistance in the pulmonary circulation. Fortunately, there are both respiratory and renal mechanisms that are brought into play to compensate for acidosis, whatever its cause.

One last word might be devoted to the accidental and often catastrophic event that follows inhalation, aspiration, or impaction of foreign material, particularly food, in the major airways. In the hospital, the accidental inhalation of gastric contents occurs once in a while in the unconscious, comatose patient. The acid gastric juices, which may contain enzymes as well as food particles, create a hemorrhagic pneumonia that, if it is not fatal, may destroy large areas of the lung. More commonly, particularly in persons who have been enjoying the fruits of Bacchus, large, incompletely masticated particles of food, especially meat, may be aspirated, and the sudden convulsive actions of the unfortunate may be mistaken for acute coronary occlusion (café coronary), whereas simple extraction maneuvers could clear the airway and save the person's life.

SYNOPSIS

The function of the lungs is to oxygenate blood, to excrete CO_2 and H_2O, and to act as a buffer. Its anatomy and physiology reflect these functions.

Infections cause the most common acute lung diseases. They may be local (abscess, tracheitis) or generalized (pneumonias), and they are caused by a wide variety of agents (virus, bacteria, fungi).

Tuberculosis is less common today than in the 1900s, but it still is an important disease of the lung, because it destroys the pulmonary tissue and is treatable.

Bronchitis and emphysema are common chronic diseases and are related to air pollution (smoke, industrial pollutants).

Carcinoma of the lung is common in smokers and may only be recognized when it has either obstructed the bronchus or metastasized. Secondary tumors to the lung from other organs are found frequently.

Vascular disease of the lung may result in increasing pulmonary arteriolar resistance and cause heart failure. Pulmonary emboli are a frequent cause of death in postoperative, debilitated, or chronically ill patients.

Dyspnea has many causes and can best be understood in the context of all the pathologic processes involving both lung and systemic circulations.

Terms

Alveoli
Bronchi
Cilia
Pleura
Surfactant
Pneumonia
Resolution

Consolidation
Dyspnea
Ghon complex
Hemoptysis
Miliary tuberculosis
Fibrocaseous tuberculosis
Emphysema

Pneumoconioses
Mesothelioma
Pulmonary edema
Pulmonary hypertension
Atelectasis
Pneumothorax
Bronchiectasis

FURTHER READING

Becklake, M.R.: Dust and emphysema. Coll. INSERM, 203:23, 1991.

Bode, F.R., Pare, J.A.P., and Fraser, R.G.: Pulmonary disease in the compromised host. Medicine, 53:255, 1974.

Brewis, R.A.L.: Respiratory failure. Br. Med. J., 1:898, 1978.

Chakrin, L.W., and Krell, R.D.: Pathophysiology and pharmacotherapy of asthma: an overview. J. Pharm. Sci., 69:236, 1980.

Comstock, G.W., et al.: The tuberculin skin test. Am. Rev. Respir. Dis., 104:769, 1971.

Cosio, M., et al.: The relations between structural changes in small airways and pulmonary function tests. N. Engl. J. Med., 298:1277, 1978.

Craighead, J.E., and Mossman, B.T.: The pathogenesis of asbestos-associated diseases. N. Engl. J. Med., 306:1446, 1982.

Doll, R., and Hill, A.B.: Lung cancer and other causes of death in relation to smoking. Br. Med. J., 2:5001, 1956.

Eller, W.C., and Haugen, R.K.: Food asphyxiation—restaurant rescue. N. Engl. J. Med., 289:81, 1973.

Fekety, F.R., Caldwell, J., and Gump, D.: Bacteria, viruses and mycoplasmas in acute pneumonia in adults. Am. Rev. Respir. Dis., 104:499, 1971.

Gazdar, A.F., Carney, D.N., and Minna, J.D.: The biology of non-small cell lung cancer. Semin. Oncol., 10:3, 1983.

Gerwitz, G., and Yalow, R.S.: Ectopic ACTH production in carcinoma of the lung. J. Clin. Invest., 53:1022, 1974.

Gracey, D.R., Byrd, R.B., and Cugell, D.W.: The dilemma of the asymptomatic pulmonary nodule in the young and not so young adult. Chest, 60:479, 1971.

Hallman, M., and Gluck, L.: Respiratory distress syndrome—update 1982. Pediatr. Clin. North Am., 29:1057, 1982.

Halkin, H., et al.: Reduction of mortality in general medical inpatients by low-dose heparin prophylaxis. Ann. Intern. Med., 96:561, 1982.

Hershfield, E.S.: Tuberculosis in the world. Chest, 76S:805S, 1979.

Huhti, E., Sutinen, S., and Saloheimo, M.: Survival among patients with lung cancer. An epidemiologic study. Am. Rev. Respir. Dis., 124:13, 1981.

King, R.J.: Pulmonary surfactant. J. Appl. Physiol., 53:1, 1982.

Lieberman, J.: Aryl hydrocarbon hydroxylase in bronchogenic carcinoma. N. Engl. J. Med., 298:686, 1978.

Light, R.W., et al.: Pleural effusions: the diagnostic separation of transudates and exudates. Ann. Intern. Med., 77:507, 1972.

Lipman, J., and Wing, J.: The adult respiratory distress syndrome. A review, some thoughts and a few new ideas. S.A. Med. J., May 23:779, 1981.

Macklem, P.T., Thurlbeck, W.M., and Fraser, R.G.: Chronic obstructive disease of small airways. Ann. Intern. Med., 74:167, 1971.

Mayo Smith, M.F., et al.: Acute epiglottitis in adults: an eight-year experience in the State of Rhode Island. N. Engl. J. Med., 314:1133, 1986.

Morse, James O., et al.: A community study of the relation of alpha₁-antitrypsin levels to obstructive lung diseases. N. Engl. J. Med., 292:278, 1975.

Niewoehner, D.F., Kleinerman, J., and Rice, D.B.: Pathologic changes in the peripheral airways of young cigarette smokers. N. Engl. J. Med., 291:755, 1974.

Robertson, B.: Basic morphology of the pulmonary defence system. Eur. J. Respir. Dis. [Suppl.], 107:21, 1980.

Roussos, C., and Macklem, P.T.: The respiratory muscles. N. Engl. J. Med., 307:786, 1982.

Sanford, J.P.: Legionnaires' disease—the first thousand days. N. Engl. J. Med., 300:654, 1979.

Sasahara, A.A., et al.: Pulmonary thrombosis—diagnosis and treatment. J.A.M.A., 249:2945, 1983.

Selikoff, I.J., et al.: Asbestosis and neoplasia (Editorial). Am. J. Med., 42:487, 1967.

Stead, W.W., et al.: The clinical spectrum of primary tuberculosis in adults. Ann. Intern. Med., 68:731, 1968.

Tobin, M.J., and Hutchison, D.C.S.: An overview of the pulmonary features of a₁-antitrypsin deficiency. Arch. Intern. Med., 142:1342, 1982.

Toomes, H., et al.: The coin lesion of the lung. A review of 955 resected coin lesions. Cancer, 51:534, 1983.

Tsao, M.-S., Schraufnagel, D., and Wang, N.-S.: Pathogenesis of pulmonary infarction. Am. J. Med., 72:599, 1982.

West, J.B.: *Respiratory Physiology—The Essentials.* Baltimore, Williams & Wilkins, 1974.

APPENDIX

Lung Structure and Function

The lung differs from most other organs in that it is supplied by 2 circulations: the pulmonary, a low-pressure, low-resistance system that perfuses the lung for purposes of oxygenation and excretion; and the bronchial circulation, which is a part of the high-pressure systemic circulation, mainly directed to keeping the branches of the bronchi alive. The differing pressures in the 2 circulations, the systemic and pulmonary, are shown in Figure A15–1. Before birth and before the lungs expand, the 2 circulations are joined by the ductus arteriosum, which normally closes within a few hours or days of birth. Should it remain open permanently, there will be a shunt of blood and pressure into the pulmonary circulation that results eventually in injury to the pulmonary arteriolar bed and causes a rise in pulmonary arterial pressures **(pulmonary hypertension)**. Other shunts between the circulations may do the same, depending on the size and duration of the shunt (ventricular septal defect, atrial septal defect).

The quantity of oxygen that could be carried in the fluid part of the blood, the plasma, would not maintain life for a second. Red blood cells (25,000,000,000,000 in the blood of

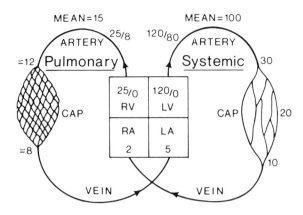

Fig. A15–1 This scheme illustrates the relationship of the systemic and pulmonary circulations and shows the difference in pressures in the two. (From West, J.B.: *Respiratory Physiology*. Baltimore, Williams & Wilkins, 1974.)

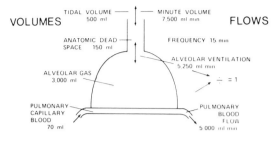

Fig. A15–2 This diagram illustrates the relationship between air exchange and blood flow in the lung. It shows the volumes and flows on which we depend for normal respiratory exchange of oxygen and C0₂. (From West, J.B.: *Respiratory Physiology*. Baltimore, Williams & Wilkins, 1974.)

a man of average size) carry oxygen because of the binding capabilities of hemoglobin. Carbon dioxide (CO_2), on the other hand, is carried mainly in the plasma combined with sodium as sodium bicarbonate ($NaHCO_3$). CO_2 is dissolved and combined with water to form carbonic acid (H_2CO_3). This process is greatly speeded by an enzyme in red blood cells known as carbonic anhydrase. The same enzyme also acts when the blood reaches the pulmonary capillaries, to break down H_2CO_3 into CO_2 and H_2O, the gas being eliminated in the expired air. The most remarkable feature of this beautiful mechanism is that it is the CO_2 in the blood flowing through the respiratory center in the medulla at the base of the brain that provides the stimulus for the muscles of respiration. Even a slight increase in the amount of CO_2 in the blood will increase the rate and depth of breathing, as becomes evident whenever you exercise. Thus a waste gas that must be removed from the body stimulates the mechanism required for its removal, surely a *tour de force* of precise automation. The amount of air exchanged and expired to blood is shown in Figure A15–2.

Each of the alveoli is lined by a film of lipoprotein called **surfactant,** so named because it lowers the surface tension and thus prevents collapse of the alveoli. The ability of the lungs to retain air depends on the special properties of this film. In the absence of surfactant, the lungs readily collapse (atelectasis) and become unable to act as a surface for exchange.

It must not be supposed that respiration is the only function of the lungs, any more than excretion is the only function of the kidneys. Both are concerned with maintenance of acid-base balance as well. When that balance is temporarily upset, it can be restored to normal much more quickly by blowing off CO_2 than by the excretion of acid by the kidneys.

Owing to the rhythmic movements of the chest during respiration, air is being continually sucked into and expelled from the lungs. One great disadvantage of this arrangement is that the interior of the lungs is in communication with the outside air, so that infectious agents are liable to enter and to cause inflammation, although most of them are held back in the nose and throat. This is not the case with any of the other organs of the body, and, for this reason, bacterial infections are far more common in the lungs than in the heart or brain.

The barriers to infection in the respiratory tract are: (1) the presence of protective enzymes in the upper respiratory tract (lysozyme); (2) the integrity of the respiratory epithelium that lines the trachea, bronchi, and bronchioles; (3) the mucus blanket that covers this epithelium; and (4) the action of the cilia, which constantly moves this blanket toward the oral cavity, where the trapped particles and mucus are shed into the gut. At the level of the alveolus (should a bacterium get that far) there is another protector, (5) the alveolar macrophage, which acts as a kind of Cerberus to tax any pneumococcus that wishes to gain access to the interstitial or vascular sanctum. Commonly, small particles and bacteria are phagocytosed and carried to regional lymph nodes if they reach the alveolar space. At the junction between the terminal respiratory epithelium and the alveolar sac is a no-man's-land, in which the protective forces seem unable to cope with the stress of pollution. This zone is where diseases of pollution often strike and cause their destruction of lung tissue, resulting in emphysema. Another reason for this localization may be that the junction of the bronchiole and alveolus is poorly supplied by clearance mechanisms (lymphatics), so that pollutants accumulate here. Alcohol and smoking have been shown to inhibit macrophages and ciliary motility, respectively, thereby allowing bacterial invaders to gain a foothold.

The lung, like the heart, is also covered by a thin membrane, the **pleura,** and a similar membrane lines the chest wall. Although a potential space, the pleural cavity, exists between the layers, in health these layers are in contact with each other. It is evident that inflammation of the lung may easily extend to the pleura and set up inflammation in that space.

16

UPPER DIGESTIVE TRACT

*Eating is touch carried to the bitter end.—*ANON.

The digestive or alimentary canal extends from the mouth, through which the food enters the body, to the anus through which residue escapes (Fig. 16–1). Its function is twofold: (1) To convert the food into a digestible form in which it can be assimilated; (2) to absorb the food thus digested. Briefly, its functions are digestion and absorption. Digestion is begun in the mouth and continued in the stomach. Absorption is accomplished by the small intestine, although digestion also takes place in the upper portion of that tube. The digestive tract has been compared to a modern factory, for it is completely automated, and the owner's job merely consists of ordering bulk supplies and of disposing of the output. Table 16–1 illustrates the sites of digestion and absorption of the different components of food, namely, protein, carbohydrate, and fats.

We may, arbitrarily, divide the alimentary canal into an upper part—the mouth, esophagus, and stomach, and a lower part—the small and large intestines. The common diseases of the upper part are inflammation and tumors.

MOUTH

The principal structures of the mouth are the lips, tongue, salivary glands, tonsils, and teeth.

The lips, especially the lower one, and the oral cavity, including the tongue, can be the site of cancer, most commonly carcinoma. There are a number of etiological factors responsible for this, factors ranging from pipe smoking to ill-fitted dentures. These carcinomas usually present as firm, raised plaques. Most of them can be cured when detected at the early stage. Cancer of the tongue and floor of the mouth are associated with a significant mortality when diagnosis is delayed.

Inflammation and infections are more common problems affecting the oral mucosa. A large number of people have aphthous ulcers which are focal, occasionally painful areas of superficial denudation of the mucosa with no demonstrable cause in most cases. There are, however, inflammatory conditions associated with specific infections. The "cold sore" lesions caused by the herpes virus were described on page 216. Most resolve spontaneously when the herpes virus retreats back to the regional nerve ganglia. In patients who are immunosuppressed, the lesions can become very extensive.

Oral candidiasis, also called thrush, is caused by *Candida albicans*, a fungus that can normally be found in the mouth. Again, in association with conditions leading to immunodeficiency, this organism can induce the typical thrush lesion which consists of a grey membrane covering an inflamed area of the oral mucosa. Oral candidiasis is the most common anatomical site affected by fungal infection. Its greatest significance is that it can be the initial focus from which candidiasis can become systemic. This is then an extremely severe complication which can usually be found as a complication in patients with uncontrolled leukemias, lymphomas, or AIDS.

Tonsillitis. The tonsils are masses of lymphoid tissue, one on each side of the throat. They are full of little recesses or crypts, and as the mouth is teeming with bacteria, it is natural that infection should be common. The infecting agent is frequently the streptococcus. As a result of the acute inflammation, the tonsils become swollen, narrowing the opening of the throat and causing great pain and difficulty in swallowing. Their surface may be covered with pus. One attack of tonsillitis predisposes to another, and a state of chronic infection may be established within the crypts. Acute or chronic sore throat, like tonsillitis, is due principally to streptococcal infection. Fortunately, the availability of antibiotics has decreased the need for tonsillectomy.

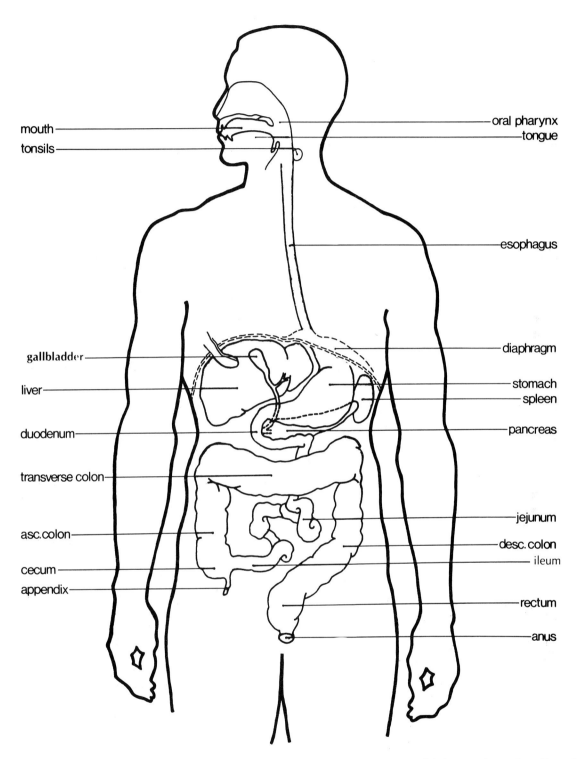

mouth
tonsils

oral pharynx
tongue

esophagus

gallbladder
liver
duodenum
transverse colon

asc. colon
cecum
appendix

diaphragm
stomach
spleen
pancreas

jejunum
desc. colon
ileum

rectum
anus

Fig. 16—1 Shown here are the anatomic relationships of the different parts of the digestive system and their approximate disposition within the body. The diagram might be referred to as disorders of different portions are discussed in this and the next chapter.

Table 16–1. Sites of Digestion and Absorption of Food Components

FOOD EATEN	ORAL DIGEST. pH≃7	GASTRIC DIGEST. pH<7	INTESTINAL DIGESTION pH>7		ABSORBED
protein	no action	⌐pepsin ├rennin └polypeptides	⌐trypsin ├chymotrypsin	⌐carboxypeptidase ├aminopeptidase dipeptidase └dipeptides	amino acids
polysaccharides disaccharides	amylase	no action	amylase	⌐maltase ├sucrase ├lactase	monosaccharides
fats	no action	⌐lipase └fatty acids, glycerin	⌐lipase ├bile salts		colloidal fats fatty acids, glycerin

Salivary Glands. Diseases of the salivary glands are frequent and are important because of the disfigurement, discomfort, and dysfunction. The most common disturbance of these glands is the inflammatory enlargement that occurs in the viral disease epidemic parotitis, commonly called mumps. Other inflammations may be due to bacterial infection of the ducts and gland, often related to ductal injury or obstruction. A more exotic inflammatory disease is the painless enlargement of one or more glands, histologic examination of which reveals only abundant lymphocytes. This inflammatory disease has been likened to other autoimmune diseases and, fortunately, is rare.

However, with the exception of mumps, the most common cause of enlargement of the salivary glands is a benign tumor called a mixed tumor. The parotid gland is often affected by this neoplasm, and over 80% of all salivary gland tumors are benign. The mixed tumor grows slowly and derives its name from its histologic appearance, which shows cartilage-like material in addition to the acinar structure, myoepithelial cells, and ducts. The slow growing benign tumors, which are covered by a well-defined capsule, are a cosmetic hazard, but they also may compress the facial nerve, which lies between the deep and superficial lobes of the parotid gland.

Mixed tumors are difficult to excise completely and therefore tend to recur locally. A few of them (not more than 2%) undergo malignant transformation which is characterized by increase in size or pain. Be-

sides, major and minor salivary glands can be the site of other types of malignant tumors appearing *de novo*. These are mostly carcinomas.

TEETH

Structures. A tooth is composed of four structures: (1) enamel, (2) dentin, (3) pulp, and (4) cementum (Fig. 16–2). The enamel is the outer covering or crown of the tooth. It is calcified and extremely hard, so that

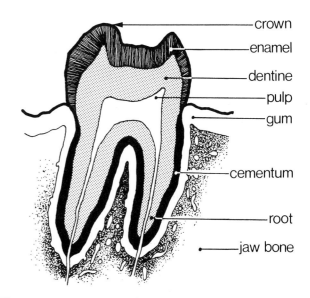

crown
enamel
dentine
pulp
gum

cementum

root

jaw bone

Fig. 16–2 Section through a tooth to show its structure.

it can stand the wear and tear of a long life and, for instance, can enable a dog to crunch bones without becoming worn away. The enamel forms a perfect covering for the dentin, but, unfortunately, it is brittle and easily cracked. Moreover, fissures may form in the course of development, and through these fissures infection may reach the underlying dentin. The dentin forms the main bulk of the tooth. Like the enamel, it is calcified. The dentin is traversed by many minute channels, the dentinal tubules, which pass from the pulp and travel to the enamel. It is along these channels that infection may find its way, once it has reached the dentin. The pulp consists of soft, connective tissue filled with blood vessels and nerves.

Caries. One of the most widespread of diseases, caries or dental caries is found in the teeth of Egyptian mummies, so that it is no new affliction of mankind, and it is worldwide in its distribution, although certain races, such as Eskimos and some African natives, are remarkably exempt. It is principally a disease of childhood and adolescence; when that period is past, the threat of caries becomes much less. Both deciduous and permanent teeth are liable to the disease, but it is most likely to attack the permanent teeth on continued exposure to refined carbohydrates coupled with inadequate hygiene. The molars are most frequently affected.

There is no single cause of dental caries, but its essence is decalcification of the inorganic salts of which the tooth is composed. Anything that endangers the integrity of the enamel covering is liable to lead to caries. The factors may be exciting or predisposing. The exciting cause is bacterial infection with acid-producing organisms, which by enzyme action cause fermentation of refined carbohydrates retained as food debris in stagnant areas around the teeth with the elaboration of organic acids that attack the enamel. Of predisposing causes, faulty diet is all-important. Caries is essentially a disease of civilization, and it is the diet of civilization, particularly finely ground white flour, sugar, and starchy food, that is the culprit.

The lesions of caries can be appreciated only when the structure of the tooth is understood. As in bone tuberculosis, caries is a gradual eating away of the tooth. All the elements of the tooth may be affected. The acids produced by the bacteria enter the enamel through cracks and defects and gradually dissolve the calcium of this hard substance. In time, the enamel is eroded away, exposing the dentin not only to the acids, but also to the bacteria themselves. Destruction of the dentin occurs much more rapidly and widely, so that a large cavity may be formed in the dentin, although there is only a small defect in the overlying enamel. The bacteria readily pass along the dentinal

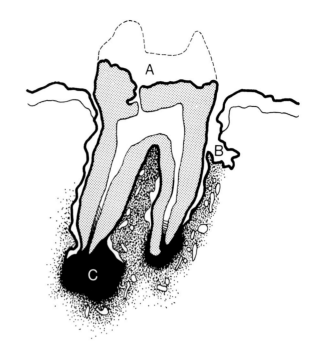

Fig. 16–3 Dental disease. *A,* Caries affecting the crown of the tooth and penetrating down to the pulp. *B,* periodontitis; shrinking of bone and gum away from tooth. *C,* root abscess.

tubules and thus reach the pulp, where they set up a true and often a violent inflammation. It is this inflammatory reaction in the pulp that is responsible for the pain of caries. The infection may pass down through the opening in the root of the tooth, through which the dental nerve enters the pulp, and may give rise to a root abscess (Fig. 16–3).

Other common conditions are periodontitis and gingivitis, but they will only be mentioned. Periodontitis, as the name indicates, is a disease of the surroundings of a tooth, not of the tooth itself. It is the greatest single cause of loss of teeth in the adult, for a gap is formed between the root of the tooth and the bone. Gingivitis is inflammation of the gingiva, the mucus membrane surrounding the neck of each tooth. The gums are swollen and inflamed and may bleed when the toothbrush is used too vigorously.

ESOPHAGUS

Considering its length and the variety of irritating fluids and solids that pass along it, the esophagus is remarkably free from disease. This is probably due to the fact that it is covered by a multilayered squamous epithelium. The only function of the esophagus is swallowing. We shall consider the lesions that interfere with this function.

Congenital Lesions. These often threaten the early days of life, because connections between the trachea and esophagus may lead to aspiration of foodstuffs and may thereby compromise both the respiratory and the digestive functions of the newborn. Failure of development of the esophagus is well recognized. Congenital lesions should be recognized promptly as most of them are surgically curable.

Inflammatory Lesions. A childhood injury to the esophagus by mechanical trauma or by chemical burns from accidental ingestion of caustic agents may lead to lifelong difficulties in swallowing. Chronic irritation or regurgitation of gastric acid may interfere with esophageal function and may lead to regurgitation of previously swallowed materials. This process is called reflux esophagitis and the mechanisms for this reflux are several including chronic alcoholism and cigarette smoking. The epithelial lining of the esophagus can be markedly altered by protracted reflux esophagitis. In time, the normal squamous epithelium is replaced by columnar epithelium resembling gastric or intestinal mucosa. This is, therefore, an example of columnar metaplasia, and the resulting condition is called Barrett's esophagus, a highly significant lesion since affected patients are at high risk for the development of adenocarcinoma at the same site.

Cancer of the Esophagus. The most serious and unpleasant disease of the esophagus is the malignant tumor that occurs most commonly in men of 50 years or more. Although relatively uncommon in North America, it is a frequent form of cancer in other parts of the world such as Northern China. Histologically, esophageal cancer is most commonly a squamous cell carcinoma and a smaller number of cases are adenocarcinomas, most commonly a consequence of Barrett's esophagus. The tumor invades the muscular tube, so that difficulty in swallowing is the chief symptom. The common site is the middle, where the esophagus is crossed by the left bronchus (Fig. 16–4). Another frequent site is the distal esophagus. The most common clinical presentation of esophageal cancer is dysphagia and patients become cachectic quite rapidly. These cancers invade locally, and it is difficult to eradicate them by surgery and irradiation. The prognosis is poor, with a mean survival time of less than three years.

Other Conditions. Another entity, particularly common in obese persons, is the occurrence of a hernia where the esophagus meets the stomach. After a large meal, while lying on the sofa, the stomach and its contents may slide into the chest because the distal esophagus is not properly anchored. This movement causes discomfort or pain and may be confused with pain arising from the heart. This entity is called a hiatus hernia.

The veins surrounding the lower portion of the

Fig. 16–4 The epiglottis is at the upper portion of the picture. The esophagus is replaced by a large, fungating eroding **squamous carcinoma of the esophagus.** The esophagus in this instance has eroded into the trachea. This tumor sometimes occurs in middle-aged men and causes symptoms of difficulty in swallowing. (McGill University, Department of Pathology Museum.)

esophagus can become dilated and eventually rupture into the esophageal lumen producing a massive hematemesis. This dramatic event is usually the result of advanced cirrhosis, a sclerotic change affecting the liver that will be described below. Liver cirrhosis decreases the hepatic blood flow and a collateral circulation develops involving the esophageal varices which are subjected to a high intravascular pressure hence the risk of rupture.

Finally, forceful, repeated and uncontrolled vomiting can occasionally cause a laceration of the mucosa at the gastro-esophageal junction. This lesion usually occurs in chronic alcoholics.

STOMACH AND DUODENUM

Structure and Function. The stomach serves several functions: it is a distensible muscular bag that can receive a seven-course meal and mix the dessert with the antipasto while waiting for a signal to proceed with further digestion, as the entry to the duodenum remains closed. It can mix all manner of foodstuffs with digestive juices and mucus (pepsin, rennin, and HCl) of a low pH (1.7), which begins the acid hydrolysis and proteolysis, key steps in all biochemical processes. The stomach also secretes a factor (intrinsic factor) responsible for the absorption of a vitamin essential to all cell maturation (vitamin B$_{12}$) (Fig. 16–5). As is well known, the stomach is exquisitely sensitive to mood, anxiety, rage, and all the expressions of personality.

The junction of the stomach with the esophagus is a sphincter, and the junction with the duodenum is another (the pylorus). In a few newborn children, the smooth muscle of the pylorus is hypertrophied, and a small olive-like mass can be felt in the infant's abdomen (Fig. 16–6). Occasionally, as in postoperative patients, or in instances of ulcer, inflammation, or tumor, the pylorus may remain contracted and the stomach will dilate, for which the simple remedy is to

pass a tube (nasogastric) to decompress the organ and to retrieve the gas and gastric contents.

Perhaps, apart from inflammations due most frequently to excessive alcohol consumption, the most important disorders of the stomach are disorders of too much or too little secretion. Excessive secretion of hydrochloric acids is related to the development of duodenal ulcers. These are described below along with peptic ulcers of the stomach.

The other side of the coin is the stomach that secretes too little or no hydrochloric acid. This condition commonly occurs in the elderly, and whenever someone identifies a patient with little or no HCl (achlorhydria), there are two diseases that should come to mind. The first is cancer of the stomach, because, for reasons that are not known, there is a high incidence of adenocarcinoma in the presence of achlorhydria. The second disease is really not of the stomach, but of the bone marrow and hematopoietic system, since it seems that patients with achlorhydria frequently have a type of anemia in which the red blood cells do

Fig. 16–5 This photomicrograph shows the **gastric mucosa.** The gastric glands at the bottom of the picture open into the pits and secrete hydrochloric acid and enzymes that are so important in the digestion of food. Four types of cells have been identified in these gastric glands. They secrete pepsin, hydrochloric acid, mucus, and 5-hydroxytryptamine. (From Bloom, W., and Fawcett, D. W.: *A Textbook of Histology,* 9th Ed. Philadelphia, W. B. Saunders Co., 1968.)

Fig. 16–6   This photograph shows the esophagus, stomach, and pylorus of an infant. At the probe the pylorus is markedly stenosed. This obstruction resulted in repeated vomiting and the untimely death of the infant. Today **pyloric stenosis** is recognized early and successfully treated in most instances. (McGill University, Department of Pathology Museum.)

not mature normally (macrocytic anemia). This particular type of disease, which also affects the spinal cord and peripheral nerves, is due to the lack of intrinsic factor secretion by the stomach and is called pernicious anemia.

The three common diseases of the stomach are gastritis, ulcer, and cancer.

Gastritis. When we consider the extraordinary assortment of substances, both fluid and solid, hot and cold, sweet and sour, alcoholic and aerated, to which the gastric mucosa is exposed, it is a wonder that we do not all have inflamed stomachs.

Acute gastritis may be caused by powerful surface irritants. The commonest of such irritants is alcohol. Acute gastritis must be present to some extent after every severe alcoholic bout, and this is largely responsible for the too familiar "morning-after" feeling. Chemical poisons swallowed accidentally by children or with suicidal intent by adults, dietary irritants, and bacterial and viral general infections may be accompanied by acute gastritis with dyspepsia. Recently, gas-

tritis has been associated with the presence of a spiral-shaped bacillus called helicobacter pylori. This organism not only enjoys the hostile low pH of the stomach but, in addition, can degrade the overlying mucus. Helicobacter is also claimed to be associated with peptic ulcer disease, although this does not necessarily imply that the association is causal. Finally, there is now an association of helicobacter with gastric carcinoma.

In gastritis the mucus membrane is red, swollen, and infiltrated with inflammatory cells. If the acute attacks are repeated, as in the habitual alcoholic, the lesions become those of chronic gastritis, and eventually gastric atrophy results.

The most serious result of acute gastritis is bleeding. This may be minor and hidden in the gastric contents, or it may be revealed in the vomitus that often accompanies acute inflammation of the stomach. The vomiting of blood is called hematemesis.

Peptic Ulcer. Excessive amounts of pepsin and hydrochloric acid are clearly related to the occurrence of ulcers in the stomach and duodenum, a disease that has been designated as the executive's "stress syndrome." Although the stimulus to excessive gastric acidity is still debated, recent insights into the various mechanisms responsible for secretion implicate at least three different routes by which the stomach is stimulated. The central nervous system (anxiety, tension, motion sickness) stimulates the stomach by the vagus nerve. The Russian physiologist, Pavlov, demonstrated in dogs that nerve input, even in the absence of stomach filling, was sufficient to initiate gastric juice secretion. Thus one of the more successful surgical treatments for ulcer has included transection of this nerve (vagotomy). Gastrin, a hormone stimulating hydrochloric acid secretion, is a powerful secretagogue, and this substance may be secreted in excess amounts by the stomach, or even by a tumor. A third stimulus to secretion is histamine. How, exactly, histamine is involved in normal and abnormal secretions is debated. Empirically, however, histamine blockers (H_2) effectively reduce the amount and acidity of gastric secretion and thereby offer some relief to ulcer patients. Current management of ulcer patients is based on attempts to diagnose the underlying reasons for the ulcer before attempting surgical treatment or relying on pharmacologic agents alone. The current treatment is the use of cimetidine or similar agents, an H_2 antagonist that seems to be particularly effective, or similar agents.

An ulcer of the stomach is called peptic, because the peptic or digestive juice plays an all-important part in its production (Fig. 16–7). A similar ulcer may occur in the duodenum next to the stomach. The mecha-

Fig. 16–7 A barium upper GI series shows a benign-appearing ulcer on the lesser curve of the stomach. The important aspects of this x-ray study are the projection of the ulcer into the wall of the stomach, and that the ulcer is on the lesser curvature.

nisms of ulcer formation are incompletely understood but appear to be quite different in the stomach and in the duodenum from the clinical and laboratory observations that are currently available. The formation of stomach ulcers is associated with a local decrease in the resistance of the mucosa to the action of acid. There is a natural barrier, in which mucin plays a major role, that normally protects the stomach from self-digestion. This barrier is focally defective at the site of gastric ulcer formation. Surprisingly, when acid secretion is measured in gastric ulcer patients, it is found to be normal, or even decreased.

By contrast, the stomachs of patients with a duodenal ulcer secrete an excessive amount of hydrochloric acid, which is a consequence of a hyperresponsiveness to the normal stimuli of acid secretion. Beyond these established facts, there is a large number of unanswered questions on the mechanisms of ulcer formation in the stomach or the duodenum, and in spite of all the theories, peptic ulcer remains a mystery. The patient with peptic ulcer is usually highstrung, restless and irritable, prone to worry, and upset by strain. These characteristics are not the result of the ulcer; they are much more probably its cause and have to be considered by the physician who undertakes the treatment of a case.

The site of the gastric ulcer is usually at the pyloric end of the stomach or along the upper border (lesser curvature). When such an ulcer is examined under the microscope, its base is found to be made of fibrous connective tissue with a variable number of inflammatory cells. Not uncommonly, blood vessels are present within this base and any further erosion can potentially trigger hemorrhage (Fig. 16–8). An excessive deposition of fibrous tissue in relation to an ulcer located near the pylorus results in partial obstruction. Hydrochloric acid acts as an acute irritant, so that the area of necrosis tends to become deeper. This necrotic tissue is in turn digested, and in time the hole may penetrate the whole thickness of the wall and may precipitate perforation into the abdominal cavity. One of the results of perforation is to permit the air that is normally in the stomach to escape into the peritoneal cavity. The presence of free air in the peritoneal cavity (Fig. 16–9), as seen in an upright x-ray examination, is an important clue to the diagnosis. Duodenal ulcers are more common than gastric ulcers and are usually located in the first portion of the duodenum (Fig. 16–10). They can penetrate quite deeply within the duodenal wall and perforate either in the peritoneal cavity or in relation to the pancreas. Differential diagnosis from cancer is much less of a concern in the duodenum, as compared to the stomach, because duodenal cancer is exceedingly rare.

Clinical Pattern. The common symptom of peptic ulcer, whether gastric or duodenal, is **pain,** relieved by the taking of foods and alkalies. The pain may be a mild feeling of discomfort, or it may be severe. It bears a characteristic relation to food, being relieved

Fig. 16–8 This large, penetrating **peptic ulcer** is in the prepyloric area of the stomach. At the base of this ulcer is an artery (at arrow). The erosion of this artery led to massive gastrointestinal hemorrhage. The specimen demonstrates two classic complications of peptic ulcer—penetration and hemorrhage. (McGill University, Department of Pathology Museum.)

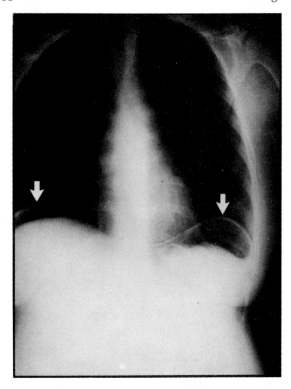

Fig. 16–9 This chest x-ray shows the presence of air under the diaphragm within the peritoneal cavity. A pneumoperitoneum (air in the peritoneal cavity) is seen with a penetrating wound of the abdomen, with a perforated stomach, as in an ulcer, or following an operation in which the wound has not been closed. The diagnostic sign is the presence of the increased contrast of air underneath the diaphragm at the arrows on both sides. If the patient is placed in another position, on his back, the air will move as in a carpenter's level to the highest place, under the abdominal wall if the patient lies on his back, or along the posterior wall if the patient lies on his stomach.

Fig. 16–10 This barium swallow shows within the circle a collar button appearance typical of a benign duodenal ulcer. The edges of the ulcer are smooth.

by the taking of food for about an hour and then coming on again. The triple rhythm of pain-food-relief shows a remarkable regularity. An alkali such as sodium bicarbonate may relieve the pain to an even greater degree. The usual explanation given for the pain and its relief by food and alkalies is that the action of the hydrochloric acid irritates the raw surface of the ulcer, the acid being neutralized by food and alkali. Muscular contraction of the stomach wall may be even more important in producing pain than is the action of the acid. A large gastric ulcer sometimes produces no symptoms until it finally perforates, a situation for which no satisfactory explanation can be offered.

It is important to distinguish gastric ulcers from gastric cancers. Modern methods of fiberoptic gastroscopy and cytologic examination are increasing diagnostic accuracy to over 90%. Most benign ulcers show healing of up to 50% of their size after two weeks of medical therapy. Most heal completely after 12 weeks, but if they do not show healing, it is likely that the ulcer is malignant.

Hemorrhage is a frequent sign, varying from a slight oozing of blood to a copious flooding that may prove fatal. Severe hemorrhage is due to rupture of a large artery in the base of the ulcer. In gastric ulcer, there may be vomiting of blood, the vomitus being not red but "coffee grounds" in appearance, owing to the action of the gastric juice on the blood. The patient may not vomit, but may pass the blood in the stools, imparting to them a blackish color (tarry stools), a condition known as **melena**.

Fortunately, the occurrence of peptic ulcer seems to be declining, as has been shown from a study of British physicians. It is of interest that peptic ulcers are more prevalent in monozygotic twins than in dizygotic twins, and there is a threefold increase of peptic ulcer among primary relatives. In addition, duodenal ulcers are more prevalent in persons with blood group O than in those with other blood groups, suggesting some heritable basis for this common, painful disorder, in which over 50% of patients have intractable pain and 30% have hemorrhage from their ulcers, which lead them often to seek surgical treatment for this disorder. It has been remarked that "surgical intervention is the substitution of one pathologic state for another, in the hope that the former is more acceptable than the latter." Surgical treatment for peptic ulceration was initiated by the great German surgeon Billroth in 1880, and has been used as a therapeutic modality with varying degrees of success ever since.

Cancer of the Stomach. This disease is much more common in men than in women. A remarkable (and unexplained) decline in gastric carcinoma in men has been taking place during the last 40 years. The usual age of occurrence is about 60 years, but it may occur much earlier. There is a curious epidemiologic pattern to stomach cancer: it is more frequent in the higher latitudes (Iceland, Finland), it is frequent in countries where smoked fish is commonly eaten, and it is more common in blood group A patients. Overall, dietary factors appear more significant than genetic factors, as is shown by the decrease in gastric cancer incidence occurring in immigrants coming from high incidence countries.

The tumor is generally situated at the pyloric end of the stomach, but it may occur in any part of the organ. It may form a large mass projecting into the cavity of the stomach, or it may merely constitute a thickening of the wall in the pyloric region. Modern gastroscopic studies in high risk populations are able to detect so-called early gastric carcinoma which involves the mucosa and has not penetrated into the thick muscle layer of the gastric wall (Fig. 16–11). Gradually, however, this thickening leads to narrowing of the opening, until finally complete obstruction may be produced, causing marked dilatation of the rest of the stomach. The tumor in the stomach is best detected by means of gastroscopy and radiologic ex-

Fig. 16–11 This photograph shows the much thickened wall of the stomach in a patient whose symptoms of loss of appetite and loss of weight had progressed for 2 years. This infiltrating tumor is called a **scirrhous carcinoma** of the stomach. (McGill University, Department of Pathology Museum.)

amination. One pattern of infiltration of the wall of the stomach by cancer gives rise to an unusual appearance which has been called the "leather bottle" stomach (Fig. 16–12).

Spread of the tumor may occur by lymphatics or by the blood stream. Cancer cells are carried to the nearest abdominal lymph nodes by the lymphatics, but sometimes the lymph nodes in the supraclavicular fossa on the left side may be enlarged by tumor growth (Virchow's node). The cancer cells may be carried by the blood to the liver, brain, and other organs. When distant spread has occurred and metastases are formed, no treatment is of any avail. It is the early spread of carcinoma, often at a time when there are no warning symptoms, that makes the operative removal of the tumor often so disappointing. In this respect, the disease resembles bronchogenic carcinoma.

Clinical Pattern. Unfortunately, pain is not an early symptom of cancer, either in the stomach or in other parts of the body, although it may be marked in the later stages, especially when pyloric obstruction has set in. Loss of appetite and a feeling of repletion before the meal is finished is much more characteristic, and should be regarded as a danger signal in a man in the cancer age who has previously had a healthy appetite, or who frequently states that up to that time he has been able to "digest nails." Absence of hydrochloric acid in the gastric contents obtained by the stomach tube is a sign of great importance. So also is the presence of blood. This blood is most easily tested for by examination of the stools. It cannot be seen with the naked eye as it is too small in amount, but it is readily detected by a simple chemical test. Blood that can be detected by such a test alone is known as occult blood, because it is hidden from the eye. Anemia is a common symptom.

When pyloric obstruction has developed, vomiting from the dilated stomach may be a distressing symptom. The vomitus may have a coffee-grounds character owing to the presence of altered blood, as in the case of gastric ulcer. It will be noticed that nothing has been said about the presence of a lump or tumor that can be felt by the doctor. Such a mass can only be felt in the later stages, when it is too late to hope for cure of the patient.

Diagnostic Tests. Historically, x-ray examination of the esophagus, stomach and duodenum after a barium meal has been the "gold standard" of diagnosis when a lesion in these organs is suspected. It is still being done, but the more recently introduced flexible gastroscope is often used first, since this powerful technique allows direct visualization and biopsies. Other tests involve the chemical analysis of gastric

Fig. 16–12 *A* and *B*, These figures show barium meal studies given 2 months apart. The barium meal shows a much smaller stomach in May 1975, due to infiltration of the wall of the stomach by carcinoma. The decrease in the normal gastric volume and the rigid wall are classic signs of this particular type of cancer.

juice which gives, for instance, useful information on hydrochloric acid secretion.

Gastrointestinal Hemorrhages. Gastrointestinal hemorrhage is a life-threatening emergency. It has a mortality of up to 30% and is often both difficult to manage and to diagnose. With the use of the fiberoptic scope, the site of bleeding can frequently be located easily. Over half the cases of gastrointestinal bleeding are due to peptic ulcer. Esophageal varices, gastric ulcer, gastritis (alcohol-induced), esophagitis, and rarely, systemic disease such as leukemia or a bleeding disorder may bring about the vomiting of blood. In at least 10% of patients, no specific source is found.

Important to the correct diagnosis are the careful noting of the patient's medical history (to identify aspirin or alcohol in particular), and a thorough physical examination (to discover signs of other disease such as cirrhosis). The immediate course is to stabilize the patient, to replace blood, and to attempt to visualize the site of bleeding. Endoscopy followed by radiology frequently solves the problem. It is characteristic of this emergency that re-bleeding may occur; the final approach may have to be surgical, although even that does not guarantee that the bleeding will not recur. One final note is that the bleeding itself, particularly in the older patient, may lead to more serious illness such as myocardial infarction and renal tubular necrosis.

SYNOPSIS

The digestive system serves three purposes: to mix/digest, to absorb, and to store/excrete foodstuffs.

The stomach secretes pepsin and hydrochloric acid in response to cerebral stimuli (vagus nerve), hormones (gastrin), and histamine.

Peptic ulcerations occur in patients with gastric hyperacidity and hypersecretion and may lead to intractable pain, massive hemorrhage, perforation and peritonitis, or obstruction.

Achlorhydria is associated with gastric carcinoma and pernicious anemia.

Gastric carcinoma may be heralded by weight loss, pain, melena, anemia, or loss of appetite.

Terms

Mixed tumor   *Gastritis*   *Melena*
Esophagitis   *Hematemesis*   *Achlorhydria*
Hiatus hernia   *Peptic ulcer*   *Pernicious anemia*

FURTHER READING

Bynum, T.E., Hartsuck, J., and Jacobson, E.D.: Gastric ulcer. Gastroenterology, 62:1052, 1972.

Cohen, S.: Motor disorders of the esophagus. N. Engl. J. Med., 301:184, 1979.

Dodd, G.D.: Genetics and cancer of the gastrointestinal system. Radiology, 123:263, 1977.

Fordtran, J.S.: Placebos, antacids and cimetidine for duodenal ulcer. N. Engl. J. Med., 298:1081, 1978.

Graham, D.Y., Malaty, H.M., Evans, D.G., et al.: Epidemiology of *Helicobacter pylori* in an asymptomatic population in the United States. Gastroenterol., 100:1495, 1991.

Griffiths, W.J., Newmann, D.A., and Welsh, J.D.: The visible vessel as an indicator of uncontrolled or recurrent gastrointestinal hemorrhage. N. Engl. J. Med., 300:1411, 1979.

Grossman, M.I., et al.: Peptic ulcer: new therapies, new diseases. Ann. Int. Med., 95:609, 1981.

Himal, H.S.: Upper gastrointestinal hemorrhage. Can. J. Surg., 21:192, 1978.

Hoey, J., Montvernay, C., and Lambert, R.: Wine and tobacco: risk factors for gastric cancer in France. Am. J. Epidemiol., 113:668, 1981.

Isenberg, J.I., and Maxwell, V.: Intravenous infusion of amino acids stimulates gastric acid secretion in man. N. Engl. J. Med., 298:27, 1978.

Ito, S.: Functional gastric morphology. In *Physiology of the Gastrointestinal Tract.* Edited by L.R. Johnson. New York, Raven Press, 1981, p. 517.

Katon, R.M., and Smith, F.W.: Panendoscopy in the early diagnosis of acute upper gastrointestinal bleeding. Gastroenterology, 65:728, 1973.

Lloyd, M.L., and Olsen, W.A.: A study of the molecular pathology of sucrase-isomaltase deficiency: A defect in the intracellular processing of the enzyme. N. Engl. J. Med., 316:438, 1987.

Mendeloff, A.I.: Dietary fiber and human health. N. Engl. J. Med., 297:811, 1977.

Meyers, W.C., Damiano, R.J., et al.: Adenocarcinoma of the stomach: Changing patterns over the last 4 decades. Ann. Surg., 205:1, 1987.

Miller, A.B.: Epidemiology of gastrointestinal cancer. In *Gastrointestinal Cancer.* Edited by J.R. Stroehlein and M.M. Romsdahl. New York, Raven Press, 1981, p. 31.

Morrissey, J.F., and Reichelderfer, M.: Gastrointestinal endoscopy. N. Engl. J. Med., 325:1214, 1991.

Moss, S., and Calami, J. *Helicobacter pylori* and peptic ulcers—the present position. Gut, 33:289, 1992.

Ottinger, L.W.: Mesenteric ischemia. N. Engl. J. Med., 307:535, 1982.

Parsonnet, J., et al.: *Helicobacter pylori* infection and the risk of gastric carcinoma. N. Engl. J. Med., 325:1127, 1991.

Sipponen, P., Seppälä, K., Äärynen, M., et al.: Chronic gastritis and gastroduodenal ulcer: case control study on risk of coexisting duodenal or gastric ulcer in patients with gastritis. Gut, 30:922, 1989.

Sipponen, P., Varis, K., Fräki, O., et al.: Cumulative 10-year risk of symptomatic duodenal and gastric ulcer in patients with or without chronic gastritis. A clinical follow-up study of 454 outpatients. Scand. J. Gastroenterol., 25:996, 1990.

Sipponen, P., Kekki, M., and Siurala, M.: The Sydney system: epidemiology and natural history of chronic gastritis. J. Gastroenterol. Hepatol., 6:244, 1991.

Stabile, B.E., and Passaro, E.: Recurrent peptic ulcer. Gastroenterology, 70:124, 1976.

Taylor, D.N., and Blaser, M.J.: The epidemiology of *Helicobacter pylori* infection. Epidemiol. Rev., 13:42, 1991.

Trier, J.S., and Madara, J.L.: Functional morphology of the mucosa of the small intestine. In *Physiology of the Gastrointestinal Tract.* Edited by L.R. Johnson. New York, Raven Press, 1981, p. 925.

Walsh, J.H., et al.: Gastrin. N. Engl. J. Med., 292:1324, 1975.

Welch, C.E., and Malt, R.A.: Surgery of the stomach, duodenum, gallbladder, and bile ducts. N. Engl. J. Med., 316:999, 1987.

Wolf, S.: *The Stomach.* New York, Oxford University Press, 1965.

Ziegler, R.G., et al.: Esophageal cancer among black men in Washington, D.C. II. Role of nutrition. J.N.C.I., 67:1199, 1981.

17

LOWER DIGESTIVE TRACT

One finger in the throat and one in the rectum makes a good diagnostician.—Sir William Osler

STRUCTURE AND FUNCTION

The lower digestive tract consists of two parts which differ in structure and function; they are called the small and the large intestine. The names apply to their diameter, not to their length; the small intestine is about 600 cm long and the large intestine is about 150 cm long. The small intestine consists of a short upper section (25 cm), the duodenum, into which open the bile duct from the liver and gallbladder and the pancreatic duct; a longer lower section, the upper part of which is called the jejunum and the lower three-fifths, the ileum. The lower end of the ileum connects with the large intestine at the ileocecal valve, situated in the lower right part of the abdomen. The vermiform appendix opens into the large bowel just beyond it. The large intestine begins as a wide pouch, the cecum, and continues as the colon, which passes up into the right flank, across the abdomen beneath the liver and stomach, and down into the left flank, to become the sigmoid, an S-shaped portion, finishing as the rectum, which is about 15 cm long and opens onto the surface at the anus.

The small intestine is concerned with the digestion and absorption of the food, and its structure is designed to perform these two different functions. The mucus membrane lining this part of the bowel contains innumerable glands in the form of simple tubes, which secrete enzymes that act on food that has begun to be digested but is not yet absorbed (Fig. 17–1). The pancreas, a flat organ that lies transversely behind the stomach, synthesizes powerful secretions (lipase, amylase, chymotrypsinogen) that enter the duodenal lumen at the same place as bile. By the emulsifying action of bile and the chemical action of enzymes on the foodstuffs in the upper bowel, digestion is enhanced and absorption can begin (Fig. 17–2).

The surface of the jejunum is arranged in small projections called villi, which look to the naked eye like velvet (Fig. 17–3). Each villus is composed of hundreds of thousands of intestinal absorptive cells that overlie the core of blood vessels and lymphatics from which they are separated by a thin basement membrane (Fig. 17–4). Each absorptive cell itself is further modified to increase its surface area by the projection of microvilli on its surface, the brush border (Fig. 17–5). It has become apparent that these adaptations, which increase the surface area over 40-fold, facilitate absorption of the molecules that have been made available by digestive processes. It seems that different sugars, fats, and amino acids are absorbed preferentially at different levels in the small bowel.

The absorption at the surface of each cell is facilitated by the presence of extracellular enzymes that lie between the microvilli. All molecules that are absorbed pass into the intestinal cell and are then released into the extracellular space, the lymphatics, or the portal vein, whence they travel to the liver and are used or stored. As food passes down the small bowel, less and less of the absorbable materials remain, and contractions of smooth muscle in the wall of the bowel (peristalsis) facilitate the transport of materials from duodenum to ileum.

At the ileocecal valve, the structure and function of the intestine become different. At this point the residue contains water and indigestible materials. The principal role of the large intestine or colon is to absorb water and to store the materials (feces) until they are excreted. Most colonic uptake of water and salts occurs in the right colon, where up to 2 liters of fluid are absorbed every day. All but about 200 ml of this absorption occurs during the passage of stool through the colon, where small amounts of sodium, potassium, chloride and bile acids are also absorbed.

Normally there are hundreds of millions of bacteria in the colon that aid in fermentation and degradation of the remaining foodstuffs. By-products include histamine and, depending on their substrate and the

Fig. 17–1 This light microphotograph shows a section of the mucosa, submucosa, and muscularis of the duodenum. The villi are seen in the upper left as projections into the lumen of the bowel. The glands that secrete material into the lumen are in this portion of the bowel called Brunner's glands. (Courtesy of Dr. H. Mizoguchi.)

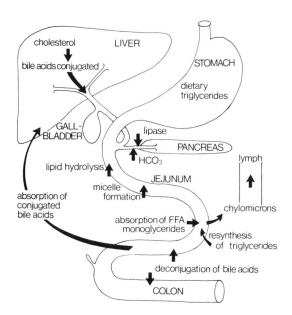

Fig. 17–2 This diagram shows a summary of fat digestion, fat absorption, and the enterohepatic circulation of bile acids in the digestive tract. It demonstrates the interrelationship of the liver, pancreas, jejunum, and circulation. A micelle is a water-soluble complex of emulsified lipid. FFA refers to free fatty acids. (Adapted from Hofmann, A.F.: The chemistry of intraluminal digestion. Mayo Clin. Proc., 48:618, 1973.)

kinds of bacteria present, gases such as methane or sulfur-containing compounds, which have distinctive odors.

The colon can be considered to have several different parts; the diseases of these different parts frequently have different symptoms and signs. For instance, inflammation or tumors of the sigmoid and rectum may signal their presence by bright bleeding, obvious pain or lesions that may be felt by the examin-

Fig. 17–3 **Intestinal mucosa.** This drawing of the surface of the jejunum shows the velvet-like structure of the epithelial mucosa which is arranged in finger-like projections or villi. The function of this arrangement is to increase the absorptive area.

Fig. 17–4 **Villus of intestinal mucosa.** This drawing shows the microscopic appearance of each villus. The epithelial cells, which cover the surface of the villus and absorb the sugars, fats, and amino acids, arise in the crypts. At the apex of each villus the cells are sloughed off. The core of each villus contains both lymphatic and blood vessels. Every molecule of substrate that is used for energy must pass across this epithelial barrier.

ing finger or seen with a short sigmoidoscope. Some degree of squeamishness to look directly at the problem makes the proctoscopic examination an often-neglected opportunity to spot trouble.

By contrast, tumors of the cecum and ascending colon may bleed silently for months until the patient has become severely anemic, with a hemoglobin of perhaps 6 instead of 13 grams.

Fig. 17–5 **Intestinal absorptive cell.** This drawing shows the electron microscope appearance of a single intestinal absorptive cell. Note at the apex of this cell there are also projections to increase the surface area of the cell. This limiting membrane has the capacity to discriminate between D and L amino acids. Extracellular enzyme is held in place between the microvilli. (After Zetterqvist, H.: The ultrastructure of the columnar absorbing cells of the mouse jejunum. Ph. D. thesis, Karolinska Institute, Stockholm, 1956.)

As we have just discussed, the mucosal lining of the small and large intestines are quite comparable but for reasons that are not entirely clear, there are significant differences in the nature and severity of the diseases affecting these two segments of the lower digestive tract. For this reason we will discuss these diseases in two sections.

DISEASES AFFECTING THE SMALL INTESTINE

Congenital anomalies of the small bowel are rare. We just need to mention the Mackel's diverticulum which is a tube or an outpouching of the terminal ileum which can have small areas of gastric mucosa and, therefore, ulcerate.

ISCHEMIC BOWEL DISEASE

This is a condition characterized by decreased oxygen delivery to the intestinal structure which can eventuate in infarction. It is a particularly dramatic condition with a high mortality rate, mostly encountered in older individuals, especially those with cardiac failure and atherosclerosis. Depending on the severity and duration of the process, bowel ischemia can involve either the entire thickness of the wall or only the mucosa. There is also a chronic form of the disease due mostly to atherosclerotic narrowing of the mesenteric vessels which leads to fibrosis of the bowel wall.

In its acute form, there is first a marked hemorrhage of the mucosa and submucosa. If the occlusion is prolonged the muscle layer can also be involved leading to transmural infarction (Fig. 4–21). After a period of one day the lesion becomes complicated with infection. Microorganisms that are normally present in the intestinal lumen penetrate the bowel wall causing an intense inflammatory reaction. One result of this complication is a perforation of the bowel wall with the dramatic picture of peritonitis. Even in the absence of this complication the typical clinical presentation consists of an acute abdomen with pain, vomiting and marked rigidity of the abdominal wall. This is accompanied by shock in a large number of cases.

Various causes are associated with ischemic bowel disease but they mostly involve arterial venous total or partial occlusion by thrombi. The occlusion itself can be attributed to atherosclerosis, extrinsic compression, embolization, or fibromuscular hyperplasia of the arteries. In addition, the low perfusion rate that accompanies a left-sided heart failure also favours the occurrence of ischemic bowel disease by creating a situation in which blood is shunted away from the intestinal structures. Of note, contraceptive pills with a high estrogen concentration are associated with a greater tendency to develop this thrombotic event especially in the venous system. Embolization usually originates from the heart, and is most commonly due to the presence of an intracardiac mural thrombus. Catheterization of the aorta can lead also to the detachment of fragments of atheromatous plaques that embolize to the mesenteric circulation.

The most common site of occlusion is the superior mesenteric artery. Ischemia of the bowel is particularly severe when the proximal segment of this artery is occluded. Ischemia can be diffuse or patchy in the small bowel and may involve the large bowel.

OBSTRUCTIONS

The symptoms of intestinal obstruction vary, depending on the site and cause. With obstruction in the small bowel, vomiting may be the principal symptom; pain and distention are evidence of large bowel obstruction. However, some obstructions are relatively silent and the diagnosis as to the nature and cause of the disease may be hidden until the postmortem examination. Hernia, volvulus, and intussusception are all entities we can consider under this heading.

Hernia. The protrusion of a loop of bowel through an opening or weak point in the abdominal wall is called a hernia, although popularly it is often referred to as a "rupture". The most common sites for these protrusions are the groin (inguinal and femoral hernia) and the umbilicus. All these occurrences depend on an anatomic weakness; hernias do not occur from lifting or from hard work. The protrusion of a loop of bowel into a space where it does not belong may recur, and with time the opening may enlarge, or the bowel may become lodged in this new cavity and become irreducible. The danger arises when the venous return is compressed, the blood supply endangered, and necrosis of the bowel becomes imminent. This situation is called strangulation.

Because of the danger of perforation and peritonitis accompanying this acute intestinal obstruction, immediate surgical intervention is warranted. The surgeon's responsibility is to determine whether the bowel is viable, to return it to the peritoneal cavity, and to repair the opening so that herniation will not recur. It is of interest to note that the most common cause of intestinal obstruction is the presence of adhesions in the peritoneal cavity, and the most common cause of such adhesions is previous surgical exploration of the bowel.

Intussusception. A much more infrequent cause of bowel obstruction, intussusception, occurs most often in children. Here, a segment of the bowel telescopes into another part, commonly at the ileocecal valve. Again, the hazards are gangrene, obstruction, rupture, and peritonitis. The preferred treatment today is to reduce the hernia with barium enema.

Volvulus. A twisting of the bowel on itself is another cause of obstruction.

Paralytic Ileus. Another name for a type of intestinal obstruction that occurs frequently after major surgery, anesthesia, or illness is paralytic ileus. The cause here is physiologic rather than mechanical: it is the absence of peristalsis, resulting in the accumulation of intestinal contents and gas, and dilatation, leading to pain and discomfort. Such obstruction is frequently relieved by the passage of a tube to drain the gas and contents.

Chronic Obstruction. This condition occurs frequently in the elderly or mentally incapable, who are often dehydrated or are unable to maintain a sufficient intake of foodstuffs, so that their feces become brittle, dry, and impacted. Tumors and old inflammatory disease may also constrict the lumen of the bowel.

MALABSORPTION SYNDROMES

The persistence of diarrhea and the occurrence of abnormal bowel movements may be due to a disturbance of absorption, rather than to inflammation such as bacillary dysentery. Many disorders can result in stools that contain poorly digested foodstuffs, and these entities have been lumped together under the title malabsorption syndrome, since they have diarrhea in common. However, these disorders may have vastly different origins, as noted in Table 17–1.

One of the most interesting diseases causing the malabsorption syndrome is called adult sprue or gluten-induced enteropathy. A relatively large number of adults plagued by diarrhea and weight loss have their complaint traced to a hypersensitivity to the wheat protein, gluten. A small bowel biopsy shows atrophy of the villi in the jejunum that necessarily results in a decreased absorptive area. When placed on a trial diet, free from wheat gluten, the absorptive area is restored and their diarrhea disappears.

Of worldwide interest is the relatively recent discovery that some persons lack the enzyme, lactase, which is necessary to digest milk. The genetically determined absence or decrease in lactase results in gaseous diarrhea and suggests that milk is an unsuitable food for such persons. However, more recent evidence has shown that, even in the absence of lactase, a considerable amount of nutritive value is still derived from the milk that is ingested. Clinical lists of the malabsorption syndrome include pancreatic diseases in which there is a loss of other digestive en-

Table 17–1. Classification of Malabsorption Syndromes

Inadequate digestion
  Following gastrectomy
  Pancreatic insufficiency
Reduced bile salts
  Liver disease
  Bile duct obstruction
  Abnormal intestinal pathways
Inadequate absorptive mechanisms
  Mechanical: intestinal resection or shunts
  Mucosal defects: genetic—enzyme deficiency
                inflammatory—tropical sprue
                infiltrative—amyloidosis
                allergic—celiac disease
  Obstructive disorders: lymphatic (intestinal lipodystrophy or
                Whipple's disease)
                cardiovascular (congestive heart failure)
Endocrine and metabolic disorders
  Hyperthyroidism
  Diabetes mellitus

zymes, but this problem may better be considered maldigestion.

Diseases that affect the liver and biliary tree result in reduced bile salts in the duodenum and are a major cause of malabsorption. In the absence of bile salts, fat cannot be absorbed. The stools are voluminous and frothy, and they float. Such a person with a gallstone in the common duct will have, in addition to other difficulties, malabsorption of fats that may result in a disorder of clotting; without adequate fat absorption, the vitamin essential to the coagulation process (vitamin K) is not absorbed either.

Other diseases of a systemic nature such as lymphomas and diabetes mellitus may result in the malabsorption syndrome by mechanical or metabolic means, and logically any obstruction to lymphatic or venous drainage may contribute to inadequate absorption.

INFECTIONS

A number of microorganisms can infect the small bowel and we will limit this discussion to the most significant ones. They typically cause diarrhea which by itself can induce severe dehydration and hypovolemia if not treated properly. Enteritis caused by viruses are extremely common in both children and adults and are usually self-limited. Bacteria cause a large number of intestinal infections. Some of them release potent toxins such as the bacterium which causes cholera, a disease affecting a large number of people around the world. The cholera toxin activates adenylate cyclase, an important enzyme of the intes-

tinal epithelial cell membrane. The activation of adenylate cyclase causes a massive secretion of water into the intestinal lumen. Profuse diarrhea is the outcome and the treatment that will save the patient is prompt rehydration with water and appropriate salts.

Recently, infections of the small bowel with *giardia lamblia*, a protozoan often found as a contaminant of mountain streams and lakes, has been determined to be a frequent cause of diarrhea in campers. The reservoir for this protozoan appears to be the intestinal tract of beavers and other forest dwellers. A second, recently discovered cause of traveller's diarrhea is bacteria of the campylobacter family (see Chapter 7) and one recent outbreak is described in Figure 17–6.

Other bacteria cause ulcers of the intestinal mucosa because of their ability to invade the epithelial lining. This is the case of shigella and salmonella. Some types of *Escherichia Coli*, the bacterium that is a normal inhabitant of our gut, can invade the mucosa and cause diarrhea, a condition often encountered in travelers who had not previously been exposed to those particular serotypes.

The incidence of intestinal tuberculosis has decreased markedly as a result of milk pasteurization. What has increased on the contrary, at least in certain parts of the world, is the incidence of fungal and protozoal infections. The typical new example is an immune-compromised patient. For this reason, the small bowel of AIDS patients is often contaminated with organisms such as cryptosporidium. Also, patients whose immune system has been severely debilitated by leukemias or lymphomas, or the chemother-

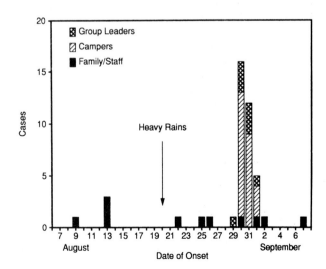

Fig. 17–6 *Campylobacter* enteritis in persons at a camp, by date of onset—Christchurch, New Zealand, August-September 1990. (From Centers for Disease Control, Morbidity and Mortality Weekly Report, 40(7):117, 1990.)

apy they receive for those diseases, are frequently affected by fungal lesions in their intestine.

The small intestine may be the site of a relatively common entity called Crohn's disease which is characterized by conspicuous inflammation. There is, however, no convincing evidence that Crohn's disease is caused by an infectious agent. Also it tends to affect not only the small bowel but the colon. It will therefore be discussed in the section on the large bowel.

TUMORS

Both benign and malignant tumors of the small bowel are rare, especially when one compares their incidence to the occurrence of neoplasms of the large intestine. The reason for this discrepancy between two organs that are so comparable in their structure is fascinating but unknown at the present time.

Benign tumors are most often found incidentally. Malignant tumors, when they occur, are usually lymphomas or carcinoid tumors. Lymphomas can affect the gastrointestinal tract by arising in intestinal or gastric mucosa with no evidence of systemic lymphoma. It has been known by histologists for a long time that the intestine contains a large number of lymphocytes; therefore we should not be surprised that lymphoma can start as easily in the gut mucosa as it does in more typical lymphoid organs such as lymph nodes.

Carcinoid tumors are derived from endocrine cells which are scattered in the normal intestinal mucosa. Although carcinoid tumors can arise in the large bowel, they are relatively more common in the small intestine. They look monotonous and "benign" under the microscope and yet most of them have the potential to behave as malignant tumors as shown by the occurrence of hepatic metastases. Indeed, a typical carcinoid syndrome with paroxysmal flushing can be observed in patients with hepatic metastases from carcinoid tumors. On the contrary, there are no characteristic symptoms when the carcinoids are confined to the intestinal mucosa.

DISEASES AFFECTING THE LARGE INTESTINE

Before describing the various diseases of this organ it is important to note that major progress has been the application of colonoscopy to observe, document, and sometimes treat colonic diseases. The colonoscope is a long, flexible tube fitted with fiber optics; with it one can observe the mucosa with almost the same elegance as the observation of the skin by a dermatologist. Shorter versions of the colonoscope are used for examination of the rectum or the sigmoid

colon only. We will also discuss appendicitis since the appendix is attached to the cecum. As in the small intestine, the number of congenital lesions of the colon are few and rare. We will mention only the imperforate anus, a failure to complete development found in a small number of newborns, and Hirschsprung's disease. This condition is characterized by a marked dilatation of the colon due to an absence of peristalsis in the rectum and sigmoid. The reason for deficient peristalsis is the lack of the autonomic nervous system cells normally present within the bowel wall.

APPENDICITIS

The vermiform appendix is a small tube about 4 inches long and as thick as the tip of your little finger. It opens out of the cecum close to the spot where the small and large intestines join. The appendix is liable to the same diseases as the rest of the bowel, but the condition of importance from the point of view of both frequency and gravity is acute inflammation.

The causal factors are infection and obstruction; it is more and more apparent that the latter is the dominant factor. As a result of the obstruction by concretions of fecal matter, the lumen becomes distended and the venous return is interfered with, so that the wall is poorly oxygenated and is then invaded by bacteria. The infecting organisms, the chief being streptococci and *Escherichia coli*, appear to invade the mucosa from the lumen. Appendicitis is undoubtedly seen more in highly developed countries and in cities than in backward countries and rural districts. Persons who live on a diet abundant in cellulose are less prone to the disease.

There are grades of acute appendicitis, from the most mild to the most severe, but for purposes of description, we shall take the severely inflamed organ that is removed just in time to prevent it from rupturing. Such an appendix is swollen and elongated, sometimes to an extraordinary degree, bright red in color, and covered by an acute inflammatory exudate (peritonitis). As the process goes on, the wall of the appendix becomes thinned at one or more points and may rupture (perforation), so that the intestinal contents are poured out into the abdominal cavity to cause generalized peritonitis. Rupture does not necessarily mean a fatal peritonitis, for adhesions to surrounding structures tend to form before the rupture occurs. These adhesions limit the inflammatory process, so that the peritonitis may remain localized and an abscess may be formed around the appendix.

The principal symptoms of a severe attack of appendicitis are pain and tenderness (in the region of the appendix), nausea and vomiting, fever, and leukocytosis. At first the pain is of a general character (a "stomach-ache"), but presently it settles in the right lower quadrant of the abdomen. Tenderness on pressure over the appendix is the most important single symptom. The pain goes on increasing in intensity until rupture occurs, when it is suddenly, completely, and most unfortunately, relieved by the cessation of tension when the pus escapes. The relief is unfortunate because it may persuade the patient and the relatives, and even the nurse, that all is well, whereas the reverse is the case. Fever and leukocytosis are general signs. Leukocytosis is a valuable means of distinguishing between the appendicitis and simple colicky pains in that part of the abdomen, unaccompanied by inflammation.

PERITONITIS

The peritoneum is the exquisitely thin layer of serous membrane that lines the abdominal cavity. It consists of 2 layers, one covering the inner surface of the abdominal wall, the other covering the stomach, intestines, and the other viscera. Between these layers lies the peritoneal cavity. Infection causing inflammation of the peritoneum generally comes from one of the hollow viscera covered by the membrane, but occasionally it is carried by the bloodstream. The most common source of the infection is an acutely inflamed appendix, but rupture of a peptic ulcer in the stomach or duodenum, or of a colonic diverticulum, or a typhoid ulcer, will flood the peritoneal cavity with septic material. The common microorganisms are streptococci and *Escherichia coli*.

Peritonitis may be local or general. Local peritonitis is inflammation limited to one region, e.g., the appendix and pelvic organs. The inflamed membrane, with its covering of fibrin, readily sticks to a neighboring part that is similarly inflamed. These adhesions are at first readily broken down and the parts separated, but they are invaluable in limiting the spread of the infection. This is particularly apparent in the case of appendicitis. General peritonitis is the result of an infection that is not limited, but rather is spread throughout the peritoneal cavity. The surface covering the intestine is red and inflamed, and becomes covered with a sticky fibrinous exudate, which glues the coils of bowel together. A large amount of fluid may collect in the cavity and between the loops of bowel. This may be thick pus or thin watery fluid, depending on the organisms responsible for the infection.

The great danger of peritonitis is intestinal obstruction and septic shock. When the wall of the bowel (the peritoneum forms the outer part of this wall) becomes inflamed, muscular movements are no longer able to pass along it, and the extremely serious condition of acute obstruction develops. The modern treatment of general peritonitis is largely directed at the acute obstruction that accompanies it along with appropriate antibiotherapy. Recently, attempts to control or prevent septic shock by the use of monoclonal antibodies have been introduced with significant success in some cases.

INFLAMMATORY BOWEL DISEASES

The colon can, of course, be inflamed as a result of various infections. Most of the same microorganisms that cause small bowel infections can also affect the colon and, therefore, the reader is referred to our discussion above. However, the colon can be the "privileged" target of specific organisms, the most common example being the protozoa *Entamoeba histolytica* which is the cause of the ulcers of amebiasis. The parasite is ingested in infected (uncooked) food or water; when it reaches the lower part of the intestine (colon) it invades the wall of the bowel, causing ulcers and the acute inflammation (colitis) known as dysentery. Amebic dysentery is a frequent disease of the tropics, but it also occurs in temperate regions.

The chief symptom is profuse and painful diarrhea, the liquid stools containing slimy mucus, pus, and blood. Large numbers of amebas leave the body in the fecal discharge. The characteristics of the ameba, together with the mode of infection, have already been discussed in connection with the protozoal parasites. In spite of modern treatment with chemotherapy and antibiotics, it may not be possible to eradicate the infection in all cases, and some amebas may remain for a long time, even for years, protected by the bowel wall. The patient may be subject to repeated attacks of dysentery.

The colon (and occasionally the small bowel) can become infected with one of their normal inhabitants, *Clostridium difficile*. The colonic mucosa is covered with pseudo membranes which are in fact patches of acute inflammatory mucosa. This happens in some patients receiving broad spectrum antibiotics.

Newborns can acquire a relatively common condition called necrotizing enterocolitis, also characterized by pseudomembranes of inflammatory exudation followed by necrosis. In this case, however, antibiotics are not involved in the cause or mechanism of the disease. Typically the disease starts in formula-fed infants. It is possible that the lack of immunoglobulins or other maternal factors creates a suitable milieu for the development of this serious disease.

ULCERATIVE COLITIS

Ulcerative colitis is characterized by severe bloody diarrhea with mucus, bowel movements up to 20 times per day, and alternating periods of worsening and improving. This disease is of unknown etiology. It may last for many years. The diagnosis is made by excluding other causes of abdominal pain, weight loss, fever, and diarrhea. The colonic mucosa is diffusely inflamed and ulcerated in patches. The most severe lesions are seen in the rectum, sigmoid, and descending colon. However, the disease extends progressively to the transverse and ascending colon. Frequently, there is a hyperplastic growth of the damaged mucosa resulting in pseudopolyps, but the muscular coats and draining lymph nodes are usually spared the disease.

Because circulating antibodies to the patient's own colonic cells have been demonstrated in some persons, an autoimmune etiology has also been suggested. Hypersensitivity to milk, foods, or bacterial by-products has been implicated also as a pathogenic factor. Since hemorrhagic necrosis of the mucosa has been found in experimentally induced Arthus reactions, a vascular etiology has been proposed. In 1922, attention was drawn to the psychologic constitution of many patients with ulcerative colitis who, while appearing calm and serene, were really anxious and hostile. It is not known whether this anxious state causes, perpetuates, or results from ulcerative colitis. The course of the disease is marked by bouts of exacerbation. Most cases are controlled by anti-inflammatory drugs but severe cases require colectomy. Of significance is the observation that about 10% of patients who have had disease for 20 years develop colon cancer. This reinforces the need for regular follow-up examination in these patients.

CROHN'S DISEASE

This disease of the bowel is as mysterious as ulcerative colitis and resembles it in many ways. The distribution of the lesions, however, is somewhat different as it involves the terminal ileum, ileocecal valve and the cecum. It was first described by Crohn of New York in 1932, and is commonly known as Crohn's disease. More distal segments of the colon become involved progressively when the disease cannot be controlled by therapy. Microscopically, the small and large bowel mucosa have deep ulcers separated by relatively normal epithelium referred to as "skip areas". The inflammatory changes involve not only the mucosa but the deeper layers of the bowel. In severe cases the bowel wall has fissures, even perforations or fistulas, communicating with other bowel

Fig. 17–7 This x-ray shows an upper GI series demonstrating the "string sign" of Crohn's disease. The terminal ileum is narrowed, its mucosa is destroyed, and there is separation of the bowel loops owing to thickening of the bowel wall, and infiltration of the mesentery. A fistula between the sigmoid colon and the ileum can be seen at the arrow.

loops. In milder forms of Crohn's disease the mural inflammation causes a marked thickening of the wall and the intestinal tube becomes very rigid and has a small lumen which gives the characteristic "string sign" on x-rays (Fig. 17–7). Another characteristic change is the presence of microscopic granulomas in the inflamed intestine. Since granulomas are often the hallmark of an infectious disease, many investigators have tried to demonstrate the presence of a microorganism. There has been consistent failure to prove an infectious etiology, and one is presently left with the same unproven theories to explain Crohn's disease as we are with ulcerative colitis. It is quite possible that the two conditions are variants of the same disease. The clinical course of Crohn's disease also has a pattern of exacerbations of bloody diarrhea. Cancer is much less frequently a complication of Crohn's disease compared to the cause of ulcerative colitis. The treatment is symptomatic in both conditions.

INTESTINAL DIVERTICULA

A diverticulum is a protrusion or herniation of the mucosa and submucosa through the muscular coat of an organ at some point of weakness (Fig. 17–8). Diverticula of the intestine may occur in any part of

Fig. 17–8 Multiple diverticula of the small intestine. Death was due to infection and perforation of one large diverticulum. (Bell, E.T.: *Textbook of Pathology*, 8th Ed. Philadelphia, Lea & Febiger, 1956.)

the bowel; the common sites are the duodenum and, more frequently, the sigmoid colon, which intervenes between the descending colon and the rectum. It is here that these herniations may cause trouble. Diverticula may be present in great numbers, a condi-

tion known as diverticulosis. The usual size of each diverticulum is that of a large pea. In the sigmoid, the contents are fecal and are sometimes in the form of concretions. Diverticulosis is sometimes complicated by bleeding but often is asymptomatic. It is often discovered incidentally in the course of a barium examination by the radiologist. If inflammation occurs in the diverticula, symptoms will be produced. Acute diverticulitis, is comparable to acute appendicitis, except that the symptoms may be on the left side of the abdomen. Chronic diverticulitis may demonstrate, characteristically, a large mass of chronic inflammatory tissue on the outside of the bowel, which may easily be mistaken for carcinoma in that region.

What is important about diverticulitis is that it may become complicated by peritonitis, which can be generalized or local; pelvic abscesses may develop; fistulas may occur; and obstruction and bleeding may be life-threatening.

NEOPLASIA

Few common cancers have taught us as much in the last 20 years about carcinogenesis as colon cancer. The mechanisms which are discussed below, typify some of the current paradigms about cancer that are presented in Chapter 11.

Colorectal cancer is among the three most numerous in terms of cancer incidence and cancer death in both men and women (Fig. 17–9). In the United States

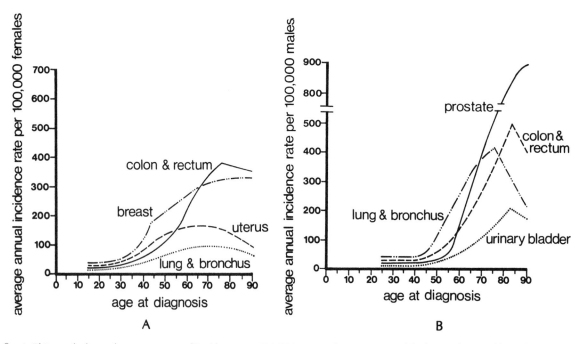

Fig. 17–9 *A*, This graph shows the average annual incidence per 100,000 women for carcinoma of the breast, lung and bronchus, and carcinoma of the colon and rectum. Note the rapid rise of carcinomas of the GI tract in ages 60 to 80. *B*, In men, carcinoma of the colon and rectum rises in a slightly older age group. (From Pitot, H.C.: *Fundamentals of Oncology*. New York, Marcel Dekker, Inc., 1978.)

60,000 people die of colon cancer every year. Not much progress has been made in its cure rate, and the 5 year survival remains at around 40%. Yet, early diagnosis is theoretically possible as we will soon discuss. These data are in contrast with the high level of knowledge that we are rapidly gaining about the cellular and molecular biology and the etiology of human colorectal cancer.

This tumor is usually found in older persons, three-quarters of the patients being more than 50 years old. This is for the "sporadic" cases in which no readily apparent genetic transmission occurs. There are, however, a number of adult patients who are much younger. Their tumors arise from one of the thousands of polyps present in their colorectum. This condition, referred to as familial adenomatous polyposis (FAP), is transmitted as an autosomal dominant trait. Within 30 years from diagnosis, all patients harboring these multiple polyps will develop cancer. There are other conditions where young patients with or without polyps develop colon cancer, and in their family colon cancer or other types of malignancies are found with a high prevalence. One of these conditions is called Lynch syndrome. Besides genetics, environmental factors are important. Here, as expected, diet plays a dominant role. Three factors that are associated with colorectal cancer are a diet poor in fiber, poor in calcium and high in fat. The mechanisms by which these diets influence the incidence of colorectal cancer are not fully understood. There are marked geographic differences in the worldwide distribution of colon cancer which is much more common in developed countries of the western world. Part of these differences are attributed to different diet habits.

To summarize, colorectal cancer results from genetic changes (as typified by the FAP) to diet factors (in the sporadic cases), and in some patients to a combination of both genetics and environment. This situation, which is not unique to colon cancer, has practical significance. Even in the absence of FAP or related genetic conditions a first degree relative of a colorectal cancer patient is three times more likely to have colorectal cancer him/herself.

An important fact learned from colonoscopy and epidemiology is that the overwhelming majority of colon cancers do not occur in isolation, or spontaneously. Most cases represent malignant transformation of pre-existing polyps. Colorectal polyps are strawberry-shaped structures attached via a stalk to the colonic mucosa, or bound directly to it. They can be removed at the time of colonoscopy. Under the microscope a large number of colorectal polyps are found to be neoplasms called adenomas. Moreover, there are dysplastic changes in them suggesting that

they could be premalignant. In fact, large adenomatous polyps sometimes already contain a carcinoma which can be limited to the mucosa or which has already involved the submucosa. Other polyps are still entirely benign and may remain so. The problem is there are no specific criteria, except size, to predict which ones already have or will harbor a carcinoma. Therefore, all colorectal polyps larger than 1 cm should be removed at colonoscopy. Patients with FAP have hundreds or thousands of these adenomatous polyps. We know that these will transform into a cancer in 100% of the patients affected by this familial condition, hence the need for prophylactic colectomy.

The overwhelming majority of cases of malignant tumors of the colon are carcinoma. Two-thirds of these arise in the rectum or sigmoid (Fig. 17–10). The remaining one-third arise in the proximal segments of the colon. This is important because it means that most colorectal cancers are within the reach of the doctor's finger or flexible sigmoidoscope. However, for unknown reasons, epidemiological studies tell us that in most countries there is a decreasing incidence of distal cancers and a rise in proximal cancers. This means that now we should not be content to limit colonoscopy to rectum and sigmoid, but that the entire colon from rectum to cecum should be examined in the symptomatic patient or in subjects belonging to high risk groups (Fig. 17–11).

Colorectal cancer grows as a fungating mass encroaching on the intestinal lumen. With time, as the tumor becomes larger, it tends to involve the entire

adenocarcinoma of sigmoid and anus

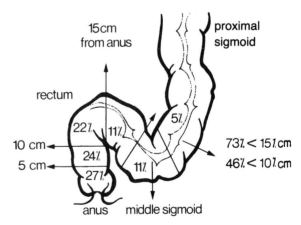

Fig. 17–10 This drawing illustrates the frequency of the sites of adenocarcinoma of the sigmoid colon and anus. The sigmoid colon and anus are divided into 5-cm, 10-cm, and 15-cm distances from the anal verge. The largest percentage of tumors of this area all lie within 15 cm and are thus detectable by proctoscopic or digital examination. (From Dionne, L.: Résultat du traitement chirurgical á visée curative des cancers recto-sigmoidiens. La vie méd. au Can. fr., 8:149, 1979.)

Fig. 17–11 This barium enema x ray of the colon shows a constricting lesion that narrows the lumen and distorts the silhouette of barium. The lesion has been likened to the core of an apple and is shown within the outline of the apple. It is a common and often surgically resectable annular carcinoma.

Table 17–2.   The Different Stages of Colorectal Cancer

DUKE'S STAGE	TNM SYSTEM	SUMMARY OF ANATOMICAL INVOLVEMENT	FIVE YEAR SURVIVAL
A	T_1, N_0, M_0	Tumor in mucosa or submucosa	
B	T_2 to T_3, N_0, M_0	Tumor in muscle wall	60%
C	T_2 to T_3, N_1, M_0	Lymph node involved	35%
D	T_2 to T_3, N_1, M_1	Distant metastasis present	

Note how the extent of disease affects survival. The Duke's and TNM classifications are the two most widely used staging systems. Although other TNM combinations are possible, the most common stages and how they relate to Duke's classification are given.

bowel circumference. These pathological features are common to both the proximal and distal tumors. However, rectal and sigmoid tumors surround and obstruct bowel relatively soon and therefore are more likely to give early symptoms such as unexplained constipation. Conversely, proximal tumors in particular cecal cancer are growing in a bowel lumen with a much larger diameter, consequently obstruction is uncommon, delaying the diagnosis. The result is that colon cancer is more common on the right side but is more difficult to diagnose.

Regardless of their location in the bowel, colorectal tumors not only grow in the lumen but, with time, will grow deeper in the bowel wall. The tumor is first present in the mucosa, or the submucosa, then penetrates through the thick muscle layer. Lymph nodes located in the mesentery near the tumor are commonly the first site of metastasis. From there the carcinoma metastasizes to distant sites such as the liver and the lungs. This progression underlies the classification of different stages of colorectal cancer summarized in Table 17–2. Staging is an important process in the management of colon cancer patients. On this note, Table 17–2 demonstrates that the diagnosis and treatment of the first stage would result in a very high

rate of cure. How could we diagnose this common disease earlier? Going back to the histopathology will tell us that like many malignant neoplasms colorectal carcinomas are highly vascularized and also that they become easily ulcerated on their luminal surface. This creates most of the conditions required for bleeding. Indeed, the discovery of red (i.e., undigested) blood in the stools is a common reason for the patient to consult his/her doctor. This blood may appear in microscopic amounts so that it is not apparent from observation of the stools. Fortunately, there is a chemical test for the demonstration of this occult blood. At the present time, however, searching for occult blood in the stools cannot be proposed as the single diagnostic method for screening asymptomatic subjects. Once the presence of a colorectal tumor has been established by various methods, surgery is the method of treatment. Unfortunately, one out of four patients is found to be inoperable at the time of diagnosis. These patients and those found to have metastatic disease are usually treated with chemotherapy, some of them with substantial benefit.

A test based on the demonstration of a protein in the serum is a very useful method to monitor if the tumor has been completely removed or if it recurs following treatment. This protein, called carcinoembryonic antigen (CEA) was identified in colon cancer tissue and intestinal embryonal cells by Gold and Freedman in 1965. It is produced in measurable amounts by the tumor cells and shed in the circulation when these cells enter into contact with adjacent blood vessels.

At the beginning of this section we mentioned that a large body of important knowledge has been obtained recently on the molecular genetics of colorectal cancer. It has been established that about half of the cases of colon cancer have a point mutation in one of the *nas* oncogenes, an important change if one recalls the significance of oncogenes described in Chapter 11. This mutation occurs early in colorectal carcinogenesis because it is found commonly in adenomatous polyps. The other cellular and molecular changes observed in polyps consist of a state of increased cell proliferation and an hypomethylation of the DNA.

However, Bodmer made an interesting additional observation in 1987. In a case of FAP he found that a copy of a gene located on chromosome 5 was missing and that the same genetic defect was also observed in some of the usual, sporadic, non-familial cases. This had occurred somatically, and not in the germinal cells, because both copies of the chromosome 5 genes were found in the normal colonic mucosa a few centimeters away from the colorectal cancer. Vogelstein extended this observation by showing that the genes located on various chromosomes (especially 17 and 18) were also lost or mutated in these tumors. The gene located on chromosome 17 codes for p53 which, you will recall from Chapter 11, is anti-oncogene. One of the gene copies is lost and the remaining one has often undergone point mutations. Therefore there are reasons to believe that the anti-oncogene properties of p53 are suppressed, and this creates the favorable condition for the development of cancer. This is confirmed by the observation that the inactivation of p53 is not present in early polyps but is found in polyps that have undergone malignant transformation. Thus, several genetic changes occur along the route whereby normal mucosa is transformed into an adenomatous benign polyp, which subsequently undergoes malignant transformation before becoming an invasive cancer. We mentioned in Chapter 11 that cancer is often the result of a multi-step process, not a single hit on our genome. Colon cancer, with these successive genetic changes occurring in normal and premalignant tissue is an example of human cancer which illustrates this concept. It is expected that these new developments in the cell and molecular biology of colorectal cancer, will soon lead to the design of new diagnostic tests and therapeutic approaches.

DIARRHEA

In our survey of some of the principal diseases of the intestine, diarrhea has been noted as a frequent symptom. It may therefore be worthwhile to review briefly this important symptom. Diarrhea, the passage of stools that are too frequent and too soft, results when the fluid contents of the small intestine are hurried so rapidly through the large intestine that there is not sufficient time for the fluid to be absorbed. It is therefore to be expected that diarrhea will be most marked in an inflammatory disease of the large bowel

such as dysentery. In this condition there is also a copious outpouring of mucus from the glands lining the colon that makes the stools still more liquid. Inflammation of the small intestine, especially when associated with ulcers, may also cause diarrhea.

Nervous diarrhea is well known, and is due to excessive nervous stimuli causing an undue amount of peristalsis. Some persons always have a looseness of the bowels when going for examinations and at other similar but equally inopportune moments.

FECES

In the course of digestion, food passes from the stomach into the intestines, where it meets in the duodenum two powerful digestive agents, the bile and the pancreatic juice, both of which are necessary for the proper digestion of fat. In the small intestine, the food becomes completely fluid, because the solid masses of food are dissolved and because of the presence of the digestive fluids of the bowel. The food now passes slowly along the large intestine, where most of the water is absorbed, so that the stools or feces that leave the body are soft, well-formed, brown, cylindrical masses. If the bowel movements are accelerated to any marked degree, there is insufficient time for the water to be absorbed, so that the stools remain fluid (diarrhea). After the protein, carbohydrate, and fat have been absorbed, there remains indigestible material, chiefly from vegetable food, which acts as "roughage" and stimulates the motility of the bowel. The feces, however, are not just residues of food that have not been absorbed, but are composed in large part of material that has been excreted from the blood. For that reason, the bulk of the feces is not totally diminished during starvation. It is surprising to learn that bacteria make up more than 10% of the bulk of the feces.

Constipation is usually due to poor habits. The passage of feces into the rectum causes a desire to defecate, which should result in the complete emptying of the rectum. If this call is neglected or suppressed, the desire passes, and water is absorbed from the fecal mass, which becomes hard and dry. If this state of affairs is continued for long, the rectum, which is only 5 inches long and should normally be empty, contains feces all the time and comes to lose its sensitivity.

An examination of the feces will reveal many facts of importance with regard to the gastrointestinal canal, the process of digestion, and the many disorders that may affect it.

Form. The normal form and consistency of the stools depend on the extraction of water during their passage through the large intestine. If the time of this passage is shortened owing to the increased irritability of the bowel, such as occurs in dysentery, water is not absorbed, and the stools are therefore fluid in character. On the other hand, the feces may remain in the large bowel for an undue length of time, owing to chronic constipation. In this case, the stools take the form of small, hard, round masses, known as scybala. When the stools are narrow and ribbon-like, it is probable that there is some marked narrowing at the lower end of the large bowel, usually due to cancer of the rectum.

Mucus and pus are found in large amounts in acute dysentery and ulcerative colitis, often associated with blood. The mucus is produced by the cells lining the mucus membrane of the inflamed large bowel, just as mucus is discharged from an inflamed nose. The presence of pus is natural in an acute inflammation such as dysentery. The mucus can be seen with the naked eye as slimy streaks or shreds. Pus is best detected by means of the microscope.

The intestinal parasitic worms causing disease and the entamoeba of dysentery have already been described in Chapter 10.

Color. The normal color varies from yellow to brown. When the stool is large and pale, it contains undigested fat, the most common cause of which is obstruction to the flow of bile into the duodenum, either by a gallstone impacted in the bile duct or by a tumor. A chemical test for bile will give a negative result. In disease of the pancreas, the stool tends to be even more voluminous and greasy, owing to complete suppression of fat digestion on account of the absence of pancreatic juice.

The stools may be colored by blood. This blood may be bright red, dark, or black. Red blood comes from the lower part of the intestine. Streaks of bright blood, especially at the end of defecation, are probably due to bleeding piles. Bright blood may come from carcinoma of the rectum or of another part of the large intestine. During the third and fourth weeks of typhoid fever, the nurse must watch the stools carefully for bright blood, because a few specks or streaks may be the forerunner of a severe hemorrhage. Acute inflammation of the colon (colitis, dysentery) is often marked by the presence of blood in the fluid stools, associated usually with mucus and pus. Dark or black blood has been altered by digestion so that it comes from high up in the alimentary canal, usually the stomach or duodenum, the lesion being ulcer or cancer. If the bleeding from the ulcer or tumor is only slight, it will not be possible to detect the blood with the naked eye; it is hidden or occult. When these lesions are suspected, a specimen is sent to the laboratory to be tested chemically for occult blood. It is important that the patient be properly prepared before this examination by the omission of all red meat, meat soups, and meat extracts from his or her diet for at least 3 days. The inclusion of green vegetables in the diet does not interfere with most of the tests for occult blood. It must be remembered that the stools may be dark and tarry in appearance for reasons other than the presence of blood, especially the medicinal use of iron or bismuth.

SYNOPSIS

The lower digestive tract is divided by the ileocecal valve into the part that absorbs sugars, fatty acids, amino acids, iron, and essential substances (the small bowel: duodenum, jejunum, ileum) and the large bowel (colon), whose function is water absorption and storage.

Diarrhea is the most important symptom of bowel disease and its causes include infectious agents (amebic dysentery, typhoid fever, cholera), inflammatory diseases of unknown etiology (ulcerative colitis, regional ileitis), and diverse disorders of the bowel that range from rare infiltrates (amyloid) or tumors to obstruction of the bile ducts.

Complications of all inflammations of the bowel include obstruction, perforation, and peritonitis.

Impairment of the vascular supply, either arterial occlusions, emboli, or venous obstruction (thrombosis or torsion), will lead to gangrene of the bowel.

The malabsorption syndromes are caused by many disorders that result in weight loss, incomplete digestion of food, anemia, and diarrhea.

Tumors of the colon are the most common tumor in man and woman, and the majority of these are within 6 inches of the anus and are amenable to early diagnosis and treatment.

Terms

Duodenum	*Sigmoid*	*Malabsorption syndrome*
Jejunum	*Dysentery*	*Polyp*

Ileum
Appendix
Villus
Brush border
Ileocecal valve
Colon

Ulcerative colitis
Crohn's disease
Diverticulosis
Diverticulitis
Peritonitis
Carcinoembryonic antigen

Familial polyposis
Hernia
Volvulus
Ileus

FURTHER READING

Almy, T.A., and Howell, D.A.: Diverticular disease of the colon. N. Engl. J. Med., 302:324, 1980.

Bayless, T.M., et al.: Lactose and mild intolerance: clinical implications. N. Engl. J. Med., 292:1156, 1975.

Bennett, R.A., Rubin, P.H., and Present, D.H.: Frequency of inflammatory bowel disease in offspring of couples both presenting with inflammatory bowel disease. Gastroenterology, 100:1638, 1991.

Bishop, D.T., and Burt, R.W.: Genetic epidemiology and molecular genetics of colorectal adenomas and cancer. Front. Gastrointest. Res., 18:99, 1991.

Bishop, D.T., and Thomas, H.: The genetics of colorectal cancer. Cancer Surveys, 9:585, 1990.

Burkitt, D.P.: Some diseases characteristic of modern western civilization. Br. Med. J., 1:273, 1973.

Dukes, C.E., and Bussey, H.J.P.: The spread of rectal cancer and its effect on prognosis. Br. J. Cancer, 12:309, 1958.

Eisenberg, B., et al.: Carcinoma of the colon and rectum: the natural history reviewed in 1704 patients. Cancer, 49:1131, 1982.

Ekbom, A., et al.: Ulcerative colitis and colorectal cancer—a population-based study. N. Engl. J. Med., 323:1228, 1990.

Erbe, R.W.: Inherited gastrointestinal-polyposis syndromes. N. Engl. J. Med., 294:1101, 1976.

Gold, P., and Freedman, S.O.: Specific antigenic similarity between malignant adult and normal fetal tissues of the human digestive system. J. Clin. Invest., 44:1051, 1965.

Gorbach, S.L., et al.: Traveller's diarrhea and toxigenic *E. coli*. N. Engl. J. Med., 292:933, 1975.

Guerrant, R.L., and Bobak, D.A.: Bacterial and protozoal gastroenteritis. N. Engl. J. Med., 325:327, 1991.

Hofmann, A.F.: The enterohepatic circulation of bile acids in man. Adv. Intern. Med., 21:501, 1976.

Kay, R.M.: Dietary fiber. J. Lipid Res., 23:221, 1982.

Mayberry, J.F., and Rhodes, J. The changing incidence of Crohn's disease in Wales and the role of heredity in its aetiology. Frontiers of Gastrointes. Res. 11:114. S. Karger, A.G. Basel, 1986.

Mettlin, C., et al.: Management and survival of adenocarcinoma of the rectum in the United States: results of a national survey by the American College of Surgeons. Oncology, 39:265, 1982.

Nishisho, I., et al.: Mutations of chromosome 5_q21 genes in FAP and colorectal cancer patients. Science, 253:665, 1991.

Nguyen, T.D., and Shaffer, N.: Cholera. In: *Gastrointestinal Infections in the Tropics*. Edited by V.K. Rustgi. Basel, Karger, 1990, p. 186.

Podolsky, D.K.: Medical progress: Inflammatory bowel disease (first of two parts). N. Engl. J. Med., 325:928, 1991.

Ransohoff, D.F., and Lang, C.A.: Screening for colorectal cancer. N. Engl. J. Med., 325:37, 1991.

Sedgwick, D.M., Akoh, J.A., and Macintyre, I.M.C.: Gastric cancer in Scotland: changing epidemiology, unchanging workload. Br. Med. J., 302:1305, 1991.

Sleisenger, M.H., and Kim, Y.S.: Protein digestion and absorption. N. Engl. J. Med., 300:659, 1979.

Stamland, J.R., et al.: Clinical presentations of diseases of the large bowel. Gastroenterology, 70:22, 1976.

Tate, H.: Plasma CEA in the post-surgical monitoring of colorectal carcinoma. Br. J. Cancer, 46:323, 1982.

Tedesco, F.J.: Pseudomembranous colitis: pathogenesis and therapy. Med. Clin. North Am., 66:655, 1982.

Willett, W.C., et al.: Relation of meat, fat, and fiber intake to the risk of colon cancer in a prospective study among women. N. Engl. J. Med., 393:1664, 1990.

Winawer, S.J., Schottenfeld, D., and Flehinger, B.J.: Colorectal cancer screening. J. Natl. Canc. Inst., 83:243, 1991.

Wirth, A., et al.: Recent advances in the treatment of colorectal cancer. Aust. N.Z. J. Med., 22:61, 1992.

Yeomans, N.D.: Pathogenesis of coeliac sprue. Lancet, 2:843, 1974.

18

LIVER AND GALLBLADDER

The liver is the lazaret of bile.—BYRON

LIVER

To the ancient Babylonians, the liver was the seat of the soul, whereas in ancient Greece it was considered the central organ of the body. The liver, tucked under the diaphragm, below the ribs on the right side of the abdomen, is the largest, warmest, and one of the most important organs of the body. Although it has remarkable regenerative powers, it also has an extraordinary reserve and can adapt to different loads of toxic substances or to nutritional excesses and deprivations. Without the liver we die quickly. One of the most interesting and puzzling things about the liver is that, although it performs many separate and distinct functions, as we shall shortly see, the cells of the liver are apparently identical and differ only in their position in the columns along which blood flows from the intestinal tract to the heart (Fig. 18–1). A diagram of the circulation of the liver is shown in Figure 18–2 and demonstrates that the liver, like the lung, receives blood from two sources. The minor component is blood from the hepatic artery, and the major (75%) is blood from the portal system, which derives its tributaries from the stomach, spleen, and small and large bowels.

Although the liver is concerned with aspects of protein, carbohydrate, and lipid metabolism, it is possible to separate arbitrarily the many functions of the liver into four categories: synthesis, secretion, detoxification, and storage. Aberrations in most or all of these functions can be determined by laboratory tests and often form the basis for distinguishing one type of liver disease from another. The reader is referred to the section on the physiology of the liver in the Appendix (p. 406).

Jaundice. "Jaundice," as William Osler said, "is the disease your friends diagnose." However, jaundice is not a disease. It is a sign of disease. Jaundice or icterus is a coloration of the skin, whites of the eyes, and

urine; in fact, all the tissues of the body are stained by excess bile pigments that circulate in the serum. Normally, as we have seen, bile is secreted into the bowel and eliminated in the feces. Three general mechanisms can disrupt this pattern of flow and may cause bile to appear in the serum, thereby causing a complexion of a yellow, orange, or even green tinge, which we recognize as jaundice. Bilirubin may circulate either as free bilirubin or as conjugated (water-soluble) bilirubin, or as a mixture of both. In order to be conjugated, bilirubin must have been acted on by liver cells. To be detectable by a laboratory test, the total serum bilirubin should be in excess of 1.5 mg/100 ml, but it usually must reach 3.0 mg/100 ml before it is obvious to an observer. Jaundice (or an increase in serum bilirubin) has been divided into three groups.

The first of these types of jaundice is easy to understand and is called **obstructive**. Since bile normally flows from liver cells to canaliculi to ductules to ducts to the common duct and to the ampulla of Vater, an obstruction may occur at any of these levels and may cause a damming of flow and backup of bile. A tumor at or near the ampulla of Vater, a stone in the common duct, a misplaced suture, or scarring of the extrahepatic ducts may each prevent the normal passage of bile into the intestine. The accompanying x-rays (Fig. 18–3) show the appearance of both the normal, intra- and extrahepatic bile ducts and the dilated ducts that occur when obstruction has taken place. When this obstruction occurs, the secretion of bile from the liver continues. Since bile cannot traverse its normal route, it seeks another path, like the waters of a stream behind a beaver dam. The bile, which has already been through the liver cell (conjugated bilirubin), leaks into the serum, since it cannot follow its rightful tributary to the gut. This reflux of conjugated bilirubin into the serum causes staining of all tissues (and is clinically apparent when the serum bilirubin is greater than 3 mg/100 ml). The serum level of conjugated bilirubin

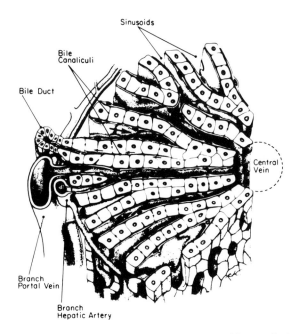

Fig. 18–1 This diagram shows the arrangement of liver cells in a hypothetical lobule, illustrating the different types of cells in the liver, namely the Kupffer cells and duct cells of the bile duct, and vascular cells. The liver cells are arranged in cords, as shown here. (From Bloom, W., and Fawcett, D.W.: *A Textbook of Histology.* Philadelphia, W. B. Saunders Co., 1968. After Ham.)

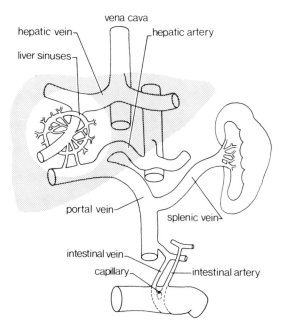

Fig. 18–2 This diagram of the circulation of the liver shows the portal vein, which is composed of veins draining from the intestine and spleen. The hepatic artery supplies blood to each liver lobule, and the blood then flows through the hepatic vein to the vena cava.

can be determined by the van den Bergh reaction, a chemical test that can be used to distinguish between conjugated and unconjugated pigments. Conjugated bilirubin is said to be "direct-reacting." Because bile fails to reach the gut, the stools become pale and are not their normal brown (they are frequently referred to as clay-colored). The bile that circulates is cleared in the kidney, causing the urine to be much darker than normal, and in fact to foam. This is because bile is a surface-active agent. If the situation lasts for any length of time (a week or 2), there is impairment of fat digestion and absorption and interference with vitamin K absorption, which interferes with synthesis of prothrombin. The jaundice will progress and the liver cells themselves will become damaged. The pattern of jaundice, with an elevated direct-reacting bilirubin, pale stools, and bile in the urine, points to obstruction in the biliary excretory systems and suggests that surgical exploration for a stone or tumor is warranted. The longer the obstruction exists, the more likely it is that complications will arise, such as hepatocellular injury, infection of the ductal system, or other problems such as bleeding.

The second type of jaundice is called **hepatocellular**, because the elevated bilirubin is not conjugated with glucuronide. Unconjugated bilirubin levels cannot be measured directly. Total bilirubin and conjugated bilirubin levels are measured directly by means of the van den Bergh test, then the conjugated level is subtracted from the total, yielding indirectly the unconjugated, or indirect-reacting, bilirubin level. This bilirubin, then, has not been acted on by the liver cells or secreted by them, usually because the liver cells have been damaged. Sometimes the circulatory system in the liver is no longer compartmentalizing the flow of pigments, and liberates bilirubin directly into the circulation. Thus an elevated serum unconjugated bilirubin can occur when many liver cells are destroyed or injured, as in infectious hepatitis (viral), or in acute toxic or vascular injury to the liver cells. It is important to recognize that if an obstruction continues, it may also injure the liver cells, resulting in an elevation of both the direct- and indirect-reacting bilirubin.

The search for the underlying cause of this type of jaundice is made more difficult when components of both obstruction and liver cell injury are present. The patient's prognosis is more guarded, because even the administration of general anesthesia, let alone the metabolic insult of a surgical operation, puts great stress on the liver.

The third type of jaundice is caused by the liberation of excessive amounts of bile pigments, that is, more than the liver can handle. The phenomenon oc-

A

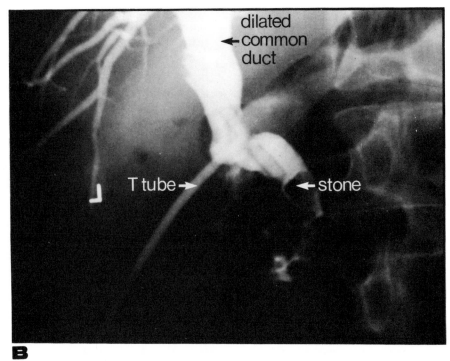

B

curs in all cases of massive hemolysis and is referred to as **hemolytic** jaundice. It appears most commonly during the first days after birth, when a transient or mild icterus should be no cause for alarm. Hemolytic jaundice is an unconjugated hyperbilirubinemia and can be expected in diseases in which hemolysis occurs (e.g., acquired or congenital hemolytic anemias), in bacterial infections, and occasionally in cases in which large areas of tissue are infarcted or bleeding. Traditionally, a mismatched transfusion is a cause of hemolysis.

With continuous excessive loads of bilirubin, as in the congenital hemolytic anemias (e.g. sickle cell disease), a complication may be the deposition of bilirubin in the form of stones that accumulate in the gallbladder, in the cystic duct, or even in the intrahepatic ducts. In this complication, two different types of bilirubin-overload intersect: the hemolytic jaundice (hemolytic anemia) may predispose a patient to a mechanical obstruction (stone), causing the obstructive type of jaundice!

Hepatic and Portal Circulation. Each liver cell is bathed in blood derived from the venous return from the intestine. This blood naturally has a lower oxygen content than arterial blood and higher content of substrates derived from the absorptive processes.

The flow of blood through the liver is estimated at 1.5 liters per minute, and the blood flows from the portal triads along the columns of cells to drain into the central veins. Thus, each liver cell is exposed to a gradient of portal blood with varying amounts of oxygen and substrate, depending on whether the liver cell is first in line (portal zone) or last at the banquet table (central zone). Should the venous pressure in the systemic circulation be raised, owing, for example, to heart failure (old myocardial infarct), then there will be stasis in the venous circulation that can be reflected as far downstream as the liver. This passive congestion may result in a slow attrition of the liver cells around the central veins of each lobule, because they are the last to receive any oxygenated blood and the last to receive any amino acids, glucose, or fatty acids. The anatomic result of long-standing congestion is a loss of functional capability that may lead to abnormalities in test dye retention, serum, bilirubin, enzyme elevations, and even in decreased synthesis of albumin. Anatomically, the liver may be smooth and enlarged. The patient complains of a dull ache in the right upper quadrant, and, if you press on the liver, a wave may be seen in the jugular veins. This chronic passive congestion of the liver is a common disorder (Fig. 18–4), and the older pathologists talk about the "nutmeg liver" because the stasis and congestion of blood in the liver resemble a sectioned nutmeg (Fig. 18–4, *inset*).

Disease upstream or in the liver may affect the intrahepatic circulation and the portal venous system below the liver. Chronic injury to the liver with scarring (cirrhosis) may lead to elevated portal venous pressure and even to thrombosis of the portal veins. Fortunately, collateral circulations may be available to return blood to the heart, but complications can arise from the use of this collateral pathway, as we shall see. The hepatic vein may also become occluded, and all the predisposing causes of thrombosis discussed earlier may be relevant in considering this uncommon circumstance.

In the liver, as in any organ, infarction may occur, but it is relatively rare, perhaps because of the dual supply of blood and because the liver cells are able to shift from aerobic to anaerobic glycolysis. The rare infarct in the liver is illustrated in Figure 18–5, and the discolored local area can be compared with the diffuse congestion seen in Figure 18–4. The most common antecedent to these infarcts in the liver, which have been called infarcts of Zahn, are episodes of profound shock associated with blood loss as in major trauma, and in surgical and obstetric accidents.

Acute Necrosis of the Liver. A more frequent occurrence than simple ischemic infarction, necrosis of the liver is most often caused by specific viral infections (hepatitis, yellow fever), by poisons that have a profound effect on the liver, such as carbon tetrachloride (CCl_4) and phosphorus (rat poison), or by special instances of unknown etiology, such as toxemia of pregnancy (eclampsia) and shock. An example of the massive injury to the liver that can occur in these instances is shown in Figure 18–6. Naturally such a widespread and extensive hepatic injury as shown in this figure may result in death. Because of the remarkable regenerative capacity of the liver, owing to the active recruitment of the pluripotential liver cells to mitosis and subsequent resumption of the organ's many functions, if the patient can be kept alive until the liver has had time to recover from such a massive injury, regeneration may restore many of the functions of this essential organ. However, following such an extensive injury, it is likely that scars will develop that will

---

Fig. 18–3   *A,* This x-ray study shows the appearance of the common bile duct and the intrahepatic bile duct, visualized by the presence of water-soluble iodinated contrast medium, which was inserted into the duct by means of a T tube following an operation. This x-ray study shows a normal, undilated, unobstructed biliary tree. *B,* Another postoperative cholangiogram shows the appearance of a markedly dilated intrahepatic biliary tree due to the presence of obstruction by a stone (arrow.)

Fig. 18–4   This gross photograph of a liver from a patient with chronic, congestive heart failure, shows the marked mottling that is typical of this condition. Its resemblance to the *inset*, a photograph of a section through a nutmeg, has caused generations of students to wonder what a nutmeg looked like. A classic cause for chronic, passive congestion in the liver is old myocardial infarctions or chronic valvular heart disease, such as mitral stenosis. (McGill University, Department of Pathology Museum.)

Fig. 18–5   Section through the liver showing an area of discoloration at the top of the liver. The portal vein is thrombosed at the arrow, and this has caused the **infarction** despite the fact that the liver has a dual circulation. (McGill University, Department of Pathology Museum.)

Fig. 18–6 This gross photograph of a section of the liver shows large, irregular, pale areas surrounded by red borders. This appearance is typical of widespread **necrosis**. Such an injury, as shown here, is so severe as to cause death, despite the remarkable regenerative capacity of the liver. This is from a case of **eclampsia**. (McGill University, Department of Pathology Museum.)

leave a permanent mark on the liver, both anatomically and physiologically. Broad bands of scar may remain to testify to the near-fatal episode of hepatic necrosis, and the portal circulation may be disordered because of the collapse of the hepatic architecture, leaving the patient with venous shunts that bypass the usual detoxifying and filtration mechanisms represented by the normal portal system. Fortunately, acute, massive, hepatic necrosis is relatively rare, as compared with the diseases we shall now consider.

Infectious Diseases of the Liver. From the worldwide point of view, infections of the liver are extremely common. Earlier we have considered schistosomiasis, yellow fever, echinococcal cysts, and amebiasis, all of which are serious and often fatal diseases of the liver (Fig. 18–7). In North America, when considering infections of the liver, we usually think first of viral hepatitis and bacterial infections of the bile ducts; the latter are a frequent complication of obstruction to the biliary tree. Abscesses, both bacterial and fungal, and tuberculous infections of the liver are becoming much less common than in the pre-antibiotic era. A solitary abscess is shown in Figure 18–8 that might have given only a mild sense of discomfort

to the patient, but it might also have provided a general feeling of illness together with a fever. The etiology of the abscess could have been related to septicemia or endocarditis, and might have occurred in someone who was debilitated by intercurrent systemic disease such as diabetes mellitus. The diffuse abscesses of the biliary tree (Fig. 18–9) are equally difficult to diagnose clinically and are more frequent, being a complication of stones and cholecystitis. In this instance, jaundice as well as a hepatic fever may point to the correct diagnosis of cholangitis with abscess formation, especially if the patient was known to have chronic inflammation of the gallbladder. Rarely, diffuse abscesses throughout the liver may arise when bacterial infections (commonly *E. coli*) from the appendix ascend to the tributaries of the portal vein and reach the liver by that route (pylephlebitis).

Currently, the most intriguing infectious disease of the liver is viral hepatitis. The term hepatitis is often misleading, since one frequently expects the suffix -itis to imply inflammation in the conventional sense, that is, inflammatory cells followed by the vascular phase of congestion and exudate. In the liver, however, the injury caused both by specific agents, such

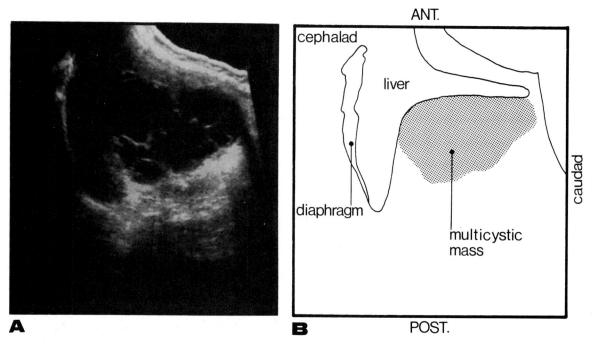

Fig. 18–7   *A,* This ultrasound scan of the liver shows a large, multicystic mass, as illustrated in *B.* This is typical of a hydatid cyst.

as the viruses of hepatitis, and by toxic agents is necrosis of hepatic cells. As suggested earlier, when the injury is slight and transient, the dead cells are removed quickly and are replaced by new liver cells, but when the injury is severe and prolonged, there is usually proliferation of fibroblasts and bile ducts, collections of macrophages, and the deposition of large amounts of collagen. These phenomena are the hallmarks of the chronic liver disease cirrhosis, but we are getting ahead of ourselves.

The term hepatitis covers a multitude of disorders. Any reader is bound to become confused by the many uses of the word in the literature. It is a little like blue jeans, which have been stretched to cover every shape

Fig. 18–8   Arrow points to walled cavity, which was an **abscess.** The remainder of the liver is normal. Such an abscess could be caused by either gram-positive or gram-negative bacteria, or by amebas, coming from the blood or gastrointestinal tract. (McGill University, Department of Pathology Museum.)

Fig. 18-9   The right half of the liver shows many small, thick-walled cavities, typical of **cholangitic abscesses** of the liver. The remaining portion of the liver is normal. This type of infection commonly arises from motile bacteria in the partly obstructed biliary tree. (McGill University, Department of Pathology Museum.)

and have been used on every social occasion. The key to successful usage of the term hepatitis is to use it with some qualifying adjective, such as acute, viral, or chronic. For example, we are now recognizing an entity that was regarded entirely differently 35 years ago. The term chronic hepatitis has been defined as "inflammation of the liver continuing for at least 3 to 6 months," and has been divided into several subsets that need not concern us here except to indicate that the causes of the inflammation may be different (viral, immunologic).

Viral Hepatitis. The major viruses that cause hepatitis have been discussed in Chapter 8, so we will only briefly review them. There are several classes: type A, type B, and type non-A, non-B.

Non-A, non-B hepatitis, which has been recognized for many years, is presently attributed to two other agents, respectively called Hepatitis C, a 10,000 nucleotide single-stranded RNA virus whose particle has not been identified, and Hepatitis E, another RNA virus of 27-32 nm size. In addition, there is an agent called Hepatitis D which is a defective virus and requires the helper function of Hepatitis B virus (see Table 18-1). In this text we will address only Hepatitis A and B.

Type A hepatitis virus (HAV) is an RNA virus which is transmitted by the fecal/oral route and may occur in epidemics (Figs. 18-10, 18-11 and 18-12). Frequently the epidemic is caused by contamination of food during preparation by an hepatitis A-infected food handler. Sometimes it is by contamination of food such as shellfish before it reaches the food service establishment. Measures to prevent food-borne hepatitis outbreaks should include training of food handlers regarding hygiene, especially good hand washing and other personal hygiene measures. Other measures include investigation of the handlers who are ill, prompt reporting to local health departments of patients with suspected hepatitis, and proper investigation by health departments of possible sources of infection. Naturally, from the incubation period, when an outbreak is identified it is usually too late to prevent further cases. The increasing number of hepatitis A cases in the United States underscores the importance of these measures. It has an incubation period of 2 to 6 weeks and usually produces mild disease without jaundice. It has no obvious chronic complications or carrier state.

Hepatitis B virus (HBV) is a DNA virus consisting of a central core and a surface coat, both of which are associated with antigens. HBV has been the focus of attention with the recognition of the importance of Australia antigen as a diagnostic tool to identify carriers and persons who have had previous infections.

Table 18–1. Comparisons of type A, type B, and non-A, non-B hepatitis

FEATURE	HEPATITIS A	HEPATITIS B*	NON-A, NON-B HEPATITIS	
			BLOODBORNE (HEPATITIS C)	ENTERIC (HEPATITIS E)
Incubation	15–45 days (mean 30)	30–180 days (mean 60–90)	15–160 (mean 50)	14–60 (mean 40)
Onset	Acute	Often insidious	Insidious	Acute
Age preference	Children, young adults	Any age	Any age but more common in adults	Young adults (20–40 years)
Transmission route:				
Fecal-oral	+++	−	Unknown	+++
Other nonpercutaneous†	+/−	++	++	+/−
Percutaneous	Unusual	+++	+++	−
Severity	Mild	Often severe	Moderate	Mild
Prognosis	Generally good	Worse with age, debility	Moderate	Good
Progression to chronicity	None	Occasional (5–10%)	Occasional (10–50%)	None
Prophylaxis	IG	Standard IG (not documented) HBIG, hepatitis B vaccine	?	?
Carrier	None	0.1–30%‡	Approximately 1%	None

* Concomitant delta hepatitis is similar in these features to hepatitis B, but more severe outcomes are favored.

† For example, sexual or maternal-neonatal contact.

‡ Varies considerably throughout the world, see text.

(From Braunwald, E.: Harrison's Principles of Internal Medicine, 12th Ed. New York, McGraw, 1990.)

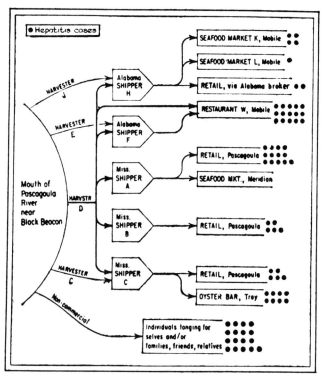

The New York Times   Nov. 19, 1961
Chart adapted from Public Health Service report shows distributors of oysters linked to 70 hepatitis cases.

The New York Times   Nov. 19, 1961
Area where contaminated oysters were harvested.

Fig. 18–10 This chart shows the distribution of oysters from the mouth of the Mississippi River and the 70 cases of hepatitis that resulted. (From *The New York Times*, November 19, 1961.)

Fig. 18–11 This figure shows the weekly clinical case rate of hepatitis in an institution for the mentally retarded during the period of an infectious hepatitis epidemic in 1972. (From Matthew, E. B., et al.: A major epidemic of infectious hepatitis in an institution for the mentally retarded. Am. J. Epidemiol., 98:203, 1973.)

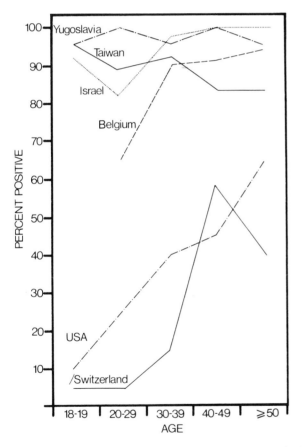

Fig. 18–12 This figure shows the age-specific prevalences of antibody to hepatitis A antigen in population samples from 6 countries. This antibody is a sensitive and specific indicator of previous hepatitis infections. The prevalence of the presence of antibody does provide valuable information about the presence of viral hepatitis A. (From Szmuness, W., et al.: The prevalence of antibody to hepatitis A antigen in various parts of the world: a pilot study. Am. J. Epidemiol., 106:392, 1977.)

Blumberg was awarded the Nobel prize in 1976 for his identification of an antigen specifically related to serum hepatitis. He had hypothesized that patients receiving multiple transfusions would receive proteins of a phenotype different from their own and would therefore produce antibodies to them. While pursuing this line of reasoning, he discovered an antigen from an Australian aborigine that was commonly present in the blood of leukemic patients. Further study soon established a closer relationship between this antigen and patients with serum hepatitis. The Australia antigen is now recognized as the surface antigen of the double-shelled hepatitis B virus (Table 18–2). One million carriers of the virus are estimated to live in the United States alone, and 100,000,000 in the world. The World Health Organization lists hepatitis B as the 9th major cause of death in the world, affecting at least 5% of the world's population. This estimate indicates that chronic hepatitis B infection may be the most important chronic viral infection of humans, but it is seen principally in Asia and Africa in the general population, while in North America it appears usually in particular high risk groups, i.e., drug users, male homosexuals, promiscuous heterosexuals, health care workers, immigrants from endemic areas, and individuals who have received blood or blood products. Hepatitis B is the chief cause of cirrhosis and hepatocellular carcinoma. In the United States, for all patients tested, at least 10% have antibodies against hepatitis B antigen, whereas in Taiwan, for example, 78% have presumably been exposed to the virus (Table 18–2). The figures are even higher for antibodies against hepatitis A antigen.

HBV can be transmitted by blood and blood products; it can also be spread sexually and in a variety of other ways because the virus is present in a number of body fluids. In Asia and Africa the most important mode of spread is vertical, i.e., from mother to infant. HBV has an incubation period of 2 to 6 months. It evokes a variety of clinical responses in infected individuals, ranging from no clinical illness to rapidly fatal hepatic failure.

Almost 90% of hepatitis cases that occur after blood transfusion are due to non-A, non-B hepatitis virus or viruses, (see Table 18–1).

Evidence of hepatitis can usually be detected early in the incubation period when levels of liver enzymes (SGOT, SGPT, and LDH) rise in the blood. Following the incubation period a mild flu-like illness may occur—probably 95% of hepatitis A cases are no worse than this. In more severe cases, regardless of the agent, the patient experiences fever, malaise, nausea, fatigue and distaste for food, cigarettes and alcohol, followed a few days later by jaundice. On examina-

Table 18–2.   Prevalence of Antibody to Hepatitis B Surface Antigen (Anti-HB's) in the Population Surveyed for HAV Infections

COUNTRY	NO. TESTED	NO. ANTI-HB's POSITIVE	% POSITIVE (CRUDE)	% POSITIVE AGE-STANDARDIZED*
U.S.A.	1,000	108	10.8	12.1
Switzerland	98	3	3.1	2.9
Belgium	133	7	5.3	4.6
Yugoslavia	97	33	34.0	32.8
Israel	112	17	15.2	17.4
Taiwan	123	96	78.0	72.8
Senegal	96	60	62.5	55.6

* Direct method; rates for Taiwan and Senegal were standardized to the 1974 Taiwan population distribution; rates for the remaining countries were standardized to the 1970 United States population distribution.

(From Szmuness, W., et al.: The prevalence of antibody to hepatitis A antigen in various parts of the world: a pilot study. Am. J. Epidemiol., 106:392, 1977.)

tion, the liver may be tender and enlarged, and laboratory tests may show evidence of hyperbilirubinemia, elevated transaminases, and other signs of disordered liver function, depending on the severity and extent of the hepatocellular necrosis. Arthritis, itching, urticaria, and thrombophlebitis have all been associated with HBV, but jaundice is the outstanding clinical feature. The symptoms of the prodromal phase usually decrease as jaundice becomes more apparent, and may last as long as 8 weeks. Abnormal liver function tests, together with specific serologic identification, confirm the diagnosis.

Biopsy may often help to determine the severity of the disease and may shed some light on the possible outcome of a particular case.

Most patients with HBV hepatitis recover completely but many remain as carriers. Some have a relatively mild persistent disease which eventually resolves and a few patients will go on to develop chronic disease, with progressive liver damage leading to cirrhosis.

Rarely, acute viral hepatitis follows a rapid and highly destructive course called **fulminant viral hepatitis** or **fulminant hepatic failure**. Acetaminophen overdose and hypersensitivity to anesthetic agents have also been known to produce this catastrophe. Fulminant hepatic failure is associated with massive necrosis of liver cells with sudden severe impairment of liver function. It is characterized by mental changes which rapidly progress from confusion to stupor and coma. Deep jaundice, prolonged prothrombin time and markedly elevated serum enzymes appear, and the whole illness from first symptom to death may take less than a week.

Treatment. Hepatitis A may be prevented by the administration of a special serum preparation containing high titres of anti-HAV antibody. If given within two weeks of exposure to HAV it reduces the frequency of the acute illness. Immunoglobulin preparations are also available for HBV infection but are usually only used in special circumstances such as accidental inoculation in a laboratory. The use of newer drugs such as interferon alfa for patients with chronic hepatitis B is now possible, but a four month course has only caused remission in about 40% of patients.

Vaccines containing the surface antigen HBsAg are currently being introduced for public use (antibody to HBsAg provides immunity). Szmuness reported a study of the effects of one vaccine on a group of homosexual males in whom the incidence of hepatitis B infection was 12% per year. Ninety-six per cent of those who received the vaccine developed anti-HBs antibody. A small number of the vaccinated group contracted hepatitis, mostly within the first 5 months after vaccination which suggests that they may have been infected before vaccination. In contrast, 27% of those who received the placebo vaccine developed hepatitis.

Hepatitis due to Other Causes. There are a few patients with enlarged, tender livers, who show accompanying laboratory disorders of elevated transaminases without jaundice. Often these persons have arthritis. The disorder is found most commonly in young women. This liver disease is of uncertain etiology, and some have claimed that the hepatic damage has an autoimmune basis. The disease is designated chronic hepatitis in some, and when evidence of connective tissue disease is present, it has also been called lupoid hepatitis.

We can also identify hepatic disease occurring in small numbers of persons who have been taking drugs such as phenothiazines (tranquilizers), or antibiotics (isoniazid), or anesthetics (halothane). This disease may take the form of acute necrosis, or of a subacute injury. Patients who take steroids such as methyltestosterone may also develop jaundice, which has been found to be due to cholestasis.

Fatty Liver. Another major classification of liver disorders is that in which most or a major portion of the liver is filled with fat in the form of triglyceride droplets. Acute fatty liver may reflect many different insults to this organ, which has only a limited repertoire of responses to injury. Excessive caloric intake, usually in the form of ethanol is the most common cause of a large, greasy, yellow liver unable to function normally because most cells have their cytoplasmic organelles displaced by the accumulated lipid droplets.

Other important causes of fat in the liver are hepatotoxins (CCl$_4$, PO$_4$) and systemic metabolic disorders such as uncontrolled diabetes mellitus and toxemia of pregnancy. The most serious of these disorders is the chronic fatty liver seen in alcoholics, who persist in taking large amounts of ethanol, which by itself is an agent that depresses glycogen synthesis and inhibits normal hepatic cell metabolism, and which provides as well a caloric fuel without some of the essential cofactors (vitamins) normally found in the diet. The fatty liver in acute alcoholism may progress, with continuing alcohol abuse, to chronic hepatitis, in which there is evidence of necrosis, leukocytic infiltration, Mallory's alcoholic hyaline bodies, and disorganization of the parenchyma. Chronic hepatitis will frequently result, eventually, in cirrhosis.

Cirrhosis. Most of the disorders we have been discussing are acute diseases of the liver. Now we shall consider a group of disorders collected under the term cirrhosis, a chronic disease of the liver. One may identify several anatomic types of cirrhosis, each of which has a differing etiology. A reasonable definition for cirrhosis is **"a diffuse structural disorganization characterized by necrosis, with nodular regeneration of liver parenchyma and fibrosis"** (Fig. 18–13). Cirrhosis inevitably produces disordered hepatic function. We should consider the respective roles played by the anatomic aberrations. First, however, it may be wise to outline some of the symptoms, signs, and physiologic abnormalities of a typical case of cirrhosis, regardless of origin.

The patient with early cirrhosis may be asymptomatic and unaware of the disorder, but physical signs such as hepatomegaly, peripheral edema, ascites, vascular hemangiomas (spider nevi), gynecomastia, and testicular atrophy may bear testimony to the diagnosis. With the progression of the disease, anasarca, splenomegaly, and other evidence of portal hypertension and a collateral circulation (hemorrhoids, esophageal varices, and collateral veins about the umbilicus) may appear. Finally, the complications of cirrhosis are full blown, and massive bleeding into the gastrointestinal tract from ruptured esophageal varices, hemorrhage, hepatic coma, and hepatic cell carcinoma may leave no doubt as to the underlying disorder.

Cirrhosis represents a morphologic response to continuing injury to the liver. Regardless of the etiology of the cirrhosis, one may generalize that the cirrhosis is a reflection of the type, location, and duration of the injury to the liver. If the injury has been a chronic inflammation of the bile ducts, the scarring will be principally in the region of the bile ducts, namely the portal area (biliary cirrhosis). If the injury has not been limited to a specific anatomic segment of the lobule, but has involved large areas of the liver, as in viral hepatitis, the scarring may consist of broad

Fig. 18–13 Liver with diffuse nodularity that is typical of **cirrhosis**. Small and irregular nodules of liver are separated by bands of scar. Within these areas of regeneration, necrosis may progress and sometimes carcinoma arises. (McGill University, Department of Pathology Museum.)

bands of collagen coursing throughout the organ (postnecrotic cirrhosis). The extent of the scarring depends on the extent and severity of the injury.

What happens when large numbers of liver cells are injured on a long-term basis? The loss of liver cells may produce ascites (due to hypoalbuminemia), jaundice (due to loss of secretory function and disturbance of excretory pathways), and hepatic coma (loss of urea synthesis and shunting). The structural disorganization and collapse distort the vascular pattern of the liver, so that the portal blood may pass directly to the vena cava without being exposed to cords of liver cells. This shunting of blood then exposes the brain to blood that contains ammonia absorbed from the colon, but is not detoxified by the liver. This shunting is believed to be a reason for the disordered central nervous system function that is such a serious complication of cirrhosis (hepatic encephalopathy). The fibrosis and nodular regeneration compress the sinusoidal spaces and the venous and portal tributaries, resulting in elevated sinusoidal and portal pressure (portal hypertension). Stasis in the circulation may even lead to portal vein thrombosis (Fig. 18–14). The lymphatic drainage is also affected and contributes additionally to the development of ascites. The continued stimulus to regeneration in the liver may be an important factor in the development of still another complication of cirrhosis, hepatocarcinoma. In North America, this disease arises rarely in the noncirrhotic liver, but is seen more commonly in cases of cirrhosis.

Although one may classify the types of cirrhosis on anatomic or etiologic bases, contemporary usage confuses these taxonomic schemes and groups cirrhosis into 5 general classes:

1. Cirrhosis due to dietary factors such as alcohol (Laennec's, portal, alcoholic).
2. Cirrhosis following massive necrosis such as viral hepatitis (postnecrotic).
3. Cirrhosis associated with pigment deposition (hemochromatosis).
4. Cirrhosis associated with disease of the bile ducts (primary and secondary biliary cirrhosis).
5. Miscellaneous cirrhoses.

Cirrhosis following congestive heart failure does not really conform to the criteria that require regenera-

Fig. 18–14   The inferior aspect of a **cirrhotic liver**, illustrating the distorted appearance of the surface of the liver, which sometimes can be palpated through the abdominal wall. At the arrow, the portal vein is thrombosed. (McGill University, Department of Pathology Museum.)

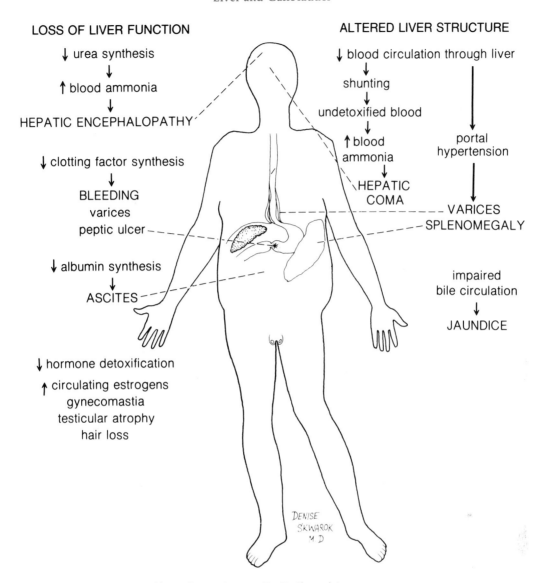

LOSS OF LIVER FUNCTION

↓ urea synthesis
↓
↑ blood ammonia
↓
HEPATIC ENCEPHALOPATHY

↓ clotting factor synthesis
↓
BLEEDING
varices
peptic ulcer

↓ albumin synthesis
↓
ASCITES

↓ hormone detoxification
↑ circulating estrogens
gynecomastia
testicular atrophy
hair loss

ALTERED LIVER STRUCTURE

↓ blood circulation through liver
↓
shunting
↓
undetoxified blood
↓
↑ blood ammonia
↓
HEPATIC COMA

portal hypertension
↓
VARICES
SPLENOMEGALY

impaired bile circulation
↓
JAUNDICE

DENISE SKWAROK M.D

Fig. 18–15 Changes in liver function caused by cirrhosis. (Courtesy Dr. D. Skwarok.)

tive nodules to be present, and it is not considered by us to be a legitimate type of cirrhosis.

For our purposes, it does not seem necessary to delve into the specific reasons for separating one type of cirrhosis from another, or to describe the morphologic features of each type. It does seem important to recapitulate the significance, in physiologic terms, of the disordered structures (Fig. 18–15). When the liver is injured and necrosis occurs, the pattern of collapse, regeneration, and new collagen formation takes place on a continuing basis; when inflammation of the bile ducts continues, or repeated episodes of alcohol excess occur, or hepatitis virus is not cleared from the liver, this organ is then unable to synthesize normal amounts of protein. In addition, the pressures in the intrahepatic and portal circulations gradually rise,

and a collateral circulation is recruited. This venous system is less well protected from the daily abrasions of life, and bleeding from unsupported veins may occur, precipitating a hemorrhage. Such a hemorrhage may plunge the patient with cirrhosis into shock and initiate new episodes of hepatic cell necrosis because of ischemia, thereby accelerating the **process of necrosis, collapse, fibrosis, and regeneration**.

Historically, the fate of most patients with cirrhosis was to die of infection, commonly of pneumonia, with gastrointestinal hemorrhage, hepatic coma, or hepatic cell carcinoma as less frequent complications. Today, hepatic coma is the most frequent and most common cause of death, as infections and hemorrhages are managed more successfully by modern methods (Fig. 18–16).

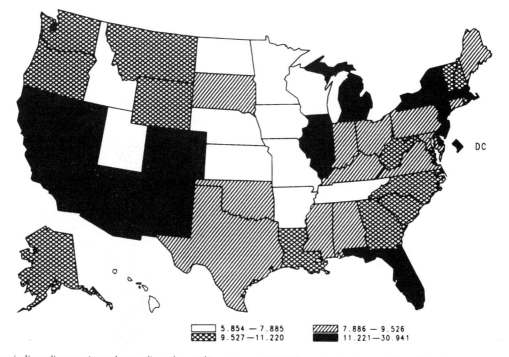

5.854 — 7.885   7.886 — 9.526
9.527 — 11.220   11.221 — 30.941

Fig. 18–16   Chronic liver disease. Annual age-adjusted mortality rates per 100,000 population by quartile—United States, 1986. (From Centers for Disease Control, Morbidity and Mortality Weekly Report, 38(46):799, 1989.)

The cause of hepatic coma is frequently debated, and no absolute answer is available to explain this fateful disorder. Explanations range from toxic effects of ammonia absorbed from the gut to the failure of metabolism of insulin by poorly functioning hepatocytes. In fact, insulin-glucagon therapy has been used with some success in the therapy of acute hepatic failure, and a low-protein diet is the rule for all cirrhotics.

Because of the intractable nature of advanced cirrhosis, liver transplants have been attempted.

Tumors of the Liver and Bile Ducts. The most common malignant tumor of the liver is metastatic tumor, most frequently arising from the lung, colon, pancreas, breast, or gallbladder (Fig. 18–17). These tumors reach the liver by hematogenous, lymphatic, or direct extension, frequently are silent, and often do not impair liver function in any recognizable way. When the metastases replace most of the liver parenchyma, as happens occasionally, signs of hepatic failure may become apparent. Even small tumors that involve the liver may give rise to signs and symptoms if they occupy such strategic points as the portal vein or bile ducts, giving rise to ascites or jaundice. The rapid increase in size of the liver, the presence of palpable nodules, and the occurrence of bloody ascitic fluid all point to the diagnosis of malignant tumor in the liver. Hepatography by liver scan has unfortunately not proved to be as reliable as hoped for, and

liver biopsy seems to be the best method to prove the diagnosis of malignancy.

In Africa and Asia, hepatic cell carcinoma is a much more common tumor than in North America and accounts for up to 30% of all malignant disease. This has been attributed to dietary habits and to the presence of carcinogens in foodstuffs or beverages. From earlier statements, the prevalence of hepatitis B virus may be a principal effector. In North America, 75% of carcinoma of the liver arises in patients with cirrhosis. Carcinoma arising in the bile ducts is also associated with cirrhosis and its first sign may be jaundice.

Benign tumors arising in the liver (hemangiomas) are common incidental findings and are seen frequently at autopsy (Fig. 18–18). Recently, a peculiar vascular tumor, an angiosarcoma, has been found in workers exposed to vinylchloride. This is another example of environmental hazards of which we were not previously aware.

Primary carcinoma of the liver, properly called hepatic cell carcinoma, but often referred to as hepatoma, is frequent in the world population. It is unusual in North America, except in patients with cirrhosis.

Hemochromatosis. Although this rare disease need not be placed in the chapter on the liver, it seems reasonable to discuss it here, as the liver is one of the principal targets affected by this disorder of iron

A

B

Fig. 18–17 *A,* More than half of this liver has been replaced by a **carcinoma**, which arose in the stomach and metastasized to the liver. One can see compression of the remaining liver parenchyma at the border of the white tumor. *B,* **Multiple metastases** to the liver are scattered randomly throughout the organ. The whitish, cauliflower-appearing material compresses the liver parenchyma. This carcinoma arose in the breast. (McGill University, Department of Pathology Museum.)

Fig. 18–18 Shown here is the most common tumor of the liver, a benign tumor of blood vessels, a **hemangioma**. It is circumscribed by a capsule at the arrow. (McGill University, Department of Pathology Museum.)

metabolism, and frequently the disordered liver functions and cirrhosis are diagnosed by biopsy as being due to some type of iron storage disease. It occurs 10 times as frequently in men as in women, usually after the age of 40, and is a classic cause of an enlarged liver and liver failure. The diagnosis is made by tissue demonstration of liver damage and of grossly increased body iron stores. The diagnosis is established when other causes for the same pattern are excluded. Hemochromatosis is not a disease of the liver alone and is sometimes diagnosed because of diabetes mellitus in a person who has an unusually darkened skin, hence the term "bronzed diabetes." Histologically, every organ can be demonstrated to contain excessive amounts of iron, from the pituitary, the pancreas, and the liver to the skin. Even the heart may be involved. These deposits of iron impair normal function of the respective organs and produce fibrosis in the liver and pancreas in particular. There is an extraordinarily high incidence of carcinoma of the liver in persons with hemochromatotic liver disease.

The causes of hemochromatosis are continually debated. It is clear that in South Africa, owing to native custom, a diet excessively rich in iron is the principal reason for the extraordinary incidence of cirrhosis and carcinoma of the liver in the Bantu. In all instances of the disease, alcohol seems to be a significant factor in increasing the iron load. Clearly, there are many persons who have a defect in red blood cell synthesis and in whom iron is diverted to body stores. All these causes are thought of as acquired instances of hemochromatosis. A second group of persons gives no history of any exogenous source. Studies have shown that their siblings have abnormally high iron levels, suggesting a congenital defect, perhaps in the intestinal mucosa, perhaps in the pancreas itself, that leads to the iron overload. It is an interesting but rare disorder in North America for which the best treatment seems to hark back to the days of Robin Hood, because bleeding, and thus depleting the body of iron, gives the best results.

DISORDERS OF THE GALLBLADDER AND BILE DUCTS

The principal diseases of the bile ducts and gallbladder are obstructions and infections. We shall consider the gallbladder and its diseases first.

The gallbladder is a small sac with a muscular wall and an epithelial lining that lies on the undersurface of the right lobe of the liver. It contains normally about 100 ml of bile, and its distal surface projects just to the free margin of the liver, so that if it is distended or inflamed, it may be palpated. In fact, a physician's name (Murphy) is associated with the presence of a palpably enlarged gallbladder. Bile flows continuously into the gallbladder from the liver by way of the cystic duct, but bile is only expelled from this small sac when a meal containing fat enters the duodenum. Bile in the gallbladder is concentrated by absorption of water. The epithelium of the gallbladder lining is a delicate series of folds filled with capillaries, much like the mucosa of the small intestine. When the gallbladder has been repeatedly inflamed due to chemical, mechanical, or infectious irritation, the ability to concentrate bile is impaired. The gallbladder wall may become markedly thickened and incapable either of responding to the stimuli to secrete or of enlarging in the face of partial obstruction.

Visualization of the gallbladder by radiographic means in the person who has experienced discomfort after a fatty meal or pain in the right upper quadrant is done by the administration of an organic iodine-containing compound, usually by mouth. This radiopaque material is selectively concentrated in the normally functioning gallbladder as water is resorbed and bile stored. If the gallbladder does not fill and cannot be visualized after repeated attempts, this failure can be interpreted as evidence of chronic disease or of obstruction. If the gallbladder fills, stones may sometimes be silhouetted against the radiopaque material (Fig. 18–19). Ultrasound is now used as a rapid diag-

nostic method to determine the presence of gallstones. The presence of small stones may then explain the reason for the discomfort and may suggest to the physician that the gallbladder could be surgically removed on an elective basis, or that an attempt to dissolve the stones may be undertaken.

Acute Cholecystitis. This most common disease of the gallbladder occurs most frequently in conjunction with obstruction at the neck of the gallbladder or in the cystic duct due to small stones. In much the same way as the appendix reacts to obstruction, the gallbladder becomes edematous and acutely inflamed. For a while, it was thought that the inflammation could be caused by some infectious agent (bacteria), but today it is generally held that the process is due to chemical injury. The edema and inflammation may impair venous return and may result in infarction or gangrene of the gallbladder. Naturally, as the small sac with its highly concentrated surface-active bile salts becomes necrotic, a great danger is rupture. The result of rupture is an abdominal catastrophe. Bile peritonitis is often fatal, since it rapidly leads to shock.

The outstanding features of both acute and chronic inflammation of the gallbladder are pain in the right upper quadrant (which sometimes masquerades as a peptic ulcer, pancreatitis, or even a myocardial infarction) and nausea and muscle guarding.

Clearly gallstones, or cholelithiasis, play a key role in the development and recurrence of cholecystitis; in fact, the diagnostic terms are used most often in conjunction. Biliary calculi, or gallstones, may be formed at any place in the biliary tree, but are most often found in the gallbladder. From many studies, estimates have been made of the frequency of gallstones in the general population, and some autopsy series give figures as high as one in every five cases. It has been estimated that 18,000,000 persons in North America have gallstones.

Gallstones are more frequent in women than in men. The old adage is that one should suspect gallstones in anyone who is "female, fat, fecund, fair, flatulent, and forty."

Recently there has been more and more evidence from studies on selected populations that heredity affects the generation of gallstones, and we have come to talk of "lithogenic" bile in certain populations such as the Pima Indians of Arizona, in whom gallstones occur in as many as 70% of adult women. A recent study shows that this highly saturated bile appears with puberty and is correlated with obesity and high levels of estrogens (Fig. 18–20).

The types of gallstones formed depend on many factors, such as heredity and certain body changes

Fig. 18–19 This x-ray shows, within the white line, the appearance of the gallbladder filled with numerous translucent stones. The gallbladder itself contains contrast from the orally administered dye.

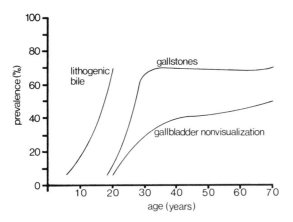

Fig. 18–20　This chart shows the prevalence of gallstones correlated with age in a population that has highly saturated bile. The first curve shows the high incidence of lithogenic bile (60% at age 10) in this population; the second curve shows that 75% have gallstones by 25 years of age. (From Bennion, L. J., et al.: Development of lithogenic bile during puberty in Pima Indians. N. Engl. J. Med., 300:873, 1979.)

(infections, pregnancy). The most common stones are composed of a mixture of cholesterol, bilirubin, and calcium. Other types are pure cholesterol and calcium-bilirubin stones, each constituting about 10% of the stones analyzed. Frequently, gallstones are multiple; they range in size from the head of a pin to a hen's egg. As it is often the little dogs that make the most noise, the same is true of gallstones. The small ones (gravel) may pass into the cystic duct and lodge there or in the common duct and cause exquisite pain and/or obstruction. Gallstones are often asymptomatic and may only be discovered by accident. Because of the complications of gallstones, the presence of a solitary silent stone in an elderly patient raises important questions about the role of elective surgery. The complications of obstruction, leading to distention of the common bile duct and the intrahepatic ducts and predisposing a person to infection (cholangitis), are

Fig. 18–21　**Two gallstones** are shown lying in a case of **carcinoma of the gallbladder** (at arrow). Surrounding this thickened wall is firm, white tumor, extending into and replacing the liver parenchyma. In the small lobe at the right of the photograph are umbilicated metastatic nodules of carcinoma. (McGill University, Department of Pathology Museum.)

Table 18–3.　Complications of Gallstones

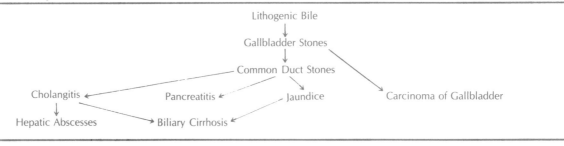

much more serious in the elderly, debilitated patient. Occasionally, large stones may erode from the gallbladder and create a fistula into the large bowel, where they may cause obstruction (ileus).

In addition to these complications, there is a much higher incidence of carcinoma of the gallbladder in patients who have had gallstones for many years, to the point where gallstones are considered a predisposing cause for carcinoma of the gallbladder (Fig. 18–21). Gallstones were present in 75% of all cases of carcinoma of the gallbladder in one study.

Table 18–3 illustrates various complications that may be caused by the presence of lithogenic bile. First, it predisposes a patient to gallstones, either in the gallbladder or in the common duct. Whenever stones occur in the common duct, a number of complications may arise: cholangitis, pancreatitis, jaundice, biliary cirrhosis. Stones in the gallbladder predispose a person to carcinoma of that organ.

All this leads to the view that this small storage bladder is not essential to health and, when there are indications, it should be removed. In every hospital, however, there should be a tissue committee that reviews all such procedures to be sure that the reason for removal was true disease, not "acute remunerative cholecystitis."

SYNOPSIS

The liver, supplied by blood from the portal veins and hepatic artery, synthesizes proteins, secretes bile, detoxifies drugs, and stores glycogen, among other functions.

Jaundice is a sign of disease. The causes of hyperbilirubinemia may be hepatocellular injury, obstruction to the bile ducts, or hemolysis.

Necrosis of liver cells is a common response to many types of injury. Acute hepatic failure may be due to viral infections, to poisons, to congestion, to ischemia, or to particular diseases such as toxemia of pregnancy.

Infections of the liver may be caused by flukes, protozoa, fungi, bacteria, and viruses, and may result in local abscess or diffuse injury, which may be either acute or chronic.

Viral hepatitis is an important public health problem in North America.

Cirrhosis is a chronic, diffuse, structural disorganization of the liver, characterized by necrosis, fibrosis, and nodular regeneration of hepatic cells.

The complications of cirrhosis are ascites, splenomegaly, gastrointestinal bleeding, hepatic coma, and occasionally portal vein thrombosis and hepatic cell carcinoma.

Carcinoma of the liver is relatively rare in North America but arises commonly in patients with cirrhosis. It is a common disease in Asia and Africa.

The principal diseases of the gallbladder and bile ducts are obstruction and infections. Cholelithiasis and cholecystitis are virtually synonymous.

Terms

Portal circulation	Hepatomegaly	Hepatic coma
Hypoalbuminemia	Cholangiogram	Hepatocarcinoma
Bilirubin	Hepatitis	Cholecystitis
Jaundice	Cirrhosis	Cholelithiasis

FURTHER READING

Bainton, D., et al.: Gallbladder disease: prevalence in a South Wales industrial town. N. Engl. J. Med., 294:1147, 1976.

Balayan, M.S., et al.: The spread of hepatitis A virus in connection with hepatitis cases in children's communities. Bull. W.H.O., 60:243, 1982.

Beasley, R.P.: Hepatitis B virus as the etiologic agent in hepatocellular carcinoma—epidemiologic considerations. Hepatology, 2:218, 1982.

Bennion, L.J., et al.: Development of lithogenic bile during puberty in Pima Indians. N. Engl. J. Med., 300:873, 1979.

Blumberg, B.S.: The Hepatitis B virus. Landmarks in American Epidemiology, 95:427, 1980.

Boyer, J.L.: New concepts of mechanisms of hepatocyte bile formation. Physiol. Rev., 60:303, 1980.

Braverman, D.Z., Johnson, M.L., and Kern, F., Jr.: Effects of pregnancy and contraceptive steroids on gallbladder function. N. Engl. J. Med., 302:362, 1980.

Cohen, A.B.: Unraveling the mysteries of alpha$_1$-antitrypsin deficiency. N. Engl. J. Med., 314:778, 1986.

Dane, D.S., et al.: Virus-like particles in serum of patients with Australia-antigen-associated hepatitis. Lancet, 1:695, 1970.

Davidson, C.S. Changing concepts in the pathogenesis of alcoholic liver disease. Alcohol. 10:35, 1986.

Fairley, C.K., et al.: Epidemiology and hepatitis C virus in Victoria. Med. J. Austr., 153:271, 1990.

Farley, T.A., et al.: An outbreak of Hepatitis A associated with swimming in a public pool. J. Infect. Dis., 165:613, 1992.

Fausto, N., and Mead, J.E.: Regulation of liver growth: protooncogenes and transforming growth factor. Lab. Investig., 60:4, 1989.

Geokas, M.C., et al.: Ethanol, the liver, and the gastrointestinal tract. Ann. Intern. Med., 95:198, 1981.

Halapin, T.J., et al.: Reye's syndrome and medication use. J.A.M.A., 248:687, 1982.

Hoofnagle, J.H.: Chronic hepatitis B. N. Engl. J. Med., 323:337, 1990.

Kaplan, M.M.: Primary biliary cirrhosis. N. Engl. J. Med., 316:521, 1987.

Klatskin, G.: Hepatic tumours: possible relationship to use of oral contraceptives. Gastroenterology, 73:386, 1977.

Lettau, L.A., et al.: Outbreak of severe hepatitis due to Delta and Hepatitis B viruses in parenteral drug abusers and their contacts. N. Engl. J. Med., 317:1256, 1987.

Lieber, C.S.: Hepatic, metabolic and toxic effects of ethanol: 1991 update. Alcohol. Clin. Exp. Res., 15:573, 1991.

Maugh, T.H.: Hepatitis B vaccine passes first major test. Science, 210:760, 1980.

Mbithi, J.N., et al.: Survival of Hepatitis-A virus on human hands and its transfer on contact with animate and inanimate surfaces. J. Clin. Microbiol., 30:757, 1992.

Mezey, E.: Liver disease and protein needs. Ann. Rev. Nutr., 2:21, 1982.

Mok, H.Y.I., et al.: Chronology of cholelithiasis: Dating gallstones from atmospheric radiocarbon produced by nuclear bomb explosions. N. Engl. J. Med., 314:1075, 1986.

Nomura, A.M.Y., and Kolonel, L.N.: Prostate cancer: a current perspective. Epidemiol. Rev., 13:200, 1991.

Omata, M., et al.: Mutations in the pre-core region of hepatitis B virus DNA in patients with fulminant and severe hepatitis. N. Engl. J. Med., 324:1699, 1991.

Piehler, J.M., and Crichlow, R.W.: Primary carcinoma of the gallbladder. Surg. Gynecol. Obstet., 147:929, 1978.

Sackmann, M., et al.: Shock-wave lithotripsy of gallbladder stones: the first 175 patients. N. Engl. J. Med., 318:393, 1988.

Saunders, K.D., et al.: Pathogenesis of gallstones. Surg. Clin. N.A., 70:1197, 1990.

Schiff, L.: Jaundice: five-and-a-half decades in historic perspective. Selected aspects. Gastroenterology, 78:831, 1980.

Southern Surgeons' Club: A prospective analysis of 1518 laparoscopic cholecystectomies. N. Engl. J. Med., 324:1073, 1991.

Starzl, T.E., Demetris, A.J., and Van Thiel, D.: Liver transplantation (first of two parts). N. Engl. J. Med., 321:1014, 1989.

Stone, W.D., et al.: The natural history of cirrhosis. Q.J. Med., 37:119, 1968.

Sveger, T.: Liver disease in alpha₁-antitrypsin deficiency detected by screening of 200,000 infants. N. Engl. J. Med., 294:1316, 1976.

Szmuness, W., et al.: The prevalence of antibody to hepatitis A antigen in various parts of the world: a pilot study. Am. J. Epidemiol., 106:392, 1977.

Tanaka, H., et al. Characteristics and significance of albumin-positive hepatocytes in analbuminemic rats. Eur. J. Cell Biol., 53:267, 1990.

Tedder, R.S., et al.: Hepatitis C virus: evidence for sexual transmission. Br. Med. J., 302:1299, 1991.

Warren, K.S.: The relevance of schistosomiasis. N. Engl. J. Med., 303:203, 1980.

Williams, R.: Problems of fulminant hepatic failure. Br. Med. Bull., 28:114, 1972.

APPENDIX

Physiology of the Liver

Synthetic Functions. Whereas the liver receives the elements of all digestive processes that arrive in the portal venous blood (a little like the groceries for the Christmas banquet arriving at the kitchen door), perhaps the most important products of the liver cell are the serum proteins.

Serum proteins (albumin, fibrinogen, prothrombin, to name 3) serve several specific functions, but collectively they contribute to the osmotic value of the serum of the intravascular fluid compartment and thereby enable the circulation to function, as was reviewed earlier.

Albumin is the most important of these proteins; the liver is the only organ that makes it. About 10 g of albumin are synthesized daily by a 70-kg man, but half this albumin will be lost in 2 weeks. A decrease in serum albumin (hypoalbuminemia) can result from increased excretion (glomerular disease), inadequate precursors (malnutrition), or decreased synthesis (liver disease). This decrease in serum albumin results in edema, ascites, or anasarca (the accumulation of fluid outside the vascular compartment).

Any acute or chronic injury to the liver may result in decreased synthesis of important protein products of the liver, such as fibrinogen and prothrombin, which are blood clotting factors. Therefore, another serious result of liver damage may be small or large hemorrhages and impairment of the normal clotting mechanisms.

The liver also synthesizes a legion of enzymes, some of which appear in direct response to a need for them, such as alcohol dehydrogenase. A teetotaler will have little of this, whereas a souse will have a high specific activity of this inducible enzyme. When liver cells are injured by toxic agents (chemicals, viruses) or impaired blood supply (heart failure), enzymes may leak into the serum, just as necrotic heart muscle leaks both muscle-specific enzymes (CPK) and nonspecific cytoplasmic or mitochondrial enzymes, such as glutamic oxaloacetic transaminase (SGOT) or lactic acid dehydrogenase (LDH). Elevations of transaminase and other isoenzymes (in the absence of necrosis of the heart tissue) are good indications of damage to the liver.

The liver also synthesizes substances other than proteins. One important class is lipids, of which lipoproteins are the form that appear in the serum. The liver takes up free fatty acids from the portal circulation and esterifies them into triglycerides that may be stored or excreted (lipoproteins). Because the preferred form for the excretion of lipid is a complex of lipid with protein, the release and secretion of lipid depends also on the protein-synthesizing capabilities of the liver. If the liver's protein-synthesizing machinery has been poisoned, then the lipids that normally would be distributed accumulate in the liver cells, which results in a fatty, enlarged liver.

Secretory Function. The principal and most obvious product of the liver is bile. This colored fluid is derived from the hemoglobin of red blood cells that have reached the end of their normal life span. The obsolete red blood cells are broken down by cells of the reticuloendothelial system (Kupffer cells), and the iron (heme) that has been separated from the protein (globin) is converted into bilirubin via biliverdin. A small proportion of bilirubin comes from other heme proteins (cytochrome, myoglobin), and from the bone marrow. Liver cells take up bilirubin and conjugate it into a water-soluble derivative, using the microsomes of their cytoplasm to do the job. The principal product of this work is a bilirubin conjugated with sugars (bilirubin diglucuronide), a step that is required for bilirubin to pass into the bile. The liver cell is able to secrete this water-soluble material into the small space between two neighboring liver cells, the bile canaliculus, which, like the tributaries of a mountain stream that join to form a river, connects with the intrahepatic, extrahepatic, and common bile ducts, terminating in the delta of the ampulla of Vater, where the bile enters the intestinal cavity and colors all the sediment a familiar muddy brown.

It is of interest that this conjugated bilirubin is not reabsorbed in the intestine, and the body is thereby permitted to excrete pigments for which it has no use. Bacteria of the large bowel have the capability, however, of converting conjugated bilirubin into urobilinogen, which can be reabsorbed and recycled, thereby conserving material if need be.

What is the function of bile? Bile contains bile salts and cholesterol as well as bilirubin. The salts in bile are surface-active substances that emulsify lipids and, by their action, permit lipids to be absorbed by the intestinal absorptive cell. In the absence of bile, fats and fat-soluble vitamins are not absorbed, and the body suffers the consequences of deficiency of vitamins D, K, and E and a lack of essential fatty acids (arachidonic, linoleic). The body has devised an ingenious mechanism for dealing with periods of famine and plenty by enabling large amounts of bile to be delivered to the intestine when a meal of seal blubber, cheesecake, or herring and sour cream has been ingested. The gallbladder is a reservoir that stores bile and can deliver relatively large amounts via the cystic and common ducts on signal from the duodenum. Normally, small amounts of bile are constantly synthesized, secreted, and delivered to the intestine. It is one of Nature's devices to combine forces whenever possible. It is of note that the ducts from the pancreas enter the duodenum at the same site (ampulla of Vater) as the bile, and pancreatic enzymes, which are concerned with hydrolysis of fats (lipases), are secreted at the same time into the duodenum as the emulsifier.

While we are on the subject of secretion of bile, it is appropriate to consider the problem of jaundice before going on to consider the other general functions of the liver (detoxification and storage).

Detoxification. The liver plays an important role in dealing with toxic and natural substances. Hormones, drugs, dietary pollutants—all are examples of substances that are excreted by the liver when they have been inactivated or converted to water-soluble materials. In order to do this job, the liver is capable of synthesizing new enzymes. Naturally, a diseased liver responds less effectively to demand than a normal one, and a dose of a drug that would be well tolerated in a normal person may be lethal in someone with severe liver disease. It has become clear that some drugs (for example, phenobarbital) may cause a change in the structure of liver cells that can even be visualized with the electron microscope. With regular doses, there is an increase in the smooth endoplasmic reticulum.

Storage. The famous experiments of Claude Bernard showed that the mammalian liver was a storehouse for glycogen, and thus provides a reservoir or physiologic buffer for serum glucose. As serum glucose is used, additional supplies may be mobilized from the liver stores, and the constancy of the serum glucose level maintained. Other substances such as iron and lipids are also deposited in the hepatic bank account, although the normal turnover is rapid and the stored balance at any given time is small (just like the average bank account). With disease, with increased loads, or from decreased mobilization, materials may accumulate in liver cells. This accumulation leads to enlargement of the liver (hepatomegaly). Rarely, foreign materials (amyloid) may be deposited among the liver cells and may also

increase the size of the liver. Moreover, in some rare hereditary disorders, such as those due to enzyme deficiencies, the liver may accumulate materials, as in the glycogen storage diseases. Naturally, with acute destruction of the liver (hepatitis), there may be a failure of normal function. For example, a patient with acute hepatitis may be in coma because of an excessively low blood sugar, since the hepatic cells are capable neither of storing glycogen nor of releasing it.

Liver Function Tests. For each of these arbitrary functions of the liver (synthesis, secretion, detoxification, and storage) there are laboratory tests that can estimate the capability of the liver.

Tests of Synthetic Function. The serum albumin in the normal human being is about 4 to 5 g/100 ml; the normal value of globulins is 2 to 3 g/100 ml. Other proteins such as fibrinogen and prothrombin are not routinely measured directly. Any decrease in serum albumin in the absence of a demonstrated loss in the urine can be attributed to decreased synthesis. This implies a disordered function of the liver cells.

If a patient has a prolonged prothrombin time, the liver may be diseased; however, if the bile ducts are obstructed, a prolonged prothrombin time will also occur because vitamin K, essential for the synthesis of prothrombin, may not be available. A simple test to see whether this disorder can be reversed is to administer vitamin K to the patient. If, in the presence of exogenous vitamin K, the bleeding tendency reverses, it is clear that the liver cells themselves are capable of using this essential vitamin. Unfortunately, the longer mechanical obstruction lasts in any system, especially the liver, the more likely there is to be damage to the cells upstream of the obstruction.

Another group of tests for the integrity of the synthetic function of the liver are those for the presence of enzymes that are not normally present in the serum, or are present in low or trace amounts only. We have already mentioned the transaminases (SGOT and SGPT), which are only present in trace amounts in the serum (less than 40 units), but which are elevated in all types of liver disease (greater than 400 units). An isoenzyme of lactic acid dehydrogenase has been traced to hepatic cells and permits necrosis of liver to be distinguished from necrosis in the heart.

Tests of Secretory Function. As outlined previously, the functions of the liver include the secretion of bile and materials that have been detoxified: hormones, dyes (bromsulfophthalein), enzymes (alkaline phosphatase, 5'nucleotidase). In order to assess liver function, it is possible to use some tests that directly and/or indirectly measure the secretory function of the liver, other than the secretion of bile.

One test is to administer a dye, bromsulfophthalein (BSP), which is rapidly taken up, concentrated, conjugated and secreted. A standard amount of dye (5 mg/kg body weight) is injected and a blood sample is withdrawn from another vein at a fixed time and analyzed for dye concentration. Normally, less than 5% of the dye remains in the serum 45 minutes after injection. Despite its nonspecificity, the test is of value in patients who do not have jaundice to assess the functional capability of the liver cells.

A second test, which complements the serum bilirubin assay, is that for serum alkaline phosphatase. This enzyme is present in the brush border of the intestine, in the kidney, in bones, and in the liver. Although its function is debated, it is well known empirically that extrahepatic biliary obstruc-

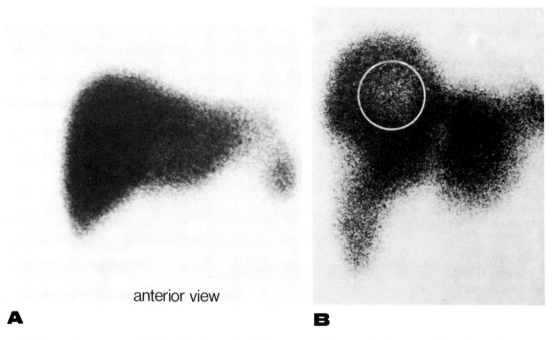

Fig. A18–1 *A,* This x-ray shows a scan of a liver 15 minutes after the intravenous injection of technitium sulfur-colloid. The uniform distribution and uptake shows the outline of a normal liver. *B,* In this instance, within the circle, there is an area of decreased uptake of the technitium sulfur-colloid. Such an absence of normal liver is compatible with the diagnosis of tumor, abscess, or cysts. The technitium is normally taken up by Kupffer's cells of the reticuloendothelial system.

Fig. A18–2 *A and B,* This ultrasound scan, using the B-mode, shows a 2-cm area in the superior aspect of the liver. This lesion is labeled in the accompanying diagram. The presence of an echogenic mass is consistent with a solid growth such as a metastasis from cancer of the colon to the liver. (The dense white line at the left of the picture is the position of the diaphragm.)

tion leads to great elevation in serum alkaline phosphatase. Perhaps hepatocellular disease leads to decreased synthesis of this enzyme, but, in any case, in the presence of obstruction such as carcinoma of the head of the pancreas, or common duct stone, the alkaline phosphatase levels are many times normal. In order to distinguish elevations of alkaline phosphatase levels that occur in bone disease from those that occur in liver disease, another enzyme, 5'nucleotidase, may be measured.

Tests of Storage and Metabolic Function. In liver disease, not only may the storage and mobilization of glycogen be impaired, but the serum glucose levels, as assayed by a glucose tolerance test, may reflect damage to the liver. The glucose tolerance test may show a rapid rise of blood glucose to abnormally high levels and an abnormally slow return to normal. The most important finding is an unusually low serum glucose level. However, a glucose tolerance test in the presence of liver disease gives variable results and cannot be considered a specific indication of the kind or amount of damage to the liver.

Other Tests of Hepatic Function. In addition to the tests outlined in the foregoing section, radiologic examination of the liver is frequently useful. A plain film of the abdomen may demonstrate calcified structures within the liver or biliary tract, and the presence of fluid (ascites) in the peritoneal cavity often points to hepatic disease. Radiopaque substances taken by mouth (oral cholecystography) or injected intravenously (IV cholecystography) or directly into the liver (transhepatic cholangiography) often outline the biliary tree, indicating an obstruction or an anatomic abnormality, guiding the surgeon to the diagnosis and treatment. Other more recent techniques take advantage of the liver's synthetic, storage, and secretory functions. When radioactively labeled substances are administered, they may be taken up by the liver and may reveal nonfunctional areas (cysts) or space-occupying lesions that may represent tumor (Figs. A18–1 and A18–2).

In the absence of any bleeding disorder, a needle biopsy of the liver can be done, yielding a small piece of tissue from which a histologic diagnosis may be made. With this background of structure, function, and possible tests of the liver's integrity, we may progress to consider the circulation of the liver before discussing important and common diseases.

19

PANCREAS *(Including Diabetes Mellitus)*

We have scientists who still pray to the gods, scientists who laugh at the gods, and some who neither pray nor laugh because they think they understand.—A.J. CARLSON

STRUCTURE AND FUNCTION

The pancreas, known in animals as the "sweetbread," is an elongated flat organ that lies behind the stomach on the left side of the abdomen. It is the most powerful digestive gland in the body, and has been called the salivary gland of the abdomen, because not only does it resemble the salivary glands in structure, being composed of tubular acini, but it pours its secretions into the digestive canal by a duct. The pancreatic duct opens into the duodenum at the same point as the common bile duct enters the bowel; indeed the two ducts usually have a common opening, the importance of which will soon become evident. The pancreas is partly exocrine, producing three digestive enzymes, and partly endocrine, releasing at least two hormones into the blood. One of the enzymes prepares carbohydrates for absorption, whereas the hormones regulate the metabolism for carbohydrates once absorbed.

Endocrine Function. The pancreatic secretions produced by the acini contain several powerful digestive enzymes, one for the digestion of proteins, one for carbohydrates, and one for fats. (1) Trypsin, like the pepsin of gastric juice, acts on the proteins, but it carries the process a step further. (2) Amylase breaks large molecules of starch into smaller molecules of maltose, which are converted into still smaller molecules of glucose in the intestinal juice. The glucose is absorbed and carried by the portal vein to the liver, where it is stored as glycogen, to be reconverted into glucose as needed. (3) Lipase splits ingested fats into fatty acids and glycerol with the aid of bile.

Endocrine Function. The endocrine part of the pancreas is not visible to the naked eye; it is represented by tiny groups of cells called the islets of Langerhans, after the man who first described them in 1869, never guessing their function. The islets are scattered among the acinar tissue throughout the length of the pancreas. Their cells are of two general types and contain granules that stain differently, so that they are known as A or alpha and B or beta cells. The alpha cells stain red and the beta cells blue. The beta cells, which secrete insulin, comprise 60 to 90% of the cells. The alpha cells produce glucagon, the other internal secretion. A third group of cells has been found to produce another hormone (somatomedin), which is discussed in the endocrine chapter.

Insulin, secreted by the beta cells, is absorbed directly into the blood that passes through the pancreas. Were it to enter the pancreatic duct, insulin would immediately be destroyed by the pancreatic enzymes. It has been known since 1889 that removal of the entire pancreas in animals was followed by fatal diabetes, but we had to wait until 1922 for the demonstration, by Banting and his co-workers in Toronto, that an extract of islets of Langerhans would control the diabetes produced by pancreatectomy (Fig. 19–1). They named the substance insulin because it came from the islets (Latin *insula*, island). The function of insulin is to regulate carbohydrate metabolism; when insufficient insulin is produced, diabetes develops. Insulin acts: (1) by making the storage of glucose possible, especially in the liver and muscles; (2) by enabling the tissues to burn glucose. When the blood glucose in the portal vein carrying blood from the pancreas to the liver is above normal (hyperglycemia), insulin is released into the vein.

Glucagon is the alpha cell hormone. It may be regarded as the opposite twin of insulin, for it is released into the portal vein when the blood sugar is below normal. It brings about the breakdown of liver glycogen into glucose, so that there is a prompt rise in the glucose content of the blood leaving the liver.

Tests of Pancreatic Function. These depend on an estimation of one or more of the three main digestive enzymes in the blood. The lipase and amylase levels in the serum give invaluable information. Lipase estimation takes longer, but serum amylase can be measured within an hour, so that it is the method of choice in acute pancreatitis, which may constitute an abdominal emergency that has to be differentiated from acute appendicitis, perforated peptic ulcer, and biliary colic. These tests are of little help in chronic pancreatitis. Tests for endocrine dysfunction will be considered in connection with diabetes.

The three most important diseases of the pancreas are acute and chronic pancreatitis, diabetes mellitus, and cancer, although others will be mentioned briefly.

Fig. 19–1　Charles Best (left) and Sir Frederick Banting (right) with their experimental animal seen in the late 1920s.

PANCREATITIS

As with all organs, inflammatory conditions of the pancreas are an important source of pain, discomfort, and dysfunction. There are two general classes of inflammatory disease in the pancreas. We shall dismiss from our consideration the chronic inflammatory conditions, which require much space and time, and instead refer the reader to a textbook of medicine or surgery. Suffice it to say that chronic pancreatitis is seen most commonly in alcohol abusers; it may occur in individuals with disease of the biliary tract, particularly where there are gallstones, and after abdominal injuries such as trauma. We shall consider here only acute pancreatitis.

Perhaps mumps virus is the most common cause of acute inflammation of the pancreas. If the other salivary glands are afflicted, the diagnosis is not difficult, and as with most viral diseases, the course is self-limited. There is little we can do except to adhere to the traditional practice of "watchful waiting."

There is another acute disease of the pancreas that is fortunately rare, but is so serious as to be life-threatening, with a mortality rate of 50% or greater. It is often seen around Christmas or the New Year, at times of gastronomic and alcoholic celebration, and is known as acute hemorrhagic pancreatitis.

The entity is an acute abdominal catastrophe and may be confused with a ruptured peptic ulcer or even with a dissecting aneurysm, because of the intense pain, coupled with shock and a rigid abdomen with guarding and tenderness. Steady, penetrating pain in the upper abdomen, which may be referred to the back and may be relieved by the patient's assuming the fetal position with the knees drawn up and the trunk folded, is typical of acute pancreatic disease. The physical signs are typical of shock, and the laboratory data will show leukocytosis, perhaps hemoconcentration, and occasionally jaundice, if the duct is compromised. A fall in the serum calcium points to fat necrosis and helps to establish the diagnosis, but the pathognomonic finding is an elevated serum amylase, which rises within a few hours of the onset of the disease. Any level above 500 Somogyi units suggests the diagnosis of acute pancreatitis.

What is the mechanism of this disease, what are the predisposing causes, and what are the complications or eventual outcome? The disease is believed to depend on the activation of pancreatic enzymes, which are normally excreted through the ducts into the duodenum. In cases in which it is anatomically possible for bile to reflux into the pancreatic ducts, this is believed to be the mechanism. Although the secreting pressure of the pancreas exceeds that of the bile ducts, and although not all ducts have a common orifice, it has been shown that a mixture of bile and pancreatic juices can produce pancreatitis.

It is well recognized that biliary tract disease, particularly the presence of stones, predisposes a person to acute hemorrhagic pancreatitis. One postulate is that a stone may obstruct the ampulla of Vater and may rechannel the bile into the pancreas, but this has not been observed in all cases. Rich and Duff found squamous metaplasia in pancreatic ducts and suggested that this led to a degree of pancreatic obstruction that set the stage for autodigestion. Alcohol in quantity, a strong stimulus to secretion, is associated with other gastrointestinal diseases, as well as with the occurrence of pancreatitis. Suffice it to say that we do not know the precise etiology of pancreatitis, but we can invoke several hypotheses, all of which require the activation of pancreatic enzymes, which then digest not only the tissues of the pancreas itself, but also neighboring structures, including blood vessels. These vessels may then rupture and bleed vigorously into the retroperitoneal space and may lead to shock. The proteolytic and lipolytic pancreatic enzymes have been implicated in the destruction of the tissues that leads to fat necrosis and destruction of the pancreas itself (Fig. 19–2).

The sequel to this acute episode depends on the

Fig. 19–2 Mottled areas of whitish material are distributed randomly throughout the pancreas. These white areas represent fat necrosis and are areas where inflammation has taken place in acute pancreatitis. (McGill University, Department of Pathology Museum.)

degree of damage. If the injury is slight (small amounts of enzymes—small areas of destruction), edema and slight sudden discomfort may be the only indication that anything is wrong, whereas a severe episode may lead to death. In between, various degrees of disability may result from loss of the exocrine and endocrine pancreas. Naturally, severe damage to the exocrine pancreas may leave the patient a digestive cripple; his or her stool may show abundant fat that cannot be absorbed and meat fibers that are not digested because of the lack of enzymes. The patient may have hyperglycemia because of damage to the islets of Langerhans; and cysts and infection in the necrotic area are always feared as results of the acute episode. Fortunately, the most severe type of pancreatitis is rare.

DIABETES MELLITUS

Diabetes means a "running through;" mellitus means "sweet" (literally, honeyed). The word diabetes is also used as an abbreviation for another disease, diabetes insipidus, in which the amount of urine is greatly increased, but contains no sugar and is therefore insipid or tasteless. The nomenclature obviously dates from the time, happily now past, when tasting the urine was a recognized part of urinalysis.

As diabetes insipidus is rare, diabetes mellitus is usually known simply as diabetes. The increases in both volume and frequency of urine and its sugar content might suggest that this was a disease of the kidneys. This is not so; the kidneys may be normal. It is

a metabolic disorder, as a result of which the carbohydrate of the food is not used by the tissues. Paradoxically, the diabetic may have adequate fuel, but may shiver, metaphorically speaking, because he cannot ignite the furnace. The cause of the disorder is a deficient supply of insulin, and the lesion responsible is in the islets of Langerhans in the pancreas.

We do know, however, that insulin in some way serves as a spark that enables the glucose carried to the tissue cells, particularly the muscles, to unite with the oxygen there and to be burned and thereby produce energy. Glucose is to the body as gasoline is to the internal combustion engine. Every time the heart beats or we move a muscle, we use glucose, and, just as a spark is necessary to fire the gasoline in the engine so insulin is necessary to burn the glucose. Insulin also enables the glucose carried from the intestine to the liver to be converted into glycogen. When insulin is lacking, it is evident that glucose will neither be changed into glycogen in the liver nor be burned by the muscles, so that it will accumulate in the blood in large amounts. When the blood reaches the kidneys, the glucose will flow out into the urine. A diagnosis of diabetes can be made by testing either the urine or the blood for sugar, remembering that some is always present in the blood. The normal fasting blood sugar level is 60 to 100 mg per 100 ml, but in diabetes it may reach 300 mg or higher.

There is an even greater danger than the failure to burn carbohydrates, namely a failure to burn fats. For the proper combustion of fat, a certain proportion of carbohydrates must be burned at the same time. In the carburetor of an automobile, the correct mixture must be present, or else the engine will "smoke" and will misfire. So also in the tissues, if the correct fat-glucose mixture is not present, it will "smoke" during combustion, the smoke representing toxic acid substances that result from incomplete combustion of the fat. These substances are known as ketone bodies, and the clinical condition is known as acidosis or ketosis. We may say then, that diabetes is initially a derangement of carbohydrate metabolism, but that this disorder leads to a perverted fat metabolism, which, if unchecked, will result in death.

It is estimated that 200,000,000 persons in the world have diabetes. In Sweden, in each of the 5 years from 1970 to 1975, there was a mean yearly incidence of 19.6 cases per 100,000 population in children, suggesting that the country could expect 330 new cases annually, with some clustering of cases in January and in the autumn, and peaks at 7 and 12 years of age. The disease is of worldwide distribution, but there are some countries that report a higher frequency than others. In the United States, it is estimated that the frequency is 1.3 diabetics per 1,000 in the population up to age 17, 17 between 25 and 44 years, 43 in the age group from 45 to 64, and 79 over 65 years of age. These numbers will continue to increase as the population grows older. Successful management of the disease prolongs life, and more diabetics live long enough to procreate.

Diabetes is 2.5 times more frequent in relatives than in the general population, and 85% of diabetics have been obese at some time. We do not know the fundamental cause of diabetes; the lesions in the islets are hardly striking, and may indeed be difficult, and sometimes impossible, to detect. There is increasing evidence that in the maturity-onset diabetic, the pancreas produces normal quantities of insulin and the problem is a reduced sensitivity of fat and muscle cells to the effects of insulin.

There are many steps involved in the action of insulin: its biosynthesis, liberation, circulation, uptake and activation, binding, and its effect on intermediary metabolism. There are just as many loci in which lesions that result ultimately in elevated blood glucose can occur. We have stated that the most obvious metabolic cause of diabetes is the lack of insulin, without specifying whether this is a lack of synthesis of insulin or of an abnormal insulin molecule, or whether it is a failure to secrete the synthesized molecule.

Clearly we may have another lesion, namely resistance to insulin. This resistance has been recognized in clinically overt diabetics who respond poorly to insulin in standard doses, but who may respond to greater than normal doses. Defects in insulin recep-

tors have been recognized recently, anti-insulin antibodies are frequently found, and accelerated rates of insulin breakdown are often discovered; these biochemical disorders can lead to diabetes.

Perhaps it is better to consider for a moment what is meant by diabetes mellitus by considering the **diabetic syndrome.** Diabetes may be defined as a metabolic disorder characterized by hyperglycemia.

Because of the body's inability to use glucose, there is starvation in the midst of plenty, and the mobilization of body fat and protein occurs, leading to acidosis. With the occurrence of hyperglycemia and the loss in the urine of glucose in large amounts, there is an obligatory water loss that leads to dehydration and consequent thirst, increased drinking of water, and more urination, as a vicious cycle continues. If the central nervous system does not receive adequate glucose, coma may ensue (Fig. 19–3). In the chronic condition, there is the classic development of changes in small blood vessels throughout the body, particularly in the retina and kidney (see Fig. 14–6). These changes can be visualized with the ophthalmoscope or in the kidney biopsy, and they result in premature visual difficulties (even blindness in some persons) and in abnormal permeability to proteins in the glomeruli, which may precipitate the nephrotic syndrome. Since it is now recognized that the basement membrane around small blood vessels is unusually thickened in diabetic patients, even biopsy is sometimes performed for diagnosis. Because of these lesions we have come to think of **diabetes as a systemic disease**, rather than simply a disorder of insulin production.

The relationship between the vascular lesions and the availability of insulin is not understood, and it may be that they are not causally related, but are simply associated, genetically determined defects.

It is convenient to regard diabetes as having four stages, implying that there may be progression from one to another (although this is an hypothesis). The stages range from the theoretic to the obvious, ending with the clinical, overt, or "decompensated" diabetes about which we have been speaking. In testing for the **potential diabetic,** we can identify the asymptomatic person whose fasting blood sugar is normal, but whose blood glucose tolerance curve shows an abnormally slow return to normal levels. A glucose tolerance curve is the serum glucose level taken at specific times after a challenge dose of glucose (Fig. 19–4), and this delayed return to normal shows an inappropriate handling of glucose. **Latent diabetes** is the term used for those persons whose random blood sugar levels are normal and whose glucose tolerance curves are normal, but who have been identified, when **under**

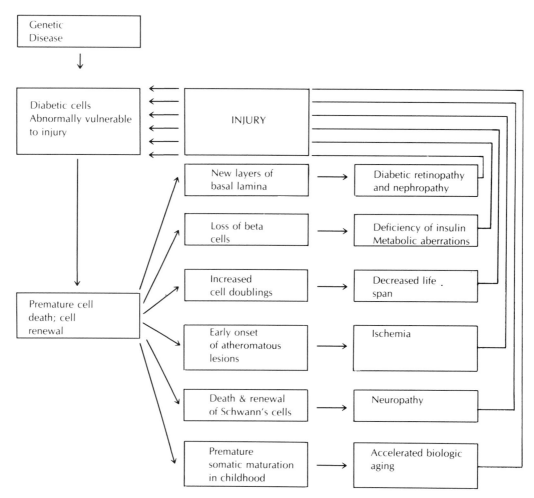

Fig. 19–3 Hypothetical flow of events in diabetes mellitus. Diabetic cells, which by the nature of a genetically transmitted defect, are more vulnerable to injury, die prematurely as a result of ordinary wear and tear. The accelerated cell turnover gives rise to (a) formation of new layers of basal lamina (the hallmark of diabetic microangiopathy), (b) loss of beta cell mass—the problem is compounded by a limited capacity of pancreas to replenish beta cells, (c) increased use of cell doublings in vivo and, consequently, decreased in vitro replicative life span, (d) lesions of atherosclerosis caused either by increased opportunity for expression of smooth muscle cell transformation or proliferation in response to release from feedback inhibition, (e) death and regeneration of Schwann's cells associated with intermittent symptoms of neuropathy, and, conceivably, (f) accelerated maturation and aging of diabetic individuals. The vascular problem, metabolic aberrations related to insulin deficiency and neuropathy, all provide additional opportunity for injurious events and probably further increase the speed and frequency of accelerated cell turnover. (From Vracko, R., and Benditt, E.P.: Manifestations of diabetes mellitus—their possible relationships to an underlying cell defect. Am. J. Pathol., 75:204, 1974.)

stress of pregnancy or serious illness or when they were obese, as diabetic. This concept is useful, as the disease may become clinically evident again. Finally, the term **prediabetes** has been introduced to describe those who can be considered to be at risk to develop diabetes, for example, a twin of a diabetic, or the child of diabetic parents. It is a concept rather than a diagnosis, because all testing shows normal metabolism of carbohydrate.

Etiology. Heredity is undoubtedly a most important factor in the development of diabetes. The genetics of diabetes are confusing at best. First, we recognize several different types of diabetes: in the child

(juvenile), in the obese middle-aged adult (late onset), and the diabetes that can be detected only by rigorous testing (latent). Of course, there is as well diabetes due to other disorders of the pancreas (pancreatitis) and diabetes as a part of another syndrome (Cushing's disease). The difficulties in perceiving the patterns of diabetes are compounded by recent studies on twins that reverse the traditional view that juvenile diabetes is hereditary, and adult-onset is acquired. In a study of 106 pairs of twins with insulin-dependent diabetes, almost half have only one member with diabetes. Dr. Pyke recalls the tragedy of a pair of female twins, of which the nondiabetic won a beauty contest

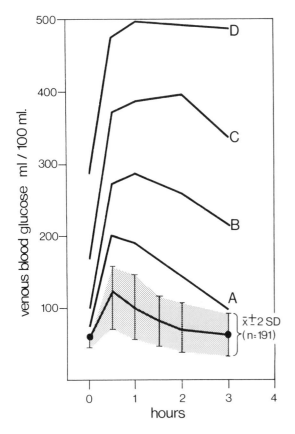

Fig. 19–4　This figure shows glucose tolerance curves for 191 normal controls (shaded area) and for 4 diabetic patients (A to D). (From Cahill, G.F., Jr.: Diabetes mellitus. In *Cecil Textbook of Medicine*, 15th Ed. Edited by P.B. Beeson, W. McDermott, and J.B. Wyngaarden. Philadelphia, W. B. Saunders Co., 1979.)

at age 20, and has a happy marriage with three children; her sister, meanwhile, developed retinopathy, became nearly blind, developed glomerular disease, and died in her early 30s from the complications of her disease. For her whole life, she had only to look at her sister to see how life would have been without diabetes. A further study of a group of adult-onset diabetics, on the other hand, has shown that there is a high concordance or frequency of diabetes in the identical twin of the adult-onset diabetic, implying a genetic predisposition for this particular form of the disease. These data reverse the widely held concept that juvenile diabetes is hereditary, and adult-onset acquired (Fig. 19–5, Tab. 19–1).

Different hypotheses to explain the confusing patterns have been put forward, but none is completely satisfactory. At this time, the most comfortable hypotheses are that diabetes is a multifactorial disease in which both heredity and environment play a significant role. Evidence that (1) there is a strong association between the HLA antigen groups, B8 and BW15, and juvenile diabetes, and that (2) infections with viruses such as Coxsackie and mumps in such persons are often followed by diabetes in children, points out the fallacy of either a hereditary or precipitating factor explanation for diabetes. Without treatment, the downhill progress is much more rapid the younger the patient is, and the untreated child will not usually survive for more than a year.

There are many other possible causes of diabetes mellitus, in addition to a deficiency of insulin. For

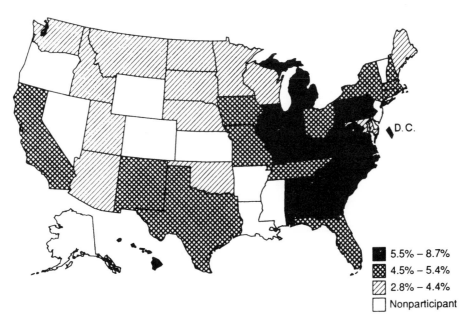

5.5% – 8.7%
4.5% – 5.4%
2.8% – 4.4%
Nonparticipant

Fig. 19–5　Age-adjusted prevalence of self-reported diabetes, by state—Behavioral Risk Factor Surveillance System, United States, 1988 and 1989. (From Centers for Disease Control, Morbidity and Mortality Weekly Report, 39(45):806, 1990.)

Table 19–1. Prevalence of Self-Reported Diabetes in 38* States and the District of Columbia, by Demographic Category—Behavioral Risk Factor Surveillance System, 1988 and 1989

CATEGORY	PREVALENCE (%)	95% CI†
Age (yrs)		
18–34	1.6	1.4–1.7
35–54	4.0	3.7–4.3
55–64	10.3	9.6–11.2
65–74	12.5	11.6–13.3
≥75	11.9	10.6–13.1
Sex		
Men	4.6	4.3–4.9
Women	5.6	5.4–5.9
Race/Ethnicity		
White	4.6	4.4–4.8
Black	8.8	7.9–9.7
Hispanic	7.4	6.0–8.8
Other	6.6	4.9–8.4
Total	**5.1**	**4.9–5.3**

* Thirty-six states participated in 1988; 38 states participated in 1989.
† Confidence interval.

example, we now know there are instances in which the presence of antibodies to insulin makes the available insulin ineffective. In some cases, the target cells of insulin are refractory to the presence of this hormone, and in others there is a pituitary-dependent insulin antagonist present. However, the generalities with which we can work are: (1) there is some decrease in the total mass of B cells in the islets (Fig. 19–6); (2) there is some decrease in extractable insulin in the majority of diabetic patients, but not in all; (3) there is a widespread tendency to differentiate two major clinical types of diabetes; and (4) etiologic factors other than insulin deficiency may play a role in early stages of diabetes.

Clinical Pattern. As shown in Table 19–2, the chief signs and symptoms of untreated diabetes are polyuria (excessive urination), glycosuria (sugar in the urine), high blood sugar, excessive thirst and hunger, marked weakness, and loss of weight. Other symptoms due to the incomplete combustion of fats are manifestations of acidosis, e.g., air hunger, coma, and ketone bodies in the urine. Still other accompaniments to the disease are itching, boils, gallstones, arteriosclerosis, and gangrene of the limbs. Nowadays, as the result of insulin treatment, most patients do not die of diabetes itself, but of complications and infections. Many of these symptoms have been alliterated by generations of students, and diabetes has been referred to as the ''P'' disease: pruritus, polyuria, polyphagia, polydipsia, and Opie, the last being the name of a pathologist who studied the pancreas.

The glycosuria is due to the excess sugar in the urine, since there is a maximum that the tubules of the kidney will resorb. The large amount of sugar dissolved in the urine raises the latter's specific gravity or density, so that it becomes 1.030 or 1.040 in place of the normal of around 1.020. Sugar acts on the kidneys as an osmotic diuretic, hence the polyuria. On

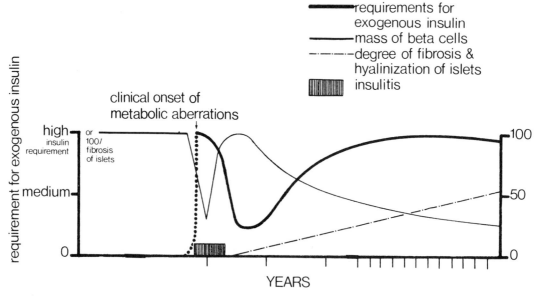

Fig. 19–6 This diagram shows the time relationships between inflammation of the islets of Langerhans and the development of diabetes (From Vracko, R., and Benditt, E.P.: Manifestations of diabetes mellitus—their possible relationships to an underlying cell defect. Am. J. Pathol., 75:204, 1974.)

Table 19–2. Pathophysiology of Diabetes Mellitus

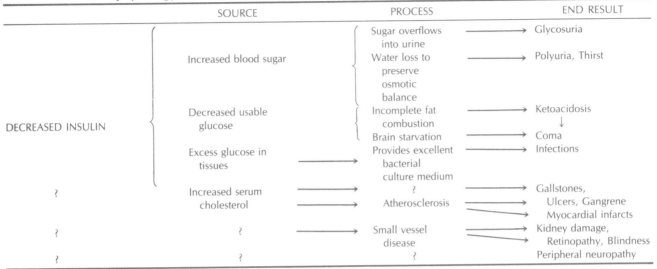

	SOURCE	PROCESS	END RESULT
	Increased blood sugar	Sugar overflows into urine	Glycosuria
		Water loss to preserve osmotic balance	Polyuria, Thirst
DECREASED INSULIN	Decreased usable glucose	Incomplete fat combustion	Ketoacidosis ↓
		Brain starvation	Coma
	Excess glucose in tissues	Provides excellent bacterial culture medium	Infections
?	Increased serum cholesterol	?	Gallstones,
		Atherosclerosis	Ulcers, Gangrene Myocardial infarcts
?	?	Small vessel disease	Kidney damage, Retinopathy, Blindness
?	?	?	Peripheral neuropathy

account of the large amount of water, the urine is characteristically pale in color. The tissues are dehydrated, which causes thirst. Because of the unavailability of glucose, there is hunger, weakness, and loss of weight. The diabetic patient draws on protein and fat reserves for nourishment and fuel. Itching, in many instances, can be traced to infections, particularly fungal infections of the genitourinary tract, but its real cause is unknown. The boils and carbuncles are also thought to arise because of the excellent culture medium provided by the excess glucose in all tissues.

Acidosis is a chief danger to life. Often, air hunger (deep respirations) signals the onset of diabetic coma, owing perhaps to the combination of acidosis, ketone bodies, and inadequate blood glucose for the central nervous system. For unknown reasons, the serum cholesterol is elevated, which predisposes a person to gallstone formation and also favors the acceleration of atherosclerosis. Characteristically, diabetics suffer from premature atherosclerosis and occlusion of blood vessels, particularly of their extremities. Gangrene of the toes and legs and ulcers that do not heal may be the first sign of diabetes in an older person. Neuropathy, numbness, tingling, and loss of motor skills are also typical for the diabetic patient (Fig. 19–7).

The treatment of the disease is directed first to the lack of insulin and second to the additional complications. The effect that "well-controlled" diabetes has on the progression of such complications as arteriosclerosis is disputed, but it is clear that thousands of patient-years have been added by good management of diabetes. The wonder of modern medicine is no-

where better seen than in the treatment of this disease, from which so many patients used to die in diabetic coma.

CARCINOMA OF THE PANCREAS

Carcinoma of the pancreas is rising rapidly in incidence in the western world and now ranks fourth among the important cancers. The prognosis of this tumor is poor indeed, with only a 2% survival rate for 5 years. Contemporary treatments such as radical surgery carry high operative mortality (20%), and chemotherapy does not seem to be much better.

Most carcinomas of the pancreas arise as epithelial tumors (adenocarcinoma) of the ductal epithelium and make their presence known by obstruction and local invasion. The pancreas is richly supplied with nerves; therefore, pain is a prominent feature of cancer of the pancreas, whether it arises in the head, the body, or the tail of that organ.

If the tumor arises in the body or tail, the prognosis is even worse than usual, because the symptoms that allow patient and doctor to suspect cancer in this centrally placed organ are so vague that the tumor has ample time to advance to a stage at which it is inoperable and will respond poorly to radiation or to chemotherapy. These tumors metastasize to regional nodes and to the liver. The only good thing that can be said about the disease is that it occurs relatively late in life, the peak incidence being in the fifth decade. Unfortunately, life expectancy after such a tumor has been diagnosed seldom exceeds a year.

What are the possible explanations for this rise in incidence? There is a clear-cut association with ciga-

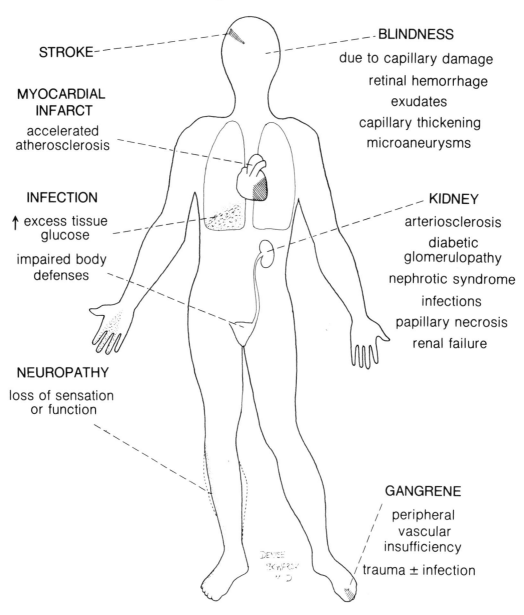

STROKE

MYOCARDIAL
INFARCT
accelerated
atherosclerosis

INFECTION
↑ excess tissue
glucose
impaired body
defenses

NEUROPATHY
loss of sensation
or function

BLINDNESS
due to capillary damage
retinal hemorrhage
exudates
capillary thickening
microaneurysms

KIDNEY
arteriosclerosis
diabetic
glomerulopathy
nephrotic syndrome
infections
papillary necrosis
renal failure

GANGRENE
peripheral
vascular
insufficiency
trauma ± infection

Fig. 19–7 **Complications of diabetes mellitus.** (Courtesy Dr. D. Skwarok.)

rette smoking, and the medium age for pancreatic cancer is 15 years earlier in smokers. Cancer of the pancreas also appears frequently in patients with diabetes mellitus. One thought is that the continued stimulus of the modern diet, rich in fat and protein, may lead to hyperplasia of the pancreas, which eventually becomes neoplasia. Of course, there is always the possibility of some unidentified carcinogen in modern processed food.

Cancer of the head of the pancreas, which accounts for more than half of tumors of the pancreas, is more apparent because of its proximity to the common bile duct (Fig. 19–8). These tumors make their presence known by jaundice, in addition to the nonspecific symptoms of weight loss, pain, anorexia, and nausea, which can be attributed equally well to biliary, hepatic or gastric causes. There is a time-honored association between pancreatic tumors and thrombophlebitis, which may herald the search for a tumor in the pancreas, but this is certainly not a universal finding, and its explanation is unclear.

Symptoms of adenocarcinoma of the head of the pancreas may be pain, or painless jaundice in a middle-aged patient without any clear-cut etiologic, environmental, or antecedent relationship of which we are aware. The patient's jaundice may be principally of

Fig. 19–8   Gross specimen of the liver, duodenum, and pancreas. The firm, white appearance in the bottom center of the photograph is typical of carcinoma. Scattered throughout the lobe of the liver are whitish nodules which are metastatic tumor from the primary, pancreatic carcinoma to the liver. This type of carcinoma frequently is associated with jaundice. (McGill University, Department of Pathology Museum.)

the direct type and his stools may be clay-colored, since bile is unable to pass into the duodenum because of the narrowed bile duct. As in the case of destruction of the pancreas by inflammation or obstruction of the pancreatic ducts from other causes, there will also be maldigestion when the pancreatic secretions do not reach the duodenum. Naturally, it is important, whenever one encounters these symptoms, to be certain that the pain, jaundice, and evidence of obstruction are truly due to a cancer, and not to a more treatable disorder such as a stone, or polyp, or inflammation, that has a much better prognosis and can often be remedied. Laparotomy and tissue diagnosis are important in such cases.

Islet Cell Tumors.   Another tumor of the pancreas is that of the endocrine portion of the islet cells. These tumors form a rare but interesting group because, although they are benign adenomas, often not more than 1 cm in diameter, they may result in the death of the patient unless a correct diagnosis is made. When that is done, the condition can usually be cured promptly. As there are two types of islet cells, alpha and beta, so there are two varieties of adenoma.

Beta Cell Tumor.   The tumor is usually a small adenoma, 1 or 2 cm in diameter, and is more readily felt than seen by the surgeon at operation, being really a gigantic islet that is easily enucleated. Occasionally, there is a general enlargement of the islets, and, still more rarely, carcinoma with metastases.

The symptoms are those of hyperinsulinism or insulin shock, with correspondingly low blood sugar owing to overactivity of the islet tissue in the adenoma. There may be attacks of weakness and unconsciousness when the interval after a meal is too long. In severe attacks, the patient may pass into a stupor, which may be followed by convulsions. The attack is at once aborted by the administration of sugar. It will be seen that the condition is the reverse of diabetes. The occupational hazard for airplane pilots, engine and taxi drivers, window cleaners, and the like is all too obvious, and the beneficial effect of enucleation of the adenoma is almost unbelievable to the despairing patient.

Alpha Cell Tumor.   In 1955, Zollinger and Ellison of Ohio State University reported two cases of curious association of (1) recurring peptic ulcers, (2) marked gastric hypersecretion and hyperacidity, and (3) an islet cell tumor that did not produce insulin. This combination is now known as the Zollinger-Ellison syndrome, and the tumor is recognized as an alpha cell adenoma which secretes the hormone gastrin, hence the tumor may be referred to as a **gastrinoma**. Severe watery diarrhea may be a feature. Other cases of this syndrome have been reported in instances in which there was only hyperplasia of the islets, and rarely, the syndrome has been reported in cases of carcinoma of the islets. The diagnosis is now made by determining the serum gastrin levels in patients with the symptom complex. Management with cimetidine has proved useful in some cases, but resection of the tumor, if possible, is desirable.

CYSTIC FIBROSIS

This condition, called fibrocystic disease of the pancreas, was not recognized 60 years ago, yet it is now identified as a cause of death in children. Cystic fibrosis is an hereditary disease involving many systems characterized by disordered secretion of mucus, salt and water. Most individuals die of respiratory complications but serious disease of the pancreas occurs as well in the majority of individuals. The disease was not understood until the 1950's and recently it has become clear that the defect in chloride secretion is due to the loss of phenylalanine at position 508 on the long arm of chromosome 7 for most of the cases.

The disease is usually diagnosed in the early postnatal period or early childhood because of acute intestinal obstruction, malnutrition, or failure to thrive. Respiratory complications come from repeated infections in partially obstructed or plugged small airways. This in turn leads to scarring, loss of respiratory exchange, and changes in pulmonary mechanics.

Chronic pancreatic disease results in malabsorption. The obstruction of small pancreatic ducts leads to recurrent pancreatitis.

In the pancreas, the small and large ducts and also the acini are dilated and converted into small cysts filled with inspissated mucus that prevent pancreatic secretions from entering the duodenum (Fig. 19–9). The child therefore fails to gain weight, although he or she develops a healthy appetite. The normal fecal matter of the newborn consists of a mixture of mucus and bile known as meconium. In mucoviscidosis, the intestinal mucus may be so sticky that it forms a plug that blocks the lumen of the bowel and leads to ob-

Fig. 19–9 Cystic fibrosis of the pancreas. (Boyd, W.: *Textbook of Pathology*, Philadelphia, Lea & Febiger, 1970.)

struction and even rupture of the ileum, a condition known as meconium ileus. This is a cause of death. If the child survives, the distended pancreatic acini become replaced by fibrous tissue, so that the term cystic fibrosis is well deserved.

In the liver, evidence of obstruction of the bile ducts is still later to develop. If the patient lives long enough, the result may be cirrhosis with portal hypertension, but this complication is exceptional.

It is evident that, despite its name, cystic fibrosis is not fundamentally a disease of the pancreas, but is one in which this organ is frequently, although not necessarily, involved. Pulmonary involvement dominates the clinical picture of cystic fibrosis and determines its outcome. The deficient pancreatic enzymes can be supplied daily, although at a cost that may well be imagined. With the aid of antibiotics, the threat of staphylococcal pneumonia may be held off, so that the child may have time to grow up.

A simple and reliable test depends on the involvement of the sweat glands in nearly every case. There is excessive perspiration with a corresponding loss of sodium, potassium, and chloride, so that the patients are unduly susceptible to heat exhaustion in hot weather. The test indicates the presence of excessive chloride on the skin. The "sweat test" has shown that adults as well as children may show the hereditary defect and may manifest mild forms of the disease.

SYNOPSIS

The pancreas secretes digestive enzymes (lipase, amylase, and chymotrypsinogen) into the duodenum through the ducts that join the common bile duct at the ampulla of Vater. It also secretes hormones into the blood, glucagon and insulin.

The exocrine function of the pancreas may be destroyed by inflammation, cancer, or surgery, or by obstruction of the ducts.

Pancreatitis may be acute, chronic, or hemorrhagic.

Tumors of the pancreas may involve the organ's head, body, or tail, or they may arise in the endocrine portion. Each type may develop a different clinical pattern.

Diabetes mellitus is systemic disease of uncertain etiology. The diabetic syndrome of polyuria, polyphagia, and polydipsia should include accelerated atherosclerosis, acidosis, neuropathy, and coma.

Terms

Diabetes mellitus   *Glucagon*   *Pancreatitis*
Insulin   *Amylase*   *Cystic fibrosis*

FURTHER READING

Avner, P.: Sweet mice, sugar daddies. Nature, 351:519, 1991.

Editorial: Death from acute pancreatitis. Lancet, 2:632, 1977.

Bank, S.: Acute and chronic pancreatitis. In *Pancreatic Disease*. Edited by T.L. Dent. New York, Grune & Stratton, Inc., 1981.

Beaven, D.W., et al.: A new international classification of diabetes mellitus. N. Zealand Med. J., 683:304, 1981.

Beger, H.G.: Acute pancreatitis—a challenge to gastroenterologists and surgeons. Hepato-Gastroenterol., 38:90, 1991.

Bennett, P.H., et al.: Longitudinal studies of the development of diabetes in the Pima Indians. In Advances in Diabetes Epidemiology. INSERM Symposium No. 22. Edited by E. Eschwege. New York, Elsevier Biomedical Press, 1982.

Boye, N.P., Skarpaas, I.J.K., and Fausa, O.: Cystic fibrosis in adult patients. Eur. J. Respir. Dis., 61:227, 1980.

Cudworth, A.G., and Festenstein, M.B.: HLA genetic heterogeneity in diabetes mellitus. Br. Med Bull., 34:285, 1978.

Davis, P.B.: Cystic fibrosis from bench to bedside. N. Engl. J. Med., 325:575, 1991.

Davis, P.B., and Di Sant'Agnese, P.A.: A review. Cystic fibrosis at forty—quo vadis? Pediatr. Res., 14:83, 1980.

Deveney, C.W., Deveney, K.S., and Way, L.W.: The Zollinger-Ellison syndrome—23 years later. Ann. Surg., 188:384, 1978.

Eisenbarth, G.S.: Type I diabetes mellitus: a chronic autoimmune disease. N. Engl. J. Med., 314:1360, 1986.

Farrow, D.C., and Davis, S.: Diet and the risk of pancreatic cancer in men. Am. J. Epidemiol., 132:423, 1990.

Fleegler, F.M., et al.: Age, sex, and season of onset of juvenile diabetes in different geographic areas. Pediatrics, 63:374, 1979.

Flier, J.S., Kahn, R., and Roth, J.: Receptors, antireceptor antibodies and mechanisms of insulin resistance. N. Engl. J. Med., 300:413, 1979.

Gabbay, K.H.: The insulinopathies. N. Engl. J. Med., 302:165, 1980.

Hägglöf, B., Holmgren, G., and Wall, S.: Incidence of insulin-dependent diabetes mellitus among children in a north-Swedish population 1938–1977. Hum. Hered., 32:408, 1982.

Hermann, R.E., and Cooperman, A.M.: Current concepts in cancer: cancer of the pancreas. N. Engl. J. Med., 301:482, 1979.

Kahn, J.C.: Insulin resistance: a common feature of diabetes mellitus. N. Engl. J. Med., 315:252, 1986.

Longnecker, D.S.: Carcinogenesis in the pancreas. Arch. Pathol. Lab. Med., 107:54, 1983.

Mahler, R.J. Diabetes and hypertension. Horm. Metab. Res., 22:599, 1990.

Malfertheiner, P., and Kemmer, T.P.: Clinical picture and diagnosis of acute pancreatitis. Hepato-Gastroenterol., 38:97, 1991.

Molsted-Pedersen, L.: Pregnancy and diabetes. A survey. Acta Endocrinologica, Suppl. 94:238:13, 1980.

Moolgavkar, S.H., and Stevens, R.G.: Smoking and cancers of bladder and pancreas: risks and temporal trends. J.N.C.I., 67:15, 1981.

Moossa, A.R., and Dawson, P.J.: The diagnosis of pancreatic cancer. Pathobiol. Ann., 11:299, 1981.

Neijens, H.J., Sinaasappel, M., deGroot, R., et al.: Cystic fibrosis, pathophysiological and clinical aspects. Eur. J. Pediatr., 149:742, 1990.

Reed, K., Vose, P.C., and Jarstfer, B.S.: Pancreatic cancer: 30 year review (1947 to 1977). Am. J. Surg., 138:929, 1978.

Reunanen, A., Akerblom, H.K., and Käär, M.L.: Prevalence and ten year (1970–1979) incidence of insulin-dependent diabetes mellitus in children and adolescents in Finland. Acta Paediatr. Scand., 71:893, 1982.

Salt, W.B., and Schenker, S.: Amylase; its clinical significance. A review of the literature. Medicine (Baltimore), 55:269, 1976.

Sarles, H.: Chronic calcifying pancreatitis—chronic alcoholic pancreatitis. Gastroenterology, 66:604, 1974.

Solow, H., Hidalgo, R., and Singal, D.P.: Juvenile onset diabetes: HLA-A, -B, -C, and -DR alloantigens. Diabetes, 28:1, 1979.

Strum, W.B., and Spiro, H.M.: Chronic pancreatitis. Ann. Intern. Med., 74:264, 1971.

Täljedal, I.B.: On insulin secretion. Diabetologia, 21:1, 1981.

Thomas, P.K.: Diabetic neuropathy—models, mechanisms and mayhem. Can J. Neurol. Sci., 19:1, 1992.

Warren, S., LeCompte, P.M., and Legg, M.A.: The Pathology of *Diabetes Mellitus*, 4th Ed. Philadelphia, Lea & Febiger, 1968.

Warshaw, A.L., and Fernandez-del Castillo, C.: Pancreatic carcinoma. N. Engl. J. Med., 326:455, 1992.

Winegrad, A.I., and Greene, D.A. The complications of diabetes mellitus. N. Engl. J. Med., 298:1250, 1978.

20

THE KIDNEY AND MALE GENITAL TRACT

The three most important things to a man are his private parts, his money and his religious opinions.—S. Butler

The genitourinary system includes the kidneys, ureters, urinary bladder, urethra, and the genitalia and accessory glands. In this chapter we consider the urinary system first and then the male genital tract. The excretion of urine is common to both males and females; the female genitalia deserve a separate chapter.

URINARY SYSTEM

Structure and Function

The urinary system removes waste products from the blood, particularly those waste substances containing nitrogen, e.g., urea. Excretion is accomplished by means of filtration and reabsorption in the kidneys. The normal glomerular filtration rate is about 125 ml per minute or 180 liters per day, but the urine output per day is less than 1% (1.5 liters for men, 1 liter for women). The urine so formed passes from each kidney in the corresponding ureter to the bladder (Fig. 20–1), and thence through the urethra to the exterior. Absorption and concentration do take place in the kidney to a marked degree; an early sign of renal disease is loss of this concentrating power. A more detailed description of kidney function is in the Appendix, p. 439.

We may classify kidney disease according to the anatomic structures involved (glomerular, vascular, interstitial, or tubular disease), or we may classify them according to origin (hereditary, neoplastic, infectious, inflammatory), but neither taxonomy is entirely satisfactory. For purposes of this chapter, we consider them arbitrarily in order of frequency, that is, the more common diseases first.

We start our consideration with the most common and treatable type of kidney diseases, those caused by infectious agents.

Pyelonephritis and Infectious Disease of the Urinary Tract

The word pyelonephritis means inflammation of the kidney and the renal pelvis, the emphasis on the pelvis indicating that infection of the kidney parenchyma often follows that of the pelvis and the lower urinary tract. The inflammation is remarkable in its sparing of the glomeruli, whereas the tubules and interstitium are markedly affected. It is usually patchy in distribution. One may use special terms to describe infections in and around the kidney, such as acute pyelonephritis, renal abscess, pyelitis, etc., as illustrated in Figure 20–2.

Urinary tract infections are common, and as many as one out of four sexually active women have pyelonephritis at some time, especially in the 15–40 age group; for men the incidence is much lower, perhaps one tenth as frequent.

The diagnosis is generally made and confirmed by examination of uncontaminated urine (clean catch) in which the colony count is greater than 100,000 bacteria per ml, with observable bacteria in the sediment.

The inflammation is caused most commonly by gram negative bacteria such E. coli, proteus, klebsiella and enterobacter, and rarely by streptococci or staphylococci. The colon bacilli ascend from the bladder in infections of the kidney, which are especially apt to occur in women and children. In men it is a common complication of enlarged prostate. The infecting organisms may also reach the kidney by the blood stream (hematogenous route). It is important to recognize that pyelonephritis can be entirely non-symptomatic and consequently patients can progress relentlessly to the chronic stage of the disease which is accompanied by significant renal failure.

The kidneys are seldom equally affected, and often only one is involved. In severe cases numerous small abscesses are scattered throughout the kidney (Fig.

Fig. 20–1 The anatomic relationships of the kidney. Its arterial blood supply, the renal arteries, break up into progressively smaller blood vessels until the afferent arteriole is reached. The renal veins, which drain blood back to the heart, are important because increased pressure or thrombosis may cause renal disease. The kidney shows to the naked eye a cortex and medulla and collecting system, the pelvis, which terminates in the ureter. The left and right ureters join the urinary bladder, which opens to the exterior through the urethra.

Fig. 20–3 This photograph of a kidney shows the cortical surface at the left, with numerous small whitish areas surrounded by a hemorrhage zone. On the right, the pelvis is opened and its mucosal surface shows a shaggy, hemorrhagic appearance. This kidney shows abscesses and inflammation of the pelvis, the diagnostic term **pyelonephritis** being appropriate. *E. coli* is a common cause of such infection. (McGill University, Department of Pathology Museum.)

20–3). These abscesses may open into tubules so that a characteristic sign is the presence of a large amount of pus in the urine, which is called **pyuria**. The progress of the disease varies, and it may end in two different ways:

1. The infection may extend; more and more renal tissue is destroyed, and the small abscesses fuse and form large ones that communicate with the renal pelvis. The clinical picture is that of an hectic, septic infection. If the patient lives long enough, one or both kidneys may become converted into large bags of pus. As so much kidney tissue is destroyed, the patient will show symptoms of renal failure and may die of uremia, if he has not already died of septic infection.

2. In other persons, the inflammatory process is much less violent, and in many of the inflamed areas healing occurs, followed by scar formation. The infection continues in other areas, until these also become scarred. In this way the kidney is gradually destroyed, but it is now a mass of scar tissue instead of a bag of pus. The scar tissue contracts, so that the kidney becomes shrunken in size and has a granular surface. In other words, the gross picture of granular contracted kidney is similar to that of chronic glomerulonephritis. If both kidneys are involved, the patient shows evidence of renal failure and dies of uremia.

Fortunately, both outcomes are rare today, when antibiotics are readily available.

Hypertension may develop in the chronic stage of pyelonephritis. Even though only one kidney is involved, there may still be hypertension. The involvement of a single kidney has suggested the possibility of curing the hypertension by removing the diseased kidney. This procedure has been done on a number of occasions, but the results have been disappointing. Although there is temporary benefit, sooner or later, and usually sooner, the hypertension returns. There is also the danger that the remaining kidney may be affected in which case the state of the patient will be worse than before.

Pyelonephritis is the commonest type of kidney dis-

A-Normal ; B-Pyelitis ; C-Cortical abscesses ; D-Diffuse pyelonephritis ; E-Infected hydronephrosis ; F-Pyonephrosis ; G-Perinephric abscess.

Fig. 20–2 This drawing shows schematically the disposition of infection in various anatomic areas of the kidney. *A*, Normal; *B*, pyelitis; *C*, cortical abscesses; *D*, diffuse pyelonephritis; *E*, infected hydronephrosis; *F*, pyonephrosis; *G*, perinephric abscess. (From Christopher, F.: *A Textbook of Surgery*. Philadelphia, W. B. Saunders Co.)

ease. It occurs particularly frequently in school-age female children and is attributed to both poor hygiene (a soiled perineum) and a short urethra. In addition, some children with cystitis often have a congenital abnormality at the attachment of the ureters to the bladder leading to a reflux of the urine from the bladder to the ureter and then to the kidney explaining why they develop pyelonephritis. It is clear, however, that pyelonephritis can be successfully treated, as can most infectious diseases, and the widespread and abundant use of antibiotics has reduced the severity and has improved the prognosis of the disease.

Recurrent episodes of pyuria (pus in the urine), fever, and flank pain should always raise the question of some underlying cause that predisposes a person to recurrent infections in the kidney. It is well established that any partial obstruction to the flow of urine makes it easier for infections to gain a foothold (another example of the dictum: obstruction leads to stasis and stasis predisposes to infection).

Important contributing factors to pyelonephritis are instrumentation or catheterization, which is frequently necessary in the aged or in persons with tumors, spinal cord injuries, obstructions, such as stones or tumors, or even pregnancy and infections elsewhere in the body (Fig. 20–4). When the urine of pregnant women is tested for the presence of bacteria it is found that 5% of them are positive, and approximately one-third of them will have symptoms of pyelonephritis if they are not treated promptly. Diabetic patients are also at increased risk to develop pyelonephritis which can be particularly severe in this group of patients. Finally, as expected, immunocompromised patients share the same risk.

In order to establish the diagnosis of pyelonephritis, microscopic examination of the urine is all-important. In the acute stage, the urine is loaded with polymorphonuclear leukocytes and bacteria, so that the diagnosis is easy. However, the same findings can be observed in cystitis and, therefore, kidney involvement has to be documented from other changes, such as flank pain and the presence of pus casts in the urine. In the chronic stage of pyelonephritis, there may be only an occasional pus cell, and the bacteriologic examination becomes particularly important. Significant bacteriuria is present when there are 100,000 bacteria or more per ml of urine.

There are specific infections of the kidneys that can be considered under the same heading. One of them is tuberculosis. Its importance arises from the difficulty in making the diagnosis on one hand, and from the extreme destruction of the kidney that it can cause on the other. Microscopic hematuria, the presence of a few mononuclear cells in the urine, and a history of low-grade fever and weight loss will suggest the

Fig. 20–4 This schematic drawing shows sources of infection that may arrive at the kidney. Frequently a predisposing cause is partial obstruction in the genitourinary tract. Additionally, infections elsewhere in the body may cause pyelonephritis because of the transient septicemia. (From Christopher, F.: A Textbook of Surgery. Philadelphia, W. B. Saunders Co.)

diagnosis, which can only be established by isolating the tubercle bacillus from the urine, not an easy task. Because the response of the host to the tubercle bacillus is often slow, the infection may smolder for months and years until all that remains of the kidney is a thin line of tissue surrounding a tennis-ball sized mass of caseous necrosis, known as the "putty kidney" (Fig. 20–5). Fortunately, the diagnosis is often made in time and the disease rarely involves both kidneys to the same degree simultaneously. Modern antibiotic therapy for tuberculosis is successful, and contemporary surgery for removal of a useless and destroyed kidney has less risk than ever.

Naturally, the tubercle bacillus had to come from somewhere, and in most instances there is pulmonary tuberculosis as well. Renal tuberculosis may also spread to the urinary bladder.

Interstitial Nephritis

In this form of nephritis which has either an acute or a chronic cause, drugs are often found to be the cause of the disease process. The acute presentation involves an immunological reaction characterized by

Fig. 20–5 This photograph shows the cortical surface on the right and the sectioned surface of the kidney on the left. The cortex and medulla cannot be perceived due to their destruction and replacement by the cheesy white material, which has given this **tuberculous** kidney the name of a "putty kidney". (McGill University, Department of Pathology Museum.)

an individual hypersensitivity to the drug. A growing number of compounds including antibiotics, nonsteroidal anti-inflammatory agents, diuretics, can induce this form of interstitial nephritis. Typically, two weeks following the use of these drugs, patients have fever, eosinophilia, a skin rash and some degree of renal failure. The interstitium of the kidneys contains numerous lymphocytes, macrophages, eosinophils and neutrophils. This is thought to represent a cell-mediated immune reaction to the drugs which somehow triggers this allergic reaction after attaching itself to the tubular epithelial cells. Discontinuing the intake of the drug reverts this condition.

A different process is involved in the form of nephritis due to analgesic abuse. This occurs in patients who over many years have absorbed kilogram quantities of analgesics containing phenacetin or aspirin. When taken in such large amounts these drugs do not induce a hypersensitivity reaction as discussed above, but are toxic to the papillae of the kidney which become necrotic and are shed into the kidney pelvis where they occlude urinary outflow. Patients who abuse analgesics are also at higher risk for the development of cancer of the renal pelvis.

Chronic injury to the kidney tubules and the interstitium can also be observed in patients who have an increased concentration of circulating uric acid or calcium, which tend to accumulate in the kidney parenchyma.

Vascular Diseases

Another common cause of impaired kidney function has its origin in disease of the blood vessels, more specifically the arterial and arteriolar supply to the kidneys. Various names have been used for these vascular diseases, ranging from nephrosclerosis, which simply means hardening of the kidney, to arteriosclerotic renal disease, or arteriosclerotic nephritis. Because the kidney has an immense reserve capacity, as do most of our organs, it is not until more than 75% of the kidney structure has been destroyed that we have any symptoms of dysfunction, but with careful testing, lesser degrees of physiologic loss can be detected. As we age, one of the targets of time is our vascular tree, and it is common to find branches of small arteries significantly narrowed, as in the coronary arteries, the cerebral vessels, and the kidneys.

Naturally, this narrowing may be partial or complete and may have varying effects. As with other vessels, if the occlusion is sudden and the area it supplies relatively large, a symptomatic infarction might occur (Fig. 20–6). On the other hand, if the narrowing is gradual, atrophy of the area will occur slowly and, if the vessel is small, the loss in function will go undetected. However, if enough small vessels are narrowed over decades, a large percentage of the nephrons will be lost, and there can be a loss in function detectable by a rising creatinine and by decreases in its clearance.

This relationship of loss of renal function to loss of anatomically and physiologically functional nephrons is shown in the accompanying graph (Fig. 20–7), in which it can be seen that the rise in creatinine as an important measure of renal failure occurs only after 75% of the kidney tissue is damaged, which is late in the progress of any disease.

The changes are focused mostly in the walls of arterioles which lose their thin, compliant, smooth muscle to be replaced by a glassy-looking layer of collagenized material, a process called hyalinization (Fig. 20–8).

There is another, less readily explainable, cause of arteriolosclerosis. From decades of observation in hundreds of cases, it is clear that narrowing of the small arterioles in the kidney follows a raised systemic blood pressure. In other words, people with hypertension (regardless of its etiology) demonstrate reactive changes in their peripheral arterioles, and, significantly, these changes may be severe in the kidneys.

It has been shown experimentally that an elevation in blood pressure can cause hyperplasia of the arteriolar smooth muscle and even an increase in the size of the endothelial cells, so that they narrow the lumen. This phenomenon is seen most dramatically in a syndrome called malignant hypertension (severe, rapidly progressive hypertension, with retinal hemorrhages, papilledema, and renal failure), a disease of uncertain etiology in which the arterioles not only become nar-

A

B

Fig. 20–6   *A,* This photograph shows (at arrow) a large depressed whitish area in the cortex of one kidney, caused by recent arterial occlusion. Such an **infarct** may arise by thrombosis or by embolism to a major branch of the renal artery. In the lower pole of the same kidney is a much larger area of discoloration, which represents an early area of necrosis. *B,* This kidney, photographed at the same magnification as *A,* shows the change in size due to the loss of substance following continued disease. Such a small, shrunken, scarred kidney can result from vascular disease, or can represent the end stage of chronic glomerulonephritis or chronic pyelonephritis. In this instance the cause is **multiple healed infarcts due to arteriosclerosis.** (McGill University, Department of Pathology Museum.)

rowed, but also undergo a peculiar fibrinoid necrosis and are prone to thrombosis and hemorrhage. These lesions are seen particularly clearly in the kidney, but they can occur in all parts of the body, especially the brain. In malignant hypertension, rapidly progressive renal failure follows the small vessel disease in the kidneys.

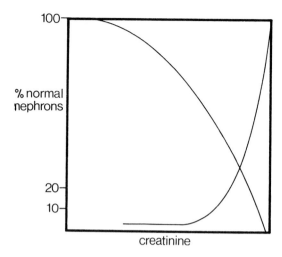

Fig. 20–7   This diagram shows the percentage of normal nephrons that must be lost before the serum creatinine level begins to rise significantly.

The corollary of these observations is the discovery by Dr. Goldblatt, many years ago, that partial occlusion of a renal artery leads to hypertension. The mechanism by which this "Goldblatt effect" is achieved is as follows: surrounding each afferent arteriole in each glomerulus is a receptor composed of a group of granule-containing cells. These granules contain renin, which may be released into the blood stream by the stimulus of a decrease in blood pressure or by hypoxia. This release apparatus serves as a mechanism to maintain the blood pressure because renin, once it is released, acts on angiotensin, a serum globulin produced in the liver. This in turn is converted to

Fig. 20–8   This light photomicrograph of a glomerulus shows the afferent arteriole (at arrow). It is a markedly thick-walled and hyalinized vessel. This is typical of **arteriolosclerosis** in the kidney, often a concomitant of hypertension. (McGill University, Department of Pathology Museum.)

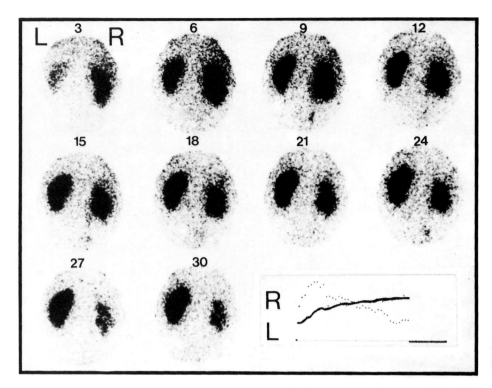

Fig. 20–9 The diagnosis of renovascular hypertension may be aided by the use of radio-Hippuran. This series of films taken every three minutes demonstrate normal function on the right but delayed uptake and excretion on the left, with no evidence of an obstructed or dilated collecting system. The curves at the bottom illustrate normal uptake and excretion in the right kidney (dotted line) and delayed uptake and secretion in the left (solid line), mirroring the information provided by the sequential films.

another substance (angiotensin II), which has powerful pressor effects on smooth muscle, causing arterioles everywhere to constrict, thereby increasing the peripheral resistance and raising the diastolic pressure.

So we have an intimate relation between arterial and arteriolar diseases and hypertension (Fig. 20–9). We have also seen how hypertension can cause vascular diseases, especially in the kidney, by narrowing small blood vessels, which in turn leads to a loss of nephrons by ischemic atrophy. On the other hand, we have heard how disease of large vessels (Goldblatt lesion) or small vessels can initiate hypertension, starting a vicious cycle of vessel disease → hypertension → small vessel disease. Thus, hypertension may both cause and result from arteriolosclerosis!

It should be noted, however, that although the Goldblatt effect helps us greatly to understand hypertension, it accounts for only 3% of the causes of increased blood pressure, and that other mechanisms are also important as discussed on p. 328.

Glomerulonephritis

The clinical picture of the nephritic syndrome with headache, puffy eyes, hypertension, and small amounts of dark urine of increased specific gravity containing blood, is quickly recognized as the pattern of acute glomerulonephritis. This disease is an acute inflammation of the glomeruli for which no infectious agent is immediately responsible. Glomerulonephritis occurs as an immunologically mediated inflammatory response.

The headache is attributed to the accompanying hypertension, the puffy eyes to edema consequent to the loss of albumin in the urine (a result of the leaky inflamed capillaries), and the oliguria (smaller than normal amount of urine, i.e., less than 400 ml/24 hours) to the damage to the glomeruli with an hypercellularity of its capillary loops.

The disease often occurs as a sequel to acute infection with certain strains of hemolytic streptococci in the upper respiratory tract or in the middle ear or following scarlet fever, after an interval of two weeks or more. This latent period, together with the absence of bacteria and the peculiar proliferative type of lesion, strongly suggests that sensitization of glomerular components is an essential feature. The glomerular inflammation is not the direct result of kidney infection by the streptococci; instead it is immunologic in character owing to an antigen-antibody complex formation in the walls of the glomerular capillary loops as shown by the technique of fluorescence microscopy. The glomerular cells enlarge and, in addition, a large number of leukocytes crowd the glomerular loops, explaining the decreased glomerular filtration rate.

It is important to recognize that most cases of acute glomerulonephritis resolve completely and the kidney returns to normal; however, a few persons develop rapidly progressive renal failure due to the formation of large crescents of proliferating cells compressing the glomerular tufts. They are left with kidneys that are anatomically scarred and physiologically incompetent (Fig. 20–10). These patients actually become uremic and are candidates for permanent dialysis or for kidney transplantation.

New methods of study by biopsy and by fluorescent and electron microscopy have permitted us to recognize several varieties of glomerulonephritis: those with minimal lesions, those with focal lesions, and those in which there are different types of structural changes in the basement membrane. It is important to recognize the various forms of acute glomerulonephritis because they each carry a specific prognosis and, consequently, a risk of evolving into terminal chronic renal failure which carries an enormous financial burden in health care. Indeed, one should not forget that even though glomerulonephritides are not the most common forms of renal disease they account for the second most common cause of terminal renal failure requiring long-term dialysis or transplantation.

As discussed above, rapidly progressive glomerulonephritis (RPGN) is a dramatic, although uncommon, complication of post-streptococcal glomerulonephritis. However, other totally different conditions can result in the same complication. For instance, systemic lupus erythematosus, which was described in the chapter on immunological diseases, very often results in various forms of renal disease from the mildest form, called mesangial, to RPGN. Recognition of this latter change is important since early treatment can often prevent chronic renal failure. Sometimes RPGN can be caused by a peculiar disease, called Goodpasture's syndrome, affecting mostly young men and characterized by the production of auto-antibodies against renal and lung basement membranes. Less commonly, various forms of vasculitis, which are inflammatory conditions targeting vascular walls, can produce RPGN. In these cases, it is unclear whether the lesions are induced by immunological mechanisms.

However, in spite of thorough clinical tests including renal biopsy and serological studies, one half of the cases of RPGN have no apparent causes and are therefore called idiopathic. These cases have an ominous prognosis.

Of course, there are other forms of glomerulonephritis which have a better outcome and are characterized by less severe lesions when seen in renal biopsies. One of them, which is the most common form of glomerulonephritis in many countries, is called IgA nephritis. It is characterized by the deposition of immunoglobulin A in the mesangium, the glomerular area at the convergence of capillary loops. A minor proportion of patients with this unexplained condition progress, although very slowly, to terminal renal failure.

The common feature of acute glomerulonephritides is a lesion that renders the glomerular capillary unusually permeable to large molecules and even to erythrocytes, resulting in an abnormal urinary sediment. The erythrocytes pile up in the tubules and are excreted in the urine as red blood cell casts, a diagnostic hallmark of acute glomerulonephritis.

Fig. 20–10   This kidney is typical of **end-stage glomerulonephritis.** Compare this photograph with Figure 20–6, an end-stage kidney caused by vascular disease. With sufficient destruction of renal parenchyma due to any chronic renal disease, the uremic syndrome appears. (McGill University, Department of Pathology Museum.)

Acute Renal Failure

Distinct from, but occasionally related to, the three principal entities we have just considered is the situation in which there is an acute episode of renal failure not directly attributable to infection, glomerulonephritis, interstitial nephritis, or vascular occlusion.

For many years, it has been recognized that in the case of a patient severely injured by trauma, as in a car accident, or after severe burns, there is oliguria or anuria in the 24 to 48 hours following the injury. Interestingly, about half of patients with acute tubular necrosis do not have oliguria which means that we have to be aware of the whole clinical picture to make the diagnosis. Examination of the kidneys in acute tubular necrosis shows that the proximal convoluted tubules have become necrotic. Tubular necrosis can be very inconspicuous in the face of an otherwise severe case of acute renal failure. We now know that the basic mechanism of most cases of acute tubular necrosis is shock following the injury. This lesion, whether it is caused by trauma, by burns, or by septicemia, fortunately, is reversible in a large percentage of cases, since the tubule cells are capable of regenerating and of repopulating the length of the nephron that has been rendered ischemic and necrotic. The principal causes of acute tubular necrosis at Montreal's Royal Victoria Hospital in 1978 were equally divided between septic conditions (28%) and shock due to cardiogenic causes (26%). Drugs, chemicals, and pigments (hemoglobin, bile) accounted for the balance.

An identical lesion can be produced by such poisons as mercury or carbon tetrachloride, which may be accidentally or intentionally taken. In this situation, the toxic material acts directly on the tubular epithelium. One result of this injury is the obstruction of the tubular lumen because of the necrotic debris, and this obstruction is a reason for the decrease in urine excretion.

Again, in situations in which a mismatched transfusion has taken place, there may be the excretion of hemolyzed red blood cells, which precipitate and obstruct the kidney tubules just as in some cases of overwhelming jaundice, bile pigments may accumulate in the tubules and directly injure its epithelial cells.

In acute renal failure the kidneys are either grossly normal or appear larger than normal, pale, and swollen. The urine, if any can be obtained, will show casts of the offending material or of tubular cells that are being shed. If the kidneys are examined microscopically, one observes, depending on the stage, patchy areas with dead tubular cells, cellular debris and casts in the tubular lumens, and evidence of tubular regeneration with a few mitotic figures.

Acute tubular necrosis is an entity with a much better prognosis today because of the life-support techniques, such as dialysis, which were not widely available 40 years ago.

Nephrotic Syndrome

The nephrotic syndrome is a clinical, not pathological, entity describing the condition of a patient either presenting with it or else complicating an established glomerular disease.

The term nephrotic syndrome is applied to the patients who demonstrate: generalized **edema** (ana- sarca), massive **proteinuria** (more than 2 g protein/24 hours), **hypoalbuminemia** (less than 2.5 g/100 ml) and **hyperlipidemia.** These abnormalities are related to either inflammatory glomerular lesions or to non-inflammatory conditions affecting the glomerular basement membrane, or to the deposition of material in the glomeruli. The mechanism by which these abnormalities exert their effect is explained in the following way.

The loss of protein in the urine is due to a defect in filtration by the glomerular capillary walls. In some conditions this defect is characterized by a loss of the negative electrical charges present on the normal structure of the capillary, which repel the plasma proteins which are also negatively charged. In other conditions the protein loss is simply due to an increase in the pore size of the glomerular basement membrane as a result of destructive mediators released by local inflammatory cells.

The loss of protein into Bowman's space and its consequent excretion (proteinuria) depletes the serum proteins, including albumin. The decreased protein level causes a decreased osmotic pressure in the serum, and the interstitial fluid fails to return to the vascular compartment at the venous end of the capillary, thus leading to diffuse edema. The explanation of hyperlipidemia is not so clear. It has been suggested that, in the race to synthesize new albumin, the liver coincidentally synthesizes lipoproteins and lipids.

Uremia

The final common pathway for a large number of renal diseases is end-stage chronic renal failure, a condition known as **uremia** (Fig. 20–11). It is estimated that 10,000 Americans develop renal failure each year, that 40,000 people are treated by means of dialysis, and that another 27,000 have received transplants. The cost of all treatment is enormous; the cost of the first year of a transplant is estimated at $50,000, an amount equal to the annual cost of dialysis in hospital.

Because the symptoms occur as the kidney reaches the limit of its function, uremia can be viewed best in the light of disorders of normal renal physiology. We have discussed the kidney's role in excretion of waste products, water balance, acid-base regulation, and regulation of electrolytes. The kidney also synthesizes erythropoietin, a hormone that helps to regulate production of red blood cells. Recently, erythropoietin has been successfully cloned and produced by recombinant DNA technology, and is now used to treat successfully the anemia of chronic renal failure patients. When a significant amount of kidney tissue has been

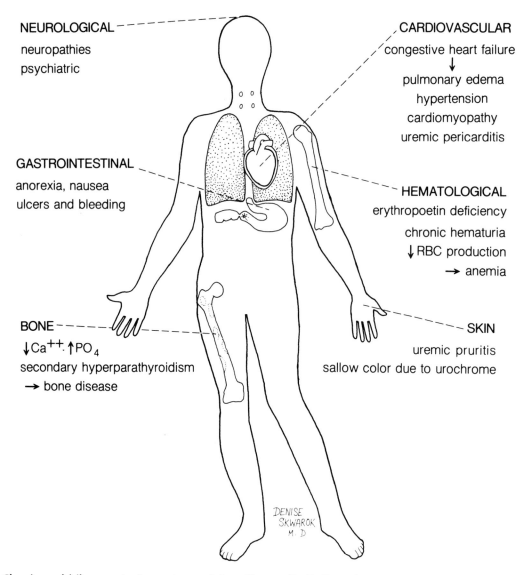

NEUROLOGICAL

neuropathies
psychiatric

CARDIOVASCULAR

congestive heart failure
↓
pulmonary edema
hypertension
cardiomyopathy
uremic pericarditis

GASTROINTESTINAL

anorexia, nausea
ulcers and bleeding

HEMATOLOGICAL

erythropoetin deficiency
chronic hematuria
↓RBC production
→ anemia

BONE

$\downarrow Ca^{++} \uparrow PO_4$
secondary hyperparathyroidism
→ bone disease

SKIN

uremic pruritis
sallow color due to urochrome

DENISE
SKWAROK
M. D

Fig. 20–11   **Chronic renal failure**—systemic symptoms and signs. (Courtesy Dr. D. Skwarok.)

destroyed by infection, by vascular disease, or by glomerulonephritis, there will be a diminished ability to excrete nitrogen-containing compounds. This leads to an increase in the number of molecules of urea, uric acid, ammonia, and creatinine, which circulate in the blood. These molecules may have specific action on the central nervous system (CNS), promoting such symptoms as irritability, insomnia or stupor, and loss of appetite. One of the major mysteries of uremia is the cause of the **central nervous system derangements,** which are debilitating to the patient.

Current explanations suggest that there is no single factor, such as creatinine, or small molecule such as urea, which could explain all the features of uremia.

The destruction of the kidney also decreases the buffering capability of the whole person, and with

retention of anion excess, he becomes **acidotic.** At the same time, the kidney fails to excrete adequate amounts of potassium, sodium, and phosphates. The elevated serum phosphate level is met with a reduction in serum calcium, which in turn leads to the muscle twitching commonly seen in uremic patients. The reduced serum calcium causes a reactive hyperplasia of all four parathyroid glands. Hyperparathyroidism will in turn induce remodelling changes in the bones, a condition called renal osteodystrophy. The retention of the sodium leads to increased water retention, and patients usually become edematous. Most important, perhaps, is the elevated serum potassium level that frequently occurs. This condition is life-threatening because hyperkalemia (high serum potassium) has a direct effect on cardiac muscle contractility. Sudden death in uremia is often due to cardiac arrhythmia traceable to abnormal serum electrolytes.

The **anemia** that occurs so often in untreated uremic patients is due mostly to the loss of erythropoietin due to destruction of kidney tissue and may be significant in the etiology of this anemia. This can now be corrected, as mentioned earlier. Another explanation of uremia is that the acidosis of uremia depresses the production of these red blood cells.

Kidney Stones

A urinary calculus is a stone that forms in the urinary tract. The common site of formation of the stone is the kidney, but it may form in the bladder. Stones in the kidney originate in the renal pelvis most frequently. Stone in the bladder may begin in the bladder, but more often it starts in the kidney (Fig. 20–12) and passes down into the bladder, where the stone continues to grow.

The causes of stone are attributed classically to infections, to irritation, and to disease of the parathyroid glands (hyperfunction). In the kidney, in addition to infection, a high concentration of crystalline salts in the urine probably plays a part, for a urinary stone is composed of such inorganic materials as uric acid, oxalates, and calcium phosphate. Some stones consist entirely of one of these materials, but usually there is a mixture of two or more. Diet may be a factor in some cases, for stones are common in some parts of India, where a large proportion of the population lives on a vitamin-poor diet. Vitamin A is perhaps the most important of the vitamins in this respect. Also the oxalates present in large amounts in the vegetarian diet set an increased risk of stone formation.

A small, benign tumor of the parathyroid glands may cause stone formation. These glands, which are four in number and lie in contact with the thyroid gland in the neck, are important regulators of calcium metabolism. When they become overactive, owing to the development of a tumor, too much calcium phosphate is removed from the bones, carried by the blood to the kidneys, and deposited there. Risk factors for stone formation are shown in Table 20–1, and the percentage of these factors that contribute to stone formation are shown in Table 20–2.

The significance of kidney stones is twofold. First, the presence of stone may cause extreme pain and may obstruct or partially obstruct some part of the "waterworks." This exquisitely painful syndrome is a relatively frequent cause of hospital admissions. This obstruction, as we have outlined before, predisposes a person to stasis and infection. Although the pain may be alleviated when the stone is removed or passed, the underlying cause of the stone raises the second and more important question, Why did the stone occur in the first place? As outlined, whenever a stone is identified in the genitourinary system, it is desirable to identify the possible physiologic disturbance that permitted the condition to develop. Such diseases as gout and cystinosis account for some

Fig. 20–12 This x-ray shows a renal calculus (kidney stone) on the patient's left side. The white mark outlines the kidney. Incidentally, there is scoliosis of the vertebral spine.

Table 20–1. Risk Factors for Kidney Stone Formation

Family history	Urinary pH
Dehydration	Diet
Medications	Hyperoxaluria
Vitamins A, D, and C	Hyperuricosuria
Acetazolamide	Hypercalcemia

Table 20–2. Causes of Stone Formation

Idiopathic hypercalciuria	20.7%
Marginal hypercalciuria	11.5%
Hyperuricosuria	14.0%
Hypercalciuria and hyperuricosuria	11.7%
Primary hyperparathyroidism	5.2%
No disorder	20.2%
Other disorders	16.2%

(From Coe, F.L.: Treated and untreated recurrent calcium nephrolithiasis in patients with idiopathic hypercalciuria, hyperuricosuria, or no metabolic disorder. Ann. Intern. Med., 87:404, 1977.)

causes of kidney stones and are treatable today, whereas 25 years ago, the recurrence of stones was a dreaded and inevitable consequence of those diseases. One has also to accept the idea that, in spite of a detailed search, no cause for stone formation can be demonstrated in a large number of patients. A major, recent advance in the treatment of kidney stones has been the introduction of lithotripsy, a large instrument which sends converging waves from external sources that can crush stones within the cavities of the urinary tract.

Malignant Tumors of the Kidney

Although tumors of the kidneys are sufficiently common to keep us aware of their existence, they are sometimes amenable to surgical treatment and can often be identified early enough to be cured. Hematuria is the most common early sign of a tumor, and the occurrence of a palpable mass in the region of the kidney suggests a new growth (Fig. 20–13). Benign tumors of the kidney are relatively uncommon. They are called adenoma and, remarkably, have the same histology as well differentiated malignant kidney tumors. Indeed, when they reach the critical size of 3

cm, adenomas have a tendency to behave like, and therefore to be, malignant tumors. Different names have been given to the most frequent form of kidney cancer, most commonly renal cell carcinoma, the latter being due to their histology which shows a large component of clear cells. They occur in older individuals. Recent molecular biology studies have documented that in some patients, renal cell carcinoma is associated with an alteration of a gene present on chromosome 3. Because of their tendency to invade the renal vein and to metastasize, kidney tumors offer a serious threat to health. Long-continued fever is a remarkable feature in some cases of kidney tumors. Removal of the affected kidney is often curative, provided metastases have not occurred. Remarkably, renal cell carcinoma is, with melanoma, one of the cancers that respond to a recently described form of immunotherapy, where the patient's lymphocytes are stimulated with a cytokine called interleukin-2 before being reinjected into the patient. Ten percent of patients have a complete remission, even of their metastases.

Wilms Tumor. This neoplasm, first described by Wilms, has a peak incidence at 15 months of age and usually occurs during the first three years of life.

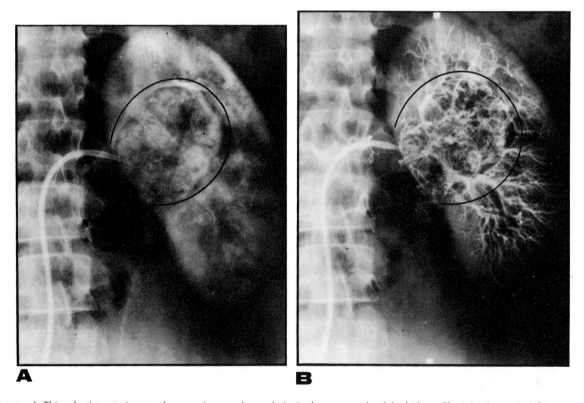

Fig. 20–13   *A,* This selective arteriogram shows an increased vascularity in the upper pole of the kidney. The injection material is present in the catheter on the left. The area of neovascularity is outlined in black. *B,* A later film from the same arteriogram shows, within the black outline, the abnormal area of small blood vessels. This is interpreted as a renal tumor.

The tumor often appears as an abdominal mass, sometimes nearly filling the child's abdomen. Surgical removal results in a cure rate of 80% when the tumor is removed under one year of age. Fever occurs in 50% of cases, and distant metastases are a common complication.

Recently, this tumor has been recognized to occur in children with the syndrome of mental retardation, other genitourinary abnormalities, and the absence of the iris of the eye. This pattern has been credited to the deletion of a small portion of the short arm of chromosome 11, thus relating the tumor to a chromosomal abnormality.

In the chapter discussing neoplasia, it was mentioned that remarkable experiments have documented that there is a gene on chromosome 2 which behaves normally as a tumor suppressor gene. Its deletion is an important causal step in the production of Wilm's tumor.

Carcinoma of the Bladder. The chief tumor of the bladder is derived from the transitional epithelium that covers the bladder mucosa, and also kidney pelvis, ureter and urethra. This cancer is therefore called transitional cell carcinoma and it is often a low grade of malignancy. In the last 50 years, epithelial bladder tumors have been found much more frequently among old persons than before. Although the tumors used to be much more common in men than in women, this pattern too is changing. Carcinoma of the bladder is also slightly more common than it used to be, but this increase can be attributed to the rise in the number of biopsies, largely owing to better techniques for visualization and operation.

This tumor usually projects into the bladder in a papillary form. Sometimes it assumes a villous form, the growth consisting of delicate fern-like papillary processes that unfold like a piece of seaweed when the bladder is filled with water and examined with the cystoscope. Each of these papillary processes contains a thin-walled blood vessel, which is readily injured when the bladder contracts during urination, so that hemorrhage is common. The outstanding symptom is therefore blood in the urine, usually unaccompanied by pain (painless hematuria). Such tumors may be removed by surgery only to recur repeatedly; in fact, it may be necessary to remove the whole bladder and to transplant the ureters into a loop of ileum.

Etiology. A number of substances are known to be carcinogenic for the bladder. Workers in aniline dye factories are liable to develop the disease, the material being inhaled and then carried to the bladder by the blood. The sharp-pointed ova of *Schistosoma haematobium* or bilharzia induces chronic cystitis and after many years can stimulate the development of cancer of the bladder. That condition has its highest incidence in Egypt, where bilharzia infection is prevalent. The latest discovery is that cigarette smoking in excess is associated with bladder tumors, carcinogenic metabolites being excreted in the urine.

Treatment. Most cases of bladder cancer can be treated by cystoscopic resection of the papillary tumors. In some cases the intravesical administration of inactivated tuberculosis bacilli, also called Bacillus of Calmette and Guerin (BCG), has proven to be an effective form of treatment by inducing a local cell-mediated immune reaction. Finally, when the tumor has invaded deeply into the wall, removal of the bladder might be required and, in this case, both ureters have to be attached to the skin of the abdomen. In spite of its high incidence, modern forms of treatment have lowered bladder cancer mortality to 3% of all cancer deaths in the U.S.

Congenital Cystic Kidney

This relatively common condition is in fact a group of diseases resulting from a congenital defect in the pre- or post-natal development of the kidney. About 30% of cases are symptomatic in infants, or are stillborn. In the remaining cases, renal cysts develop much more slowly and symptoms are noted in early adult and middle life. The condition is nearly always bilateral. The kidneys are converted into a series of cysts, and may be enormously enlarged (Fig. 20–14). The contents of the cysts are watery, but hemorrhage may occur from intervening vessels, so that, should the cyst rupture into the renal pelvis, there will be hematuria. Hardly any renal tissue may be left, so that the occurrence of hypertension, renal insufficiency, and uremia is easily understood. Polycystic kidney has a large hereditary component. The most common form of adult polycystic kidney disease has an autosomal dominant form of inheritance due to a genetic defect found mostly on chromosome 16. In infants and children the mode of inheritance of the severe forms of cystic disease is autosomal recessive. In this disorder, small cysts may also be found in the liver, and there is also an association with aneurysms of the cerebral vessels (berry aneurysms).

Summary

A reflection on the variety of syndromes that occur in kidney disease of different types indicates the wide spectrum of complaints that can be traced to these organs. We have seen that flank pain, chills, and fever—signs of infection—can often be traced to acute abscess or pyelonephritis in one or both kidneys. At another extreme, nonspecific signs of loss of appetite,

Fig. 20–14   This photograph of a **congenital cystic kidney** shows the absence of any normal renal parenchyma. It is no wonder that the uremic syndrome eventually occurs with this progressive, slow destruction of the kidney. (McGill University, Department of Pathology Museum.)

weakness, and muscle twitching are traceable to the uremic syndrome, a terminal phase in any renal disease. In between, signs such as hematuria, oliguria, edema, proteinuria, or palpably enlarged kidneys can herald such diverse entities as glomerulonephritis, tubular necrosis, stones, tumors, or congenital cystic disease of the kidney.

The correct diagnosis is arrived at when careful history-taking and physical and laboratory examinations have been carried out, and when such special studies as are warranted, e.g., pyelograms (Fig. 20–15), ultrasound, CAT scans, arteriography, and biopsy may have been undertaken. Examination of the urine as a routine is described in the Appendix, p. 439. The most heartening thought, however, is the recent success in managing serious kidney disease by a combination of dialysis and transplant. Table 20–3 and Figure 20–16 illustrate the rehabilitation rates for dialysis and transplant patients, and also show the improvement during three periods of patient and cadaver kidney transplants. More than in any other organ system, modern medical and surgical advances offer the patient with severe renal failure hope for a reasonable life.

MALE GENITAL TRACT

Prostate

The prostate is a gland about the size of a horse chestnut situated at the neck of the bladder, sur-

A

B

Fig. 20–15   *A,* This film shows a normal intravenous pyelogram after one minute. The kidneys are normal in position, size, shape, and contour. This is called the renal phase. *B,* This is the 5 minute film, which shows the excretion of dye into the pelvis and ureters. Again, this is a normal film.

rounding the urethra. It really belongs to the male reproductive system, but, when diseased, it produces symptoms associated with the urinary system on account of its position at the outlet of the bladder. Three diseases of the male accessory gland, the prostate,

Table 20–3.   **Rehabilitation Rate for Dialysis Patients and Cadaver Kidney Recipients**

	HEMODIALYSIS	TRANSPLANTATION
Total patients	359 (100%)	272 (100%)
Complete rehabilitation	179 (50%)	205 (75%)
Partial rehabilitation	79 (22%)	14 (5%)
No rehabilitation	101 (28%)	53 (20%)

(From Kreis, H.: Selection of hemodialysis versus cadaveric transplantation. Kidney Int., 13, Suppl., 8:S–91, 1978.)

Fig. 20–16 These graphs show the improvement in survival from the time of operation of patients who received transplanted cadaver kidneys between June 1962 and January 1977. The graphs illustrate both the survival rates of the patients and the success of the kidney transplants. (From Kreis, H.: Selection of hemodialysis versus cadaveric transplantation. Kidney Int., 13, Suppl. 8S-91, 1978.)

deserve mention in this brief section: prostatitis, benign hyperplasia, and carcinoma.

Prostatitis. As in other organs that are hidden in the body, inflammation may frequently occur, but the predisposing causes and etiologic agents are not always discovered or understood. Whenever there is inflammation in a glandular structure that eliminates its secretions by a duct or a system of ducts, and when the controls over secretion include nervous stimulation, hormones, and a variety of other agents, there are legitimate theories as to the importance of each factor in causing the inflammation.

Inflammation of the prostate can also arise as a result of infection by bacteria from neighboring structures such as the urethra (gonococcus) or bladder (*E. coli*). Sometimes, a history of exposure to venereal disease or of urinary tract infection can be elicited, and the prostate secretions can be stained and cultured to show the offending organism. Treatment with appropriate antibiotics usually limits the disease, although the prostate does not always respond rapidly to

chemotherapy because of the difficulties some drugs have in reaching the site of inflammation. Naturally, an abscess in the prostate is anatomically a different matter from a boil of the buttock. The prostate is a favorite site for occult or hidden infections to smolder, causing fever of obscure origin and a long-term feeling of ill health.

Another frequent cause of prostatitis is the occurrence of acute, sterile inflammation in young or middle-aged men who have indulged in high living with lots of sex, alcohol, coffee, spiced foods, cigars, and little sleep, as is common at a convention or on a holiday. The symptoms of urgency, frequency, and retention of urine lead one to suspect cystitis and/or prostatitis. The absence of discharge, fever, and flank pain, combined with the history of fatigue and dietary excess, point to this diagnosis. It is not clear why the prostate should be the target for such inflammation but it is well known to urologists that this small gland is a kind of Achilles heel.

Prostate Hyperplasia. When the gland becomes enlarged and can be felt through the rectum as being increased in size, the most common cause of this is an increase in the number of glandular and stromal cells. Enlargement of the prostate is common in men over 60 years of age, but fortunately, it only produces symptoms in about 8% of these cases. The disease is hardly ever seen in early life. It is really an hyperplasia or over-growth rather than an hypertrophy. Its cause is unknown and its mechanism involves an increased proliferative responsiveness of the prostate cells to sex hormones which otherwise are not secreted in abnormal amounts.

The effects of prostatic enlargement are partial obstruction to the outflow of urine and an inability to empty the bladder completely (Fig. 20–17). The residual urine retained in the bladder tends to become infected. Two great dangers that threaten the man suffering from enlargement of the prostate are (1) urinary retention with back-pressure on the ureters and kidneys, and (2) infection that ascends from the bladder to the kidneys. The result is accompanied by distension of the bladder, cystitis, dilation of the ureters, hydronephrosis (Fig. 20–18), and pyonephrosis.

Treatment has entirely changed the outlook for the man in declining years whose last days used to be made pitiable by prostatic enlargement. The enlarged gland can be removed by various non-invasive, transurethral, surgical measures. Non-surgical treatment has even been introduced recently with significant benefit in some cases.

Cancer of the Prostate. In 1991 it is estimated that there will be 122,000 new cases diagnosed in the U.S.,

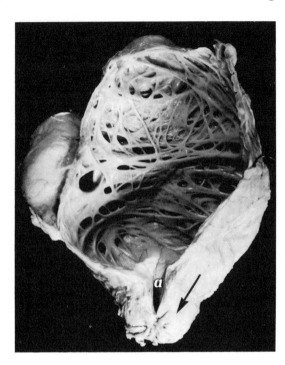

Fig. 20–17   The **prostate,** a small walnut-sized organ, can be recognized at the arrow. Most of the photograph shows the interior wall of the urinary bladder, which is markedly trabeculated. This is the result of the partial obstruction at the level of the prostate. A prominent posterior lobe is apparent at a. Benign prostatic hyperplasia is a common disease in men over 60. (McGill University, Department of Pathology Museum.)

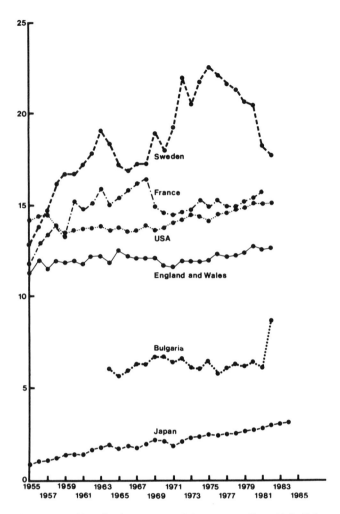

Fig. 20–19   Mortality from cancer of the prostate. (From Muir, C.S., et al.: The epidemiology of prostatic cancer. Acta Oncol., 30:133, 1991.)

Fig. 20–18   This x-ray shows the collection of dye in the kidney, displaying an extraordinary amount of material. This illustrates right-sided hydronephrosis due to obstruction in the ureter.

and that 32,000 men will die of prostate cancer, making it the second leading cause of cancer deaths in males (Figs. 20–19 and 20–20).

With carcinoma the prostate becomes enlarged and hard and may cause symptoms of urinary obstruction. The tumor infiltrates the surrounding structures early and extensively, and, on that account, surgical treatment is far from satisfactory. The blood vessels and lymphatics are also invaded at an early date, and metastases are found in various organs, particularly in the bones. When an elderly man is found to be suffering from bone pain, carcinoma of the prostate should always be suspected.

However, carcinoma of the prostate depends in part on the male hormone of the testicle (Fig. 20–21). Castration (removal of both testicles) before puberty prevents development of the prostate, and castration in adult life causes regression of the normal gland.

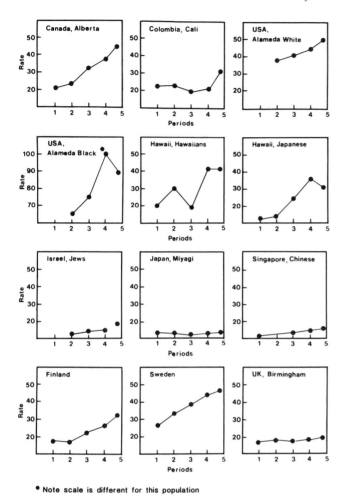

• Note scale is different for this population

Fig. 20–20 Time-trends of prostatic cancer incidence for certain cancer registries from 1960 to 1980. (From Muir, C.S., et al.: The epidemiology of prostatic cancer. Acta Oncol., 30:133, 1991.)

This knowledge has been applied to the problem of the control of cancer of the prostate with remarkable results, for castration often leads to shrinking of the tumor and to relief of the severe bone pains caused by metastases in the skeleton, particularly in the spine. The administration of stilbestrol, a synthetic form of the female sex hormone, also affords relief, probably because of interference with the male hormone. This form of therapy has largely replaced castration. Sometimes both approaches are combined.

One means of observing any improvement produced by these methods is afforded by determining the serum concentration of a protein produced by the prostate epithelium, called Prostate Specific Antigen (PSA). This protein is greatly increased when cancer of the prostate develops, and especially when secondary tumors are formed in bones. Under these circum-

stances there is a marked rise in the level of PSA, which disappears if the treatment is successful. The word "success" is used in a relative sense only, for it is not claimed that cancer of the prostate can be cured by these means. This approach is not limited to the follow-up of documented cases of prostate cancer. Indeed, recently, the measurement of serum PSA has been proposed as an efficient adjunct, along with digital rectal examination, in the screening of males for prostate cancer.

Testis and Epididymis

One word before considering the diseases of the testis. Jules Verne described a marvelous journey in *Around the World in 80 Days*, which is known to many, but the sperm of man makes what seems to us to be an equally incredible journey, as shown in the accompanying Table 20–4. Surely, to take a voyage of 7.84 meters within the real distance of something significantly less than 0.3 meters requires remarkable engineering!

The maturation and migration of sperm cells are two functions that persist even in very old men.

Epididymis. The epididymis is the convoluted excretory duct of the testis and although it lies separate from, although attached to, the testis, it may be considered with the latter in connection with disease. By far the most common causes of inflammation of the epididymis are chlamydia and the gonococcus. The epididymis becomes enlarged, hard, and tender. Minute abscesses are formed, but there is no extensive breaking down of tissue, such as might be expected. The inflammation is acute and subsides quickly, but often leaves fibrous scars that obliterate the seminiferous tubules. When the condition is bilateral, complete sterility may result. The epididymis can also be the target of tuberculosis, usually as a complication of pulmonary disease (Fig. 20–22).

Orchitis. The two common causes of inflammation

Table 20–4. Sperm Journey

Seminiferous tubule	30 to 80 cm
Straight tubule	0.2 cm
Rete testis	1.0 cm
Efferent ductule	4 to 6 cm
Common lower vas	15 to 20 cm
Epididymis	400 to 600 cm
Vas deferens	40 to 45 cm
Ejaculatory duct	1.9 cm
Urethra	20 cm
Uterus	2.5 cm
Uterine tube	7.1 cm
	7.84 m

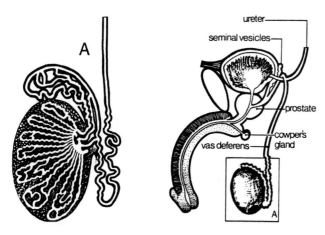

Fig. 20–21   *Left*, This diagram shows the anatomy of the testicle and epididymis. *Right*, The urinary bladder and external genitalia are shown schematically. (Redrawn from Christopher, F.: *A Textbook of Surgery*, 5th Ed., Philadelphia, W.B. Saunders Co.)

Fig 20–22   This section of a testicle shows a large area of white material, which is caseous necrosis caused by the tubercle bacillus. Tuberculosis usually starts at the lower pole of the epididymis (at arrow) and involves the whole epididymis. (McGill University, Department of Pathology Museum.)

of the testis (orchitis) are injury and mumps. Traumatic orchitis, caused by a blow, is often followed by acute inflammatory edema of the organ. Mumps orchitis is usually unilateral, and is rarely seen before the age of puberty, being most common in young men. It may follow or may precede the enlargement of the parotid gland or involvement of the pancreas, which are characteristic of mumps.

Tumors. In the testis, tumors are overall fairly rare (0.5% of all cancer deaths) except in the 15–35 year age group. Although there are several single and complex types of testicular cancers, one need be preoccupied mostly by the distinction between seminomas and non-seminomatous tumors. Although both groups derive from germ cells, they have markedly different clinical presentations and prognoses. Overall, seminomas have a much better prognosis with a 90% cure rate.

SYNOPSIS

The kidneys filter blood and excrete urine; they act as excretory organs for catabolic waste products, as water-regulating organs, as electrolyte monitors, as buffering agents, and as stimulators of the bone marrow.

Infectious diseases of the kidney and bladder are the most common. Partial obstruction along the urinary tract leads to stasis and is an important predisposing cause to kidney infections.

Renal vascular diseases may be of large or small vessels and may be either the cause or result of hypertension.

Glomerular diseases are often of immune etiology and may result in the nephrotic syndrome and end-stage renal failure.

Acute renal failure may have diverse etiologies, should be differentiated from other causes of little urine output, and may require hemodialysis.

Chronic renal failure (uremia) may be caused by any renal disease. Usually more than 80% of the kidney is diseased anatomically. The symptoms and signs are diverse and are sometimes difficult to recognize.

Examination of the urine is the most important laboratory approach to kidney disease.

Three diseases of the prostate, prostatitis, hyperplasia, and cancer, occur frequently.

Terms

Glomerulus	*Arteriolosclerotic nephritis*	*Nephrotic syndrome*
Pyelonephritis	*Arteriolonecrosis*	*Uremia*
Arteriosclerotic nephritis	*Glomerulonephritis*	*Hematuria*
	Acute tubular necrosis	*Hypernephroma*

FURTHER READING

Bakir, A.A., and Dunea, G.: Current trends in the treatment of uraemia: a view from the United States. Br. Med. J., 1:914, 1979.

Biesecker, G. Membrane attack complex of complement as a pathologic mediator. Lab. Invest. 49:237, 1983.

Brenner, B. M., and Humes, H.D.: Mechanics of glomerular ultrafiltration. N. Engl. J. Med., 297:148, 1977.

Broadus, A.E., and Thier, S. O.: Metabolic basis of renal-stone disease. N. Engl. J. Med., 300:839, 1979.

Campbell, J.D., and Campbell, A.R.: A patient's perspective of end-stage renal disease. N. Engl. J. Med., 299:386, 1978.

Catalona, W.J., Smith, D.S., Ratliff, T.L., et al.: Measurement of prostate-specific antigen in serum as a screening test for prostate cancer. N. Engl. J. Med., 324:1156, 1991.

Coe, F.L., Keck, J., and Norton, E.R.: The natural history of calcium urolithiasis. J.A.M.A., 238:1519, 1977.

Daifuku, R., and Stamm, W.E.: Bacterial adherence to bladder uroepithelial cells in catheter-associated urinary tract infection. N. Engl. J. Med., 314:1208, 1986.

Davis, C.P., and Cohen, M.S.: Biology and management of bladder cancer. N. Engl. J. Med., 324:125, 1991.

Debré, B., et al.: Epidemiology of prostatic cancer. J. Intl. Med. Res., 18:3, 1990.

DeKernion, J.B., and Berry, D.: The diagnosis and treatment of renal cell carcinoma. Cancer, 45:1947, 1980.

Denis, L., and Mahler, C.: Prostatic cancer, an overview. Rev. Oncol., 3:665, 1990.

Dixon, F.J., Feldman, J.D., and Vasquez, J.J.: Experimental glomerulonephritis. J. Exp. Med., 113:899, 1961.

Fawcett, D.W.: The cell biology of gametogenesis in the male. Perspect. Biol. Med., 22:S56, 1979.

Ferris, T.F.: The kidney and hypertension. Arch. Intern. Med.,142:1889, 1982.

Freeman, R.B.: Does bacteriuria lead to renal failure? Clin. Nephrol., 1:61, 1973.

Freeman, S.: The evolution of the scrotum: A new hypothesis. J. Theor. Biol., 145:429, 1990.

Gitter, R.F.: Carcinoma of the prostate. N. Engl. J. Med., 324:236, 1991.

Gottschalk, C.W. History of the urinary concentrating mechanism. Kid. Intl. 31:507, 1987.

Groth, C.G.: Kidney transplantations in the Nordic countries 1956–1980. Scand. J. Urol. Nephrol., Suppl. 64:12, 1981.

Guttmann, R.D.: Renal transplantation. N. Engl. J. Med., 301:975, 1979.

Horvath, J.S., et al.: The detection of renovascular hypertension: a study of 490 patients by renal angiography. Quart. J. Med., 202:139, 1982.

Kunin, C.M.: Natural history of lower urinary tract infections. Infection 18:S44, 1990.

Leaf, A., and Cotran, R.: Renal Pathophysiology. New York, Oxford University Press, 1976.

Lemley, K.V., and Kriz, W.: Anatomy of the renal interstitium. Kidney Intl., 39:370, 1991.

Levinsky, N.G.: Pathophysiology and acute renal failure. N. Engl. J. Med., 296:1453, 1977.

Mauer, S.M., Ellis, E.N., et al. The pathology of diabetic nephropathy. Transplant. Proc. 18:6:1629, 1986.

McCluskey, R.T. Modification of glomerular immune complex deposits. Lab. Invest. 48:241, 1983.

Merrill, J.P.: Glomerulonephritis. N. Engl. J. Med., 290:257, 1974.

Mettlin, C., et al.: American Cancer Society National Prostate Cancer Detection Project. Cancer, 67:2949, 1991.

Michael, A.F., et al.: The glomerular mesangium. Kidney Intl., 17:141, 1980.

Muir, C.S., Nectoux, J., and Staszewski: The epidemiology of prostatic cancer. Geographic distribution and time-trends. Acta Oncologica, 30:133, 1991.

Nordenstam, G.R., et al.: Bacteriuria and mortality in an elderly population. N. Engl. J. Med., 314:1152, 1986.

Ober, W.: Boswell's gonorrhea. Bull. N.Y. Acad. Med., 45:587, 1969.

Platt, R. et al.: Mortality associated with nosocomial urinary-tract infection. N. Engl. J. Med., 307:637, 1982.

Roberts, J.A.: Pathogenesis of pyelonephritis. J. Urol., 129:1102, 1983.

Rouffignac, C.: The urinary concentrating mechanisms. Comparative Physiol., 2:31, 1990.

Silverman, D.T., et al.: Epidemiology of bladder cancer. Hematol. Oncol. Clin. North Am., 6:1, 1992.

Smith, L.H., Van Den Berg, C.J., and Wilson, D.M.: Nutrition and urolithiasis. N. Engl. J. Med., 298:87, 1978.

The Canadian Multicentre Transplant Study Group: A randomized clinical trial of cyclosporine in cadaveric renal transplantation: Analysis at three years. N. Engl. J. Med., 314:1219, 1986.

White, W.I.: A new look at the role of urinalysis in the history of diagnostic medicine. Clin. Chem., 37:119, 1991.

Zbar, B., et al. Loss of alleles of loci on the short arm of chromosome 3 in renal cell carcinoma. Nature 327:721, 1987.

APPENDIX

Physiology of the Kidney

The mechanism for filtration is elegant. Each kidney, with an average weight of around 150 g, is composed of over 1,000,000 units or nephrons (Fig. A20–1). They all function independently as minute filters and resorbers (Fig. A20–2). The nephron is a complex tube, partly coiled (convoluted tubule) and partly straight (collecting tubule), the upper end of which is formed by a spherical structure, the glomerulus. The lower end opens into the chamber or pelvis of the kidney, from which the urine passes to the bladder. In the glomerulus, which contains the filter, a small artery, the afferent arteriole of the glomerulus, breaks up into a little cluster of capillary loops that project like a bunch of grapes into the dilated upper end of the tubule. As the blood passes through the loops, water and solutes diffuse across a highly selective membrane into the space around the capillaries and pass down the various segments of the tubule, where reabsorption and secretion of water, low molecular weight

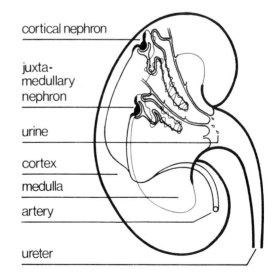

Fig. A20–1 This figure shows the relationship of the nephron to the cortex of the kidney. Note the two different types of nephrons, those that arise in the cortex and those that arise in the corticomedullary junction.

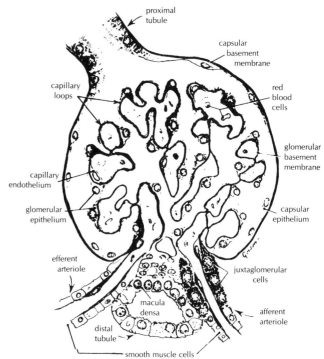

Fig. A20–2 The nephron is the fundamental unit of the kidney. Shown here is the glomerulus and the respective parts of the tubular epithelium, the proximal and distal convoluted tubules that proceed to the collecting ducts.

Fig. A20–3 The glomerulus, or filtration bed for the kidney, is composed of a convoluted capillary loop, which lies within Bowman's space. Outside the cells of the capillary are epithelial cells. Between the capillary and the epithelial cell is a complex basement membrane, which frequently reflects inflammatory injury to the glomerulus. (From Ham, A. W.: *Histology*, 7th Ed. Philadelphia, J. B. Lippincott Co., 1974.)

proteins and electrolytes take place before excretion into the pelvis of the kidney. Table A20–1 outlines the function of different portions of the nephron.

The process of filtration or secretion of urine depends to a large extent on the pressure with which the blood is forced through the glomerular capillaries. If the blood pressure falls markedly, the secretion of urine diminishes or stops.

Under normal conditions, water, urea, and salts pass from the blood through the walls of the glomerular capillaries into the tubules, while albumin and other large mole-

cules of blood plasma are not allowed to escape (Fig. A20–3). Indeed, the glomerular basement membrane present in all capillary loops has a very selective filtering system which exerts strict conditions on the passage of molecules depending on their size and electrical charges. Detection of protein in the urine indicates disease of the glomeruli.

It is evident that in the formation of the urine there are two opposite factors at work, glomerular filtration and tubular reabsorption. Were it not for reabsorption in the tubules, the body would soon be drained of its fluid, for only 1% of the fluid that passes through the glomeruli appears as urine. The normal amount of urine passed is about 1,000 ml per day, but this will vary with, for example, the amount of water drunk or the amount lost in perspiration, as well as with body size.

One important indication that all is not well with the kidneys is any serious departure from average excretion, particularly in the direction of too little (oliguria). However, frequency of urination, that is, an increase in the number of voidings in any given time, is a common sign of some urinary tract disorder. The accompanying chart shows how the clinician might evaluate a problem involving frequency of urination (Table A20–2). As illustrated by this table, frequency (frequent urination, usually with some pain, i.e., dysuria) is a common symptom of urinary tract disease. Obstructions may be due to stones, strictures, tumors, or other causes as shown in the left-hand columns of Table A20–2.

Table A20–1. Functions of the Nephron

SEGMENT OF NEPHRON	FUNCTION
Glomerulus	PRODUCES ultrafiltrate of PLASMA (120 ml/min)
Proximal Tubules	REABSORBS 66% of filtered Na, Cl, H_2O
	REABSORBS HCO_3, glucose, K, P, amino acids, uric acid, and some proteins
Loop of Henle	REABSORBS Na, Cl
Distal Tubule	REABSORBS Na, Cl, H_2O
	SECRETES H^+, K^+, NH_4
Collecting Duct	REABSORBS Na, Cl, H_2O
	SECRETES H, NH_4, K

Table A20–2. Assessment of Urinary Frequency

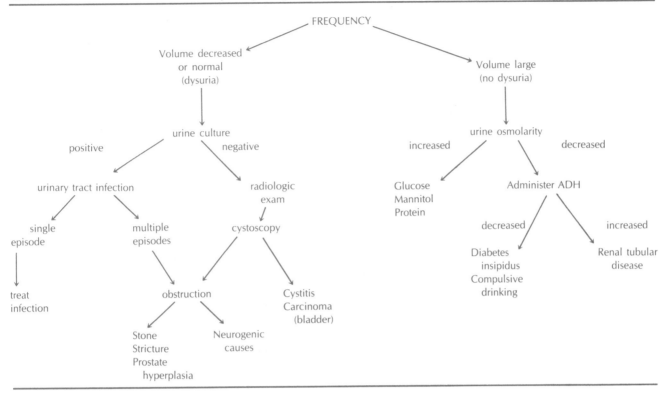

Large volumes of urine may be due to the presence of osmotically active substances in the urine, such as occurs in diabetes mellitus (glucose), or in therapeutic treatment (mannitol), or in diabetes insipidus (either the loss of antidiuretic hormone due to pituitary surgery, for example, or tubular unresponsiveness to ADH).

Although we have spoken of the kidneys as excretory organs, it is known that the regulation of the acid-base balance of the body fluids and the maintenance of the normal concentrations of electrolytes are functions of equal importance. Indeed, acid-base balance is tightly regulated by the excretion/reabsorption of important solutes. This regulation, as readers will recognize, represents one aspect of the preservation of the internal environment. The acid-base balance is preserved by the formation of carbonic acid by the epithelium of the convoluted tubules and by the reversal of the proportion of acid and alkaline phosphates with the exchange of hydrogen for sodium ions. As the result of these interchanges, the alkaline serum filtrate of the blood that is excreted by the glomeruli becomes the acidic urine that enters the bladder.

The concentrations of solutes and substances in the urine contribute to its specific gravity. Depending on the dilution of urine or the dehydration of the person, the specific gravity of urine from normal kidneys varies between 1.015 and 1.025. If a solute is filtered in excessive proportion by the glomerulus and/or is insufficiently reabsorbed, the specific gravity will be greater than normal, as is the case of the diabetic patient's urine, which, in the absence of effective treatment, may contain significant amounts of glucose. If the nephrons have been injured by disease, their ability to

secrete and to resorb will be impaired; therefore, the specific gravity of the urine may be fixed at a low value and the kidney cannot respond to such a physiologic challenge as the need to conserve water by excreting a concentrated urine.

Examination of the Urine

Urinalysis serves to show the presence of disease in the kidneys and in the bladder. It also indicates the presence of systemic diseases such as diabetes, metabolic disorders, or vasculitis. In a complete urinalysis, the following points are noted: color, pH, specific gravity, examination for protein and sugar, and a microscopic examination for blood, pus, and casts. Most of these parameters can be easily tested by simple immersion of a dipstick in a sample of urine. If an anomaly is found, then it is imperative to observe a spun down sediment of urine.

Color. The normal color of the urine is yellow or amber and its intensity depends on the amount of water the urine contains. If the patient is drinking a large amount of water, the urine is dilute and pale. On the other hand, if much water is lost by perspiration in hot weather or as the result of fever, the urine becomes darker. The same is true of chronic nephritis, in which the kidneys lose their normal power of concentrating the urine. A smoky red or brown color is usually due to the presence of blood.

pH. Although the blood is slightly alkaline, the normal pH of the urine is acidic. In infections of the bladder, it tends to be alkaline, owing to the action of bacteria. It is

Table A20–3.   Observations in the Normal Urine and in Different Kidney Diseases

NATURE OF RENAL LESION	PROTEIN EXCRETION G/24 HR	R.B.C. MILL/24 HR	EPITHELIAL & w.b.c. MILL/24 HR	ABNORMAL CELLS	CASTS MILL/24 HR	BLOOD CASTS	R.B.C. CASTS	FATTY CASTS	BROAD CASTS	WAXY CASTS	OTHER CASTS
Normal	male 0 to 0.060 female 0 to 0.090	0 to 0.130	0 to 0.650	—	0 to 0.002	–	–	–	–	–	–
Glomerulitis	0.5 to 5.0	1 to 1,000	1 to 400	—	0.1 to 0.5	+	+	–	–	–	+
Tubular necrosis	5.0 to 40.0	1 to 100	20 to 1,000	oval fat bodies	0.1 to 2.0	–	–	+	–	–	+
Malignant arteriolitis	2.0 to 10.0	1 to 100	1 to 200	—	0.1 to 1.0	–	+	+	–	–	+
Renal failure	2.0 to 7.0	1 to 10	1 to 50	—	0.5 to 4.0	–	–	–	–	–	–
Infection	0.5 to 7.0	0 to 1	20 to 2,000	pus cells	0 to 0.1	–	–	–	–	–	–
Neoplasm	0	0 to 1,000	0	tumor cells	0						

important to remember that if the specimen of urine is allowed to stand for many hours in a warm room, the normal pH may be changed to alkaline because of the action of contaminating bacteria. The urine should therefore be fresh and sent at once to the laboratory.

Specific Gravity. The concentration or specific gravity of the urine depends on the amount of solids (waste products of the tissues) held in solution. When the urine is secreted by the glomeruli, it is of low concentration, but during its passage along the convoluted tubules a large amount of water is absorbed; this normal process is known as the concentrating power of the kidney. Extensive kidney disease, particularly chronic nephritis, results in destruction of many of the renal tubules, with corresponding interference with the concentrating power. This loss of the normal concentrating power of the kidneys, along with a rise in the concentration of serum creatinine, are the most valuable evidence of the presence of chronic diffuse renal disease.

Protein. When protein is present in large amounts in the urine it is an indication of a glomerular lesion, as a result of which the permeability of the capillaries is increased. This is best tested by measuring the total amount of protein excreted during a 24 hour period.

Sugar. In nearly all cases, the presence of glucose in the urine (glycosuria) indicates diabetes mellitus. The rare exceptions need not be discussed here. At the onset of diabetes the kidneys are normal but the blood sugar is so high that some of it leaks out into the urine. Later on during the course of the disease, glycosuria persists but other abnormalities associated with renal damage, such as proteinuria and a rise in serum creatinine, develop. In addition, uncontrolled, insulin dependent diabetes is characterized by ketonuria, i.e., the presence of diacetic acid and acetone in the urine.

Blood. Hematuria, the presence of blood in the urine, is due to a large number of causes with a significance ranging from jogging while being dehydrated to kidney or bladder cancer. Hematuria is either macroscopic or microscopic. In the latter case, the presence of blood is first detected using a dipstick, and needs to be confirmed by microscopic examination of a centrifuged specimen for red cells and red cell casts. Blood in the urine (hematuria) with rare exceptions indicates disease of the kidney, ureter, or bladder. The disease may be inflammation (acute or chronic nephritis), tuberculosis, stone, or tumor. Hematuria, characterized by red blood cell casts, is particularly significant as it signals the presence of glomerulonephritis. Painless hematuria without any other symptoms suggests a malignant tumor of the kidney or bladder.

Pus. Pyuria or pus in the urine gives a cloudy or turbid appearance. Microscopically, large numbers of pus cells (polymorphonuclear leukocytes) are readily recognized. Pus in the urine may be caused by an infection anywhere in the urinary system or the bladder. If pus is found in female urine, a second specimen should be obtained from the bladder by means of a catheter.

When tuberculosis of the kidney is suspected, a search must be made for tubercle bacilli.

Casts. A urinary cast is a composed of intact or degraded cellular material molded in the lumen of a renal tubule for some time before being flushed out of the kidney. Red blood cell casts are the hallmark of glomerulonephritis.

The accompanying Table A20–3 summarizes findings in normal urine and in different diseases.

21

FEMALE REPRODUCTIVE SYSTEM
(Including Breast)

Natural man has only two primal passions: to get and to beget.—OSLER

FEMALE REPRODUCTIVE SYSTEM

Structure and Function

The female genital system includes the external genitalia or vulva, vagina, uterus, fallopian tubes, and ovaries (Fig. 21–1).

The external genitalia or vulva include the mons pubis, the labia majora and minora, the clitoris, the openings of the urethra and vagina, and the perineum.

The vagina or birth canal connects the opening of the uterus with the vulva, and is the usual mode of exit of menstrual fluids and the products of conception.

The cervix is the neck of the uterus. Its funnel shape connects the uterine cavity with the upper vagina.

The uterus proper is called the corpus or body and is a pear-shaped organ, about the size of a large spoon, that sits in the lower pelvis between the bladder and the rectum. It provides the crucial environment for the growth and development of the fetus. It is lined by a complex layer of cells, the endometrium, which changes remarkably during the course of a menstrual cycle (Fig. 21–2). The myometrium (uterine wall) is a thick layer of muscle. The outer surface (serosa) is covered by smooth peritoneum. The uterus grows tremendously in shape and volume during pregnancy, and then returns almost to its original size like a deflated balloon within 6 weeks after the birth of an infant.

The fallopian tubes extend from the upper corners of the uterine cavity to the ovaries. They are suspended by folds of the broad ligament and tend to fall back behind the uterus. Each tube is 8 to 12 cm long. The portion near the uterus (the isthmus) is narrow. The diameter increases gradually toward the fimbri-ated (fringed) end, next to the ovary. The fallopian tubes receive mature ova from the ovary, provide the site where fertilization occurs, and transport the fertilized ovum to the uterine cavity, where it will implant and continue its growth.

The ovaries are two almond-sized organs on the pelvis at the fimbriated end of each fallopian tube. They are attached to the broad ligament, and also to the posterior wall of the uterus. Each ovary releases mature ova and steroid hormones, mainly estrogen and progesterone.

Menstrual Cycle

An average menstrual cycle lasts 28 days and can be divided into the follicular or proliferative phase, ovulation, and the luteal or secretory phase.

During the follicular (proliferative) phase, the ovarian follicle which contains the ovum begins to grow under the influence of FSH (follicle-stimulating hormone, released from the anterior pituitary on orders from the hypothalamus) (Fig. 21–3). The hypothalamus issues its orders for the release of FSH when it senses a declining level of estrogen in the blood, which has occurred at the end of the previous menstrual cycle and during the days of endometrial shedding or menstruation. As follicles grow, the cells around them produce estrogen, which acts on target organs to induce growth. The main target organ is the endometrium. Endometrium responds to estrogen by growth of epithelium and connective tissue, by reformation of its connective tissue, and by growth of the small spiral arterioles that supply it with blood. Although several follicles begin to grow under the influence of FSH, usually only one becomes fully mature.

At approximately the fourteenth day of the cycle, a sudden increase in estrogen and FSH stimulates the hypothalamus to release a surge of luteinizing hormone (LH) from the anterior pituitary. LH travels to the ovary and releases a mature ovum into the fallopian tube. This is called **ovula-**

443

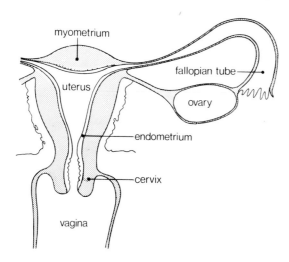

Fig. 21–1   This drawing shows the relationships of ovary, fallopian tube, and uterus. The muscular wall of the uterus is called the myometrium, the lining is called the endometrium, and the junction and entrance to the uterus is called the cervix. The vagina is shown at the bottom.

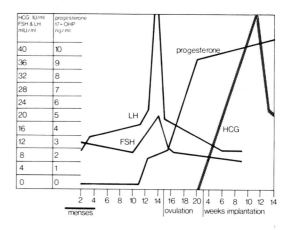

Fig. 21–3   This chart shows the relative amounts of the differing hormones, luteinizing hormone (LH), follicle-stimulating hormone (FSH), progesterone, and human chorionic gonadotropin (HCG) during the menstrual cycle. (From Speroff, L., Glass, R. H., and Kase, N. G.: *Clinical Gynecologic Endocrinology and Infertility,* 2nd Ed. Baltimore, Williams & Wilkins, 1978.)

tion. It is signalled by rise in body temperature that can be detected by daily measurement. The follicle that contained the maturing ovum is transformed into a corpus luteum by the action of LH. The corpus luteum produces large amounts of progesterone that cause the endometrium to undergo changes that characterize the secretory phase of the cycle.

The ovum should be fertilized within 48 hours of its release from the ovary (Table 21–1). If this does not occur, the ovum disintegrates, the corpus luteum wanes and collapses, hormone production declines, and the endometrium breaks down and is shed during menstruation. When

the hypothalamus senses the low level of estrogen in the blood, it begins again to order the anterior pituitary to release FSH, which starts a new cycle of follicular growth in the ovary.

If the ovum is fertilized, it spends 2 to 3 days passing through the fallopian tube, where it begins to divide. When it reaches the endometrial cavity, it spends another 2 to 3 days dividing before it implants itself in the endometrium on the wall of the uterus (Fig. 21–4). By this time, the secretory activities of the endometrial glands are at a peak and are able to provide a wealth of nutrients, which the tiny conceptus needs. Already, the conceptus has divided itself into a portion that will form the embryo and a portion that

Fig. 21–2   This drawing shows the size and appearance of the endometrial epithelium in the middle of the picture, at the days of the menstrual cycle shown as numbers at the top. The appearance of the ovum follicle and corpus luteum is shown above the top line. At day 14 of the cycle the ovum is released from the follicle. The relative levels of the two hormones, estrogen and progesterone, are indicated at the bottom of the figure. (From Bloom, W., and Fawcett, D. W.: *A Textbook of Histology.* 10th Ed. Philadelphia, W. B. Saunders, 1975.)

Table 21–1. Risk-Benefit Ratio of Contraceptives

METHOD	FAILURE RATE OR EFFECTIVENESS	MAJOR SIDE EFFECTS	MINOR SIDE EFFECTS	APPROXIMATE COST $
Female sterilization	1 in 200–1 in 1000	post-tubal syndrome	none	850
Male sterilization	1 in 1000	possible atherosclerosis	none	175
Oral contraceptives	0.5 per 100 woman years	thrombophlebitis, pulmonary embolus, cerebral thrombosis	pseudopregnancy	75/yr
Intrauterine devices	2–3 per 100 woman years	uterine perforation, pelvic infections	uterine bleeding and cramping	75/yr
Barrier methods	3–20 per 100 woman years	none	allergic reaction, nuisance to use	30/yr

(From Droegemueller, W., and Bressler, R.: Effectiveness and risks of contraception. Annu. Rev. Med., 31:329, 1980.)

will form the placenta (the trophoblast cells). The trophoblast cells begin to produce human chorionic gonadotrophin (HCG), which is released into the mother's blood, travels to the ovary, and causes the corpus luteum to continue full production of progesterone. The detection of HCG in the urine forms the basis of pregnancy tests. This process insures that the endometrium will not break down and shed, and that the endometrial gland will continue to secrete nutrients for the embryo until the placenta has developed sufficiently to take nutrients directly from the mother's blood. This development is fully established by 17 days after fertilization. The entire sequence of the menstrual cycle, fertilization, and implantation, is an amazing achievement of neatly synchronized events.

In the 1950s a method of interfering with the menstrual cycle for the purpose of contraception was developed. The oral contraceptive prevents ovulation by interfering with hormonal feedback control: in women taking the "pill" the preovulatory LH surge (see Fig. 21–3) does not occur. Oral contraceptives also alter vaginal pH, cervical mucus and uterine and tubal motility, which converts the reproductive tract into a hazardous obstacle course for the incoming sperm.

Epidemiologic studies have shown that oral contraceptives increase the risk of venous thrombosis, gallbladder disease, cerebrovascular accidents, myocardial infarcts and liver tumors. Of these the vascular diseases have attracted the most attention. Oral contraceptives elevate blood pressure in most women, although this rise is quite small on average. In addition, they increase the coagulability of the blood by enhancing platelet activity and altering the coagulation system. As the reader will know by now, all of these are important in the development of thrombi and emboli.

It appears that the contraceptive pill multiplies the effects of risk factors for myocardial infarcts and stroke. Thus any woman with hypertension, diabetes mellitus, or a heavy smoking habit, or any older woman (age is also a risk factor) is at increased risk (see Fig. 21–14). In women without such risk factors the risks of the pill must be compared with the risk of pregnancy, i.e., failure rates of various contraceptive methods (Fig. 21–5).

There is considerable evidence that the time of conception after ovulation affects the gender of the offspring. Studies on two populations of women have confirmed that the proportion of male babies is higher in the offspring of women who have sexual intercourse two days after ovulation. The proportion is lower on or near the day of ovulation than on the previous day or so.

VULVA

Inflammations and Infections

The vulva may be the site of many skin diseases that occur elsewhere on the body.

The most common inflammations in this area are contact dermatitis from use of soaps, deodorant sprays, or dyes in clothing; fungal infections, particularly candida; herpes simplex type II; and condyloma acuminatum or venereal warts.

Candida vulvitis often occurs with a concomitant candidal vaginitis, and is particularly frequent in women with diabetes mellitus. Other predisposing conditions include pregnancy, use of oral contraceptives, and recent treatment with broad-spectrum antibiotics. The vulvar skin itches intensely and is red, edematous, weeping, and may show small, white patches on the labial folds. The diagnosis can be established by microscopic examination of skin scrapings, vaginal secretions, or by culture. Prompt relief is obtained when appropriate medication is given.

Herpes simplex type II causes painful, vesicular lesions on the vulva and vagina that ulcerate to form small craters filled with necrotic gray-white material surrounded by a red rim. The diagnosis can be confirmed by cytologic examination of scrapings from the crater base. The modern treatment of herpes infection includes the use of antiviral drugs which shorten the duration of the disease.

Condyloma acuminatum is a warty, papillary growth caused by the human papilloma virus (HPV). They occur on the labia, perineum, perianal skin, vagina, or cervix, and are usually several millimeters in diameter. As discussed above in the chapter on neoplasia and below, there is a correlation between

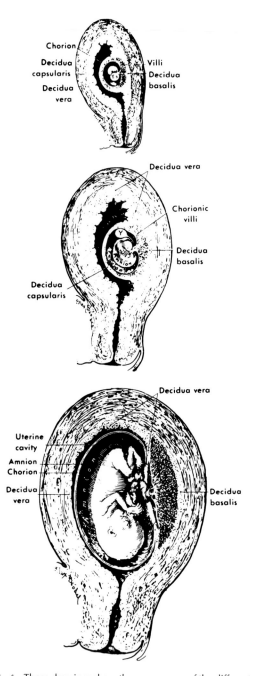

Fig. 21–4 These drawings show the appearance of the different components of the implanted, fertilized egg in the wall of the uterus. These are shown at different stages of growth. The fetus lies within the amniotic cavity in the bottom figure. (From Bloom, W., and Fawcett, D. W.: *A Textbook of Histology*, 10th Ed. Philadelphia, W. B. Saunders, 1975.)

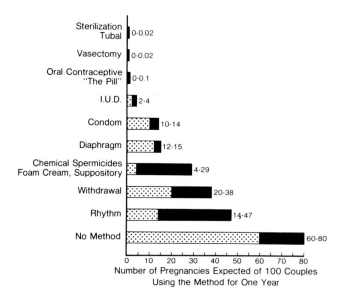

Method	Number of Pregnancies
Sterilization Tubal	0-0.02
Vasectomy	0-0.02
Oral Contraceptive "The Pill"	0-0.1
I.U.D.	2-4
Condom	10-14
Diaphragm	12-15
Chemical Spermicides Foam Cream, Suppository	4-29
Withdrawal	20-38
Rhythm	14-47
No Method	60-80

Number of Pregnancies Expected of 100 Couples Using the Method for One Year

Fig. 21–5 Failure rates of various birth control methods. (Wyeth Limited.)

the presence of condylomas caused by HPV and the occurrence of vulvar carcinoma.

Other inflammations of the vulva are gonorrhea, syphilis, chancroid, granuloma inguinale, and lymphogranuloma venereum (LGV). Gonorrhea is particularly significant because its causal agent, the gonococcus, can infect not only the vulvar tissues, but also migrate up to the fallopian tubes where it can induce chronic pelvic inflammatory disease leading to infertility in a significant number of cases.

Cysts

The most common cystic lesion affecting this region is the Bartholin's gland cyst or abscess. Bartholin's glands are located in the deep tissues on each side of the vaginal opening. They frequently become infected with gonococci, and less commonly with other microorganisms. When the duct draining the Bartholin's glands becomes infected, cysts develop which are treated by surgery. Clinically, the patient has an enlarged, tender, red, fluctuant mass at the base of the labia majora on one side that may make sitting or walking difficult. Treatment is by incision and drainage and by administration of antibiotics. Sometimes, the duct that normally drains these glands becomes obstructed, leading to retention of the gland secretions. In this case, a Bartholin's gland cyst develops. These are usually nontender, unilateral swellings at the base of the labia majora brought to the physician's tion when the patient notices a lump. The treatment for these cysts is surgical.

Dystrophy

In some women, the vulvar skin may undergo changes of atrophy or hyperplasia. These changes usually occur in older women and often present clinically as intense itching. The skin may appear thin, shrunken, or thickened, with red, pink, white, scaling, or weeping patches. Microscopically, one sees variable patterns of atrophy of hyperplasia of the skin structures. These changes are called vulvar dystrophy and are benign. They are treated medically.

It is important to realize that it is not possible to distinguish between the types of dystrophy (i.e., atrophic or hyperplastic), or between these benign conditions and early cancer (carcinoma in situ), without a small biopsy. Only then can the correct medical therapy or need for further surgery be determined.

Carcinoma

Cancer of the vulva is the fourth most common cancer of the female genital tract. It usually affects elderly women (over age 60). Histologically, the majority are squamous cell carcinomas. A smaller proportion of vulvar cancers are melanoma.

The patient may notice a small lump or sore on the vulva that begins to itch or to ulcerate and bleed. Often she is embarrassed or afraid to seek medical advice and will treat the lesion with assorted creams and other preparations for many months. By the time the patient comes to the physician's attention, the lesion is often greater than 2 cm in size and it may have caused extensive destruction of the vulvar skin and spread to the lymph nodes of the groin decreasing the chance of successful surgical management.

Unfortunately, there may also be an element of delay by the physician in establishing the diagnosis. In early cancers, the skin changes may not be so obvious. The skin may appear similar to that described for vulvar dystrophy, and itching may be a prominent complaint. The physician may treat the patient with various lotions or creams, and only after some months have passed without improvement will a biopsy be done. By this time, an early, in situ cancer may have become invasive, with the danger of lymph node metastases and a decreased chance of successful surgical treatment.

The treatment of invasive cancer of the vulva is radical surgery in which all the vulvar skin, subcutaneous fat, and lymph nodes of the groin are removed and submitted for microscopic analysis. The 5-year sur-

vival rate depends on the size of the lesion at the time of surgery, and on the presence or absence of lymph node metastases. It ranges from more than 80% for a lesion under 2 cm in size with negative lymph nodes, to 15 to 30% for a large lesion (greater than 3 cm) with positive lymph nodes. The importance of early diagnosis is therefore obvious.

VAGINA

Inflammations

The most common causes of vaginitis are candida and trichomonas. Inflammation with discharge often occurs after insertion of a foreign body—such as a forgotten tampon, or an object inserted by a child.

In candidal vaginitis, the vagina appears red and edematous. The discharge may be thick, white, and may resemble cheese curds, or it may be thin with small, white patches stuck to the mucosa. Diagnosis and treatment are as described in the section on the vulva.

Trichomonas vaginalis is a single-celled protozoan which commonly causes vaginal discharge and itching. The discharge may be heavy and watery, or it may appear greenish and frothy. Diagnosis is established by demonstration of the organism on a wet smear of the vaginal secretions. Treatment is with metronidazole (an antifungal agent). The vaginitis may recur if the woman's sexual partner is not treated, because the organism survives well in the male genital tract and is transmitted during sexual intercourse.

Hemophilus vaginalis causes a grayish discharge with a disagreeable odor. It gives little inflammation of the underlying tissue, in contrast to candida and trichomonas. The diagnosis may be suspected by finding so-called ''clue cells'' in the vaginal secretions (epithelial cells filled with bacteria). Treatment is with antibiotics.

The thin vaginal mucosa of postmenopausal women is prone to infection by various bacteria from the gastrointestinal tract. Treatment with intravaginal antibiotics and estrogen creams kills the offending bacteria and promotes growth of a thicker, more resistant vaginal mucosa.

Cysts

Sometimes, benign cysts develop from embryologic remnants located deep in the side walls of the vagina. These growths are called Gartner's duct cysts and may be small or large. They may be asymptomatic, or the patient may notice a bulging mass in the vagina. Most vaginal cancers are squamous cell carcinomas but, overall, vaginal malignancies are very uncommon.

Intrauterine DES Exposure

During the 1940s and 1950s, patients with certain pregnancy complications, such as threatened abortion, were treated with diethylstilbestrol (DES), a synthetic estrogen compound. In the early 1970s, it became apparent that 1 to 2% of the daughters of these patients were developing cancers of the vagina and cervix during their teenage and young adult years. Cancer of the vagina is almost unheard of in young women, and these cancers were of a particularly rare type: clear cell adenocarcinoma. A frantic attempt to find other offspring of these DES-treated mothers began, so that the former could be examined and treated if a cancer was found.

Since the first reports on this subject appeared, it has been learned that, although there are many young women who had been exposed to DES prenatally, particularly in the United States, the vaginal and cervical cancers occur in only about 1 to 2% of them. There are only 300 cases reported worldwide. Careful examination of these women has revealed that many have developmental abnormalities of the vagina and cervix. Some of these abnormalities are areas of persistent columnar epithelium and gland formation, called vaginal adenosis (the vagina and exocervix are normally covered by squamous epithelium), partial or complete blockage of the vagina by excess tissue (vaginal septa), and an abnormal shape of the cervix. These abnormalities may be detected by careful pelvic examination, including Pap smears and colposcopy.

It is not known whether these women will have an increased risk of developing other cancers at the sites of adenosis as they grow older, so it is important that these patients be identified and undergo regular follow-up examinations.

The male offspring of DES-treated mothers may also show certain genital tract abnormalities (epididymal cysts and small testes), and some of these young men have low sperm counts.

Cervix

There are a number of ways by which the cervix, and the vagina leading to it, can be examined. These include digital examination and visualization through a speculum. However, more precise information can be gained by using the colposcope. The colposcope is a stereoscopic magnifying instrument that looks like a pair of binoculars on a stand. It magnifies from 2 to 50 times. Through it, the external surfaces of the vagina and cervix can be carefully studied. Abnormali-

ties such as adenosis, dysplasia, carcinoma in situ, and invasive cancer show specific changes in the contours of the epithelium that are too small to be seen without the aid of this magnifying instrument. Its chief benefit is to help the physician to determine the location of abnormal areas, which should be examined by biopsy.

Inflammatory Conditions

The cervix may become infected by a variety of agents. These are bacterial (e.g., gonorrhea or syphilis), fungal (e.g., candida), protozoan (e.g., *Trichomonas vaginalis*), or viral (e.g., papilloma virus, herpes simplex type II). Commonly also, the cervix can become acutely inflamed by infection with bacteria normally found in the vagina.

The cervix appears boggy, red, and inflamed. A characteristic type of lesion or discharge may be present, which aids the physician in making the diagnosis.

A common finding is a small, yellow cyst protruding from the surface. This growth is called a nabothian cyst, and results when an endocervical gland becomes obstructed and material collects behind the obstruction. This obstruction may be caused by inflammation or by active metaplasia in the area.

Polyps

Endocervical polyps are benign and result from a localized overgrowth of endocervical glands. The polyps vary in size and often will protrude from the external os (opening), where they appear as a soft, red, raspberry-like mass, attached by a stalk. They are composed of delicate blood vessels and of fibrous tissue covered by endocervical glands. Because the vessels are fragile, these polyps are relatively frequent and may cause abnormal bleeding, i.e., bleeding between menstrual periods, postcoital bleeding, or postmenopausal bleeding.

Dysplasia (Cervical Intraepithelial Neoplasia)

The reader will recall that when we discussed the development of a cancer in Chapter 11 the emphasis was on the current concept whereby cancer arises through multiple steps, not *de novo*. Cancer of the cervix is, with colon cancer, a paradigm of this hypothesis. In addition, a virus, HPV, plays a determinant role in the development of cervical cancer.

Concerning the progression through multiple steps there is ample evidence that overt cancer of the cervix is preceded by dysplasia.

Dysplasia is an abnormal growth pattern in which some of the epithelial cells have features of malignancy. In the normal maturation sequence of squamous epithelium, the most common immature cells (basal cells) occupy a single layer just above the basement membrane, which separates the surface epithelium from the connective tissue (stroma) of the cervix. Above the layer of basal cells are multiple layers which differentiate in an orderly fashion, into a fully mature squamous epithelium. In dysplasia, some of these basal cells take on malignant criteria and begin to involve more of the cell layers above it.

Although exact definitions of dysplasia have not been set down, the condition is usually graded as mild, moderate, or severe, depending on how much of the epithelial thickness is replaced by abnormal cells. In the mildest forms, up to about 25% of the epithelium is made up of abnormal cells. In severe dysplasia, only a thin rim of nonmalignant, nondysplastic cells are left at the surface. When the entire epithelial thickness is replaced by these cytologically malignant cells, it is called carcinoma in situ (CIS). At this point, the disease has still not broken through the basement membrane, i.e., it is still confined to the epithelium.

The current terminology for the spectrum of dysplastic lesions is **cervical intraepithelial neoplasia,** and it is graded I, II, and III, corresponding to mild (CIN I), moderate (CIN II), and severe dysplasia, which is clinically equivalent to *carcinoma in situ* (CIN III). The three grades refer to whether the abnormal cells are present respectively in one-third, two-thirds, or the full thickness of the squamous epithelium. This terminology helps to emphasize that these lesions do form a continuous spectrum and that the process is, in fact, a type of neoplasia. Severe dysplasia and CIS are grouped together because the dividing line between the two is often difficult to decide, and because CIS is still a disease confined to the epithelium, i.e., it is not invasive.

CIN is usually asymptomatic and is diagnosed initially by an abnormal Papanicolaou test, so-called "Pap" smear—the cervix usually appears normal to general inspection. The abnormal cells tend to be less cohesive than normal squamous cells, and are readily detached when a "Pap" smear is performed. Further examination of the cervix is recommended with the colposcope, with which it is possible to see abnormalities of color, surface contour, and a vascular pattern too small to be noticed with the naked eye. These abnormal patterns are then examined by biopsy so that an exact diagnosis can be made and appropriate treatment can be given to destroy the abnormal cells. The exact type of treatment depends on the degree of the abnormality and on the patient's desire to keep her uterus. After definitive therapy, it is important for the patient to be followed closely by regular examination and cytology, because she is at increased risk for developing other areas of CIN.

Microinvasive Carcinoma

This is a special category of invasive cervical carcinoma in which small groups of malignant cells break through the basement membrane into the cervical stroma, but penetrate less than 3 mm below the point of the rupture in the basement membrane. These patients are usually treated by simple hysterectomy, but a small proportion of them (less than 5%) will have microscopic metastases to regional lymph nodes.

Invasive Carcinoma

Invasive carcinoma of the cervix is now the seventh most common cancer in females after cancer of the lung, breast, colorectum, endometrium, lymph nodes and pancreas, and is ranked as the eighth most common cause of cancer death. Compared to figures from a few decades ago, these figures might represent a significant improvement since at that time advanced cancer of the cervix was a common cause of cancer-related deaths. Invasive squamous carcinoma of the cervix was the most common female genital tract malignancy until recent times. In the past 25 years, Pap smear examinations have permitted detection of the disease in early, potentially curable, stages. The middle-aged woman who suddenly visits her physician because of abnormal vaginal bleeding, not having been examined since the birth of her last child 20 years before, and who is found to have a far advanced cervical cancer, has largely become a thing of the past in developed countries.

Unfortunately, we are now observing an increase in the incidence of cervical cancer even though death from it remains relatively low (Fig. 21–6). This is explained in large part by the notion that women are exposed, both earlier and more often, to the risk factors associated with colon cancer. Indeed, epidemiologists have documented that there is a correlation between the risk of developing cervical cancer and the number of male sexual partners, the sexual promiscuity of these partners and the age of the female patient at the time of first intercourse. These notions tell us that cancer of the cervix behaves as a sexually transmitted disease. To support this concept it has been established that close to 100% of patients with this disease have evidence of prior infection by HPV, a virus with oncogenic properties, as discussed in Chapter 11. HBV is also found in the CIN lesions and could well be the initiator of cervical neoplasia. Of note is the fact that there are a large number of HPV types and that discrete types are prognostically associated with progression to carcinoma. To be complete, it is thought that co-factors participate in the promotion of cervical cancer once the determinant effect of HPV infection has been exerted.

The average age of patients with invasive cervical carcinoma is 45, versus age 30 for those with CIS, and under 35 for CIN. There is good epidemiologic

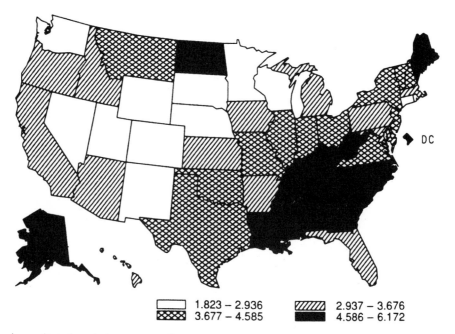

Fig. 21-6   Mean annual age-adjusted cervical cancer mortality rates per 100,000 females, by quartile—United States, 1984–1986. (From Centers for Disease Control, Morbidity and Mortality Weekly Report, 38(38):652, 1989.)

evidence to support the belief that this spectrum of disease is related to sexual intercourse, i.e., early age of beginning sexual activity, multiple sexual partners, and prior infection with agents known to be sexually transmitted, notably herpes simplex type II (Figs. 21-7, 21-8).

The usual presenting symptom is abnormal vaginal bleeding, particularly postcoital bleeding. Inspection of the cervix shows an obvious lesion that may be cauliflower-like and friable, or deeply ulcerated. A portion of the cervix, or its entirety, may be replaced by the tumor. Microscopically, one sees nests and

cords of malignant squamous cells infiltrating the cervical stroma. The major routes of spread are to the vaginal mucosa, to the pelvic and para-aortic lymph nodes, and by growth directly into the soft tissues around the uterus with further extension out to the pelvic side walls. As the tumor grows, it may entrap the ureters as they pass close to the cervix, or it may invade the bladder and rectum. It may also spread to distant sites. The usual cause of death is entrapment and blockage of the ureters by tumor, causing uremia and death over a period of months.

The treatment and prognosis for survival depend

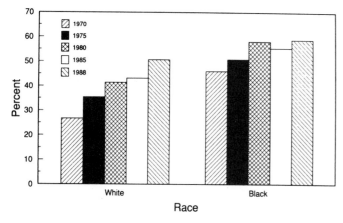

Fig. 21-7   Percentage of women 15–19 years of age who reported having had premarital sexual intercourse, by race and year—United States, 1970–1988. (From Centers for Disease Control, Morbidity and Mortality Weekly Report, 39(51,52):931, 1991.)

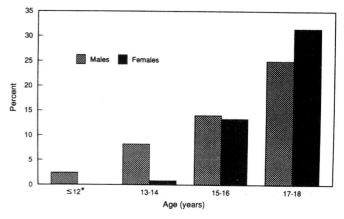

Fig. 21-8   Percentage of high school students who reported having had sexual intercourse, by sex and age of initiation—Frascati, Italy, 1990. (From Centers for Disease Control, Morbidity and Mortality Weekly Report, 40(13):215, 1991.)

on the stage of the disease at the time of diagnosis. Staging includes a careful pelvic exam, radiologic investigations, and sigmoidoscopy and cystoscopy to determine the extent of disease (see Table 21–2). The primary treatment is radiation therapy. Radical hysterectomy with pelvic lymph node dissection is a formidable operation reserved for the younger patient with a small, localized lesion.

Five-year survival figures range from 90% for stage I lesions which are confined to the cervix, to less than 15% for stage IV which has extended beyond the true pelvis or has invaded the bladder or rectum.

Finally, one out of ten cervical cancers is an adenocarcinoma instead of the usual squamous cell carcinoma. The mode of spread to neighboring organs is comparable in both forms of malignancy.

Endometrium

The endometrium is unique in that each month it undergoes a complex series of structural changes in response to hormonal signals from the ovary, in order to receive and to nourish a fertilized ovum, and is broken down and shed if conception has not occurred. This is discussed in detail at the beginning of this chapter.

The endometrial pattern depends on the proper sequence of hormonal stimuli from the ovary. The ovary, in turn, cannot put forth the proper stimuli unless it receives accurate signals from the anterior pituitary. The anterior pituitary receives its orders from the hypothalamus, which receives stimuli from higher centers in the brain, such as the cerebral cortex, thalamus, and limbic system. We can see that any disturbance along the complex pathway of the menstrual cycle may result in an abnormal endometrial response. The patient will then experience what is for her an abnormal menstrual period—too scanty, too heavy, delayed in onset, or skipped altogether. These abnormal bleeding episodes are not caused by a specific structural abnormality of the endometrium, but reflect a derangement in the hypothalamic-pituitary-ovarian control system. The derangement may exist for a single cycle only, or it may be the dominant feature of all the woman's menstrual cycles. This derangement is called **dysfunctional uterine bleeding** (DUB).

DUB is most common in the teenage years just after the onset of menses and in the several years just before menses stop (perimenopausal age group). Irrespective of the age at which it occurs, DUB is often accompanied by either anovulation or an inadequate secretion of progesterone, both resulting in transient infertility. This common disorder can also occur at any other time in between those two age groups. The young woman who leaves her family to attend college or to take a job in another city, and who then begins to have menstrual problems, is the classic example of DUB. Because DUB is a reflection of alteration in the normal, orderly transfer of hormonal signals between the parts of the reproductive control system, it is a frequent finding in women who are infertile because of absent or infrequent ovulation.

Contraceptive pills have a characteristic hypoplastic effect on the endometrium. Intrauterine devices (IUD) also produce a characteristic picture. There is indentation of the endometrial surface and inflammatory changes (acute and chronic) at the places where the intrauterine device touches the endometrial surface. Sometimes, areas of ulceration or of squamous metaplasia may occur.

Inflammation

Acute inflammation of the endometrium is uncommon. When it occurs, it usually follows abortion or delivery, especially when fragments of the placenta remain in the uterus, when the delivery has followed a long labor with multiple vaginal examinations, or when cesarian section was required. A mild degree of acute inflammation is frequent following insertion of an intrauterine device.

Chronic endometritis is found in association with retained products of conception, pelvic inflammatory disease (see section on fallopian tubes), and the presence of an IUD. Antibiotics are successful in treating both acute and chronic endometritis after the retained products of conception or the IUD have been removed.

Table 21–2.   Clinical Stages in Carcinoma of the Cervix

Stage I.	Carcinoma strictly confined to the cervix (extension to the uterus should be disregarded).
Stage Ia.	Microinvasive carcinoma (early stroma invasion).
Stage II.	The carcinoma extends beyond the cervix but has not extended onto the pelvic wall. The carcinoma involves the vagina, but not the lower third.
Stage III.	The carcinoma has extended onto the pelvic wall. On rectal examination there is no cancer-free space between the tumor and the pelvic wall. The tumor involves the lower third of the vagina. All cases with a hydronephrosis or nonfunctioning kidney.
Stage IV.	The carcinoma has extended beyond the true pelvis or has clinically involved the mucosa of the bladder or rectum.

(Adapted from DiSaia, P.J., et al.: Definitions of different clinical stages in carcinoma of the cervix uteri. In *Synopsis of Gynecologic Oncology.* New York, John Wiley and Sons, 1975.)

Hyperplasia

When the endometrium has been subjected to prolonged stimulation by estrogen, unopposed by the effects of progesterone, it becomes hyperplastic.

The unopposed estrogen stimulation may be the result of the use of estrogen-containing drugs commonly given to perimenopausal age women to control symptoms such as hot flushes; noncyclic activity of the hypothalamic-pituitary-ovarian axis, which causes anovulation and a lack of progesterone production by the ovary; some steroid-secreting neoplasms of the ovary or adrenals; or the conversion of certain steroid compounds made in the ovary and adrenal to estrogens by the body's fat tissue.

When hyperplasia is neither severe nor grossly atypical, it can be removed by endometrial curettage and prevented from recurring by eliminating the sources of excess estrogen. When severe and atypical, hysterectomy is usually recommended. Although the number of women with hyperplasia that progresses to adenocarcinoma is only 5 to 10%, the chances increase when the hyperplasia has been untreated for a long time, or when it is severe and atypical.

Polyps

Endometrial polyps are covered with either functioning or hyperplastic endometrium. They result from small areas of endometrial hyperplasia. They are usually located near the top of the endometrial cavity. These glands do not usually respond to hormonal stimuli. Endometrial polyps may become large and are a common cause of postmenopausal bleeding. They may ulcerate, become infarcted, or protrude through the external cervical os. Rarely, adenocarcinoma develops in a polyp.

Carcinoma

Adenocarcinoma of the endometrium has now become the most common invasive cancer of the female genital tract (Fig. 21–9). It usually occurs in postmenopausal women (over age 50). The typical patient is described as an obese, diabetic, hypertensive woman who has never had children. She occasionally has a family history of endometrial carcinoma and a personal history of breast cancer.

Recent studies have indicated that women taking estrogens for relief of menopausal symptoms have an increased risk (4 to 8 times) of developing carcinoma of the endometrium. Because the use of these drugs is so widespread today, and because the Pap smear is not a reliable detector of endometrial carcinoma, aspiration biopsies of the endometrium are frequently

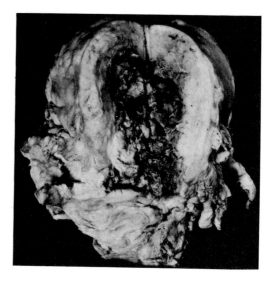

Fig. 21–9 This uterus shows an irregular outer surface, a thick wall, and a fungating necrotic mass occupying the endometrial cavity. (McGill University, Department of Pathology Museum.)

performed to follow these patients. This biopsy is an office procedure done on an annual or semiannual basis. If any abnormality is seen in the biopsy, or if the patient develops postmenopausal bleeding, a curettage is done.

The common routes of spread of this tumor are downward growth to involve the cervix, paracervical lymphatics, and vagina, penetration into and finally through the myometrium, with implantation of tumor on the pelvic and abdominal organs, spread to pelvic and para-aortic lymph nodes, and distant metastases, especially to the lung.

The tumor is staged as shown in Table 21–3. Treatment consists of hysterectomy with or without radio-

Table 21–3. Clinical Stages in Carcinoma of the Corpus Uteri

Stage I.	The carcinoma is confined to the uterus.
	The Stage I cases should be subgrouped with regard to the histologic type of the adenocarcinoma, as follows:
	Grade 1. Highly differentiated adenomatous carcinomas.
	Grade 2. Differentiated adenomatous carcinomas with partly solid areas.
	Grade 3. Predominantly solid or entirely undifferentiated carcinomas.
Stage II.	The carcinoma has involved the uterus and the cervix.
Stage III.	The carcinoma has extended outside the uterus, but not outside the true pelvis.
Stage IV.	The carcinoma has extended outside the true pelvis or has obviously involved the mucosa of the bladder or rectum.

(Adapted from DiSaia, P.J., et al.: Definitions of different clinical stages in carcinoma of the corpus uteri. In *Synopsis of Gynecologic Oncology.* New York, John Wiley and Sons, 1975.)

therapy depending on the stage of the disease. A good prognosis with a 5-year survival of more than 90% is expected when the cancer is restricted to the uterus, dropping to 20% when it has extended beyond the true pelvis or involved the bladder or rectum.

Endometriosis

Endometriosis is the presence of normal-appearing endometrium in sites other than their normal location inside the uterus. The most common locations are the ovaries and tubes, pelvic peritoneum, other pelvic organs such as large bowel, and soft tissues, for example, abdominal scars, episiotomy scars, and the umbilicus. Occasionally such distant sites as the lung and pleura may be involved.

Several theories have been put forth to explain how the endometrial tissue appears in such unusual locations. Some of these are: reflux of endometrial fragments backward through the tubes during menstruation with implantation in the pelvis, metaplastic transformation of multipotential cells on the abdomen and pelvis, implantation of endometrial fragments during surgery or delivery, and blood or lymphatic spread to distant places.

The patients are usually in their late 20s or early 30s. The presenting complaints depend on the organs involved. The more common symptoms include pelvic pain, dysmenorrhea, and infertility, whereas more unusual implantation sites may lead to monthly episodes of bloody sputum production or partial bowel obstruction.

Myometrium

The two common conditions affecting the uterine muscle mass are adenomyosis and leiomyomas.

Adenomyosis is the presence of normal-appearing endometrial glands and stroma deep in the muscle wall of the uterus. The uterus may appear grossly normal or round and globular in shape, with tiny areas of hemorrhage surrounded by bands of smooth muscle.

The patient is usually a middle-aged woman complaining of pelvic pain, abnormal menstrual bleeding, and dysmenorrhea. This condition is usually not associated with endometriosis. Treatment is by hysterectomy.

Leiomyomas are benign smooth muscle tumors that are present in at least 20% of all women. They have been misnamed fibroids or fibroid tumors, although they are composed of interlacing bundles of smooth muscle and not of fibrous tissue. Leiomyomas may be either small or very large, and a patient may have one or many. They vary in location from submu-

cus (which distort the endometrial cavity and often produce menorrhagia), to intramural (the most common), to subserous (which lie just beneath the outer surface of the uterus).

Leiomyomas are frequently asymptomatic. However, they may become large enough to distort the shape of the uterus completely. When symptoms do occur, they consist of abnormal bleeding, pelvic pressure, frequent urination because of compression of the bladder, constipation due to rectal pressure, or infertility. The patient may also notice a mass in her lower abdomen. Leiomyomas tend to grow under the direct or indirect influence of estrogens.

The cut surface of these tumors is characteristic. They are white, solid, rubbery, and have a whorled pattern. Sometimes they contain small areas of hemorrhage or of cystic degeneration. They may be densely calcified. Rarely, the tumors may have undergone malignant transformation and in this case they are called leiomyosarcomas.

The treatment of leiomyomas depends on the size of the uterus and on the patient's symptoms. Small, asymptomatic tumors may be left alone, whereas larger, symptom-producing ones will often require hysterectomy.

Fallopian Tube

The major conditions that affect the fallopian tube are acute and chronic salpingitis, **pelvic inflammatory disease**, and ectopic pregnancy.

Acute salpingitis is most often the result of infection with the gonococcus (Figs. 21–10 and 21–11), which is thought to travel along the mucosa from its portal of entry at the endocervical glands to the fallopian tubes. Other organisms, such as *chlamydia*, streptococcus, *E. coli*, and anaerobes, can also cause acute salpingitis. Acute salpingitis may result from an unsterile abortion or delivery, or it may follow the insertion of an IUD. Salpingitis is usually bilateral, but in cases associated with an IUD, it is often unilateral.

The fallopian tube appears red and swollen, may be covered with exudate, and is often leaking pus from the fimbriated end. The patient has a fever, lower abdominal pain, nausea, and vomiting. There is often severe pain on pelvic examination. Treatment is with high-dose antibiotics and bed rest.

Chronic salpingitis frequently follows one or several episodes of acute salpingitis. The delicate mucosal folds may be damaged or destroyed by the inflammatory process, and adhesions frequently occur both in and around the fallopian tube, causing it to bind to neighboring structures. Often, the fimbriated end of the tube becomes occluded by adhesions and

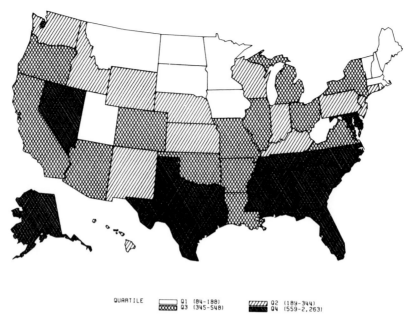

QUARTILE   Q1 (84-188)   Q2 (189-344)
            Q3 (345-548)   Q4 (559-2,263)

Fig. 21-10   **Gonorrhea**—reported cases in civilians per 100,000 population, by area, United States, 1981. (Centers for Disease Control, Morbidity and Mortality Weekly Report, 30(54):40, 1982.)

the tube fills with fluid (hydrosalpinx). Repeated flare-ups of salpingitis are common. When a hydrosalpinx becomes infected, the fallopian tube may become filled with pus and greatly distorted in shape and size. If the ovary is also involved, this mass is called a tubo-ovarian abscess. Rupture of such an abscess is a serious emergency that requires high-dose intravenous antibiotics and surgical drainage. Pelvic inflammation accompanied by chronic salpingitis is an important disease because it can cause pain, sterility and ectopic pregnancy. Although mild flare-ups of salpingitis may be treated with antibiotics, the long-term complications of this condition, chronic pelvic pain, infertility, and ectopic pregnancy, frequently require surgery.

Tuberculosis as the cause of salpingitis is uncommon and may manifest as infertility. It is usually brought to the fallopian tube by hematogenous spread from a tuberculous focus in the lung.

Ectopic pregnancy is described under disorders of pregnancy.

Ovary

The ovary is a small but complicated organ with two functions:

1. To release a mature egg at a specific time of the menstrual cycle.
2. To receive signals from the anterior pituitary (by means of the gonadotrophins FSH and LH), to

interpret the signals, and to translate them into the production of steroid hormones (mainly estrogen and progesterone), which are then released into the blood and cause characteristic changes in the other female reproductive organs.

It is easier to understand the abnormalities of ovarian structure and function if we divide the ovary into four compartments:

1. the surface epithelium
2. the germ cells
3. the follicles
4. the stroma or interstitial tissue

Surface Epithelium. The ovary is covered by a single, thin layer of cells, the same cells that form the linings of the fallopian tube, the endometrium, and the endocervical canal. The most common types of ovarian tumors develop from these surface epithelial cells, which will change as they grow from their usual cuboidal shape to resemble endometrial- or endocervical-type cells.

Germ Cells. The mature germ cell is called the ovum and is released at ovulation. The germ cells come to the ovary from the yolk sac during early embryologic life and populate the cortex (located just beneath the surface epithelial cells).

Follicles. After each germ cell arrives in the ovarian cortex, it is surrounded by a double layer of specialized cells that are important in the production of estrogen and progesterone. This unit of germ cell surrounded by a special double cell layer is called a follicle. The inner ring of cells is

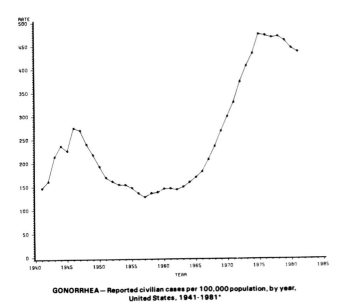

GONORRHEA — Reported civilian cases per 100,000 population, by year,
United States, 1941-1981*

*1941-1948 Fiscal Years: Twelve-month period ending June 30 of the years specified.
1947-1981 Calendar Years.

Fig. 21-11 **Gonorrhea** is the most frequently reported communicable disease in the United States. Beginning in 1966, reported gonorrhea cases increased at about 12% per year until 1973, when 842,621 cases were reported. The sharp increase of reported cases in the late 1960s and early 1970s is thought to represent an actual increase in the occurrence of disease as well as improved case-detection procedures. Since 1973, when federally assisted state and local programs were implemented to control gonorrhea, the number of reported cases has plateaued at about 1 million cases per year: 990,864 cases were reported for 1981, about 1.3% fewer than the number reported for 1980. The case rate per 100,000 population decreased from 443.3 for 1980 to 435.2 for 1981. The leveling-off of reported cases since 1975 is thought to be due to disease-intervention activities initiated in 1973.

Pelvic inflammatory disease (PID) is the most common serious complication of gonorrhea and is considered a major public health problem. It is estimated that about 1 million cases of PID occur annually in the United States and about 25% of the patients require hospitalization. After initial cases of PID, women often experience recurrences and are at elevated risk for infertility and ectopic pregnancy. (Centers for Disease Control, Morbidity and Mortality Weekly Report, 30(54):38, 1982.)

called the granulosa cell layer. This is surrounded by an outer layer, called the theca cells. During development of the follicle on days 1 to 14 of the menstrual cycle, these cells (especially the theca cells) are actively producing estrogen. When the egg is released at ovulation, the granulosa and theca cells remain behind on the ovary. The granulosa cells, lining the cavity in which the ovum matured, become bright yellow, plump, and full of vacuolated cytoplasm. This change is called luteinization and the cavity is called a corpus luteum (CL). It is here that progesterone, which causes the secretory changes in the endometrium, is made. If fertilization of the ovum does not occur, the CL regresses, hormone production wanes, and a small, white scar, the corpus albicans, is left. The ovary repeats this cycle in response to FSH and LH signals from the anterior pituitary.

Stroma (Interstitial Tissue). The ovarian follicles sit in a bed of dark, spindle-shaped cells, called the stroma. During early embryologic life, the primitive gonad is bipotential. It will develop into a definite male or female gonad only after certain influences push it in one direction or the other. The ovarian stroma retains some of this bipotential ability. It produces a full range of steroid hormones, including androgenic and estrogenic compounds. When tumors develop from these cells, they may also produce these hormones, leading to rare, but clinically striking, pictures.

Functional Cysts

The ovary forms small cystic structures (i.e., the follicle and corpus luteum) during a normal menstrual cycle. Sometimes, these cysts become much larger than usual. They can cause symptoms such as pain or pressure on the bladder, or they may be discovered at a routine pelvic examination. Characteristically, their size changes quickly and they may be 4 to 5 cm in size when first examined, only to disappear completely within a few weeks. Because they are related to the normal small cystic structures (follicle and CL) in the ovary, these growths are called functional cysts. Cysts derived from the *corpus luteum* may rupture around the time of ovulation, and when this occurs in the left side the pain that is produced can mimic acute appendicitis.

Polycystic Ovaries

A common cause of female infertility is anovulation. Some infertile women have polycystic ovaries (Stein-Leventhal syndrome). These individuals have absent or infrequent ovulations, and they suffer from oligomenorrhea, amenorrhea or DUB, infertility, and often some signs of virilization, such as increased facial hair and acne.

The ovaries are usually bilaterally enlarged with a smooth and thick surface capsule. The cut surface shows multiple small cysts just below the thickened external capsule, an absence of corpora lutea, few corpora albicantia, and hyperplasia of the ovarian stroma.

The hypothalamus of these women fails to send its signals to the anterior pituitary. The proper amounts of FSH and LH are not released in time to promote the normal maturation sequence in an ovarian follicle and to cause ovulation to occur. The primary treatment is by drugs to induce ovulation.

Tumors of the Ovary

In this section we will discuss both the benign and malignant neoplasms of the ovary because most types have, at least initially, comparable gross characteristics. In addition, there are intermediate forms which are called ovarian tumors of borderline malignancy.

Neoplastic cysts and tumors of the ovary are described according to their compartment of origin. Ovarian neoplasms may be totally cystic, totally solid, or a mixture of both. Up to 65% of ovarian tumors, especially the malignant ones, are bilateral. Such tumors cause symptoms such as pressure in the pelvis, frequent urination, rectal pressure, increasing abdominal size (if large), or they may be asymptomatic.

Tumors from the Surface Epithelium. This forms the largest group of ovarian tumors. The benign types grow as cystic masses to a very large size. There is generally one or a few cystic cavities. On the contrary the malignant tumors derived from the surface epithelium have a large number of complex cystic cavities separated by solid areas.

Under the microscope there are three possible types of epithelial lining around the cystic spaces: serous, mucinous, or endometriod. The serous cystadenomas and the serous cystadenocarcinomas are the most common of the three types and tend to have papillary growths inside the cystic cavity which is otherwise filled with a clear serous fluid. The mucinous cystadenomas and mucinous cystadenocarcinomas contain a viscous mucin fluid. In the latter, malignant version the mucinous fluid can escape and massively invade the peritoneal cavity where it will create the proper milieu for further malignant growth. In its endometriod type, the ovarian tumor is malignant and, as the name implies, the neoplastic epithelium resembles endometrium.

This group of ovarian tumors is rare in patients under 40. Because these tumors are often asymptomatic in the early stages, patients tend to have widespread disease by the time a diagnosis is made. Here, once again, because of the delay in diagnosis, we are faced with a situation in which the tumor incidence is quite low as compared to cancers from anatomical sites, and yet the mortality is relatively high. Such cancers invade their capsule and sow tumor cells all around the pelvis and abdomen. These cells grow into tumor nodules that eventually encase the pelvic organs, small bowel, omentum, stomach, and liver. Ascites and pleural effusions are common. The usual presenting symptoms are abdominal swelling, abdominal discomfort, or vague pain, and nonspecific gastrointestinal symptoms such as bloating, nausea, anorexia, or heartburn. Sometimes, abnormal vaginal bleeding alerts the patient. Rarely, the first symptoms may be shortness of breath due to a malignant pleural effusion.

Treatment consists of surgery, to remove the uterus, tubes, ovaries, and as much tumor bulk as possible, followed by chemotherapy or radiation. Recently, improved survival rates have been obtained by the use of multiple-drug chemotherapy. Survival depends on the stage of the tumor, on the degree of differentiation of the cells, and on the amount of residual tumor left behind after surgery.

Germ Cell Tumors

Tumors derived from the germ cells of the ovary are rare. (They usually occur in children or in young adults.) Except for the benign cystic teratoma or dermoid cyst, they are malignant. They are microscopically the same as the germ cell tumors that arise on the testis.

The benign cystic teratoma or dermoid cyst is the most common germ cell tumor. It contains mature tissues derived from all three germ cell layers—ectoderm, endoderm, and mesoderm. Grossly, this is a smooth cystic tumor that contains an unforgettable, greasy mixture of keratin, sebaceous material, and hair. Occasionally teeth are found and, if present, give a diagnostic x-ray picture. Microscopically, many tissues such as skin, cartilage, bone, nerve, brain, and thyroid are seen. The malignant variant in this category is quite rare but tends to occur in children and young women. There are even more uncommon germ cells of the tumors, called endodermal sinus tumor, dysgerminoma, and embryonal carcinoma. Interestingly, they tend to have their counterparts in the germinal tumors of the testes.

Tumors of the Gonadal Stroma

These tumors are rare, but remarkable because they may produce hormones that cause characteristic clinical estrogenic or androgenic manifestations.

The granulosa cell tumor is composed of granulosa cells alone or mixed with theca cells. These are the same cells that form the lining of the ovarian follicle, and many of these tumors produce estrogens. They can cause precocious puberty when present in a child, or postmenopausal bleeding in an elderly woman, because the estrogen produced by the tumor stimulates the endometrium.

The Sertoli-Leydig cell tumor contains cells resembling those seen in the testis. It should be remembered that in the embryo, the primitive gonad is bipotential. These tumors are thought to arise from cells of the ovarian stroma that suddenly begin to differentiate along the lines of a testicle. When these tumors are steroid-forming, they make androgenic hormones, which cause a striking degree of masculinization in the patient—including acne, growth of facial and chest hair, clitoromegaly, and deepening of the voice. The tumors are extremely rare.

Metastatic Tumors

This type of tumor frequently involves the ovaries. The most common primary sites are the colon, the stomach, the pancreas and the breast.

Metastatic tumors are bilateral in 50 to 60% of cases and are often asymptomatic. Microscopically, the general architecture of the ovary is preserved, but tumor cells are seen infiltrating in nests or cords between the ovarian structures.

A special type of metastatic ovarian tumor is the Krukenberg tumor, in which the ovary contains mucin-secreting cells which represent metastatic deposits, usually from a cancer of the stomach or the colon.

Placenta

The placenta is a temporary organ that accomplishes the transfer of nutrients and oxygen to the fetus and the passage of metabolic waste products back to the mother for excretion. It is composed of numerous arborizing villi through which fetal blood circulates. The placenta attaches itself to the wall of the uterus, and these villi penetrate into the maternal endometrium (called decidua in pregnancy). The decidua at the site of implantation contains many sinuses into which maternal blood flows. The villi are bathed in the blood of these sinuses, and the exchange of nutrients, oxygen, CO_2, and waste products occurs at this point. Although the blood of the mother and the fetus pass close to each other, they usually do not mix.

Except at the implantation site, the placenta is surrounded by a double layer of membranes—the inner

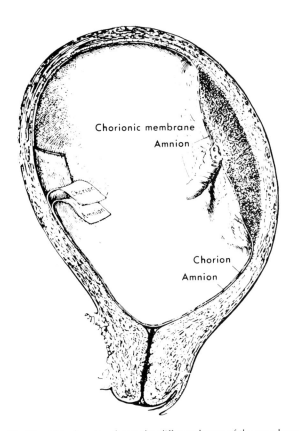

Fig. 21–12 This drawing shows the different layers of the envelope containing the fetus, namely the **amnion**, the **chorion**, and the **umbilical cord**. It demonstrates the placenta at the upper right. (From Bloom, W., and Fawcett, D. W.: *A Textbook of Histology.* 10th Ed. Philadelphia, W. B. Saunders, 1975.)

and the outer chorion (Fig. 21–12). Inside the membranes, the fetus floats in a bath of amniotic fluid. (The fetus is attached to the placenta by the umbilical cord, which ranges from 35 to 120 cm in length, and contains 2 arteries and 1 vein.) It has now become commonplace when there is a gestational problem to remove a sample of amniotic fluid using a needle inserted through the mother's abdominal wall (amniocentesis). By this means, chemical analysis of the fluid can determine fetal lung maturity, can detect certain congenital abnormalities, or can follow the course of Rh-induced hemolytic disease. Fetal cells in the fluid can be cultured and examined for evidence of chromosomal abnormalities such as Down's syndrome, certain inborn errors of metabolism, and determination of the fetal sex.

Abnormalities of the Cord

The umbilical cord contains only 1 artery and 1 vein in about 1% of cases (about 7% of twins). Up to 25% of infants with a 2-vessel cord have other congenital anomalies. The cord may occasionally contain a true knot, but this usually does not tighten enough to cut off the blood supply to the fetus.

Abnormalities of the Placenta

The placenta may contain an accessory lobe, connected to the main placenta by blood vessels. Accessory lobes are important chiefly because they may be left behind in the uterus after delivery and may cause a postpartum hemorrhage.

Placenta previa is insertion of the placenta near or covering the cervical canal. It usually causes bleeding in the latter part of pregnancy.

Placenta accreta is an abnormal adhesion of the placenta to the uterine wall. At the implantation site, there is thin or absent decidua, so that the placenta villi are directly in contact with the myometrium. In more severe degrees of this abnormality, the villi invade the myometrium (placenta increta), or perforate the uterus (placenta percreta). In these rare situations, the placenta does not separate from the uterine wall after the baby is born, heavy bleeding results, and immediate hysterectomy is usually necessary.

Sometimes a portion of the placenta separates from the implantation site prematurely. This is called **placental abruption** and may be severe enough to cause fetal death. Usually the size of the abruption is small (less than 20% of the surface of the placenta). Inspection may show a depressed area on the maternal surface of the placenta filled with clotted blood.

Abnormally large placentas are found with severe Rh incompatibility (erythroblastosis fetalis), syphilis, cytomegalic inclusion disease, toxoplasmosis, and polyhydramnios. Abnormally small placentas are seen with prematurity, severe maternal diabetes, hypertension, or renal disease, some fetal chromosome abnormalities, and rubella.

Twins

The placenta should be carefully examined in cases of twin pregnancy possibly to determine whether the twins resulted from a cleavage of the ovum within the first days after fertilization (monozygotic or identical twins) or from the simultaneous fertilization of two separate ova (dizygotic, nonidentical, or fraternal twins).

The possibilities are shown in Figure 21–13.

Ectopic Pregnancy

The fertilized ovum may implant outside of the endometrial cavity. Such a condition is called **ectopic pregnancy**. The implantation occurs in the fallopian tube (most cases), on the ovary, cervix, or in the abdominal cavity (rare).

The etiology of tubal implantation is usually delayed or obstructed passage of the ovum through the tube because of adhesions from previous salpingitis, endometriosis, or previous surgery on the fallopian tube. The ovum implants and penetrates the wall of the fallopian tube while growing, which will either rupture or attempt to abort the pregnancy through its fimbriated end. Both situations cause serious intra-abdominal hemorrhage.

Chorion	Amnion	Incidence (%)	Gross Configuration	Twin Type
2 (separate)	2	35.2		Monozygotic or dizygotic
2 (fused)	2	34		Monozygotic or dizygotic
1	2	29.6		Monozygotic
1	1	1.2		Monozygotic

Fig. 21–13.   This drawing shows the possible varieties in the appearance of the placenta in twins. (From Benirschke, K., and Driscoll, S. G.: *The Pathology of the Human Placenta.* New York, Springer-Verlag, 1967.)

Clinically, the patients often present as an emergency with severe lower abdominal pain, menstrual abnormalities, a tender mass on one side of the uterus, fainting, or shock from loss of blood. The patient may not even be aware that she is pregnant. The pregnancy test might even be negative. Ectopic pregnancy must be distinguished from salpingitis, a ruptured or twisted ovarian cyst, appendicitis, and threatened abortion. An uncertain diagnosis is confirmed by laparoscopy, which requires the insertion of a viewing scope through a small incision just below the umbilicus. If an ectopic pregnancy is found, the affected tube must be excised.

Abortion

An abortion is the termination of pregnancy before fetal viability, either spontaneously or electively. The risk of abortion at different ages is shown in Figure 21–14, which also illustrates the risk of other forms of contraceptive control. Viability is usually set at 500 g (about 20 weeks gestation) even though infants weighing less than 1,000 g at birth usually do not survive.

Spontaneous abortions are said to occur in about 20% of all conceptions. The incidence may be higher than this, because some conceptions abort before the pregnancy is diagnosed. Most spontaneous abortions occur in the first trimester (first 14 weeks) of pregnancy, and often reflect chromosomal or developmental abnormalities in the fetus that are incompatible with life (blighted ovum). If a careful search of the aborted material is performed, one usually finds only an empty gestational sac, or a sac containing a malformed portion of fetal tissue.

Spontaneous abortions are clinically categorized as threatened, incomplete, or missed. In **threatened abortion**, there is vaginal bleeding and cramping, but the cervix remains closed and no tissue is passed. **Incomplete abortion** occurs when the cervix opens and the patient spontaneously passes some of the products of conception. However, some pieces of placental tissue remain behind on the uterus and must be removed by curettage. In **missed abortion,** the fetus dies, but for some reason is retained in the uterus for 6 weeks or longer. The products of conception

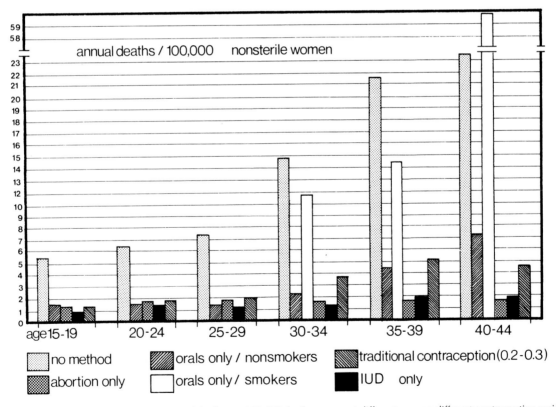

Fig. 21–14 This figure shows the annual number of deaths per 100,000 fertile women at different ages on different contraceptive regimens, and with different smoking histories. The graphs show that the number of deaths in the 15 to 19-year-old age group is highest in those who are on no contraceptive regimen, whereas the death rate in the 40 to 44-year-old age group is 60/100,000 for women who smoke and take oral contraceptives. (Adapted from Kase, N.: The ovaries. In *Cecil Textbook of Medicine.* 15th Ed. Edited by P.B. Beeson, W. McDermott, and J.B. Wyngaarden. Philadelphia, W. B. Saunders, 1979.)

may abort spontaneously after several weeks, but curettage is often required to remove them. Microscopically, a missed abortion usually shows degenerated, hyalinized villi with chronic inflammation. Fetal parts are usually not seen. **Septic abortion** occurs when there has been contamination of the uterine cavity by bacteria with acute inflammation of the products of conception and decidua. Before safe, elective abortions were widely available, sepsis was common after attempted illegal abortions, which were frequently done under unsterile conditions. Septic abortion may be life-threatening to the mother. It requires aggressive antibiotic therapy and prompt evacuation of the uterus.

Trophoblastic Disease

Trophoblast is the name given to the cells that form the placenta. These are the light-staining cytotrophoblast and the smaller, dark-staining syncytiotrophoblast. These cells are characterized by rapid growth and by their tendency to invade the maternal endometrium and myometrium as part of the normal course of pregnancy. Trophoblastic tissue also manufactures human chorionic gonadotropin hormone (HCG). Detection of this hormone in urine or in blood forms the basis of tests for pregnancy. HCG also provides a "marker" by which the physician may follow the course of patients who have recently been treated for one of the three types of trophoblastic disease. In these situations, a falling or absent titer of HCG in the blood indicates eradication of the abnormal trophoblastic tissue.

Hydatidiform Mole

Hydatidiform mole is an abnormal product of conception in which there is usually no fetus. The uterus is filled with cystically dilated chorionic villi that look like a bunch of grapes (Fig. 21–15). It is felt that hydatidiform mole may represent the missed abortion of a blighted ovum in which the only genetic material present is derived from the father. The villi then continue to absorb fluid and become swollen. Microscopically, one finds edematous villi that contain no fetal blood vessels, and degrees of overgrowth of the trophoblastic tissue ranging from mild to marked.

Hydatidiform mole occurs in about 1 in 2,000 pregnancies in North America, but the incidence rises to about 1 in 300 in parts of the Far East. The reason for this geographic difference is unknown.

Molar pregnancy is more common in older women. The patient has vaginal bleeding early in pregnancy. The uterus is often found to be larger than expected for the length of the pregnancy. No fetal heart tones can be found, and a characteristic pattern is seen on ultrasound. The HCG titer remains elevated, instead of showing the expected decline after the first trimester.

A molar pregnancy usually aborts spontaneously early in the second trimester. Sometimes, however, this does not occur, and suction curettage must be done. The patient is

Fig. 21–15   This drawing shows the appearance of an hydatidiform mole. The grape-like clusters of edematous villi without fetal blood vessels appear as tiny grape-like cysts. (From Eastman, N. J.: *Williams Obstetrics*, 10th Ed. New York, Appleton-Century-Crofts, 1950.)

followed closely with serial measurements of the HCG blood titer. After complete evacuation of a molar pregnancy, the titer should be normal within 8 weeks. Follow-up is continued for 6 to 12 months because, although more than 80% of patients require no further treatment after evacuation of the mole, about 10% develop invasive mole and 2 to 3% have choriocarcinoma.

Invasive Mole

An invasive mole is one in which molar tissue is found deep in the uterine wall. It appears grossly as a circumscribed, hemorrhagic nodule deep in the uterine wall. Microscopically, one sees the edematous mole villi surrounded by overgrown trophoblastic tissue mixed with hemorrhage. An invasive mole can be thought of as a molar pregnancy with placenta increta. It is not a malignant proliferation but is nevertheless significant because of the risk of uterine rupture.

It is impossible to diagnose invasive mole from uterine curettings. The diagnosis can be established if the uterus is received after hysterectomy, or, more commonly, by an HCG titer that remains elevated after evacuation of a molar pregnancy by curettage.

Invasive mole responds quickly to treatment by chemotherapy, with prompt return of the HCG titer to normal.

Choriocarcinoma

Choriocarcinoma is a malignant tumor of the trophoblast. In choriocarcinoma, the trophoblast grows wildly, without production of villi. This tumor deeply invades the myometrium and rapidly spreads to distant organs. The most common sites of metastasis are lungs, vagina, brain, and liver.

Aside from the 2 to 3% of patients, mentioned previously, with hydatidiform mole who develop choriocarcinoma, the disease can also rarely occur following a normal term delivery and after spontaneous abortion of a nonmolar pregnancy. Typically, patients present with a mild amount of hemorrhage per vagina and their uterus is not enlarged.

If patients with choriocarcinoma are considered as a group, 50% have had a prior hydatidiform mole, 25% give a history of spontaneous abortion, and 25% have had a normal term delivery.

Foci of choriocarcinoma are located deep in the myometrial wall, surrounded by hemorrhage and cavitation of the tissue.

Microscopically, one sees sheets of cytotrophoblast and syncytiotrophoblast cells growing together uncontrollably in a plexiform, double-layer arrangement. Chorionic villi are almost never present.

The diagnosis is usually not made on the basis of uterine curetting, but because of persistently elevated HCG titers and evidence of distant metastases.

Before the discovery in 1956 that choriocarcinoma is sensitive to methotrexate, death from widespread disease occurred in under a year. Now, aggressive chemotherapy with methotrexate and actinomycin D have greatly improved this dismal prognosis.

BREAST

Diseases of the breast are frequent, and breast biopsy is a common surgical procedure. The differential diagnosis of lumps felt in the breast in these cases is essentially "cancer or not cancer."

In the section to follow, the most common breast conditions are described.

Structure and Function

The breast is a special type of secretory gland derived from the skin sweat glands. It is made up of about 12 lobes arranged around a central nipple. The lobes are composed of lobules, or clusters of epithelial cells arranged in gland formations. These gland spaces are drained by a system of ducts that join to form a main excretory duct for each lobe. The main excretory ducts radiate out from the central nipple like the spokes of a wheel. Just beneath the nipple, they dilate into lactiferous sinuses, which act as small reservoirs. Each duct is surrounded by a layer of myoepithelial cells that contracts the ducts and expels the milk when suckling occurs (Fig. 21–16). The ducts are themselves connected to lobules which are composed of ductules ending in blind-end acini.

The lobules and ducts of the breast are supported and held in place by connective tissue, called the stroma. The contour of the breast is filled out by fat tissue. It is largely the amount of fat that determines the size of the breast.

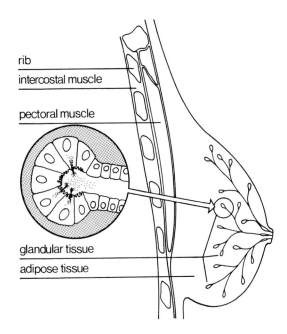

Fig. 21–16 This drawing shows the appearance of the tissues of a normal breast, illustrating the relationship of the lobular architecture to the ducts and to the nipple.

During pregnancy, maternal hormones cross the placenta and stimulate the fetal breast tissue. After delivery, the baby may show mild enlargement of the breast with secretion of small amounts of milk (witch's milk). This condition disappears after a few days.

Up to the time of puberty, the breast structure is similar in males and females. At puberty, hormones produced by the ovaries stimulate an increase in breast size and development of the pigmented areola around the nipple. Estrogen causes the ducts of the breast to elongate and to branch out. Progesterone is thought to act mainly on the lobules and promotes gland formation.

The breast is sensitive to estrogen and progesterone. It responds to the hormonal fluctuations of the menstrual cycle by growth and regression of its epithelial and stromal components. Many women notice increases in breast size and tenderness just before each menstrual period.

Pregnancy provides the major stimulus for growth and complete development of the breast (Fig. 21–17). In addition to elevated levels of estrogen and progesterone, prolactin from the anterior pituitary and special hormones from the placenta (placental lactogen) are present in large amounts. During the early months of pregnancy, further growth of ducts, and particularly lobules, occurs. The breasts become larger and firmer. During the latter part of pregnancy, secretion of nonmilk colostrum begins. Following delivery of the baby, the influence of prolactin is dominant. This hormone causes the lobular epithelial cells to produce milk, which is then secreted into small ducts. When suckling occurs, the posterior pituitary is stimulated to release oxytocin. Oxytocin causes the milk to be propelled along the duct system and to be ejected out of the nipple to the infant. Suckling also stimulates the anterior pituitary to continued prolactin secretion, so that the production of milk will be maintained. Thus, suckling the infant insures a continuous milk supply

Fig. 21–17   A, This histologic section shows the glandular tissue of **normal breast** surrounded by a large area of connective tissue. The dark cells surround a small ductule cavity in this resting state. B, This section is from a **lactating breast.** Here a lobule of secretory epithelium secretes milk into the ductule cavities of each acinus. Compare the relative amount of cell per square unit of surface area in the resting and lactating breasts.

by releasing the hormones that cause milk production (prolactin) and milk ejection (oxytocin) from the pituitary gland.

Breast milk is a unique blend of proteins, lactose, and fatty acids. It also contains immunoglobulins that guard the newborn against certain types of infections. The exact "formula" of breast milk has never been duplicated in the laboratory. Because its mixture of proteins, sugar, and fatty acids is specifically designed to nourish human infants, is

easy to digest, and does not cause allergies, breast milk is the best possible food for newborn babies.

When breast-feeding is stopped (or if the woman did not breast-feed after delivery), the secretory lobules and ducts regress and become less prominent. The breast is again composed mainly of connective tissue, stroma, and fat.

After menopause, the lack of hormonal stimulation by estrogen and progesterone causes a gradual atrophy of the lobules, ducts, and stroma. The breasts become smaller and flattened.

Developmental Conditions

Sometimes an imbalance of hormones causes one or both breasts to become very large. This phenomenon occurs in the adolescent age group and is called virginal hypertrophy. The hypertrophy is mainly due to increased fibrous tissue. The breast ducts show hyperplasia of their epithelial cells. The hypertrophy is permanent and reconstructive surgery is necessary to restore the breast or breasts to their normal size.

Gynecomastia is the name given to hypertrophy of the male breast. It is due to hormonal imbalance in which a relative increase in estrogen as compared to testosterone occurs. Gynecomastia is found in adolescents, and in old age, in patients with cirrhosis of the liver, testicular atrophy, decreased gonadotropin levels (i.e., Klinefelter's syndrome), and in some men receiving estrogen as part of the treatment for carcinoma of the prostate.

The breast ducts become elongated and branching. The surrounding connective tissue undergoes a pale bluish change, and inflammatory cells are present about the ducts. Pronounced gynecomastia must be treated surgically.

Inflammatory Conditions

The most common inflammation of the breast is puerperal mastitis, a bacterial infection occurring in the first few weeks after giving birth. The organisms involved are usually *Staphylococcus aureus* or streptococci. These bacteria invade the breast tissue through cracks or fissures in the nipple, which are common in the early weeks of breast-feeding. The breast appears red, swollen, hot, and tender. The woman may develop chills, fever, and malaise. Treatment consists of antibiotics, local application of heat, and frequent emptying of the affected breast. With prompt treatment, formation of a breast abscess can usually be avoided.

Fibrocystic Disease

Fibrocystic disease or cystic mastitis is a spectrum of common, benign breast abnormalities that occur because the breast tissue is out of phase with the ovarian hormone cycle.

Instead of an orderly pattern of growth and regression, many of the breast elements (the lobules, ducts, myoepithelial cells, intralobular stroma, or general connective tissue) overgrow. The exact pattern produced depends on which of these elements is dominant. Thus one may see multiple dilated ducts or cysts, growth of cells inside ducts, duct structures on an area forming a mass (adenoma), or increased fibrosis around and between lobules. It is usual to see more than one pattern in different areas of the breast.

Fibrocystic disease is common and affects women in the middle and late reproductive years. It may affect one or, more commonly, both breasts. The patient usually notices discomfort in the breast and may feel a lump. The physician may palpate a discrete lump or notice only a poorly defined "thickening." If a cyst is present, aspiration and cytologic examination of the fluid may be helpful in establishing the diagnosis. Mammography or xerography (both x-ray techniques) may better define the abnormal area. However, the best way to identify the nature of these breast "lumps" is by direct observation through the microscope. The breast tissue can be sampled either by fine needle aspiration cytology or, more accurately, by excisional biopsy. It is not always possible to distinguish a lump of fibrocystic disease from a small lump of carcinoma using only palpation or x-ray studies (Figs. 21-18, 21-19, and 21-20). All breast lumps should be suspected of being cancer until proven otherwise, and only microscopic examination can give the answer.

A commonly asked question is whether fibrocystic disease predisposes to breast cancer. There is no easy answer because fibrocystic disease itself has several facets. What is known is that the presence of cysts or microcysts inside the breast is not a premalignant change. However, when there is a marked and atypi-

Fig. 21-19   This mammogram shows the normal appearance of blood vessels and tissue.

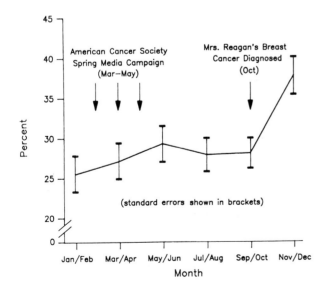

Fig. 21-18   Percentage of women ≥ 50 years of age who had a screening mammogram in the last year, by interview month, 1987. (From Centers for Disease Control, Morbidity and Mortality Weekly Report, 38(9):138, 1989.)

cal hyperplasia of cells within the ducts, the risk for subsequent development of cancer can be as high as 5 fold.

Neoplasms

Fibroadenoma

The fibroadenoma is a benign breast tumor formed by an overgrowth of connective tissue and haphazardly branching ducts. It is found in young women and is usually small although it may grow rapidly during pregnancy.

The fibroadenoma is a well-defined nodule; typically, it can easily be "shelled out" at the time of surgery. It is rubbery, white, moist, and lobulated.

Papilloma

A papilloma is a small epithelial mass growing inside a large duct lumen or cyst cavity, where it looks

Fig. 21–20 Mammogram *A* shows dysplasia, a diffuse abnormality, otherwise called fibrocystic disease. *B* shows a carcinoma of the breast.

like a raspberry attached to the wall. Because of its location, the papilloma frequently causes a cloudy or bloody nipple discharge that brings the patient to the physician.

Although most intraductal papillomas are benign, some may become malignant, and these lesions should be excised.

Carcinoma

Carcinoma of the breast is the most common cancer in women. About 140,000 new cases are diagnosed, and 40,000 patients die from breast cancer each year in the United States. Not so long ago breast cancer used to be the leading cause of cancer deaths in women. Now, as in men, lung cancer has taken the lead. This does not mean that the incidence of breast cancer has decreased. Indeed, it is estimated that 1 of 15 North American women will develop breast cancer in her lifetime. The disease also occurs rarely in men.

Breast cancer is more frequent in women who have never been pregnant, in sisters and daughters of breast cancer patients, and in patients who have previously had certain types of benign breast disease—particularly the types of fibrocystic disease where the duct epithelium shows hyperplasia or atypia. Women who have had a carcinoma in one breast are at risk for developing carcinoma in the other breast. This risk is estimated at about 1% per year. Pregnancy before age 30, frequent pregnancies, and early menopause seem to decrease the risk of breast cancer. Use of oral contraceptive pills has not been found to increase the risk. Breast cancer is much more common in the United States than in Far Eastern countries.

Many breast cancers are sensitive to estrogen and grow more rapidly under its influence. It is possible to determine which tumors are estrogen-dependent and to use this information to help plan subsequent therapy.

The etiology of breast cancer in humans is not known. This is different from breast cancer in mice which is due to a virus. More is known about the mechanisms that control the growth of breast cancer.

Fig. 21–21 This photograph of an elderly patient with **adenocarci-noma** of the right breast shows the indrawing of the nipple and dimpling of the skin. (The Evans Collection, Osler Library, McGill University.)

Besides the growth-promoting effects of estrogen, a number of proto-oncogenes have been found to play a significant role. The most important one is the c-erbB-2 oncogene, also called neu. This is discussed in more detail in Chapter 11. The disease is most common after age 45, but it can also occur in younger women. It is usually discovered by the patient herself as a firm lump. Some cancers are discovered by mammography and are not palpable by the patient or her doctor. These tumors are usually small, are efficiently treated by limited surgery, and most have a good prognosis. This gives a rationale for recommending a routine examination and mammography every year or in alternate years in all women above the age of 40.

The typical patient has a single, hard, non-mobile lump. If the lump is located in the central part of the breast, the nipple may be deformed or inverted (Fig. 21–21). The tumor may be fixed to the overlying skin, causing retraction or ulceration (if advanced). The lump may be fixed to the pectoral muscle lying beneath the breast. Sometimes the skin over a breast cancer resembles the skin of an orange (peau d'orange), owing to infiltration of the connective tissue by tumor.

The tissue is firm and cuts with the same gritty consistency as that of an unripe pear. The cut surface shows an ill-defined opaque mass surrounded by radiating translucent lines of connective tissue containing yellow-white dots and streaks (Fig. 21–22). The tumor is depressed below the cut surface. Its infiltrating nature and the pronounced fibrous tissue response around the tumor cells give it the name "scirrhous" carcinoma.

Other gross appearances of breast cancer are less common and include the soft, large, hemorrhagic medullary carcinoma, papillary carcinoma, and come-

Fig. 21–22 This section of a surgically removed breast shows the firm, whitish tissue in the center, which is **adenocarcinoma.** (McGill University, Department of Pathology Museum.)

docarcinoma (a cancer-filled duct containing a central necrotic area). Paget's disease of the breast is a variant of infiltrating duct carcinoma in which the skin of the nipple and areola covering the tumor shows a red, weeping, scaly appearance. Microscopically, the epidermis contains large vacuolated, so-called Paget's cells.

Most cancers of the breast are carcinoma arising from the epithelial cells of the ducts. Cancer may also arise from the breast lobules (lobular carcinoma), or, rarely, from the connective tissue (sarcomas).

The major route of metastasis is to the lymph nodes, particularly of the axilla. It is estimated that more than 50% of patients have axillary node metastases at the time of initial surgery. Other patients already have deeply located metastatic lymph nodes along the internal mammary arteries. The skin lymphatics may be involved, or the disease may spread across to the opposite breast. Tumor cells can also disseminate via the blood vessels to distant sites, most commonly in the lungs and pleura (more than 50% of cases), and in the liver, bones, brain, adrenal glands, and ovaries.

The standard treatment for breast carcinoma used to be radical mastectomy, in which the breast, pectoral muscle, and axillary contents were removed. Currently the treatment consists of the modified radical mastectomy which includes breast and axillary lymph nodes. More recently, surgery consists of excision of the lump, with or without x-ray therapy or chemotherapy. Patients with estrogen-dependent tumors and known metastases are often also treated with hormonal manipulations using hormone analogues that block the growth-promoting effects of endogenous estrogens. The exact method of treatment depends on the type and size of the lesion, on the presence of known metastases, and the efficacy of combined therapy. Clinical studies are currently in progress in an attempt to determine the best approach to this disease. That the overall 10-year survival rate (about 50%) has not changed significantly in the past 40 years reflects the need for continuing research in this area.

SYNOPSIS

Bleeding from the uterus in excessive amounts or at unusual times should always be investigated.

Carcinoma of the cervix is common and can be diagnosed early either by smear or biopsy. Carcinoma of the endometrium is less common and occurs at an older age.

Infections of the female genitourinary tract occur most commonly in the urinary bladder (cystitis), fallopian tubes (salpingitis), and occasionally in the endometrium (endometritis). Puerperal sepsis used to be much more significant as a life-threatening disease than it is today.

Benign tumors of the female genitourinary tract include leiomyomas of the uterus and cysts of the ovary of different designations.

Malignant tumors of importance are carcinoma of the cervix and adenocarcinoma of the endometrium. Tumors of the ovary are less common.

Mammary dysplasia is the commonest disease of the female breast. Biopsy is the surest way to confirm the diagnosis.

Carcinoma of the breast is a common important lesion with a tendency to early local metastases and generalized metastases. All single nodules of the breast should be regarded as malignant until proven otherwise.

Terms

Menorrhagia	Cervical intra-epithelial neoplasia	Carcinoma of endometrium
Metrorrhagia	Chorionepithelioma	Salpingitis
Amenorrhea	Choriocarcinoma	Dermoid cyst
Leiomyoma	Human papilloma virus	Teratoma
Endometrium	Hydatidiform mole	Fibroadenoma
Endometritis	Carcinoma of cervix	Adenocarcinoma of the breast
Endometriosis		

FURTHER READING

Adami, H.O., et al.: Chapter II. Breast cancer etiology. Intl. J. Cancer, Supp. 5:22, 1990.

Adami, H.O., et al.: The incidence of ovarian cancer in Sweden, 1960–84. Am. J. Epidemiol., 132:446, 1990.
Editorial: Genital herpes and cervical carcinoma. Br. Med. J., 1:807, 1978.

Blaustein, A. (Ed.): *Pathology of the Female Genital Tract*. New York, Springer-Verlag, 1977.

Bottoms, S.F., et al.: The increase in the cesarean birth rate. N. Engl. J. Med., 302:559, 1980.

Brinton, L.A., and Fraumeni, J.F. Epidemiology of uterine cervical cancer. J. Chron. Dis. 39:1051, 1986.

Broadbent, R.V., and Reid, M.H.: Mammography—misunderstood and underutilized. Mammography, 7:93, 1981.

Bronson, F.H., and Manning, J.M.: The energetic regulation of ovulation: A realistic role for body fat. Biol. of Reproduction, 44:945, 1991.

Cates, W., and Wasserheit, J.N.: Genital chlamydial infections: Epidemiology and reproductive sequelae. Am. J. Obstet. Gynecol., 164:1771, 1991.

Chiapetta, C., Kirkland, J.L., Loosemitchell, D.S., et al.: Estrogen regulates expression of the jun family of protooncogenes in the uterus. J. Ster. Biochem. Molec. Biol., 41:113, 1992.

Cowan, B.D., and Morrison, J.C.: Management of abnormal genital bleeding in girls and women. N. Engl. J. Med., 324:1710, 1991.

Crile, G., Jr.: The case for local excision of breast cancer in selected cases. Lancet, 1:549, 1972.

Curran, J.W.: Economic consequences of pelvic inflammatory disease in the United States. Am. J. Ob/Gyn., 138:848, 1980.

DeBuono, B.A., et al.: Sexual behavior of college women in 1975, 1986, and 1989. N. Engl. J. Med., 322:821, 1990.

DiSaia, P.J., Morrow, C.P., and Townsend, D.E.: *Synopsis of Gynecologic Oncology*. New York, John Wiley & Sons, 1975.

Dorfman, S.F.: Maternal mortality in New York City. Obstet. Gynecol., 76:317, 1990.

Faro, S.: *Chlamydia trachomatis*: Female pelvic infection. Am. J. Obstet. Gynecol., 164:1767, 1991.

Galloway D.A., McDougall J.K.: HPV and carcinomas. Adv. Virus Res., 37:125, 1989.

Goldfarb, J.M., and Little, A.B.: Abnormal vaginal bleeding. N. Engl. J. Med., 302:666, 1980.

Goldzielier, J.W., and Dozier, T.S.: Oral contraceptives and thromboembolism: a reassessment. Am. J. Obstet. Gynecol., 123:878, 1975.

Goodman, M.J.: Breast cancer in multi-ethnic populations: the Hawaii perspective. Breast Cancer Research and Treatment, 18:S5, 1991.

Haagensen, C.D.: *Diseases of the Breast*, 2nd Ed. Philadelphia, W.B. Saunders Co., 1971.

Hall J.M., Zuppan P.J., Anderson L.A., et al.: Oncogenes and human breast cancer. Am. J. Hum. Genet., 44:577, 1989.

Harlap, S.: Gender of infants conceived on different days of the menstrual cycle. N. Engl. J. Med., 300:1445, 1979.

Hendersen, B.E., and Bernstein, L.: The international variation in breast cancer rates: An epidemiological assessment. Breast Cancer Research and Treatment, 18:S11, 1991.

Henderson, I.C., and Canellos, G.P.: Cancer of the breast: The past decade. N. Engl. J. Med., 302:17, 1980.

Herbst, A.L. (Ed.): Intrauterine exposure to diethyl stilbestrol in the human. American College of Obstetricians and Gynecologists, Proceedings of Symposium on DES, 1977.

Holmes, K.K., Eschenbach, D.A., and Knapp, J.S.: Salpingitis: overview of etiology and epidemiology. Am. J. Obstet. Gynecol., 138:893, 1980.

Houlston, R.S., McCarter, E., Parbhoo, S., et al.: Family history and risk of breast cancer. J. Med. Gen., 29:154, 1992.

Jensen, E.V.: Hormone dependency of breast cancer. Cancer, 47:2319, 1981.

Kritchevsky, D.: Nutrition and breast cancer. Cancer, 66:1321, 1990.

LiVolsi, V.A., et al.: Fibrocystic breast disease in oral-contraceptive users: histopathological evaluation of epithelial atypia. N. Engl. J. Med., 299:381, 1978.

Mack, T.M., et al.: Estrogens and endometrial carcinoma in a retirement community. N. Engl. J. Med., 294:1262, 1976.

Maguire, Jr., H.C., Greene M.I.: The neu (c-erbB-2) oncogene. Semin. Oncol., 16:148, 1989.

McCormack, W.M., et al.: Sexually transmitted conditions among women college students. Am. J. Obstet. Gynecol., 139:130, 1981.

McKenna, T.J.: Current concepts: Pathogenesis and treatment of polycystic ovary syndromes. N. Engl. J. Med., 318:558, 1988.

McKinlay, S.M., Brambilla, D.J., and Posner, J.G.: The normal menopause transition. Maturitas, 14:103, 1992.

Ogra, P.L., and Greene, H.L.: Human milk and breast feeding: an update on the state of the art. Pediatr. Res., 16:266, 1982.

Perez, R.P., et al.: Ovarian cancer biology. Semin. Oncol., 18:186, 1991.

Piver, S.M., et al.: Epidemiology and etiology of ovarian cancer. Semin. Oncol., 18:177, 1991.

Popkin, D.R.: Early diagnosis of ovarian cancer. Can. Med. Assoc. J., 120:1106, 1979.

Pytkowicz Streissguth, A., et al.: Teratogenic effects of alcohol in humans and laboratory animals. Science, 209:353, 1980.

Resnick, S.D.: Toxic shock syndrome: Recent developments in pathogenesis. J. Pediatr., 116:321, 1990.

Schachter, J.: Sexually transmitted infections and cervical atypia. Sexually Transmitted Dis., 8(Suppl):353, 1981.

Schindler, A.E., and Schmidt, G.: Post-menopausal bleeding: a study of more than 1000 cases. Maturitas, 2:269, 1980.

Schuchat, A., and Broome, C.V.: Toxic shock syndrome and tampons. Epidemiol. Rev., 13:99, 1991.

Skolnick M.H., Marshall C.J., Schumann G.B., and Eyre H.J.: Inheritance of proliferative breast disease in breast cancer kindreds. Science, 250:1715, 1990.

Smith, D.C., et al.: Association of exogenous estrogen and endometrial carcinoma. N. Engl. J. Med., 293:1164, 1975.

Spencer, J.D., Millis, R.R., and Hayward, J.L.: Contraceptive steroids and breast cancer. Br. Med. J., 1:1024, 1978.

Speroff, L., Glass, R.H., and Kase, N.G.: *Clinical Gynecologic Endocrinology and Infertility*, 2nd Ed. Baltimore, Williams & Wilkins, 1978.

Stadel, B.V.: Oral contraceptives and cardiovascular disease. N. Engl. J. Med., 305:612, 1981.

Staffa, J.A., et al. Progestins and breast cancer—an epidemiologic review. Fert. Steril., 57:473, 1992.

Thomas, D.B.: Rapporteur's report—epidemiology. Breast Cancer Research and Treatment 18:S31, 1991.

Trussell, J.T., Hatcher, R.A., Cates, Jr., W., et al.: A guide to interpreting contraceptive efficacy studies. Obstet. Gynecol., 76:558, 1990.

Ziel, H.G., and Finkle, W.D.: Increased risk of endometrial carcinoma among users of conjugated estrogens. N. Engl. J. Med., 293:1167, 1975.

Zur Hausen H., et al.: Papillomaviruses. In *Advances in Viral Oncology*, Edited by G. Klein. New York, Raven Press, 1989, p. 1.

22

ENDOCRINE SYSTEM

The heart has its reasons, and the endocrines have theirs.—A. Huxley

The body has two major communication networks that enable its many parts to operate in a coordinated, efficient manner. One of these is the nervous system, in which messages are passed from neuron to neuron, as a network of wires connects all the telephones of a city. Communication depends on the integrity of these neurons, and if the wires were cut, communication would cease just as in our telephone system.

The other major communication network is the subject of this chapter, namely, the endocrine system. Endocrine communication is not like telephone communication; it generally does not depend on wires. It is more like radio communication, of which the essential elements are transmitter, signal, and receivers. The signal is not transmitted by wires to a specific destination, rather it is carried through the blood all over the body, just as any radio in the general area will receive a radio message. Thus endocrine signals may come into contact with cells throughout the body; however, some cells, like radio receivers tuned to the right frequency, are particularly sensitive to and dependent on the signals, and these are referred to as the "target organ." For example, the pituitary secretes adrenocorticotropic hormones (ACTH) into the blood, which carries the hormone all over the body. However, the cells of the adrenal cortex appear to be the principal ones to respond to this signal, as far as we know. Like radio receivers, organs have "receptors" which are becoming increasingly well characterized.

Endocrine organs were commonly referred to as glands, a term that connotes secretion of a substance. Endocrine glands secrete their products into the blood (as opposed to exocrine glands, which secrete onto a surface, e.g., sweat glands).

The products of endocrine organs are called **hormones;** these are the chemical signals we have mentioned. Hormones are substances of different kinds: steroids (cortisone), proteins (growth hormones), peptides (antidiuretic hormone), amino acids (thyrox-

ine), or amines (epinephrine). They range from large to small molecules and have chemical structures of varying complexity. The term hormone (which means "to set in motion") was introduced at the turn of the century from the work of Bayliss and Starling, who demonstrated that there were substances that could initiate secretion in a distant organ.

The endocrine system includes all endocrine organs and their products, the hormones. This system is composed of anatomically and histologically distinct parts, possessing many individual functions. However, the system as a whole is regarded as having a regulatory function. It is the system that, on orders from above, regulates and coordinates many of the functions of the organism.

Historically, we came to understand the function of endocrine organs largely through the effects of their destruction. Disorders of the endocrine system are the result of lesions in the transmitting organ (or occasionally in the target receptor; Fig. 22–1). Whereas a lesion in the wires of the nervous system may have disastrous results, this kind of signal disruption is not possible in the endocrine system. However, lesions in the endocrine system may have lethal ramifications. This situation may be compared with that of an army general whose radio transmitter breaks, which causes all troops, who depend on his orders, to fail to function in an orderly way. The troops may simply not act, or they may act in an unregulated fashion.

There are three important principles of endocrine disease that should be kept in mind:

1. Endocrine disease can arise from a malfunction of control mechanism (a breakdown in the transmitter).
2. Such a malfunction may lead to insufficient, excessive, or inappropriate emission of signal. Any of these alternatives leads to disordered function. For example, when the anterior pituitary

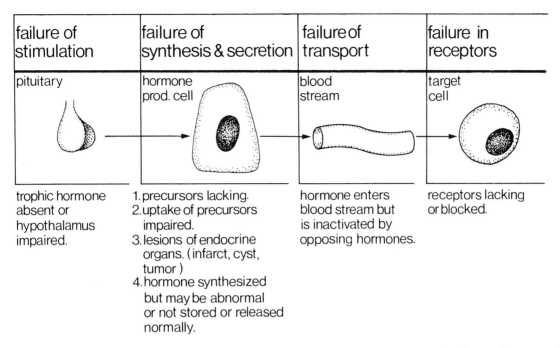

failure of stimulation	failure of synthesis & secretion	failure of transport	failure in receptors
pituitary	hormone prod. cell	blood stream	target cell
trophic hormone absent or hypothalamus impaired.	1. precursors lacking. 2. uptake of precursors impaired. 3. lesions of endocrine organs. (infarct, cyst, tumor) 4. hormone synthesized but may be abnormal or not stored or released normally.	hormone enters blood stream but is inactivated by opposing hormones.	receptors lacking or blocked.

Fig. 22–1 This diagram illustrates different reasons for the **failure of hormone action**. Failure of stimulation, of synthesis and secretion, of transport, and in receptors are all easy to understand conceptually, but each may be difficult to prove in an individual patient.

is destroyed by necrosis, all the target organs, whose functioning depends on pituitary hormones become atrophied. Conversely, when a tumor of the eosinophilic cells of the anterior pituitary produces excess growth hormone an afflicted child may grow up to be a great basketball player, with a height of 7 or 8 feet. Finally, a diseased endocrine gland may secrete more or less or the right amount of hormone, but at the wrong times. Acromegaly, which is a syndrome caused by excessive secretion of the growth hormone, is an example of this last type of disorder.

3. Although most hormones may demonstrate their effects on a single target most obviously, since hormones are chemical messengers that circulate to all tissues and cells, the absence or excess of their effects may be seen in all tissues. To be more specific, whereas endocrine disorders such as hyperthyroidism may be viewed as a disturbance of the control mechanisms of thyroid hormone production, the effects of excessive thyroxine can be detected not only in skeletal and cardiac muscle, but also in biochemical and submicroscopic lesions in the liver, as well as in the general behavior of the patient. Conversely, the destruction of the thyroid gland causes many symptoms that are manifest in the attitude of the torpid patient.

Thus endocrine diseases may be best viewed as **multisystem disorders,** that is, their effects cut across anatomic boundaries and create disorders of function in many different parts of the body. They are not confined to one system alone.

In this chapter, we first consider the pituitary, its relationship to the hypothalamus and its target organs, then the adrenal, thyroid, and parathyroid glands, and, finally, the islets of Langerhans (Table 22–1). The testes and ovary have already been considered in chapters on the male and female genitourinary system, respectively.

PITUITARY

This small organ, about the size of a cherry pit, is hidden deep in the skull. It develops from an outpouching of the oral cavity during embryonic life and comes to rest dead center at the base of the brain, attached to it by the most slender stalk (Fig. 22–2). This stalk carries nerves from the hypothalamus to the posterior part, but only blood vessels to the anterior portion. The blood supply of the anterior pituitary is curious because, unlike any other in the body (usually a simple extension of the arterial blood supply, with the standard arrangement of capillaries and veins), it consists entirely of venous blood from the hypothalamus (the anterior pituitary receives no arterial blood),

Table 22–1. Endocrine Glands, Hormones, and Their Effects

ENDOCRINE GLAND	HORMONE	EFFECT
HYPOTHALAMUS	Thyrotropin releasing factor (TRF)	Stimulates the anterior pituitary to secrete thyrotropic hormone (TSH).
ANTERIOR PITUITARY	Thyrotropic hormone (thyroid stimulating hormone, TSH)	Stimulates thyroxine formation and release from the thyroid gland.
	Adenocorticotropic hormone (corticotropin, ACTH)	Stimulates the adrenal cortex to secrete cortisone.
	Follicle-stimulating hormone (FSH)	♂: Stimulates development of germinal epithelium in testes and, therefore, spermatogenesis as well. ♀: Induces maturation of ovarian follicle.
	Interstitial cell-stimulating hormone (ICSH, luteining hormone, LH)	♂: Stimulates interstitial cells of testes to produce testosterone. ♀: Develops corpus luteum.
	Prolactin	♂: No known action. ♀: Maintains activity in fully developed corpus luteum and stimulates milk secretion.
POSTERIOR PITUITARY*	Oxytocin	Stimulates pregnant uterus to contract.
	Vasopressin (antidiuretic hormone ADH)	Promotes reabsorption of water from distal tubule in the kidney.
THYROID	Thyroxine (T_4) Triiodothyronine (T_3)	Increases metabolism in most tissues of the body.
PARAFOLLICULAR CELLS OF THYROID	Calcitonin	Inhibits reabsorption of calcium from bone (lowers serum calcium level).
PARATHYROID	Parathormone	Mobilizes calcium and phosphorus from bone (increases serum calcium level).
ADRENAL CORTEX	Aldosterone	Stimulates sodium and chloride reabsorption in the kidney. Promotes potassium excretion.
	Cortisone	Regulates carbohydrate metabolism (and is used clinically to suppress inflammation).
	Androgens	Promote masculinization.
ADRENAL MEDULLA	Epinephrine and Norepinephrine	Neurotransmission. Preparation for "flight or fight."
PANCREAS: B CELLS	Insulin	Lowers blood glucose. Mobilizes glycogen from liver.
TESTIS	Testosterone	Develops male secondary characteristics.
OVARY	Estrogen	Develops female secondary characteristics. Helps to regulate menstruation.
CORPUS LUTEUM	Progesterone	Prepares uterus for implantation of fertilized ovum during "luteal" phase of menstrual cycle.

* Hormones secreted by the posterior pituitary are not in fact produced there. They are formed in the hypothalamus, in nerve cells that have long axons extending down into the posterior pituitary (hence the synonym: *neuro*hypophysis). The pituitary stores and secretes these hormones.

so the blood to the pituitary has already been circulated to a part of the brain.

This venous blood divides into a second capillary network that arborizes around the cells of the anterior pituitary. The arrangement is elegantly suited to the transport of chemical messengers arising in the brain itself, for this is how the pituitary receives its signals. It is not by a system of wires, but by a hydraulic waterway. It is now clear that the anterior pituitary produces its hormonal products intermittently, in spurts that are greatly dependent on the functioning of the central nervous system. Figure 22–3 shows the rhythmic and pulsatile secretion of a variety of hormones from the anterior pituitary, each of which is modulated, if not governed, by stimuli from the hypothalamus through the mechanism of releasing hormones.

The hypothalamus itself receives signals from the afferent or incoming pathways such as sight, smell, temperature, even hunger, and especially rage and fright. Its connection to the pituitary thus makes it possible for the experience of the world to be interpreted and reacted to, preparing the individual by grading and stimulating or by inhibiting the hormone production from the pituitary by its own products, those small polypeptides known as releasing or inhibitory hormones. These polypeptides are secreted into the vascular system just described, and are received and reacted to by anterior pituitary cells. Hormonal products of the anterior pituitary cells are quickly cir-

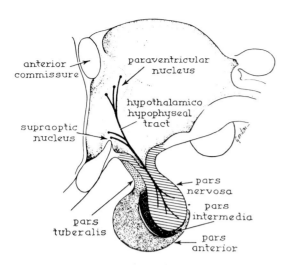

Fig. 22–2 This drawing shows the **relationship of the pituitary to the hypothalamus.** The tracts joining the hypothalamus to the pituitary are illustrated as heavy black lines. The anterior pituitary is shown in the stipple, the pars intermedia in the dark shading, and the pars nervosa or posterior pituitary by the cross-hatching. (From Ham, A. W.: *Histology*, 7th Ed. Philadelphia, J. B. Lippincott Co., 1974.)

culated in the blood stream to all parts of the body, where they may signal for more testosterone, more thyroxine, or more cortisone, for example.

A second and important aspect of the blood supply to the anterior pituitary is that the cells are also exposed to direct chemical messengers from the rest of the body, so that signals of hypoglycemia, high serum sodium levels, and the feedback hormones from the peripheral endocrine organs are all constantly perfusing these cells. These signals are received simultaneously, together with those from the hypothalamus. This arrangement permits a finely graded tuning that makes the life of an air traffic controller at a major international airport seem simple by comparison.

The secretion of the releasing hormones from the hypothalamus depends in turn on biologic rhythm such as the sleep-waking cycle, but it may be modified by anxiety, stress, exercise, and diet. For an outline of the principal hormones turn to the Appendix, p. 491.

Hyperfunction of the Anterior Pituitary

Despite the fact that at least 5 important hormones (growth hormone, ACTH, FSH, LH, and TSH) are synthesized and secreted by anterior pituitary cells, there is a good correlation between structural abnormality and evidence of overproduction for only the first two of these hormones. In most cases of gigantism, there is an adenoma of the eosinophilic cells of the pituitary (Fig. 22–4), as there is in most cases of the adult form of excess growth hormone production,

commonly called acromegaly. Excessive ACTH production causes a pattern of abnormalities collected together under the term Cushing's syndrome, named after the neurosurgeon who recognized the relationship to the adenoma of basophils of the pituitary. Oddly, overproduction of FSH, LH, and TSH are clinically rare, and tumors responsible for their production have not been recognized. The occurrence of galactorrhea (milk secretion without pregnancy) is being found more frequently, and adenomas of prolactin-producing cells are seen often, thanks to newer diagnostic methods (radioimmunoassay), and to developments in the surgery of the anterior pituitary.

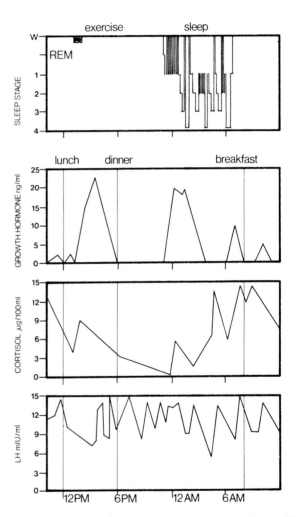

Fig. 22–3 This set of graphs illustrates human activities during a full 24-hour day. The top graph illustrates the levels of growth hormone at different times, illustrating the intermittent nature of the secretion of growth hormone and its relationship to exercise and sleep. Meals, exercise, and sleep are illustrated in the second graph. Cortisol has a diurnal cycle with two peaks, and luteinizing hormone is secreted discontinuously in small amounts throughout the 24-hour period. (From Federman, D.D.: Endocrinology. In *Scientific American Medicine*. Edited by E. Rubinstein and D. D. Federman. New York, Scientific American Illustrated Library, 1979, Vol. I.)

Fig. 22–4 This photograph shows the effect of **hyperfunction of the anterior pituitary**. The woman is of normal height and the giant could be suspected of having a growth-hormone secreting adenoma of the anterior pituitary.

Acromegaly

This term designates the clinical syndrome that arises in adults when there is continuing excessive secretion of the growth hormone. The principal clinical manifestations and their frequency are outlined in Table 22–2. The principal significant abnormalities arise from growth within the pituitary of a clone of cells designated an adenoma. These cells appear to be eosinophilic on routine histologic examination in

Table 22–2. Acromegaly: Frequency of Manifestations

MANIFESTATION	PERCENTAGE OF CASES
Enlarged sella turcica	93
Headache	85
Visual impairment	62
Secondary to growth hormone excess:	
Weight gain	39
Hypermetabolism	70
Excessive sweating	60
Impaired glucose tolerance	25
Clinical diabetes mellitus	12
Growth of flat bones	100
Prognathism	Common
Arthritic complaints	Common
Osteoporosis	Common
Soft tissue growth	100
Hypertrichosis	53
Pigmentation	40

most cases. The patient with acromegaly produces only small amounts of growth hormone, but does it continually, unlike normal persons, whose growth hormone secretion is triggered by the many stimuli we have outlined. Sleep is the usual principal signal to growth hormone secretion, and the sleep need not be long. Thus the catnap or regular afternoon snooze has a valuable endocrinologic result. This only underscores the wisdom of our parents who used to insist on an afternoon nap for all growing children, which we thought was only to give the parents some time away from looking after us.

Acromegaly is probably less often diagnosed than it might be, since, as with many insidious and slowly progressive disorders, the diagnosis does not become evident until the suspicion of its existence has crossed the mind of the consulting physician. This discovery is usually long after the patient has become symptomatic. Typically, this disorder of too much growth hormone in the adult appears in his or her 40s or 50s with headaches, sweating, weakness, fatigue, and lethargy. These symptoms are all nonspecific in themselves. The presence of disturbances in vision should always suggest that the structures around the optic chiasm be investigated. Although x-ray studies of the pituitary fossa may be normal in up to one quarter of acromegalics, most patients show abnormalities of the sella turcica, that small pocket in which the pituitary sits. In one study, 138 of 140 patients examined by x-ray showed abnormalities!

The expression of acromegaly in the features and extremities of the unfortunate patient is memorable, as the accompanying photos demonstrate (Fig. 22–5), but the family, friends, and attending physician, as well as the patient, may all be oblivious to the slow changes that finally culminate in the coarsened facial appearance, prominent forehead, widened teeth, and change in hat size. A husky voice, a need for new and larger gloves, and increasing deafness all may be signs of acromegaly. The prognosis of the untreated acromegalic is guarded, since many of them die with heart failure before the age of 60, for unknown reasons. One suggestion is that the constant secretion of excessive amounts of growth hormone requires unusual protein synthesis from heart muscle, and that this departure from normal leads to the increased size and eventual failure of this organ. Other complications of acromegaly are atherosclerosis, hypertension, and diabetes mellitus.

The diagnosis of the disease can now be easily confirmed by growth hormone assay (particularly of the cerebrospinal fluid) and treated by surgery to remove the adenoma, or with such drugs as bromocriptine.

Fig. 22–5   The progression of **acromegaly** is illustrated in these photographs: *A*, normal, age 9 years; *B*, age 16 years with possible early coarsening of features; *C*, age 33 years, well-established acromegaly; *D*, age 52 years, end-stage acromegaly with gross disfigurement. (Clinical Pathological Conference. Am. J. Med., 20:133, 1956.)

Prolactin Overproduction and Galactorrhea

The result of hypersecretion of prolactin is milk secretion in individuals, either male or female. The hormone prolactin may have physiologic effects in addition to causing milk secretion, but we do not yet know what they are. Many persons, however, may have overproduction of prolactin without milk production. The commonest cause of excess prolactin secretion is the presence of a chromophobe adenoma. Its appearance may be signaled by the involvement of the optic chiasm by the slowly growing tumor. The presence of an enlarged sella turcica is the warning to search for excess prolactin or growth hormone in the serum of the patient. However, in an era of drug therapy for every illness, real or imagined, another common cause of elevated prolactin levels and/or of abnormal milk secretion is the use of drugs that influence the hypothalamus (methyldopa, reserpine), or drugs such as monoamine oxidase inhibitors, phenothiazines, or estrogens. Thus the presence of an excessive amount of hormone in response to testing or the recognition of milk secretion may not, in fact, be due to a tumor.

Cushing's Disease

Although this subject is normally considered under diseases of the adrenals, since adrenal cortical hyperfunction is responsible for the excessive hormone production that leads to the signs and symptoms described by Harvey Cushing, he correctly ascribed the disorder to a functional basophil adenoma of the anterior pituitary. Thus the disorder should at least be mentioned as we consider disorders of hyperfunction of the anterior pituitary. For a further discussion of Cushing's disease and of Cushing's syndrome, we refer the reader to the sections on the adrenal in this chapter.

Hypofunction of the Anterior Pituitary

The pituitary may fail to produce hormones in two ways. The most common deficiency is called panhypopituitarism, since it is a deficiency of all the functions and may be caused by a variety of means, such as tumors that compress or destroy the gland from within or without, necrosis, or cysts. The less common deficiency is the absence of a single pituitary hormone, which is conventionally called monotropic deficiency. These deficiencies may be gonadotropic (usually both FSH and LH hormones are lacking, generally owing to a congenital deficiency of hypothalamic-releasing hormone). A lack of TSH may occur rarely; a lack of ACTH alone has been reported, but it is also rare and difficult to prove.

We might venture that the anterior pituitary is the only endocrine gland in which destruction by tumor is a significant or relatively common cause of hypofunction. The adrenal cortex and thyroid are rarely, if ever, so destroyed by the common metastatic tumors. The commonest cause of panhypopituitarism is compression by a tumor known as the chromophobe adenoma, discussed more completely in the chapter on the nervous system. Another tumor is the craniopharyngioma, a tumor of childhood, and the third commonest cause is metastasis, usually from breast or lung cancer.

Panhypopituitarism

There are some different clinical manifestations of panhypopituitarism, depending in part on the age of the patient (if it occurs before growth is completed, the person may be dwarfed), his or her sex (since menstrual irregularities may be the most prominent feature), or whether the pituitary function is lost gradually or suddenly.

The general rule for the deficiencies of hormone production, particularly when several hormones are lacking as in panhypopituitarism, is that the person may complain of some problem that is not obviously central to the loss of these several normal, human drives. Thus a male patient with panhypopituitarism may complain of being mistaken for a woman on the telephone, rather than complain directly about impotence. A peculiar apathy and listlessness of which the patient may not be aware may characterize panhypopituitarism. The woman may first recognize something is amiss when she has no menstrual period, owing to the lack of gonadotropic hormones (FSH and LH). The absence of growth hormone, thyroid-stimulating hormone, and ACTH may go unnoticed, as these hormones lead more slowly to changes that may be nonspecific. The man may notice as his first complaint in addition to lassitude, weakness, and fatigue, a loss of sexual desire and function. Of course, if the cause of pituitary destruction is a tumor growing in the optic chiasm, the symptoms may not be referable to the loss of endocrine function, but rather to headaches and interference with vision.

One type of panhypopituitarism, pituitary dwarfism, occurs in children. The lack of hormone produces a mentally alert, normally intelligent, but small and sexually underdeveloped individual, who is much like a graceful and attractive child, and who never grows up, similar to Peter Pan (Fig. 22–6). This type of panhypopituitarism usually results from the presence of a cyst or tumor, which must be distinguished from a genetically determined dwarfism and from congenital hypothyroidism. The genetic dwarf has normal secretion of all hormones except growth hormone, whereas the cretin, or congenital hypothyroid, is condemned to subnormal mentality, and the appearance of the body remains infantile.

Simmonds' disease is the term given to panhypopituitarism occurring in the adult, which results in the absence of all pituitary secretion. The classic cause of this used to be the occurrence in young women of excessive blood loss at the time of delivery. The shock that accompanied this blood loss found a particularly sensitive target in the large, vascular pituitary of pregnancy, which may be 2 or 3 times normal size, and is particularly susceptible to hypotension. Sheean described the occurrences of panhypopituitarism in such young women (Fig. 22–7) and discovered that there was necrosis of the pituitary due sometimes to

Fig. 22–6 Hypophyseal infantilism. Girl on left, age 15 sexually infantile, next to normal sister on right, 2 years younger and fully matured. Striking example of pituitary dwarfism plus sexual infantilism. (Lisser and Escamilla: *Atlas of Clinical Endocrinology,* 2nd Ed. St. Louis, C. V. Mosby Co., 1962.)

Table 22–3. Average Size of Organs in Simmonds' Disease and Acromegaly Compared with Normal

BODY WEIGHT ORGAN	SIMMONDS' DISEASE (4 CASES) 95 LB. GM.	NORMAL GM.	ACROMEGALY (5 CASES) 194 LB. GM.
Heart	175	300	448
Liver	866	1500	2462
Kidney	89	155	247
Spleen	144	200	353
Pancreas	43	100	135
Thyroid	10	40	76
Adrenals (together)	6.4	12	26
Gonads	small	—	normal or large
Thymus	—	—	sometimes enlarged

thrombosis and sometimes simply to ischemic necrosis. The onset of symptoms appeared insidiously during the postpartum period, and months and years later they were found to be changed persons, without thyroid or adrenal function (Table 22–3). Thus to the list of causes of panhypopituitarism, which include tumors (craniopharyngioma, chromophobe adenoma, metastatic tumor), cysts, and granulomatous lesions such as tuberculosis and sarcoid, we may add postpartum necrosis, which carries the eponym **Sheean's syndrome.**

Fig. 22–7 Simmonds' disease. The photograph on the left shows the patient with one of her children taken just before her last pregnancy. At this time she was 32 years old and weighed 140 lbs. The picture on the right was taken 9 years later following a pregnancy accompanied by a massive hemorrhage. Her weight at the time of this photograph was 85½ lbs. She died of panhypopituitarism 3 years later. These photographs were taken before the availability of replacement therapy.

Posterior Pituitary

Any surgical trauma, inflammation, hemorrhage, or tumor may injure the posterior pituitary as well, and may interfere with the exquisite balancing mechanisms that control the tonicity of our blood plasma by regulating water and sodium absorption at the level of the kidneys. This regulation is effected through the secretion of the substance vasopressin. The posterior pituitary also secretes oxytocin. These hormones are synthesized and are secreted in the hypothalamus and are transported along axons that terminate in storage vesicles in the posterior pituitary. Any interference with this mechanism may lead to the syndrome of **diabetes insipidus,** which consists of polyuria (passing large volumes of urine, more than 2,000 ml per day) and polydypsia (the drinking of large volumes of water). This syndrome must be distinguished from the polyuria and polydypsia that accompany the presence of excessive serum glucose in diabetes mellitus and the occurrence of psychogenic water drinking.

ADRENALS

The adrenals are two small glands, each shaped like a cocked hat, one on either side of the aorta, located just above the kidney. Each adrenal consists of two parts, an outer portion or cortex, and an inner portion or medulla. These are not merely two parts; they are two different organs joined together, different in origin, in structure, in function, and in the diseases that visit them. The function of the adrenal gland is difficult to summarize. It does many things, but if one tried to generalize, one might say that it controls the body's adjustments to changes in posture by regulating the tone of blood vessels and the volume of blood, in conjunction with other organs such as the kidney and the heart. It also modulates the intermittent, rather than constant, intake of nourishment. It does this in conjunction with the liver. Finally, the adrenal gland acts as a storehouse for hormones that are used in times of emergency, such as hemorrhage, infection, and shock. The loss of these adrenal functions is a life-threatening phenomenon, as we shall see.

The cortex is essential to life, since, when it is removed, death occurs in a few days. For over 100 years, it has been known that patients with adrenal insufficiency often die from minor infections and stresses that patients with normal adrenals will survive. More than 20 different steroids with different types of physiologic action have been isolated from the adrenal cortex. Roughly, they may be divided into three general groups: (1) those that regulate salt and water metabolism; (2) those that regulate carbohydrate metabolism; and (3) those that modify sexual functions. For persons with a desire to memorize things easily, the three functions may be represented by the letter S, as salt, sugar, and sex. For the others, these categories are the mineralocorticoids, the glucocorticoids, and the androgenic hormones.

Mineralocorticoids. Aldosterone, produced by the cells of the more superficial layer of the cortex, is a hormone that governs sodium and chloride retention and potassium excretion, and thereby controls the amount of water retained in the body. The exogenous administration of aldosterone leads to edema and increase in body weight due to sodium retention. Persons with aldosterone-secreting tumors also complain of fatigue and show electrocardiographic abnormalities because of the depletion of potassium that accompanies sodium retention. Normal levels of aldosterone are essential for life, and the loss of aldosterone production contributes significantly to the syndrome of adrenal cortical insufficiency, known by the name of its discoverer, Addison.

Under normal circumstances, the production of aldosterone is regulated largely by the secretion of renin from the kidney. The small, specialized area of cells, called the juxtaglomerular apparatus discussed in the kidney chapter, detects pressure changes in the blood that perfuses the kidney. Any reduction in blood volume, for example as occurs in hemorrhage, results in decreased perfusion and, therefore, in decreased pressure. This reduction is perceived by the juxtaglomerular apparatus, and its response is the secretion of small granules containing a protein that is converted in the serum and eventually results in increased aldosterone secretion from the adrenal cortex. Teleologically, this is a convenient means of retaining more salt and water, thus increasing the fluid volume that has been lost in the hemorrhage.

Glucocorticoids. Carbohydrate metabolism is regulated by a number of factors. Amino acids may be converted into glucose instead of into protein, raising the supply of serum glucose and contributing to the store of glycogen in the liver by the presence of glucocorticoids. Cortisone and hydrocortisone are produced by the inner layers of the adrenal cortex and are under the regulation of ACTH from the anterior pituitary.

Cortisone has been synthesized and available for over 40 years as part of the physician's equipment. In man, cortisone has an inhibitory effect on lymphoid tissue. Cortisone therefore suppresses the inflammatory response to practically all forms of injury. This anti-inflammatory reaction may relieve the pain and discomfort of inflammation, and is of value in noninfectious inflammation as exemplified by rheumatoid arthritis, but, unfortunately, whereas cortisone relieves the symptoms of disease, it does not influence the cause. It does not put out the fire, nor does it repair the damage after the fire. It could be thought of as providing the tissues with some kind of asbestos suit, which may itself be only temporary. We must remember that inflammation helps the body to mobilize its defenses against infection. When a patient is taking high doses of steroids, inflammation against bacterial invaders is also suppressed. The patient may appear well and show few signs of infection, although he may be experiencing a fulminating bacteremia.

Cortisone is a two-edged sword that must be used with respect and understanding.

Androgens. These hormones tend to masculinize the body, to retain amino acids, and to enhance protein synthesis. Androgenic hormones are used (illegally to be sure, and unwisely in most cases) by weight lifters and those interested in increasing their body strength for questionable purposes. When androgens have been metabolized, the 17-ketosteroids are excreted in the urine. The breakdown products of androgens form the basis for the doping tests used at Olympic events, but the tests are also used in cases of virilism in which some disorders of the adrenal is suspected. Naturally, in adrenal cortical deficiency, the 17-ketosteroid level will be low.

Medulla. The adrenal medulla is derived from the sympathetic nervous system. Unlike the cortex, its secretory products are epinephrine and norepinephrine. These substances have a direct effect on the smooth muscle in the walls of arterioles. They may also have an effect on glycogenolysis, liberating glucose from the stores of glycogen in the liver into the serum. In severe stress, such as rage or fear, surgical operations, or any life-threatening event, epinephrine is poured into the blood; in the words of Cannon, the person is prepared for "flight or fight" and may be enabled to perform extraordinary feats during this emergency.

Hypoadrenalism

Adrenal cortical insufficiency should be thought of in two general ways. First, it may be a medical emergency that, if not recognized, could result in the patient's death within hours. However, the commonest form is a chronic and insidious adrenal cortical insufficiency, which is often not recognized. The second general idea is that adrenal cortical insufficiency can either originate in the adrenals (and it is necessary for both adrenals to be involved), or it may be due to absence of the tropic hormone ACTH, owing to destruction or disease of the anterior pituitary. We have come to talk about primary adrenal insufficiency—that originating in the adrenals, and secondary adrenal insufficiency—that which is not due to disease of the adrenals themselves, but rather to disease of the anterior pituitary (lack of ACTH) and which therefore causes atrophy of the adrenal glands.

Today, the causes of adrenal insufficiency are different from those recognized by Addison 130 years ago. They are also different from those recognized 50 years ago. The three most important causes of adrenal insufficiency in Addison's day were tuberculosis, tuberculosis, and tuberculosis. With the control of this disease, the most common finding in Addisonian patients now is a lymphocytic infiltration of the adrenal cortex with patches of fibrosis, seen in three-quarters of such patients. Two-thirds of these cases show immunofluorescent antibodies to an antigen derived from adrenal cell cytoplasm. These observations are interpreted as evidence for an autoimmune adrenalitis, the initiating cause of which remains obscure. We need not go into other associations that have been made with this discovery, such as the occurrence of autoimmune thyroiditis, but pass on to other causes of adrenal insufficiency before discussing their clinical manifestations.

Today, tuberculosis is still a significant cause of Addison's disease, but it probably accounts for chronic adrenal insufficiency only about 1 case in 10. It used to be far and away the most common cause.

A third cause of chronic adrenal insufficiency is the atrophy that occurs with the long-term administration of exogenous corticosteroid for such disorders as arthritis and regional ileitis. The adrenal cortex becomes smaller and, if the steroids are withdrawn, the patient is unable to meet the normal requirements of hormone, which inability may precipitate a crisis. Alternate-day therapy with cortisone seems to be a way to attempt to resolve this atrophy. The cause of adrenal atrophy is called iatrogenic, naturally. There are also other instances in which there is no apparent reason for the adrenal failure, and we call those cases idiopathic. At present, autoimmune, tuberculous, and iatrogenic causes lead the list of causes of chronic adrenal failure.

The patient with **Addison's disease** (usually a woman) complains of weakness, loss of appetite, nausea, irritability, and orthostatic hypotension. These nonspecific symptoms are so universal that almost anyone might think that he has Addison's disease. However, two other observations should suggest the diagnosis as well as the appropriate laboratory examination to confirm the suspicion. Increased pigmentation of the skin occurs in almost all patients with primary adrenal cortical failure, since the feedback inhibition of the anterior pituitary is lacking. Owing to decreased cortisol production or lack of it, the anterior pituitary continues to secrete ACTH, and with it there is an excess of melanocyte-stimulating hormone, which causes the pigmentation. Of course, in cases of pituitary failure with secondary adrenal atrophy, the pigmentation does not occur. The second observation is the recognition of a low systolic and diastolic blood pressure. The person with Addison's disease may have a decreased blood volume and a loss of regulation of the normal responses that control blood pressure, because of the absence of the hormone that regulates salt and water retention. Thus hypotension and the sudden occurrence of life-threatening shock are all part of the syndrome of hypoadrenalism.

Acute adrenal cortical insufficiency is a problem with different causes and different clinical manifestations and implications. The person with adrenal insufficiency is in immediate danger of death. It is a medical emergency that often produces shock with prostration, hypoglycemia, and nausea and vomiting. Thus the explanation for the crisis may be confusing, because of the apparent gastrointestinal symptoms. Laboratory diagnosis is helpful, but the delay in waiting for the results of the serum sodium and potassium could be fatal. The appropriate treatment in cases of collapse from suspected acute adrenal cortical insufficiency is immediate administration of cortisol and other supportive measures.

The pathogenesis of acute adrenal cortical insufficiency is best understood in terms of two ideas. First, it may be superimposed on chronic disease, by which the adrenal cortical reserve has been eroded by chronic destruction and replacement or by atrophy of the gland. When a sudden challenge such as infection or a trauma occurs, the unfortunate patient has no ability to manufacture or to secrete supplemental steroids. Thus the crisis is due to a marked discrepancy between the need and the ability to respond. The second setting is the one in which the adrenal has been functioning normally, but is the site of sudden destruction. Most commonly, this phenomenon occurs because the highly vascular adrenal is the site of massive hemorrhage and necrosis. The causes of this pathologic process are usually septicemia, often from the meningococcus. This second type of insufficiency occasionally occurs with anticoagulant therapy, or after an operation. The name for this catastrophe is the Waterhouse-Friderichsen syndrome, named after the physicians who described death in cases of patients with meningococcemia, vascular collapse, and the presence of purpuric hemorrhages all over the skin.

Addison's disease, whether primary or secondary, can be managed today by replacement therapy. Daily oral doses of steroids can restore the metabolic equilibrium, just as insulin manages to restore the appropriate physiologic pathways in the diabetic. It is important, however, to remember that the patient with Addison's disease is still physiologically crippled and cannot adjust to increased demands for adrenal hormones as occur during infections or operations. Thus the dose needs to be adjusted to the circumstances. A medical alert card, bracelet, or notice greatly enhances his chance of survival in the event of an accident.

Hyperadrenalism

Hyperfunction of the adrenals may be either cortical or medullary. Many conditions have been described that result from the overproduction of 1, 2, or all 3 hormones. Each of the following syndromes represents an overproduction of a single hormone primarily.

Cushing's syndrome refers to the clinical features caused by excess glucocorticoid hormones, but it does not imply a particular cause. It may have already occurred to the thoughtful reader that the mere administration of cortisone may cause Cushing's syndrome, which is true and is probably the most common contemporary cause of this extraordinary change from normal. First, we shall consider the appearance of persons with this syndrome, and then we shall discuss the possible causes of it.

The clinical expression of Cushing's syndrome is unforgettable, as is seen in Figure 22–8 A and B. A round, moon-shaped face, often with an acne-like eruption, and the presence of excess hair attract one's attention at once. The body and trunk may be grossly exaggerated, compared with the thin, stick-like arms and legs. The presence of truncal obesity, a hump at the back of the neck, and purplish bruises are all classic findings on examining a patient with Cushing's syndrome. When the physician asks, the patient usually will speak of weakness, loss of strength, amenorrhea, impotence, and, sometimes, bone pain. Frequently, psychiatric symptoms are included. Weakness and diabetes mellitus are also part of the pattern. This pattern is unforgettable, and has many and complicated explanations, but it should suffice to attribute them to the excess of cortical hormone secretion.

Now the problem is to distinguish the different origins of this torrent of hormones. Since we know these hormones come from the adrenal cortex, a rare cause (10%) is the presence of a tumor of the adrenal cortex. Even in this small number of cases, it is far more common for a benign tumor (adenoma) than for a carcinoma to produce Cushing's syndrome. A second and more common cause is Cushing's disease, which is the presence of an ACTH-secreting tumor in the anterior pituitary that stimulates the adrenal cortex to secrete excess amounts of hormone. The association of this basophil adenoma of the pituitary with bilateral adrenal cortical hyperplasia was described in the 1920s by Harvey Cushing, a neurosurgeon, and accounts for 80% of the cases of Cushing's syndrome (excluding iatrogenic causes and those rare cases of ectopic hormone production). This latter cause (ectopic hormones) is a much more recent discovery. It was observed that in a few cases of Cushing's syndrome, there was neither an adrenal tumor nor a basophil adenoma, and yet there was adrenal cortical hyperplasia in patients with carcinoma (frequently of the lung). Such tumors have now been shown to secrete ACTH or ACTH-like hormones, which achieve

C

Fig. 22–8 *A*, Face of a patient with **Cushing's syndrome** due to bilateral hyperplasia of the adrenals. This 45-year-old patient underwent a 2-stage bilateral total adrenalectomy. *B*, Disappearance of all signs and symptoms 8 months after the second adrenalectomy, during which period patient received complete substitution therapy. (A and B from Williams: *Textbook of Endocrinology,* 4th Ed. Philadelphia, W. B. Saunders Co., 1968.) C, Adrenal virilism in boy 4½ years of age.

the same result, namely, excessive ACTH production, and to stimulate the adrenal to produce glucocorticoids in its own turn. Thus we have four significant causes of Cushing's syndrome: (1) iatrogenic administration of cortisone, (2) Cushing's disease, (3) adrenal tumors, and (4) ectopic hormones (lung).

Androgen excess (adrenal-genital hyperplasia) usually arises at any time between birth and early adolescence. The excess androgens tend to make little boys little men (Fig. 22–8C) and little girls little boys. This syndrome is most often caused by a decrease in one of the enzymes leading to the production of cortisol. Therefore, low levels of cortisol feed back to the pituitary and adrenal synthesis is increased in efforts to achieve normal levels of cortisol. However, because of the partial block, many cortisol precursors are shunted into the synthesis of sex steroids.

This syndrome, with all its psychologic as well as physical ramifications, should be recognized because the whole pathway of overproduction of androgens can be turned off by giving the patient daily oral doses of cortisol.

Aldosteronism is an overproduction of aldosterone, the powerful mineralocorticoid produced by the most superficial layer of the cortex. Aldosterone serves to regulate fluid balance and the excretion of electrolytes; overproduction of this mineralocorticoid causes retention of sodium and increased loss of potassium. The biochemical picture of aldosteronism, then, is opposite to that of Addison's disease. The adrenal lesion is much more likely to be an adenoma than it is cortical hyperplasia or carcinoma.

The clinical picture (known as **Conn's syndrome)** is characterized by periodic, severe muscular weakness amounting to paralysis, by arterial hypertension, and by renal dysfunction. The serum potassium level is low, which explains the muscular weakness, whereas the sodium level in the blood is raised. The urinary aldosterone level is high. Surgical removal of the cortical tumor is followed by a dramatic and complete disappearance of the clinical signs and symptoms, including the hypertension.

The **adrenal medulla** is the second portion of this essential organ. The adrenal medulla is of neuroectodermal origin and consists of cells and tissue that stain with chromium salts. It is part of a system distributed throughout the body, principally along the arterial network, and its role is to modulate and to control, by endocrine means, the peripheral resistance. Epinephrine, a small molecule synthesized from tyrosine, is the principal vasoactive product of the adrenal medulla and other chromaffin tissues. It is of interest that the adrenal cortical hormones control the secretion and the liberation of the adrenal medulla indirectly.

The effect of epinephrine on the body is not limited to increasing peripheral resistance. It also increases the liberation of glucose from glycogen storage in the liver, inhibits release of insulin, and inhibits the synthesis of new glycogen in the liver. Epinephrine also directly affects the heart, increasing its rate and strength of contraction.

The principal effect of disease of the adrenal medulla is to produce excess epinephrine-like hormone. The tumor most commonly seen, although it is rare itself, is called a **pheochromocytoma.**

This is an important tumor to know about because it is a treatable cause of hypertension, and it is sometimes hereditary, and it appears in association with other syndromes. However, most important is that the diagnosis can be difficult to make, because the presence of excess episodic or continuous amounts of epinephrine may be mistaken for other kinds of disease.

Most patients with pheochromocytoma have hypertension, sweating, palpitations, weight loss, and may appear with a chief complaint such as headache. In all patients with hypertension, pheochromocytoma should be suspected, if only to be ruled out.

The diagnosis of these rare tumors can be guessed at from the clinical situation in which the patient may be able to evoke the hypertension and the secretion of norepinephrine and epinephrine. I recall an instance in which the distressing episodes occurred when the patient bent his body sharply to one side; the adrenal mass was compressed on that side between the diaphragm and the kidney, and it squeezed out hormones like juice from an orange. Usually, the disease is one of many possible diagnoses and is established by laboratory findings of the catecholamines and their metabolic breakdown products in the urine. There are, in addition, challenge tests, using drugs that provoke the discharge of hormones from the adrenal (histamine, glucagon) or that block the effect of these pressor amines (Regitine [phentolamine]). Such pharmacologic experiments must be done with great care, with all the proper antidotes available, lest the blood pressure either skyrocket or disappear, leaving the patient at risk. Of course, direct (surgical) and indirect (radiologic) attempts to visualize the adrenal are also used.

There is an additional note about pheochromocytoma. We now recognize the increasing frequency of these tumors in families that have other endocrine tumors. In these instances, the pheochromocytoma is usually bilateral.

THYROID GLAND

The thyroid gland, shaped like a small shield, lies under the strap muscles of the neck at the level of the larynx. When it becomes enlarged or nodular, it can be visualized or felt easily in most persons (Fig. 22–9). The cells that compose it are arranged in vesicles called follicles, surrounding a central core of colloid, the storage form of the active material known as thyroxine, which is the only natural iodine-containing substance in the body. Each follicle of cells surrounding the colloid itself is enmeshed in a rich network of capillaries. From this network the amino acid tyro-

Fig. 22—9   This photograph shows a group of persons in the Philippines, all of whom demonstrate some thyroid abnormality. The large masses in the neck in 6 of the 7 persons are typical of **nontoxic goiter**. The seventh shows another abnormality characterized by the prominent **exophthalmos** and evidence of weight loss.

sine, which exists in most proteins, is continually extracted, iodinated, and sequestered in the form of a large molecule, thyroglobulin. When a person's energy requirements call for thyroxine, thyroid-releasing factor (TRF) from the hypothalamus stimulates the anterior pituitary to release the thyroid-stimulating hormone (TSH). This release, in turn, signals cells of the colloid follicles. They reach into their bank of colloid and withdraw from their savings account the active hormone, thyroxine, a small molecule that may contain either three iodine molecules (T3) or four iodine molecules (T4). This sequence of events, the uptake of iodine, its organification, and its subsequent release, depends on a number of enzymes, and different steps in the sequence may be blocked by drugs (thiouracil, lithium). More rarely, different enzymes may be congenitally absent. If iodine is absent from the diet, the important and necessary hormone is not made in adequate amounts, either; although the pathway is there, the essential iodine is not. The thyroid is unique among the endocrine glands in that it stores large amounts of hormone and releases it slowly. There is enough thyroxine in the normal adult gland for about 100 days. Thus there are several potential reasons for a lesion responsible for an inadequate amount of effective thyroid hormone: lack of iodine, blocked uptake, failure to manufacture thyroglobulin,

or inappropriate release. These lesions can be thought of as being in the thyroid (primary failure), being in the anterior pituitary, or being in the hypothalamus.

What is the function of this hormone thyroxine? Without it, the body, and in particular the nervous system, fails to grow. In the adult, all the essential functions lose their normal tempo, and there is a slowing of the pulse of life, a coarsening of the features, and a general torpor which we shall discuss further under hypothyroidism.

The thyroid hormones, T3 and T4, are essential to maintain the cadence and tempo of normal metabolic processes in all tissues. Like the damper on the furnace door, thyroxine controls the draft or rate of oxidative metabolism. An excess of thyroxine uncouples oxidative phosphorylation and has the effect of a runaway furnace, burning up the patient with too rapid pulse rate, fever, increased respiratory rate, and diarrhea. At the cellular level, mitochondria in all tissues from muscle to liver suffer from not having the correct amount of hormone. Without it, they cannot provide the normal amount of energy for cellular metabolism; with too much, they are like the out-of-control furnace just described.

During normal development in many forms of life, such as amphibia, thyroxine is the factor that initiates metamorphosis and enables liver cells to synthesize albumin, so that the amphibian can survive the transition onto land by having an intravascular pool of protein that protects the animal from immediate dehydration. Thyroxine starts the conversion from a fetal hemoglobin to an adult type, and initiates the remodeling that results in the development of limbs and in the resorption of the tail.

Exactly how thyroxine functions at the cellular level is a matter of dispute, but it is agreed that the hormone is essential for normal cellular health. One major function seems to be the stimulation of adenosinetriphosphatase (ATPase), which regulates sodium transport across cell membranes. Thus thyroxine directly affects cellular permeability and metabolism. A second observation is that there are thyroxine-binding sites in the nuclei of liver, kidney, and other cells, and the implication is that thyroxine also modifies the transcription of genetic information.

In the blood, thyroxine has been liberated from the colloid of the thyroid follicle and is bound to a serum protein, thyroid-binding globulin. A small fraction circulates free or unbound, and it is this fraction that is the active material. It seems that triiodothyronine (T3) rather than T4 is the more active form. We have methods today of measuring all these important substances: T3, T4, thyroid-binding globulin, thyroid-stimulating hormone, and thyroid-releasing factor.

Free or unbound T3 (8 to 10 times greater than T4 in normal serum) correlates most closely with the metabolic state of the person, rather than with the total concentration of T3 and T4. Thyroxine may be bound to thyroid-binding globulin, to prealbumin, or to albumin.

TSH, a glycopeptide secreted by the basophilic cells of the anterior pituitary, stimulates the thyroid follicle cells. Within minutes, these cells begin to reabsorb colloid from the follicle and to internalize it as colloid droplets, in which the thyroglobulin is broken down to release thyroxine, which in turn is liberated into the circulation. TSH stimulates the metabolism of nucleic acid and of protein; in fact, it stimulates all steps leading to the synthesis and secretion of thyroglobulin as well as its release. These effects can be seen histologically by the change from the normal cuboidal cells to tall columnar cells in the follicle following administration of this hormone. Conversely, in the absence of TSH, the cuboidal cells may become attenuated and may even appear squamous. Little activity takes place in these follicles.

TSH secretion, in turn, is regulated by thyrotropin-releasing hormone from the hypothalamus. There is a second antagonistic hypothalamic hormone that acts in the opposite way, but this process is more complex than we need to discuss here, except to indicate that the central nervous system control of these hormones, which in turn release thyroxine, underscores the possible effects of emotional and psychologic factors in governing our health. An example of such an effect is thyroid disease, which has been known to follow times of emotional turmoil and stress.

Hypothyroidism

The general term for a deficiency of thyroid hormone is hypothyroidism, regardless of the cause. The term **myxedema** is usually used to refer to the fully developed syndrome of this deficiency. Hypothyroidism is a systemic disorder affecting all tissues in the body, and it may be congenital or acquired. It may result from dysfunction of the thyroid gland itself, or from disease of the anterior pituitary or of the hypothalamus.

Congenital hypothyroid disease can be due to agenesis of the thyroid gland, to insensitivity of the thyroid gland and the thyroid-stimulating hormone, or to a variety of rare enzymatic defects, and the thyroid dysfunction may not necessarily be all or none. However, the significance of congenital hypothyroidism, whatever its cause, is that the failure to recognize the disorder in an infant condemns the child to mental retardation. As we have said, all the tissues of the body (the central nervous system in particular) require thyroxine for normal growth and development

The cretin is a dwarf physically and mentally. The mind, the skeleton, and the sexual organs do not develop. Like Peter Pan, the cretin never grows up, but (unlike the child with panhypopituitarism) he has none of Peter Pan's vivacity, because the vitalizing influence of the thyroid is lacking. He is a sad, old child. Osler described the cretin: "No type of human transformation is more distressing to look at than an aggravated case of cretinism. The stunted stature, the semi-bestial aspect, the blubber lips, retroussé nose sunken at the root, the wide-open mouth, the lolling tongue, the small eyes half closed with swollen lids, the stolid expressionless face, the squat figure, the muddy dry skin, combine to make the picture of what has been termed, the pariah of Nature" (Fig. 22–10).

In the adult, the disease **myxedema** begins usually without forewarning and may progress for decades

Fig. 22–10 A **cretin**.

before it is perceived as the pathologic pattern we now describe. Weakness, fatigue, lethargy, sleepiness, cold intolerance, menorrhagia, little appetite, but a gradual and steady increase in weight, may all suggest the disorder. The voice becomes deeper and husky, hair coarsens and may fall out, the skin becomes stiff and dry and the patient may become deaf. All of these changes may be mistaken for the decay of age.

The florid, full-blown case shows someone with a dull, expressionless face (Fig. 22–11), who sits immobile, moving little and talking, if at all, with a lethargy that signals an effort for each word. It is as if the pendulum on life's clock were lengthened from a yard to a mile, and the ticking of time took an hour for each minute. There is periorbital puffiness, a swollen tongue that barely fits the mouth, and pale, dough-like skin that feels rough. The heart is enlarged and fails to function normally, the bowel dilates and accumulates stool, and the patient may lapse into coma.

One unusual complication of thyroid deficiency is called **"myxedema coma."** This rare phenomenon can be likened to the complication of hyperthyroidism called "thyroid storm." In myxedema coma, which usually has a serious prognosis because it has been overlooked as the underlying cause of the unresponsiveness, hypotension, hypothermia, hypoventilation, bradycardia, and convulsions, the suspicion of the diagnosis is the key to successful management. If the physician waits for laboratory tests to come back, the patient may be lost. The obese patient is the one in whom the suspicion should be raised, particularly

someone in whom infection or trauma have occurred. A surgical procedure may precipitate this acute hypothyroid crisis, which may be masked by the other things that are happening. A low basal temperature may be the feature that prompts the laboratory diagnosis, and the lifesaving treatment is intravenous administration of short-acting thyroxine.

The laboratory manifestation that best confirms the diagnosis is the elevation of the patient's level of TSH. This elevation occurs because the feedback loop in thyroxine is inhibited and fails to depress secretion of the stimulating hormone from the pituitary gland. Serum T4 is more reliable than T3 in this disease.

The explanation for all these changes is simple, in that thyroxine is not available to keep normal metabolism going, and every tissue suffers. There is a peculiar material that accumulates in the interstitial spaces and contributes to the coarsening of the skin and features, in addition to clogging up the larynx and heart and mechanically altering the structure and function of every organ, so that it does not move. Recently there is some evidence to support the idea that the edema derives from a disorder of the capillaries themselves.

Supportive treatment to manage the carbon dioxide narcosis and the administration of thyroxine rapidly reverse the progressive torpor and restore the patient to a normal state. The causes of hypothyroidism are shown in Table 22–4, and we shall consider here only the chronic and subacute inflammatory conditions, as the others seem self-explanatory.

Hashimoto's disease is probably the most common

Fig. 22–11   *A,* **Myxedema** of 20 years' duration; patient bedridden and imbecile. *B,* After treatment with thyroid extract; the same patient 30 years later, aged 94 years. (Harrington: *The Thyroid Gland—Its Chemistry and Physiology.* Oxford University Press.)

Table 22–4. Causes of Hypothyroidism

MECHANISM	CAUSE
Deficiency of TRH	Hypothalamic disease
Deficiency of TSH	Pituitary tumor or infarction
Thyroid destruction	Chronic inflammation
	Surgical ablation
	Radioiodine ablation
	Irradiation of the neck (usually for malignant disease)
Thyroid deficiency	Iodine deficiency (i.e., substrate lack)
	Iodine excess (i.e., interference with hormone release)
	Antithyroid drugs
	Biosynthetic defects

cause of hypothyroidism, except for iodine deficiency. This disorder would be better called chronic thyroiditis or chronic lymphocytic thyroiditis, since that is the nature of the lesion. Its cause may be debated by some, but the bulk of the evidence points to an autoimmune process. The disorder is far more common in women than in men (7:1), and can usually be perceived by the clinician as a diffuse swelling of the thyroid gland in a patient who may be hypothyroid. Nearly all such patients can be shown to have circulating thyroid antibodies. Biopsy of the thyroid shows marked lymphocytic infiltration with atrophy and loss of thyroid follicles. This process is progressive. It is of interest that the relatives of these patients frequently may have a history of thyroid disease, and they may also have antithyroid antibodies. Whether the disease arises from an earlier infection with some virus has not yet been shown. The patient with chronic lymphocytic thyroiditis is treated with thyroid replacement, and this is usually a lifelong requirement.

Hyperthyroidism

Excess circulating thyroid hormone arises from a variety of causes. The commonest cause is **Graves' disease** (70 to 90%), which goes by many names (e.g., toxic diffuse goiter). The second commonest cause is **toxic nodular goiter.** The third cause is a single adenoma or **toxic adenoma** of the thyroid. There are some other rare causes, and, except for the important concept that a pituitary tumor producing TSH has been reported, they are all so unusual as to be out of place here.

The clinical manifestations of hyperthyroidism usually begin in early adult life, more frequently in women (5:1), and the onset is often sudden and acute, sometimes following some serious emotional event or illness. The patient's complaints may vary, in that

different presentations ranging from acute psychosis to muscle weakness to diarrhea alone are all well recognized. Perhaps the most common problem is a cardiac arrhythmia or palpitations. Sometimes the problem is heart failure.

The diagnosis is based on classic physical findings: prominent, bulging eyes, a staring gaze, a diffusely enlarged thyroid gland, tachycardia, and marked fine tremor of the outstretched hands. The history is also classic: insomnia, irritability, frequent bowel movements, a good appetite but weight loss, and increased perspiration. The patient likes winter more than summer and cannot sleep with blankets. These observations leave little room for alternate explanations, especially when the pulse rate is 100 and there is a venous hum in the neck and a systolic murmur. Laboratory tests will confirm elevated T3 and T4 levels and an increased radioactive I^{131} uptake (Fig. 22–12). The serum cholesterol will be lower than normal. The basal metabolic rate is elevated, if the test is done. When the diagnosis is made, the problems begin, because the etiology of Graves' disease is poorly understood, and the correct treatment for the patient is a matter of debate and of individual consideration.

Graves' disease (toxic diffuse goiter) shows uniform enlargement of the thyroid follicle cells histologically (Fig. 22–13), and is diagnosed as we have indicated from the clinical pattern. Laboratory data will confirm the diagnosis. Whereas the etiology of the disease is a matter of current investigation, Mackenzie showed that the disease is mediated by an immunoglobulin antibody to the TSH receptor. This antibody stimulates increased production of thyroxine in an autonomous manner. The material present in the serum of many patients with Graves' disease has been called

Fig. 22–12 This **nuclear medicine scan** of the thyroid gland shows the outline of the thyroid gland 24 hours after the administration of I^{131}. In a hyperactive gland, the iodine is taken up rapidly and sequestered in the thyroid gland, as shown here.

Fig. 22–13 Histologic appearance of thyroid of Graves' disease undergoing involution under iodine treatment. The papillary processes are being withdrawn from the enlarged acini, and colloid is reappearing. Above and below there is still dense hyperplastic tissue. × 150. (Boyd: *Textbook of Pathology*. Philadelphia, Lea & Febiger.)

long-acting thyroid stimulator (LATS). The origin of this LATS appears to be the lymphocytes of these patients, so the disease, like Hashimoto's disease, can be thought of as an autoimmune disorder. It used to be thought that excess thyroid-stimulating hormone was the offending agent, but this is not so in all but a few cases.

Exophthalmos in patients with Graves' disease is a serious and often complicated management problem. Its etiology is poorly understood. The marked prominence of one or both eyes, with a staring gaze and a retraction of the lids, is an unforgettable sight. Examination of the retro-orbital tissues shows increased mucopolysaccharides, inflammatory cells, and connective tissue that collect to push the eye forward, often making it impossible to close the eyelids, and thereby exposing the cornea to abrasions and inflammation. The muscle weakness of the hyperthyroidism may contribute to difficulties with the eyelids. In the worst cases, exophthalmos can result in the loss of vision. The current view of this disorder is that it also is of autoimmune etiology, but that it is unrelated to the presence of LATS or TSH. It has been recognized that exophthalmos may occur by itself or with other endocrine disorders.

Toxic nodular goiter differs in several ways from Graves' disease. First, it occurs in persons who have had a goiter for many years, and in those who are older (40 to 65). Malignant exophthalmos is rare, and the serum T4 levels are usually not markedly elevated. The radioactive iodine uptake level can be within the normal range. Finally, it is a diagnosis best understood by the statistic that it probably occurs in about 15% of all those with simple goiter. The best way to think of it is that it occurs within the gland that has undergone hyperplasia. After many years (and countless efforts), a group of thyroid cells have been able to free themselves from the controls imposed by the anterior pituitary and thus to function on their own, without regard for the inhibitory signals from thyroxine or stimulatory signals from TSH. To be sure of the diagnosis, a radioactive scan should show areas of increased uptake against the background of normal radioactive iodine uptake. In addition, the T3 level should be elevated.

Toxic adenoma is a single focus of cells in the thyroid that produces symptoms of hyperthyroidism. The remainder of the thyroid gland is suppressed, as is production of TSH by the anterior pituitary, since the autonomous group of cells produces more T3 and T4 than the patient needs. Toxic adenoma is identifiable because there is only a single nodule in an otherwise normal or atrophied gland. This occurs naturally in a hyperthyroid patient. Radioactive scans confirm that the "hot" nodule is present (Fig. 22–14) in a gland that is physiologically depressed and yet responds to TSH. This can be done as a diagnostic test by giving TSH and by repeating the scan, which should now show an increased uptake in the thyroid around the "hot" nodule. The treatment of this cause of hyperthyroidism is uncomplicated, as either surgical removal of the nodule or the administration of radioactive iodine will cure the disease.

Whether the cases of hyperthyroidism should be treated with antithyroid drugs such as propylthiouracil, with or without the beta blocker propranolol, by

Fig. 22–14 This **nuclear medicine scan** of the thyroid following administration of I^{131} shows the appearance of a hot nodule. The rest of the gland is suppressed.

subtotal thyroidectomy, or by radioactive iodine therapy is a matter of debate and is beyond the scope of the present volume.

Before leaving hyperthyroidism, however, it would be well to comment on the hyperthyroid counterpart of myxedema coma, namely, **thyroid storm.** This condition is a severe, life-threatening extension of hyperthyroidism in which the symptoms become increasingly severe and incapacitating, with prostration, high fever, marked tachycardia, restlessness, and shock. Heart failure and possibly death may supervene. In short, it is the exaggeration of all we have been describing under the hyperthyroid state, and is usually seen as a complication of simple hyperthyroidism. The issue, of course, is to recognize it for what it is, and to treat it with emergency antithyroid drugs.

Goiter

This term is most confusing. It is typical of terms that have been used through the ages for different purposes, that are continually redefined and used, but that have different meanings for different people. Goiter is synonymous with enlargement of the thyroid gland and does not imply the reason for the enlargement. The enlargement is diffuse rather than nodular, and there are three forms of thyroid enlargement that can be recognized. First, as we have outlined, enlargement due to **Graves' disease,** which has

been referred to also as diffuse toxic goiter. Second, as we have indicated in our discussion of chronic inflammatory disease of the thyroid, the gland may be diffusely enlarged, but the patient may be hypothyroid. **Hashimoto's disease** is an example of this condition. Third, the gland may be enlarged, and the patient may have normal thyroid function, or the patient may be hypothyroid. This diffuse enlargement is called *endemic goiter,* colloid goiter, or **simple nontoxic goiter.** We may understand it best as a hyperplastic response to a deficiency of iodine. The iodine deficiency may be due to different factors. There can be a relative lack because the body needs more iodine than is available from the diet, as occurs during periods of rapid growth. It may be due to inadequate amounts of iodine from the diet.

Endemic goiter typically appeared in regions such as the alpine districts of Switzerland and the Himalayas, or the area of the Great Lakes in North America before the commercial addition of iodine to salt and bread. The incidence of endemic goiter has been greatly diminished because of this supplement. In part of Ohio, a mass experiment was performed, giving the school children a small amount of iodized salt for 1 or 2 weeks twice a year, and by this simple expedient there was an astonishing reduction in the incidence of goiter in that community.

The symptoms of goiter are related to the local enlargement of the gland (Fig. 22–15) or to the long-term results of continuing inadequate ability to make thyroxine. Compression of the surrounding structures may cause difficulty in swallowing and noisy breathing.

The administration of iodine will make up for the dietary lack, and the gland may regain its normal small size. If the gland is massively enlarged, surgical removal may be appropriate.

Tumors of the Thyroid

This subject is of great interest for two reasons. The first is that 5% of the adult population have a nodule in the thyroid that can be felt by an examiner, and there is a remote chance that this nodule could be cancer. The other more likely possibility is that the mass represents a cyst or a benign, nonfunctioning group of cells, a benign adenoma. Of course, the nodule could be an inflammatory lesion. Unfortunately, there is no test other than a biopsy to establish the diagnosis.

The incidence of carcinoma of the thyroid is greater in persons who have a family history of such tumors, who have had irradiation to the neck, or who have a nodule that is either hard or fixed, or is growing rap-

A   B

Fig. 22–15   *A*, **Diffuse multinodular colloid goiter**, showing the compressed veins and congested appearance of the face. *B*, Same patient 15 days after removal of the goiter. Note rapid relief of congestion of the veins of the face. (From de Quervain: *Goitre and Thyroid Diseases*. New York, William Wood & Co., 1924.)

idly. The likelihood of the nodule's being cancer is small, but every case must be judged individually. It is of interest that whereas benign nodules are more common in women over 40 (10 times more frequent than in men), the incidence of cancer of the thyroid is twice as frequent in men.

The clinical signs of thyroid carcinoma are related to the type. The different types are not an important part of our discussion here. However, it is easy enough to delineate three general types, because they differ radically in their biologic behavior. Carcinoma of the thyroid may appear as a palpable mass or, as we have said, as a nodule that is either fixed or growing rapidly.

Of malignant tumors of the thyroid, the rarest, lethal type (5%) is an undifferentiated tumor that grows like wildfire and has a guarded prognosis, with a life expectancy of a year or less. The most common type of malignant tumor (60%) shows both follicular and papillary appearances on histologic examination. The better developed it is generally, the better the prognosis. This means a survival rate of 10 years for 70% of patients with well-differentiated carcinoma. The well-differentiated tumors respond to TSH and, if they are follicular, may take up radioactive iodine as well, allowing the physician both to suppress their function and to stimulate it, and to treat the tumor medically or surgically, or in both ways.

A few (15%) well-differentiated papillary carcinomas grow slowly and are compatible with a long sur-

vival rate for the patient. If you insist on having a tumor of the thyroid, this is probably the one to have.

A rare tumor, medullary carcinoma of the thyroid, only deserves mention because of its association with adenomas of other endocrine organs, and I refer you to other texts for a discussion of this disease.

PARATHYROID GLANDS

In the volume of endocrine romance, there are few more thrilling chapters than that which deals with the story of the parathyroids. For more than 70 years, these four tiny glands, each smaller than a lentil, have been identified, but their function was not understood. Normally, they lie in the neck, two on each side, behind the upper and lower poles of the thyroid gland. In 1925, Collip succeeded in preparing an extract of parathyroid glands that he called **parathormone**. Injection of this extract mobilized calcium and raised the serum calcium level. Normally the serum calcium is closely controlled between 9 and 11 mg%. The principal pathway of calcium metabolism is absorption from the gut and deposition in the bone. Parathyroid hormone has been shown to affect the absorption from the gut, the resorption from the bone, and the reabsorption from the urine. Calcium is a divalent cation essential for function of all cell membranes, and it must be present in just the right amount. Medically, there are emergencies of both too much and too little serum calcium.

Parathyroid hormone acts directly to change the osteocyte into an osteoclast, which secretes a collagenase that breaks down the fully mineralized collagen and liberates both calcium and phosphate into the serum, as well as the hydrolytic products of the collagen breakdown. One can identify hydroxylysine or hydroxyproline excretion in the urine, as testimony to the lytic effect on bone of hyperparathyroid disease.

Serum phosphate, which normally ranges from 3 to 5 mg%, is also maintained in inverse proportion to the amount of serum calcium. Thus the product of the calcium times phosphorus is kept at a constant. Normally, the calcium/phosphorus ratio is maintained by intestinal absorption, renal excretion, and/or bone deposition or mobilization.

A second hormone that plays a role in calcium homeostasis was identified in the early 1960s, and this hormone has been called **calcitonin.** The role of this hormone seems analogous to that of glucagon in the pancreas, so that for the regulation of blood glucose levels we have two hormones, insulin and glucagon, and for the regulation of serum calcium and phosphate levels we have parathyroid hormone and calcitonin.

It is too complicated to describe the parathyroid hormone's mechanism on the absorption of calcium in the gut. The primary effect of calcitonin is to reduce the resorption of calcium from bone when the serum calcium level begins to rise. Calcitonin is an antihypercalcemic factor, and seems to be much more active in young, growing animals than in adults.

Hyperparathyroidism

This term is applied to any disorder in which an elevated level of effective parathyroid hormone occurs, and, as we shall see, its effect may be to raise the serum calcium under some circumstances. However, the serum calcium level may be normal or low. Hyperparathyroidism has been divided into three types: primary hyperparathyroidism, an excess that arises from an adenoma or hyperplasia of the parathyroid glands; secondary hyperparathyroidism, which represents an adaptive excess of parathyroid hormone in response to hypocalcemia, hyperphosphatemia, or, occasionally, hypomagnesemia; a third type of hyperparathyroidism is due to the ectopic production of hormones with parathyroid hormone-like activity.

Primary hyperparathyroid disease is due to a single or solitary adenoma occurring in 1 of the 4 parathyroids in 80 to 90% of cases. This adenoma is a clone of cells that have undertaken autonomous growth and secretion, and are independent of normal control mechanisms. They synthesize and secrete excessive, active parathyroid hormone. There is no knowledge of any particular stimulus or cause for their growth or secretion, and, short of surgical removal of the enlarged, hyperfunctioning parathyroid adenoma, there is no other satisfactory treatment.

Clinical patterns of hyperparathyroid disease range from the full-blown description by von Recklinghausen in 1891 of a patient with a deformed skeleton and bone pain, who showed cystic areas of rarefaction and fibrotic patches in the bone, owing to the extreme calcium loss, to the contemporary patient who is completely asymptomatic, but whose routine multiphasic analysis of serum turns up an elevated serum calcium. Generally, there are two patterns for patients with overt primary hyperparathyroidism. These patterns seem to relate to the size and duration of the hyperfunctioning gland. One group, like von Recklinghausen's patient, has bone pain and may even show collapse of vertebrae; these patients have high serum calciums and a short history of being ill; large adenomas are found at surgery. The second group, with smaller adenomas, have kidney stones and a longer history of illness with only modest hypercalcemia. We have always said that whenever kidney stones occur, a possibility that must be investigated is hyperparathyroid disease, disappointing as it may be to uncover high serum calcium in fewer than 10% of patients with kidney stones.

A second cause for primary hyperparathyroidism is the presence of what is called **chief cell hyperplasia,** or four-gland enlargements. This variant is more perplexing, because it implies some regulating factor that is unidentified. Such patients may have lower parathormone levels than the patients with solitary adenoma. Again, surgery is the treatment of the illness, leaving half of one parathyroid gland to maintain homeostasis.

In all patients with primary hyperparathyroidism, the symptoms may be vague and nonspecific. Weakness, weight loss, fatigue, and muscle atrophy, in addition to bone pain, gastrointestinal distress, pancreatitis, or kidney stones are common.

Hypercalcemia has come more and more to be the single finding around which the diagnosis of hyperparathyroidism revolves, and forces us to discuss the other causes of elevated serum calcium levels in order to avoid jumping to the conclusion that it is inevitably due to hyperparathyroid disease. Whereas more than 95% of patients with hyperparathyroidism have elevated serum calcium levels, there are other causes of a high serum calcium, as shown in Table 22–5. The serum calcium level is the product, as we have outlined, of reabsorption of calcium by the renal tubular cells from the glomerular filtrate (conservation), increased absorption from the gut of calcium (under vitamin D control), and mobilization of calcium from bone (due to parathyroid hormone). In each of these mechanisms, parathyroid hormone plays a crucial role.

Increased mobilization of calcium from bone that

Table 22–5.   Etiology of Hypercalcemia

Excess bone resorption	Excess absorption from gut
Hyperparathyroidism	Sarcoidosis (other
Malignant tumors	granulomas)
Producing PTH	Vitamin D intoxication
Producing other hormonal	? milk-alkali syndrome
agents	? adrenal insufficiency
Immobilization	Excess renal reabsorption
Thyrotoxicosis	? thiazide diuretics

(From Goltzman, D.: Parathyroid hormone and hyperparathyroidism: current concepts. Can. J. Surg., 21:285, 1978.)

raises serum calcium levels occurs frequently in various neoplastic diseases, particularly in multiple myeloma, a tumor of plasma cells. Occasionally, other cancers secrete ectopic parathyroid hormone, making the problem more complicated until the presence of the malignant neoplasm is recognized.

Hypercalcemia can represent a medical and surgical emergency when it rises above 18 mg%. The patient may lapse into coma, and emergency treatment should be instituted while preparing the person for the necessary surgical exploration of the neck to remove the functional parathyroid adenoma that causes the hypercalcemia.

Secondary hyperparathyroidism is an adaptive response to parathyroid hormone secretion. It occurs most commonly in chronic renal disease, in which the kidney is no longer able to excrete phosphate normally. Because of renal disease, the kidney also may have lost the ability to create the active form of vitamin D. In the absence of this vitamin, the gut absorbs less calcium than it would normally, thus contributing to a lower than normal calcium level. Either a lower serum calcium or a raised serum phosphate level may act as a stimulus to the parathyroid glands to increase the secretion of parathyroid hormone. (It is well to remember that there is a homeostatic drive to keep the calcium times phosphate ratio constant.) Thus in chronic renal failure, it is common to find hyperplasia of all four parathyroid glands, but the serum calcium may not necessarily be elevated. Rather, it is a normal serum calcium level in persons in whom one suspects a low serum calcium that suggests the diagnosis of secondary hyperparathyroidism. This situation represents the epitome of adaptation with respect to calcium homeostasis. Since the serum phosphate level is raised, it acts as a stimulus to the secretion of the parathyroid hormone which in turn calls out more calcium from the bone depot. The restoration of the serum calcium level (which had been low) toward normal represents a relative hypercalcemia in such patients with chronic renal failure. If the serum calcium level is abnormally high, and the serum phosphate

level is, too, one occasionally finds metastatic calcification throughout the body.

Hypoparathyroidism

This deficiency of parathyroid hormone results in hypocalcemia. Of course, it is not the only cause of hypocalcemia, just as a high serum calcium level is not only attributable to excess parathyroid hormone. Most instances of hypoparathyroidism are the consequence of surgical operations of the neck, removal either of the thyroid or of the parathyroids. There are, in addition, rare disorders such as pseudohypoparathyroidism, which we shall not consider.

The clinical pattern of hypocalcemia, whatever its cause, is interesting and important because of the ease with which the disorder may be treated. Numbness and tingling of the extremities and around the mouth are common complaints. Cramps of individual muscles, particularly in the hands and feet, are a result of inadequate calcium. Occasionally, convulsions occur. A host of nonspecific aberrations of thought, such as irritability, emotional lability, depression, are reported. To confirm the clinical impression of hypocalcemia, Chvostek's sign of twitching of the muscles about the mouth, nose, or eyelids can be evoked by tapping the facial nerve. Trousseau's sign (carpal spasm) occurs when a blood pressure cuff is inflated above systolic pressure for more than two minutes. These signs are evidence of the irritability of muscle and nerve in the absence of calcium.

Calcium replacement by oral or intravenous route is a readily available cure to the immediate problem.

This abnormal irritability is called tetany, and may also occur in other disturbances of calcium metabolism, such as in cases of alkalosis.

ISLETS OF LANGERHANS

The islets of Langerhans are small groups of cells scattered throughout the pancreas, particularly in large numbers in the tail of that organ. Together the islets of Langerhans constitute another endocrine organ. Their principal product is insulin, and their subsidiary product is glucagon. Recently, it has been shown that there are cells in the islets that also secrete somatostatin. Like other endocrines, there may be under- or overproduction of the hormones of these tissues. **Hypoinsulinism** (otherwise known as diabetes mellitus) has been discussed in an earlier section. Replacement therapy by insulin is the standard approach to this insufficiency.

Hyperinsulinism is caused by the presence of a tumor of the islets of Langerhans. This tumor is rarely malignant. More commonly, it is simply an adenoma with functional excess of hormone. The clinical pattern is distinctive, in that the person with an excess continuous secretion of insulin is continually hypoglycemic. This hypoglycemia leads to constant hunger, and that patient may not only be subject to hypoglycemia with fainting, convulsions, and loss of consciousness, but he also may be meeting his need by continuous feeding. Occasionally, a patient with an insulinoma may be grossly obese. Today, the diagnosis of an insulinoma should be suspected whenever someone has convulsions, syncopal attacks, and/or a remarkably low level of blood sugar. Modern assays for serum insulin will confirm the diagnosis.

SYNOPSIS

Endocrine disorders can generally be considered to be instances of too much or too little secretion by respective endocrine glands. The anatomic lesions generally are functioning adenomas or hyperplasia of a particular type of cell, although there are rare examples of malignant tumors of nonendocrine tissue that secrete substances with hormone-like activity.

Hyperpituitarism results in gigantism or acromegaly; hypopituitarism may appear as dysfunction of all the endocrine glands (thyroid, adrenal, gonads, etc.), or it may be symptomatic because of a particular dysfunction.

Benign and malignant tumors without endocrine function may occur in any endocrine gland.

Hyperadrenalism may result in Cushing's syndrome, Conn's syndrome, or the adrenogenital syndrome. Hypoadrenalism is called Addison's disease. It has several causes.

Hyperthyroidism and hypothyroidism each may have many causes.

The parathyroid gland's relation to calcium and phosphate metabolism is complex, and current views still do not explain the original stimulus to adenoma or hyperplasia.

The stimuli to adenoma and hyperplasia of the endocrine organs remains a riddle deserving more attention.

Terms

Hypophysis
Growth hormone
Luteinizing hormone
Thyrotropin
Acromegaly
Simmonds' disease
Mineralocorticoid
Glucocorticoid

Pheochromocytoma
Goiter
Hashimoto's thyroiditis
Hyperthyroidism
Prolactin
ACTH
Oxytocin
Vasopressin

Androgen
Addison's disease
Cushing's syndrome
Myxedema
Cretin
Parathormone
Calcitonin
Thyroidism

FURTHER READING

Addison, T.: Disease of suprarenal capsules. Lond. Med. Gaz., 43:517, 1855.

Ahérn, B.: Regulatory peptides in the thyroid gland—a review on their localization and function. Acta Endocrinol. (Copenh), 124:225, 1991.

Allison, A.C.: Self-tolerance and autoimmunity in the thyroid. N. Engl. J. Med., 295:821, 1976.

Bartalena, L., Marcocci, C., Bogazzi, F., et al.: Use of corticosteroids to prevent progression of Graves' ophthalmopathy after radioiodine therapy for hyperthyroidism. N. Engl. J. Med., 321:1349, 1989.

Beckers, C. Endemic and sporadic nontoxic goiter. In *Physiopathology of Endocrine Diseases and Mechanisms of Hormone Action*. New York, Alan R. Liss, Inc., 1981, p. 153.

Bergland, R.M., and Page, R.B.: Pituitary-brain vascular relations: A new paradigm. Science, 204:18, 1979.

Bloom, S.R., and Polak, J.M.: Somatostatin. Brit. Med. J., 295:288, 1987.

Collier, J., and Vallance, P.: Physiological importance of nitric oxide. Br. Med. J., 302:1289, 1991.

Copp, D.H., et al.: Calcitonin. Endocrinology, 70:638, 1962.

Crichton, M., Christy, N.P., and Damon, A.: Host factors in "chromophobe" adenoma of the anterior pituitary: a retrospective study of 464 patients. Metabolism, 30:248, 1981.

Cushing, H.: The basophil adenomas of the pituitary body and their clinical manifestations. Bull. Johns Hopkins Hosp., 1:137, 1932.

DeLuca, H.F.: Vitamin D endocrinology. Ann. Intern. Med., 85:367, 1976.

De Meyts, P., and Rousseau, G.G.: Receptor concepts. A century of evolution. Supp. I, Circ. Res., 46:I-3, 1980.

Duncan, G.A., Hill, F.M., and Ezrin, C.: Acromegaly: a review of 100 cases. Can. Med. Assoc. J., 87:1106, 1962.

Editorial: The pathogenesis of autoimmune thryoid disease. N. Engl. J. Med., 325:278, 1991.

Etkin, W.: Logic versus imagination in an experimental analysis. Perspect. Biol. Med., 20:394, 1977.

Favus, M.J., et al.: Evaluation of 1056 patients. Thyroid cancer occurring as a late consequence of head-and-neck irradiation. N. Engl. J. Med., 294:1019, 1976.

Gold, E.B.: Epidemiology of pituitary adenomas. Epidemiol. Rev., 3:163, 1981.

Goltzman, D.: Parathyroid hormone and hyperparathyroidism: current concepts. Can. J. Surg., 21:285, 1978.

Guillemin, R.: Control of adenohypophysial functions by peptides of the central nervous system. Harvey Lect., 71, 1978.

Heath, H., III, Hodgson, S.F., and Kennedy, M.A.: Primary hyperparathyroidism: incidence, morbidity, and potential economic impact in a community. N. Engl. J. Med., 302:189, 1980.

Hedberg, C.W., et al.: An outbreak of thyrotoxicosis caused by the consumption of bovine thyroid gland in ground beef. N. Engl. J. Med., 316:993, 1987.

Jones, H.W.: A long look at the adrenogenital syndrome. Johns Hopkins Med. J., 145:143, 1979.

Kidd, A., et al.: Immunologic aspects of Graves' and Hashimoto's diseases. Metabolism, 29:80, 1980.

Krieger, D.T., and Liotta, A.S.: Pituitary hormones in the brain: where, how and why? Science, 205:366, 1979.

Lane, M.D.: The regulation of insulin receptor level and activity. Nutrition Rev., 39:417, 1981.

Li, C.H.: β-endorphin. Cell, 31:504, 1982.

Lippe, B.: Turner syndrome. Endocrinol. Metabol. Clin. N.A., 20:121, 1991.

Mallette, L.E.: Primary hyperparathyroidism, an update: incidence, etiology, diagnosis and treatment. Am. J. Med. Sci. 293:239, 1987.

Masi, A.T., Hartmann, W.H., and Shulman, L.E.: Hashimoto's disease: an epidemiological critique. J. Chronic Dis., 18:1, 1965.

McKenzie, J.M.: Does LATS cause hyperthyroidism in Graves' disease? (A review biased towards the affirmative.) Metabolism, 21:883, 1972.

Melmed, S.: Medical Progress: Acromegaly. N. Engl. J. Med., 322:966, 1990.

Moncada, S. Palmer, R.M.J., and Higgs, E.A.: Nitric oxide: Physiology, pathophysiology, and pharmacology. Pharmacol. Rev., 43:109, 1991.

Nelson, D.H., Meakin, J.W., and Thorn, G.W.: ACTH-producing pituitary tumors following adrenalectomy for Cushing's syndrome. Ann. Intern. Med., 52:560, 1960.

O'Malley, B.W.: Studies on the molecular mechanism of steroid hormone action. Harvey Lect., 72, l978.

Ord, W.M.: On myxoedema: a term proposed to be applied to an essential condition in the "cretinoid" affection occasionally observed in middle-aged women. Med. Chir. Trans., 61:57, 1878.

Rechler, M.M., et al.: Hormonal regulation of human growth. N. Engl. J. Med., 316:941, 1987.

Roti, E., and Emerson, C.H.: Postpartum thyroiditis—a clinical review. J. Clin. Biochem. Endocrin. Metab., 74:3, 1992.

Rudman, D., Feller, A.G., Nagraj, H.S., et al.: Effects of human growth hormone in men over 60 years old. N. Engl. J. Med., 323:1, 1990.

Russell, C.F., and Edis, A.J.: Surgery for primary hyperparathyroidism: experience with 500 consecutive cases and evaluation of the role of surgery in the asymptomatic patient. Br. J. Surg., 69:244, 1982.

Schwartz, I.D., and Root, A.W.: The Klinefelter syndrome of testicular dysgenesis. Endocrinol. Metabol. Clin. N.A., 20:153, 1991.

Talmage, R.V.: Discovery, physiology and chemistry of calcitonin. Bone and Mineral, 16:155, 1992.

Valentin, J-P., et al.: Modulation of endothelin effects on blood pressure and hematocrit by atrial natriuretic peptide. Hypertension, 17:864, 1991.

Wilkins, L., Lewis, R.A., and Klein, R.: The suppression of androgen secretion by cortisone in a case of congenital hyperplasia. Bull. Johns Hopkins Hosp., 81:249, 1950.

APPENDIX

Principal Hormones of Anterior Pituitary

As we have said, the **anterior lobe** secretes hormones in response to releasing and inhibitory factors of the hypothalamus and in response to the hormones produced by the glands that they stimulate. This form of regulation can be likened to a thermostat and furnace. On a warm day, the heat, the product of the furnace, signals to the thermostat to turn off the furnace, just as a high blood level of thyroxine turns off the thyroid. Similarly, when the temperature falls, the thermostat turns on the furnace, and, despite changes in the weather, the house remains at a given temperature. However, the thermostat can be regulated just as the hypothalamus regulates, and at times resets, the pituitary. The principal hormones of the anterior pituitary are:

Growth hormone (GH), as its name implies, regulates growth; therefore, its target is the whole body. An animal that has undergone hypophysectomy (removal of the pituitary) cannot grow unless growth hormone is replaced. The secretion of growth hormone is usually regulated through somatomedin, a substance made in the liver. A tropic hormone that might govern the release of growth hormone has been postulated, but not identified. Instead, many other signals, such as exercise, amino acids, hypoglycemia, sleep, all promote its secretion. Growth hormone also helps to protect the body from hypoglycemia during fasting. The secretion of this hormone is triggered by hypoglycemia and is increased in response to a rise in amino acids (particularly arginine) or following either stress or the administration of alpha-adrenergic stimuli (such as L-DOPA). Growth hormone is secreted shortly after sleep starts, even during the day. Its secretion is suppressed by a newly discovered substance called somatostatin. Growth hormone has a short half-life in the peripheral blood of about half an hour. The amount of circulating growth hormone is constantly fluctuating in the normal individual. GH and insulin combine to provide tissues with a continuously available source of fuel. This function of GH explains why patients with hypopituitarism are subject to severe hypoglycemia after a small injection of insulin, which could be easily tolerated by a patient with an intact pituitary. When the function of a patient's anterior pituitary is uncertain, insulin or arginine is administered to see whether the gland can secrete growth hormone normally.

Gonadotropic follicle-stimulating hormone (FSH) and **luteinizing hormone** or interstitial-cell-stimulating hormone (LH, ICSH) are necessary both for the proper development of the male and female reproductive organs and for the menstrual cycle, since the hormones stimulate the ovaries to monthly activity, which in turn produces hormones responsible for the changes in the uterus that result in menstruation. One of the first signs of pituitary disease in the female is cessation of the normal female menstrual function.

Thyrotropin (TSH) signals for the release of thyroxine from the thyroid gland and is essential for normal wellbeing. Thyrotropic hormone occasionally occurs in excess, and the normal serum values are a sensitive indicator of the integrity of the feedback mechanism between the liberation of thyroxine and the availability or inhibition of TSH.

Prolactin stimulates the production of milk in the female animal. Its effectiveness depends on the previous effect of adrenal hormones on breast tissue. Suckling initiates the release of prolactin. Prolactin is a large peptide hormone that has many functions in lower animals, but apparently only one in man. It shows physiologic variations, as does growth hormone, in association with sleep, stress, and other stimuli. The secretion of prolactin seems to be regulated by an inhibitory factor, secreted from the hypothalamus. Prolactin secretion rises progressively during pregnancy, reaching its maximum at term, coincident with the delivery of the fetus.

Adrenocorticotropin (ACTH) is the hormone that indicates to the adrenal cortex that it should produce a number of hormones. Hyperproduction of ACTH is the most common cause of Cushing's syndrome, which we discussed in this chapter.

Melanocyte-stimulating hormone. In lower animals, this hormone is produced in the intermediate lobe of the pituitary, and it stimulates melanocytes (pigment-producing cells). In man, it is produced in the anterior lobe and has some melanocyte-stimulating properties.

The posterior lobe, called the neurohypophysis, produces two hormones: oxytocin and vasopressin (antidiuretic hormone).

Oxytocin derives its name from its ability to cause contraction of smooth muscle, principally in the uterus (Greek *oxys*, swift, and *tokos*, birth). This hormone is used clinically to induce uterine contractions during ineffective labor, and to cause tonic constriction of the uterus following delivery to control postpartum bleeding. Oxytocin also seems to have an effect on the mammary gland and aids in the ejection of milk.

Antidiuretic hormone (ADH), or vasopressin, increases the rate of reabsorption of water and electrolytes by the renal tubules, so that it reduces the output of urine. It thus performs the important function of guarding the organism against excessive water loss. In the absence of antidiuretic hormone, continued loss of fluid and accompanying thirst lead to the syndrome called diabetes insipidus.

23

BLOOD AND LYMPH NODES

Half the secret of resistance to disease is cleanliness; the other half is dirtiness.—ANONYMOUS

The hematopoietic system includes the circulating blood, lymphoid tissue, and its site of origin, the bone marrow. For most purposes, the spleen is included in any consideration. Whereas marrow of long bones is yellow and is partially composed of fat in adult life, in childhood it is red and full of active precursors of both red and white blood cells. One may regard the hematopoietic system as a tissue whose cells include the red blood cell and white blood cell series and platelets. The interstitial space is the plasma. Thought of in that way, the hematopoietic system is a large organ of from 4,000 to 8,000 grams, depending on the size of the person. The normal liver weighs 1,200 grams and is the largest single organ of the body.

We may separate diseases of blood into three general categories: those of the red cells (erythrocytes), those of the white cells (leukocytes), and those of platelets. There may be too few cells (anemia for red blood cells, leukopenia for white blood cells), or too many (polycythemia for red blood cells, leukemia for white blood cells), but this classification is an oversimplification.

We shall consider the normal structure and function of each of these elements before going on to discuss their diseases.

The **erythrocyte** is a biconcave disc about 8 μ in diameter and has no nucleus in man. The shape has been a source of much discussion; like most successful packages, it does its job well, for a biconcave disc presents the largest interface between the surface of the cell and the plasma. This shape permits efficient absorption and release of gases. In health, there are 5 to 6 × 10⁶ red blood cells per mm³ in men, and 4.5 to 5 × 10⁶ in women. The mature erythrocyte is derived in a sequence of steps from a primitive stem cell which, according to the unitarian hypothesis, is the progenitor of all blood cells. The erythroblast contains no hemoglobin, but as one line of differentiation takes place through **normoblasts** to **normocytes,** the ribosomes of this cell begin to make hemoglobin, that quintessential pigment of all animal forms. The normocyte loses its nucleus in man, becomes a

reticulocyte, and then a mature erythrocyte, which lives for about 120 days under normal conditions.

The mature erythrocyte is easily deformed, which allows it to pass through narrow capillaries, and normally it has an average diameter of 8.4 μ, which can be used as a standard for estimating the size of other cells seen under the microscope. The normal erythrocyte appears uniformly stained with routine hematoxylin and eosin or Wright's stain, as distinct from abnormal erythrocytes, which are present in some of the congenital or acquired anemias. The erythrocyte is a simple bag of hemoglobin designed to transport this iron-containing pigment around and around, giving up oxygen in the microenvironment, taking on CO_2, only to release it later in exchange for oxygen. The living hemoglobin molecule is made of 574 amino acids in four chains, totaling 10,000 atoms with a molecular weight of 64,500. Each hemoglobin molecule can carry four molecules of oxygen at a time. It is estimated there are 280,000,000 hemoglobin molecules in each erythrocyte.

As told in a most enthralling way by Horace Judson in *The Eighth Day of Creation,* Max Perutz was able to demonstrate that the hemoglobin molecule changes its shape as it takes up oxygen and gives it off. This observation confirms the hypothesis of Monod that the conformation of proteins is directly related to their function, and that this structure/function relationship exists at the molecular level as well as at other levels of biologic action. Monod called hemoglobin an ''honorary enzyme because it acts like one'' (Tab. 23–1).

In the normal human adult male, there are about 15 g of hemoglobin per 100 ml, and in the adult female there are

Table 23–1. Red Cell Values in Adults: Normal Range

	MEN	WOMEN
Red blood cells	4.5–6.3	4.2–5.4 × 10⁶/mm³
Hemoglobin	14–18	12–16 g/dl
Packed cell volume	42–45	37–47 ml/dl
Mean corpuscular volume	83–97	83–97 fl
Mean corpuscular hemoglobin	27–31	27–31 pg
Mean corpuscular hemoglobin concentration	32–36	32–36 g/dl
Reticulocytes absolute	0.2 to 2.0	0.2 to 2.0 × 10⁶l

493

about 14 g per 100 ml. Packed cell volume is measured by the **hematocrit.**

It must be emphasized that a well-stained blood smear, studied by an educated eye and brain, still affords one of the best means of arriving at an accurate hematologic diagnosis. The smear provides the observer with information as to the size and shape of the red cells, the concentration of the hemoglobin in these cells, and the presence of nucleated cells and reticulocytes. The size and shape of the red cells demand special attention. Anisocytosis (variation in size) and poikilocytosis (variation in shape) are indications of disease (Fig. 23–1).

The **leukocytes** or white blood cells number from 6,000 to 8,000 per cubic millimeter of blood. Large numbers, however, are trapped in unused capillaries, and as physical exertion causes great numbers of these capillaries to become opened, the leukocyte count shows a corresponding rise after exercise. Unlike erythrocytes, white blood cells are not uniform in type, but are of several kinds. In one variety, the granules are large and stain bright red with eosin; this type is known as the **eosinophil.** Eosinophils form only 2% of the total leukocyte count. The neutrophil constitutes about 70% of the leukocytes, but this figure varies considerably. Another type has granules that stain blue, hence the name **basophil.**

These types of cells are formed in the sinusoids of the bone marrow, in much the same way as the erythrocytes are formed, i.e., they go through immature stages before the adult form is reached. These stages are the **myeloblast** and the **myelocyte.** Granules appear for the first time in the myelocyte, and these cells are present in large numbers in the marrow, but they do not enter the blood stream under normal conditions. Polymorphonuclear leukocytes defend the body against bacteria by phagocytosis, a process dis-

cussed in connection with inflammation. PMNs in the blood are enormously increased in acute infections, because the depots in the bone marrow pour their reserve into the blood stream, and at the same time speed the rate of production. The function of eosinophils is uncertain, but their number may be markedly increased in allergic and parasitic conditions.

Lymphocytes form about 20% of the total leukocyte count. They are small, plain-looking, mononuclear cells, with little cytoplasm around the spherical nucleus. Large numbers of lymphocytes appear at a focus of chronic inflammation, some derived from the blood, others from the tissues. Lymphocytes have been divided into two classes, on the basis of their site of origin and their surface markers. We now recognize T cells (thymus-derived) and B cells (bursa-derived). These cells and their function have been discussed in the chapter on immunology.

Monocytes (large mononuclear cells), are actively phagocytic, and play an important part in the inflammatory process. In acute inflammation, they form the second line of defense, arriving later than the polymorphonuclear leukocytes and serving the useful purpose of scavengers. They are formed in the bone marrow and constitute about 8% of the leukocytes. Monocytes secrete a large number of cytokines and enzymes. The most important cytokine is interleukin-1 which has a multiplicity of effects, including stimulation of lymphocytes.

In a blood examination, the leukocytes may be examined in two ways: (1) leukocyte count and (2) differential count. The object of the leukocyte count is to estimate the total number of leukocytes, and to determine whether there is a leukocytosis (increase in the number) or leukopenia. This useful procedure is simple and takes only a few minutes. In a differential count, several hundred leukocytes are exam-

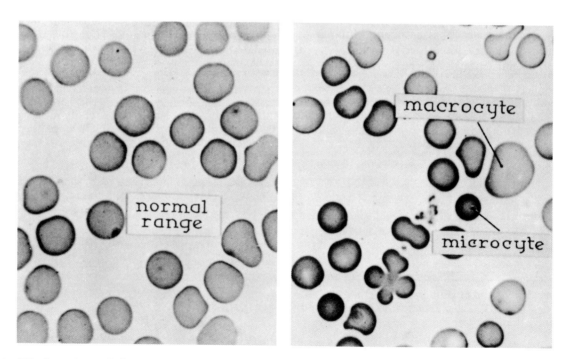

Fig. 23–1   This photomicrograph shows the smear of **normal erythrocytes** on the left and **erythrocytes with variable size** on the right. A large red blood cell or macrocyte, and a small red blood cell or microcyte are both shown on the right. (From Ham, A.W.: *Histology*, 7th Ed. Philadelphia, J. B. Lippincott Co., 1974.)

ined, note being taken of whether each cell is a polymorphonuclear leukocyte, an eosinophil, a lymphocyte, or a monocyte. In this way, the percentage of the various cells is determined. In selected cases, this count may prove of great use. It is essential in the leukemias, where one or more white cell lines may predominate in blood.

Platelets are the third type of cell of the blood, but the last to have had their function recognized.

The electron microscope has revolutionized our concept of the platelet, which used to be regarded as an inert particle, structureless, and possibly an artifact. Now it is known to possess abundant metabolic equipment, microtubules, three types of granules, and 80 enzymatic activities.

The platelet is the first element to appear at a break in the lining of a blood vessel. Within 1 to 3 seconds, platelets adhere to the damaged wall, surely the promptest first aid we could imagine. By their adherence and agglutination, they initiate the coagulation cascade. And this is the element of the blood that we used to consider structureless, without function, and possibly an artifact!

Blood Groups. The red cells of a person may clump together when mixed with blood of another person, with fatal results if transfusion is done. Landsteiner showed in 1900 that all persons can be divided into four major blood groups, depending on the reaction of the serum of one on the red cells of another. Red blood cells and serum of each person are perfectly adapted to one another, but the cells of one person may be incompatible with the serum of another.

When two bloods are incompatible, the red cells from the donor clump together (agglutinate) in the serum of the recipient, owing to the presence of agglutinins in the serum of the latter. The incompatibility lies in that, in human blood, the red cells contain either no antigens or one or both of two antigens, known as A and B, which may produce agglutination, whereas the serum contains corresponding antibodies or agglutinins known as beta or anti-B and alpha or anti-A. Under natural conditions, an antigen and its corresponding agglutinin cannot be present simultaneously in the same blood. If, however, blood containing antigen A or B is introduced by transfusion into a person whose blood contains the corresponding antibody, agglutination occurs. Moreover, hemolysis as well as agglutination of the transfused red cells may occur. This hemolysis is the real danger of the blood transfusion, because breakdown products of blood provoke a hypersensitivity reaction and collect in the kidney and may lead to renal failure.

Depending on the presence of the two antigens, the blood of all persons can be divided into four major groups, known as O, A, B, and AB. Group O contains no antigen, group A contains A antigen, Group B contains B antigen, and group AB contains both A and B antigens (Table 23–2). As group O contains no antigen, it does not react with the blood of other groups, even though they contain agglutinins. Therefore, persons belonging to this group are called universal

Table 23–2. Determination of Blood Groups

Cells agglutinated by serum from a known:		Person belongs to:
Group A	Group B	
No	No	Group O
No	Yes	Group A
Yes	No	Group B
Yes	Yes	Group AB

donors because their blood is compatible with that of any of the four groups. Fortunately, this is the largest group, comprising over 40% of persons. A person in any group may receive blood from anyone in the same group. The AB group, having no agglutinins in the serum, is a universal recipient. The term "universal" unfortunately ignores the Rh and other factors, to be discussed.

Specific antigens and agglutinins (antibodies) are hereditary, a fact that is sometimes made use of in cases of disputed parentage.

The suitability of a donor is determined by two methods, known as grouping (or typing) and matching (or cross-matching). The blood group to which someone belongs can be decided by testing his red cells against serum from both a known group A (which contains anti-B agglutinins) donor and a known group B (which contains anti-A agglutinins) donor, and by noting whether any agglutination occurs. When the cells and serum of the prospective donor have been cross-matched for ABO blood group against the serum and cells of the patient, there still may be incompatibility. One factor we have not yet accounted for is the **Rh factor,** so called because it was first discovered in the blood of the *rh*esus monkey. About 85% of persons possess this factor or antigen, so they are said to be Rh-positive, whereas 15% lack the antigen and are Rh-negative. Anti-Rh agglutinins are not normally present in the serum, but may be formed in Rh-negative persons following transfusion by Rh-positive blood. Thus the first transfusion of Rh-positive blood into an Rh-negative person will **not** cause a reaction, because there are no antibodies yet. After this transfusion, the Rh-negative person will begin to synthesize antibody to this new antigen he has just encountered. The next time he receives an Rh-positive transfusion, the antibodies will attack the donated blood and cause a transfusion reaction. You will recall from Chapter 6 that this immunological reaction can also be encountered in the case of an Rh-negative mother who becomes pregnant for the second time from a Rh-positive man. Today, all persons who donate or receive blood are "typed" with regard to the Rh factor, as well as A, B, and O; so this type of transfusion reaction is rare.

The chief value of transfusion is replacement of blood after a severe, acute hemorrhage, when it is truly a lifesaving procedure. Transfusion is also useful for combating shock following surgical operations, especially those associated with much loss of blood. Repeated transfusions are sometimes used in the treatment of chronic anemias and in severe infections.

Unfortunately, it is not possible to use the blood of all and sundry for the purpose of transfusion. It should be clear that the blood of some persons carries infectious agents such as syphilis, the hepatitis viruses, or HIV.

If the bloods of the donor and the recipient are incompatible, there may be immediate signs of shock, as evidenced by restlessness, pallor, shortness of breath, feeble rapid pulse, and fall in blood pressure. There may also be a more delayed type of reaction, marked by chills, fever, pain in the back, jaundice, and the presence of hemoglobin in the urine. These delayed symptoms are all due to the breaking down of the red blood cells. About 40% of the patients showing these symptoms of hemolysis make a complete recovery. In the remaining 60%, symptoms of renal failure develop in the course of a week, and the patient may die if left untreated. From a consideration of these facts, it is evident how important it is to prevent reactions to transfusions, and how necessary are the preliminary laboratory tests to determine the question of blood incompatibility. It is essential that blood for cross-matching be correctly and adequately labeled, so that there can be no doubt about the identity of the person from whom it was collected. For many purposes, particularly in the treatment of shock, blood plasma can be used instead of whole blood. As the plasma contains no red cells, the question of incompatibility does not arise, and the dangers of using unsuitable blood are thus avoided. Plasma has a great advantage over whole blood in that it can be dried, and can be kept in the dry form for an indefinite period, but, unfortunately, it may be contaminated with infectious agents.

For the purposes of this chapter, we divided disorders of the red blood cell series into considerations of too little (anemias) and too much (polycythemias). We then consider platelet disorders and abnormalities of coagulation. Finally, we turn to disease of the lymphoid system: namely, increase in circulating white blood cells (leukemias), and infiltrations of the lymphoreticular system (lymphomas).

ANEMIAS

Anemias are defined as a **"decrease in the total amount of hemoglobin in a given volume of whole blood."** This reduction can be due to a decrease in the number of red blood cells in a given volume, or it may be due to a decrease in the amount of hemoglobin per red blood cell. It may also, much more rarely, be due to a decrease in the amount of blood, as in acute blood loss. The basic defects can be understood best in terms of (A) defects in synthesis of components of the red blood cell, (B) increased destruction of the red blood cell, or (C) loss that is greater than synthesis. Anemia should not be regarded as a disease, but rather as evidence of a disease, which can reside in a red blood cell or can be caused by some other abnormality.

Any consideration of anemias is complicated by the existence of so many different causes that some conceptualization of the problem is the only way to deal with the vast number of possibilities. Two general attempts to classify anemias as morphologic and as etiologic are shown in Tables 23–3 and 23–4. Neither of these classifications is the complete answer, any more than other attempts to impose schemes of organization on biologic phenomena satisfy all people, but the

Table 23–3. Anemias: Morphologic Classification

1. Macrocytic (MCV 93 mm³)
    a) Megaloblastic erythropoiesis (deficiency of vitamin B_{12} or folic acid)
    b) Liver disease and obstructive jaundice
    c) Reticulocytosis
2. Normocytic
    a) Acute blood loss before reticulocytosis
    b) Hemolytic anemia when not associated with spherocytosis
    c) Anemia of chronic disease
3. Microcytic and hypochromic
    a) Iron deficiency
    b) Thalassemia
    c) Sideroblastic anemia

(From Brain, M. C.: (The anemias.) Introduction. In *Cecil Textbook of Medicine*, 15th Ed. Edited by P. B. Beeson, W. McDermott, and J. B. Wyngaarden. Philadelphia, W. B. Saunders Co., 1979.)

advantage of recognizing both classifications is that often recognition of the anemia is made on examination of the smear, and the approach to diagnosis is facilitated by using a cross-reference.

We shall consider the different types of anemias after we reflect on the signs and symptoms common to all anemias.

The first fact that emerges from any experience with

Table 23–4. Anemias: Etiologic Classification

I. Principally caused by impaired production
    A. Disturbances of the proliferation and differentiation of stem cells
        1. Aplastic anemia
        2. Anemia of chronic renal failure
        3. Endocrine deficiency (pituitary, thyroid, adrenal, or testicular hormones)
    B. Disturbances of proliferation and maturation of differentiated erythroblasts
        1. Defective DNA synthesis (vitamin B_{12}, folic acid, and metabolic defects in purine and pyrimidine metabolism)
        2. Defective hemoglobin synthesis
            a. Deficient globin synthesis (thalassemia)
            b. Deficient heme synthesis (iron deficiency)
        3. Protein malnutrition
        4. Anemia of chronic disease
        5. Myelophthisic anemias due to bone marrow infiltration
II. Principally caused by increased rate of destruction
    A. Intrinsic or red blood cell abnormalities
        1. Membrane disorders
        2. Congenital or inherited enzyme deficiencies
        3. Disorders of hemoglobin
    B. Extrinsic or extraerythrocytic abnormalities
        1. Plasma factors
        2. Physical factors
        3. Chemical or toxic agents
III. Anemia of blood loss (acute or chronic)

(From Brain, M.C.: (The anemias.) Introduction. In *Cecil Textbook of Medicine*, 15th Ed. Edited by P. B. Beeson, W. McDermott, and J. B. Wyngaarden. Philadelphia, W. B. Saunders Co., 1979.)

patients who are truly anemic is the extraordinary variability of their symptoms. The significant majority of these patients may have no appreciation of any physiologic disability. The reason for this unawareness is that anemias usually evolve over months and years, and the gradual development of the significant decrease in hemoglobin may be so insidious that adaptive mechanisms completely compensate for concentrations of hemoglobin as low as 6 g (normal 14). We have seen several elderly patients with hematocrits of 15% (normal 45%) who are totally without symptoms at rest, and for whom the physiologic embarrassment of shortness of breath is credited simply to old age. The awareness of a gradual loss of oxygen-carrying capacity goes unnoticed, particularly in the aged and sedentary patient. Severe blood loss, on the other hand, is accompanied by other alarming symptoms, and the anemia is usually of less significance than such problems as shock, collapse, dyspnea, or the appearance of blood in the stool or vomitus.

Typically, however, anemia causes nonspecific symptoms of decreased oxygen in the tissues: weakness, fatigue, shortness of breath on exertion, pain in the chest, awareness that the heart is beating rapidly (palpitations), irritability, headache, and lightheadedness, all of which can be caused by other diseases, and most of which are often misinterpreted.

The physical examination of an anemic patient may show only the pallor of the mucus membranes, although this may be inconspicuous and overlooked.

For the purposes of this discussion, anemia will be grouped into four categories: normochromic and normocytic (normal size and color); hypochromic and microcytic (reduced color and size); hemolytic; and macrocytic.

Normochromic, Normocytic Anemias

The easiest form of anemia to understand is that in which there simply is not enough blood because of blood loss. The clinical patterns of this blood loss are shown in Table 23–5 and are appropriate and consistent with the volume of the loss. We do not ordinarily regard this situation as an anemia, because usually the explanation is obvious and it does not represent a puzzle to be solved, as many anemias usually do.

One of the commonest and most difficult clinical problems to solve, however, is the presence of a **normochromic** (normal amount of hemoglobin per cell), **normocytic** (normal and regular size of red blood cells) anemia in a person who may have a number of predisposing causes. The traditional explanations offered for the occurrence of this simple chronic anemia are: decreased life span of the erythrocytes, a failure of the bone marrow to compensate for the mild hemolytic process, or an impairment of iron release from the reticuloendothelial cells. Each and all of these lead to failure in maintaining the normal numbers of red blood cells. This disorder is seen usually in persons with one of the following: infection, arthritis, liver disease (cirrhosis), endocrine disorders, cancer, or renal failure. Because the anemia is often mild, and the underlying disease is severe, emphasis is on the management of the underlying disease. If treatment is successful, the anemia usually disappears.

Another cause of normocytic, normochromic anemia is malnutrition in which protein deficiency is a serious component. Worldwide, anemia is of great economic importance, especially in those parts of the world where protein is in short supply and is often unavailable for growing children.

A third, but much more general, cause for this type of anemia is the failure of the bone marrow to produce all (not only red blood cells) cellular elements. This disease is called **aplastic anemia** and it may occur without apparent cause, or it may be related to exposure to chemical agents, cytotoxic drugs, infections, irradiation, or be associated with such diverse etiologies as invasion of the bone marrow by cancer.

Whereas the etiology of aplastic anemia in simplest terms is interference with the normal maturation and

Table 23–5. Clinical Manifestations of Acute Blood Loss

VOLUME OF BLOOD LOST		CLINICAL MANIFESTATIONS
% OF BLOOD VOLUME	ML	
10	500	Usually none; rarely vasovagal syncope
20	1,000	Few changes supine; upright or with exercise, tachycardia and mild hypotension are often present
30 to 40	1,500 to 2,000	Marked postural hypotension and tachycardia; central venous pressure, cardiac output, and arterial blood pressure are reduced; pulse is thready; skin is cold and clammy; thirst, air hunger, headache, and syncope are frequent
50	2,500	Severe shock, often leading to death

(From Brown, E.B.: Acute hemorrhagic anemia. In *Cecil Textbook of Medicine*, 15th Ed. Edited by P.B. Beeson, W. McDermott, and J.B. Wyngaarden. Philadelphia, W.B. Saunders Co., 1979.)

development of the pluripotent hematopoietic stem cell, resulting in a decreased number of red blood cells, white blood cells, and platelets, the mechanism by which this occurs is not entirely clear.

Regardless of its etiology, aplastic anemia has been treated successfully with bone marrow transplants.

Normochromic, normocytic anemia is diagnosed in the laboratory by finding simply too few normal red blood cells, as distinct from the other types of anemias (hypochromic, microcytic, and macrocytic), in which the appearance of the red blood cells suggests the diagnosis. Aplastic anemia is diagnosed by the paucity of all elements and not just of the red blood cells (pancytopenia).

Hypochromic, Microcytic Anemias

The commonest cause of anemia, world-wide, is **iron deficiency,** because of the increased iron loss due to intestinal parasites coupled with inadequate dietary intake. In much of the world (Asia, Africa) more than half the adult population may suffer from serious iron-deficiency anemia. Estimates range from 60% of pregnant women to 30% of all women, and 5% of all men. The reason for the difference is monthly loss of blood in the menses, coupled with the requirements for fetal iron during pregnancy. Repeated pregnancies and excessive menstrual loss are great drains on the body stores. A prolonged milk diet for children fails to supply them with iron. In the western world, inadequate meals of young mothers and hidden gastrointestinal bleeding in men of all ages are additional common causes that contribute to this particular type of anemia. Iron-deficiency anemia is most easily diagnosed by finding small, poorly stained red blood cells on a good smear of peripheral blood. The red blood cells show variation in size (anisocytosis) and shape (poikilocytosis). A calculation of the mean corpuscular volume and of the mean corpuscular hemoglobin concentration shows these values to be low. These values can be determined by knowing the number of red blood cells, the hemoglobin concentration, and the hematocrit. The mean corpuscular volume (MCV) is $\dfrac{\text{HCT}}{\text{RBC number}}$ which gives a number that normally ranges between 80 and 105 μ^3. It is spuriously elevated with some of the newer counting methods because of trapping of serum, so that the value should be suspected from the examination of the smear.

The mean corpuscular hemoglobin concentration (MCHC) is determined by dividing the hemoglobin by the hematocrit. It is normally between 32 and 33 g per ml and is never elevated. Values of less than 30 g per ml indicate iron deficiency, and the mean corpuscular volume is unusually less than 80.

Two other determinations to confirm the suspicion of iron deficiency as a cause of anemia are the plasma iron concentration and the total plasma iron-building capacity.

When someone has been either losing iron or taking it in inadequate amounts, the next thing that happens is mobilization of iron stores from such cells as the reticuloendothelial system in the liver. When these iron stores have been used up, a signal is given to the small intestine to increase the rate of iron absorption. As the iron requirements for the biosynthesis of hemoglobin (and myoglobin, particularly in growing children) increase, the plasma iron concentration falls. The concentration of the serum protein responsible for transporting iron (transferrin) increases and the saturation of this protein by iron is decreased. When the demand for iron is not met, blood cells are liberated into the peripheral blood that show this lack; on smear they are distorted and contain too little hemoglobin.

Iron is an essential element in man largely for its role in hemoglobin and myoglobin maintenance and production. With increased loss, as in bleeding from a peptic ulcer, decreased intake, or extra requirements (pregnancy), there may be insufficient iron. This lack may be visible in the red blood cell itself, which appears as a pale, small shadow of its normal self. This manifestation of iron deficiency is a late result of the process, because the body, in its wisdom, tends to use up all the other stores before it circulates a physiologically unfit cell.

The symptoms of this type of anemia are no different from those of the previous types. They begin insidiously and are nonspecific. The tiredness, shortness of breath on exertion, headache, light-headedness, palpitations, and irritability are all part of the syndrome. Physical findings may show pallor alone. The diagnosis is made only by laboratory examination of the smear and calculation of the red blood cell indices. The treatment is twofold: short-term, to treat the anemia if necessary, even by transfusion, and to replace iron. Second, to determine and treat the underlying cause of the iron deficiency, be it nutritional or blood loss.

Macrocytic Anemias (Megaloblastic)

The term megaloblastic (Greek *megas*, large, and *blastos*, germ) or macrocytic is used because the common abnormality is gigantism of all proliferating cells, most obvious in examinations of the smear of the peripheral blood, but also exfoliated cells of the gastrointestinal and genitourinary tract. The defect common to all these cells is delayed synthesis of DNA.

Macrocytic anemias are caused by inadequate ingestion of factors on which DNA synthesis depends **(folic acid and vitamin B_{12})**; inadequate absorption (due to interference with factors on which B_{12} depends for absorption, intrinsic and extrinsic); or increased requirement, excretion, or destruction of these factors.

A poor diet, such as strict vegetarianism, in which there are no sources of vitamin B_{12}, or long-term alcoholism, in which no folic acid is available, or simple poverty will often lead to macrocytic as well as other types of anemias. A gastrectomy or invasion of the stomach by cancer will bring about macrocytic anemias, just as atrophy of the gastric mucosa, associated with autoimmune disease, is a predisposing cause. **Pernicious anemia** is the name given to the particular type of macrocytic anemia that is due to deficiency of intrinsic factor, which is essential for B_{12} effectiveness. This factor is a carrier that is secreted by the gastric mucosa and permits the passage of the large molecule of B_{12} across the mucosa of the ileum. Lack of carrier molecules, usually caused by atrophic gastritis, leads to B_{12} deficiency. This disease is age-related. It has a worldwide incidence of 1 per million at 1 year, 1 per 10,000 at age 10, 1 per 5,000 at age 35, and 1 in 200 at age 60. In some instances there are circulating antibodies to intrinsic factor, which implies an autoimmune etiology for this disease.

Other causes of macrocytic anemias may occur if the small bowel is affected by disease, such as sprue, or by granulomatous lesions, or if the patient is taking drugs that impair normal mucosal renewal (e.g., methotrexate), or if the bowel has been resected. These conditions reduce absorption.

Another major cause is the competition for vitamin B_{12}, such as occurs with intestinal parasites or bacterial overproduction. The fish tapeworm (*Diphyllobothrium latum*) and the presence of loops of bowel that do not empty properly and in which bacteria grow abundantly (blind loop syndrome) are such examples.

It is important to remember that normal adult body stores of B_{12} last 3 to 6 years after absorption of B_{12} ceases. However, symptoms may not occur for 20 years or more after B_{12} is no longer ingested, because the body jealously guards its storehouse of B_{12} by continuing to reabsorb it from the bile.

Clinically, the symptoms are those of anemia in general, with the additional and important neurologic manifestations of B_{12} deficiency, such as parasthesias,

numbness and tingling, and loss of vibration and position sense. Other changes affect the tongue which becomes smooth and shiny (Fig. 23–2), and the stomach with a dramatic decrease in the number of parietal cells. Examination of the bone marrow shows clusters of large cells called megaloblasts.

One of the most important points in diagnosing macrocytic anemia is to distinguish between those anemias caused by folate acid deficiency and those due to B_{12} deficiency, because the latter form has serious neurological complications affecting the spinal cord (Fig. 23–3). Neurologic changes of B_{12} deficiency may be irreversible. It is unwise to treat macrocytic anemia without clearly establishing the correct etiology. A patient whose lack of intrinsic factor causes his or her B_{12} deficiency would be on a monthly maintenance dose of B_{12} for life. Vitamin B_{12} deficiency impairs myelin formation and is followed by axonal degeneration and finally destruction of the neurons.

The distinction between folate deficiency and B_{12} deficiency is made now by measuring serum levels of both B_{12} and folate, and it is wise to recognize that both deficiencies may occur in the same patient, for example, in an alcoholic with intrinsic factor deficiency.

Hemolytic Anemias

This is a large and heterogeneous group. A shortened life span of the red blood cells with resulting hemolysis, that is to say, lysis or solution of the red cells either in the circulation or in the spleen, is the

Fig. 23–2 Smooth tongue in a case of **pernicious anemia**. (Wintrobe, M.: *Clinical Hematology*. Philadelphia, Lea & Febiger.)

Fig. 23–3 These two photographs show sections from the thoracic and lumbar spinal cord of a patient dying with **pernicious anemia** in 1926, before treatment was available. The central pallor in the ascending and descending tracts of the posterior columns is typical of the irreversible neurologic lesions that accompany untreated pernicious anemia. (From Follis, R.H.: *Deficiency Disease.* Springfield, Ill., Charles C Thomas, 1958.)

feature common to all. The mechanism by which this process occurs may be one of two profoundly different types. In the first, the defect is hereditary, and in the second it is acquired, being commonly caused by circulating antibodies. (These antibodies are frequently the product of autoimmune reactions.) Thus the red cell may either be born vulnerable or it may become so, owing to acquired external factors. In the

congenital (hereditary) form, the fault lies in the red cells, whereas in the acquired form it lies in the environment. For this reason, removal of the spleen, the graveyard of the erythrocytes, may be beneficial in the congenital type of this disease. ACTH or cortisone may also benefit the acquired form. The two types are differentiated in the laboratory by means of the Coombs test, which is designed to show the presence

Blood and Lymph Nodes

501

of antibodies (agglutinins) absorbed to the surface of the red cells in the acquired but not in the congenital form.

We must also recognize that increased hemolysis does not necessarily result in anemia. Bone marrow activity may compensate for destruction of the erythrocytes. Under these circumstances, a person is said to have hemolytic disease, but not to suffer from hemolytic anemia, which only occurs when the bone marrow is unable to compensate for the shortened life span of the erythrocytes. The best signpost of hemolytic anemia is a persistent increase to 5% or more in the number of reticulocytes (immature red blood cells). Other evidence of bone marrow overactivity is leukocytosis, the presence of nucleated red cells in the peripheral blood, and increased platelets.

The hereditary defect may involve abnormal red cells or abnormal hemoglobin. The outstanding example of a red cell defect is spherocytic anemia; corresponding examples of hemoglobin defect are sickle cell anemia and thalassemia.

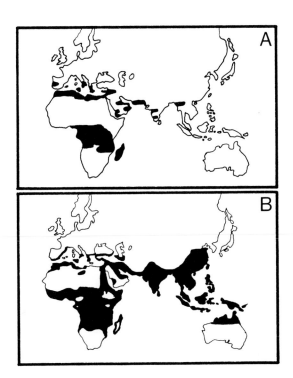

Fig. 23–4 These 2 maps show A, the distribution of **sickle cell disease**, and B, the **distribution of malaria**. One can superimpose maps A and B and identify the distribution of malaria and sickle cell disease in Africa. The sickle cell gene is not a significant part of the gene pool in Asia. Since the presence of the sickle cell trait (heterozygous) appears to confer some immunity to malaria, it is thought that the sickle cell trait is an evolutionary adaptation to malaria in the environment. (From Motulsky, A. G.: Metabolic polymorphisms and the role of infectious diseases in human evolution. Human Biol., 32:43, 1960.)

Congenital spherocytic anemia, as the name implies, shows a spheroidal shape of the erythrocytes in place of normal biconcave discs. Their shape is due to a defect in spectrin which is filamentous cytoskeletal protein organized in a network underneath the red cell membrane. This results in increased rigidity leading to excessive red cell destruction or hemolysis. The disease is transmitted as an autosomal dominant trait.

The blood shows anemia, usually mild, but severe in crises. Two chief characteristics of the blood film are microspherulocytes and reticulocytes. A spherocyte is smaller than a normal erythrocyte and spherical instead of biconcave. Reticulocytes are more numerous than in any other disease. In place of the usual 1%, they may constitute 20%. There is an increased fragility of the red cells when placed in a salt solution of a strength that leaves normal cells untouched. This is the basis of a simple laboratory test for spherocytic anemia.

The disease may remain latent for many years, although the fragility is there, hanging like the sword of Damocles over the head of the person carrying the defective gene. For some unknown reason, there may be occasional crises, in which there is increased blood destruction with attacks of pain referable to the abdomen, fever and low blood pressure.

Jaundice is the characteristic feature of the crises, although a mild degree of jaundice, often unrecognized, may be present all the time. Jaundice (French *jaune,* yellow) results from increased hemolysis, which produces an increase in circulating blood breakdown products, one of which is a pigment, bilirubin. It is, of course, the result of the increased fragility of the red cells, the actual destruction taking place in the spleen, which becomes enlarged, and which appears to assume a function of overactivity, known as hypersplenism. On this basis, splenectomy has become the recognized treatment for congenital spherocytic anemia, often with dramatic and satisfying results.

Sickle cell anemia is a genetic anomaly in the formation of the hemoglobin molecule; it has much in common with spherocytosis. Both conditions are hereditary; in both there may be active disease (anemia), or merely the fingerprints (spherocytes or sickle cells, as the case may be); and both are characterized by hemolytic anemia and by the appearance of large numbers of reticulocytes in the peripheral blood. A major difference is that the genetic defect in sickle cell anemia is largely confined to Africans (Fig. 23–4). It is transmitted as a dominant mendelian characteristic by either sex. Sickle cell anemia is observed in homozygous individuals, whereas the **sickle cell trait** represents a heterozygous state. The biochemical defect is a point mutation resulting in the substitution of one amino acid for another in the hemoglobin protein. This is the prototypic "molecular disease."

Based on this knowledge, a test has been designed to screen fetuses using a molecular hybridization technique which can be performed on a tiny biopsy of chorion sampled through the cervix of pregnant women, or on cells collected by amniocentesis.

The blood presents a striking picture in the active phase of the disease. There is marked anemia as well as leukocytosis, and the blood smear shows an extraordinary change in the shape of the red cells, for large numbers of these are crescentic or sickle in form (Fig. 23–5).

In the latent phase, sickle cells are not present in the circulating blood, but they can be readily demonstrated in the presence of a decrease in the oxygen tension.

This causes the hemoglobin inside the red blood cell to polymerize, forcing the cell to have a sickle shape. This unusual shape is associated with markedly diminished deformability and the cells pile up in blood capillaries. The net result is a decreased oxygen supply in the tissues that are dependent on these capillaries, with microinfarctions being the ultimate consequence.

Acute crises occur in sickle cell anemia. Not only is the anemia intensified, but the patient suffers from attacks of abdominal pain that may be confused with acute appendicitis or with ruptured peptic ulcer. Infarcts of the spleen are common, owing to thrombosis in that organ.

Overall, in the absence of intense therapy, patients with sickle cell disease usually die in their third decade.

Thalassemia is another of the hereditary group of hemolytic anemias. The gene responsible for the defect in hemoglobin formation is distributed among the peoples of the eastern Mediterranean basin. For this reason, it has long been known as Mediterranean anemia or thalassemia (Greek *thalassa*, sea, i.e., the Mediterranean). The trait has now been carried far and wide throughout the world by the migration of peoples. This hemoglobin defect also results in a decreased life span of the circulating red cells.

There are several forms of thalassemia and the basic molecular defect has been identified for a good num-

A   **B**

Fig. 23–5 *A*, This smear shows red blood cells, some of which are slightly distorted. *B*, Following anoxemia, many cells appear to have an elongated sickle form with pointed ends. These cells cause the sickled erythrocytes to fill the capillary bed. (From Herrick, J.B.: **Peculiar elongated and sickle-shaped red corpuscles** in a case of severe anemia. Arch. Intern. Med., 6:517, 1910.)

ber of them. Normal adult hemoglobin is made up of two α chains and two β chains. The fundamental disorder of thalassemia is decreased or absent α or β chains. The reason is, most often, either a mutation that interferes with the normal processing of the corresponding m-Rna, or simply a deletion of the gene.

Because thalassemia is genetically diverse, its clinical manifestations are also quite variable. Besides hemolysis, patients often have hepatomegaly and splenomegaly. Facial bones can be deformed as a result of active erythropoiesis in the marrow. The pigment leaking from hemolytic red blood cells favors the formation of gallstones. In the forms of thalassemia where synthesis of one of the globin chains is completely suppressed, death occurs either *in utero* or at birth.

Many acquired hemolytic anemias are caused by extraneous agents. Among these may be mentioned chemicals and drugs, bacterial toxins such as those of hemolytic streptococci, and the malaria parasite, which, as we have seen, specializes in destroying the red cells in which it resides.

In **hemolytic disease of the newborn,** the hemolysis with resulting anemia is caused by antibodies transferred across the placenta during pregnancy. Hemolytic disease of the newborn occurs once in every 200 pregnancies worldwide and used to account for 2 to 3% of all neonatal deaths.

The immune mechanisms of hemolysis are discussed in Chapter 6.

The clinical picture varies. The child may be born dead in a condition of extreme general edema or hydrops. About 7% of those who survive are mental defectives. Jaundice may or may not be present. The blood picture is that of congenital anemia and **erythroblastosis fetalis,** that is to say, with great numbers of nucleated red cells (erythroblasts), owing to compensatory activity of the bone marrow. The mortality rate formerly was 70 to 80%, but with modern treatment and prenatal care, the incidence has dropped markedly. Exchange transfusion was given at birth when there was evidence of disease, but now Rh immunization is the treatment of choice.

POLYCYTHEMIAS

The term polycythemia means an increase in the number of the cells of the blood. **Polycythemia vera,** as the name indicates, is a true or primary increase in the number of red blood cells; its etiology is unknown. Primary polycythemia is considered to result from a clonal expansion of myeloid stem cells. There is also a secondary form of polycythemia as found in people living at high altitudes or in patients with chronic lung disease and congenital heart disease. Rarely, one observes an association of polycythemia with tumors of the kidney. This observation is interesting because a hormone, **erythropoietin,** which stimulates the bone marrow, has been found to be synthesized in the kidney.

Whatever the form of polycythemia, its cardinal manifestation is due to the presence of a markedly increased cell mass. The result is an augmented viscosity of the blood resulting in thrombosis and infarction.

In polycythemia, red blood cells are greatly increased in number, usually from 7,000,000 to 10,000,000 per cubic millimeter. Blood volume is also increased, and the blood becomes viscid, owing to the disproportionate decrease in serum. This predisposes the patient to thrombosis and infarction, particularly of the spleen, a frequent finding in polycythemia, whether it is primary or secondary. There is moderate leukocytosis, and occasionally primitive red and white cells are present in the circulating blood. As might be expected, the bone marrow is markedly hyperplastic, so that the condition may be regarded as a type of neoplasia, being comparable to leukemia in this respect. Perhaps it is significant that occasional cases have changed from erythremia to leukemia of myelogenous type.

The clinical picture is striking, for the skin and mucus membrane of the mouth are red and the conjunctiva is bloodshot. The color is due to the increased number of red cells. The spleen is always enlarged. At autopsy, the visceral vessels are greatly distended and are often thrombosed. The disease may be treated and the blood volume may be effectively reduced by repeated blood letting.

Secondary polycythemia is a compensatory increase of red cells in conditions of insufficient oxygenation, such as congenital heart disease, emphysema, and residence at high altitudes. It will be obvious that the condition is in no sense one of disease, but rather it represents a compensatory adaptation. There is no increase in leukocytes, a diagnostic point of value in distinguishing erythrocytosis from polycythemia vera.

HEMORRHAGIC DISORDERS

These disorders have been called by many names (bleeding disorders, purpuras), and have many causes, but the principle common to all is some perturbation in the mechanisms that normally control hemorrhage and maintain blood where it belongs, namely in the blood vessels. Bleeding disorders can result from such different causes as heredity, tumors, taking of drugs, or exposure to toxic chemicals. We shall consider first the normal hemostatic mechanisms, then heritable disorders characterized by bleeding, and finally a few assorted causes of increased bleeding tendencies.

Everyone knows that a characteristic of blood is its ability to clot. This is one of the most important homeostatic mechanisms of the body, for without the ability to clot, as we shall see, this essential juice of man oozes away from tiny nicks and scratches. Paradoxically, blood must be a liquid in order to circulate and it must rapidly become a coagulum in order not to be wasted.

Three different mechanisms are responsible for staunching the flow of blood when a vessel is severed, as in any traumatic injury. First, the blood vessel wall, which contains smooth muscle, will contract and narrow the orifice. There are abundant tales of severance of a limb after which arteries go into spasm and act virtually as a tourniquet. This is more likely to happen in small than in large arteries. When there is a disorder of small blood vessels, as occurs in scurvy, and old age, for example, all other hemostatic mechanisms are intact. The basic defect is in the collagen support of the blood vessel. Bleeding may occur from slight trauma, and the application of a tourniquet, such as a blood pressure cuff, may lead to hemorrhages. This is called a positive tourniquet test. The second hemostatic mechanism is the formation of a platelet plug at sites of endothelial injury. When platelets are decreased in number in the peripheral blood (**thrombocytopenia),** or have a defective function, the first signs of the abnormalities may be the spontaneous appearance of small hemorrhages in the skin (**petechiae).** The third hemostatic mechanism is coagulation proper. Before going on to consider the clotting mechanisms themselves, we shall digress for a minute to consider the platelet and its disorders.

Platelets. The normal platelet count in man varies from 150,000 to 400,000/mm^3 in the peripheral blood. Platelets are formed in the bone marrow from large cells called megakaryocytes and represent fragmentation or subdivisions of large cells. They are not complete cells in that they have no nuclei and cannot replicate. Currently, we regard platelets as performing three general functions. The surface is covered with a mucopolysaccharide that is involved in adhesion. Platelets are the first line of defense in vascular injury and adhere to the lining of blood vessels whenever structures such as collagen and basement membranes are exposed to the circulating blood. Platelets also contain large numbers of membrane-bound granules containing substances that are released on contact with such an injured surface. These secretory granules have been shown to contain serotonin, catecholamines, and a heparin-neutralizing factor, as well as lysosomal enzymes such as acid phospha-

tase and cathepsin. There are also many filaments and microtubules in platelets that enable the platelet to change its shape and to participate in clot retraction. Finally, platelets can liberate a growth factor which affects the neighboring tissue. Platelets live for about 10 days, and it is estimated that 80% of all platelets are in the circulation at any given time and that only 20% are in the spleen.

In addition to acting as a mechanical plug, the most important function of platelets is their release of a number of physiologically active substances when the platelets have become arrested on the wall of a blood vessel. The result of this release is the continued aggregation of platelets at the site of adhesion, and the progress of the coagulation process, which involves the conversion of fibrinogen to fibrin. Because platelet plugs stop bleeding from damaged capillaries, any deficiency in the number or function of platelets can be estimated by measuring the bleeding time. Conventionally, this is determined by the time it takes for bleeding to stop from 3 incisions 1 mm deep in the forearm. Bleeding time is normal in disorders of the coagulation system, but prolonged if there is a decrease in the number of platelets and in disorders of platelet function. It is also prolonged when there is a total absence of fibrinogen. Table 23–6 illustrates the clinical distinctions between capillary and platelet deficiency and defects in the coagulation mechanism.

Thrombocytopenia, or a platelet count of less than 100,000/mm^3 often leads to bleeding, which may occur after an operation or trauma. When the count is less than 40,000, bleeding may occur spontaneously. A low platelet count may result from defective production, defective maturation, disordered distribution (sequestration), or accelerated destruction. Defective production can be due to direct injury to the bone marrow by drugs or chemicals, or it may be due to invasion of the bone marrow by carcinoma or lymphoma. With deficiency of B$_{12}$ for example, there may be a defective maturation of megakaryocytes, the platelet precursor.

Other conditions that lead to a decrease in platelets are disseminated intravascular coagulation (DIC), which captures platelets in aggregates of thrombi, idiopathic thrombocytopenic purpura (ITP), and a disorder of unknown etiology that leads usually rapidly to death, called thrombotic thrombocytopenic purpura (TTP).

Disseminated Intravascular Coagulation

This pathologic phenomenon was described relatively recently and has become a well-known entity in the last 20 years, although it is difficult both to diagnose and to treat. Because it may occur as a complication of many disorders, ranging from cancer to infections, as well as in many situations in which bleeding occurs (obstetrical or operative hemorrhage, and allergic reactions), one should keep it in mind as a possible explanation for the lack of response after hemorrhage to first-line defense transfusions.

Table 23–6. Differential Considerations of Bleeding Disorders

FINDINGS	DISORDERS OF COAGULATION	DISORDERS OF PLATELETS OR VESSELS—"PURPURIC"
Petechiae	Rare	Characteristic
Deep dissecting hematomas	Characteristic	Rare
Superficial ecchymoses	Common—large and solitary	Characteristic—small and multiple
Hemarthrosis	Characteristic	Rare
Delayed bleeding	Common—cannot maintain clot	Rare
Bleeding from superficial cuts and scratches	Minimal	Persistent, often profuse
Sex of patient	80 to 90% of hereditary forms only in males	Relatively more common in females
Family history	Common	Rare

Disseminated intravascular coagulation (DIC) is characterized by abnormal clotting mechanisms and by generalized hemorrhage. As its name implies, there is an activation of the clotting mechanisms with the consequent consumption of fibrinogen and platelets and other coagulation factors of the circulatory system, particularly in the capillary vessels. This activation is usually the result of such triggering mechanisms as the presence of a large clot in the uterus, for example. The successful treatment of the underlying disorders (evacuation of the clot) will interrupt the vicious cycle of fibrinolysis and thrombosis. The sequence of fibrinolysis and thrombus formation leads to obstruction of the microcirculation by a fibrin meshwork. This fibrin meshwork, in turn, leads to the rapid breakdown of erythrocytes, due to the knife-like effect of the fibrin strands on red blood cells as they try to move through the partially obstructed capillary. To make the diagnosis, one should test for fibrinogen-fibrin degradation products (fibrin split products) in the laboratory, or see damaged red blood cells on the smear of the peripheral blood. Levels of less than 100 mg/100 ml of fibrinogen, thrombocytopenia (less than 100,000/mm^3), and decreased coagulation factors V and VII all confirm this diagnosis. Treatment with heparin is sometimes successful, but the underlying disorder such as septicemia must be the principal target for the therapeutic efforts.

Idiopathic thrombocytopenic purpura is a typical example of autoimmune disease. Antibodies become absorbed on the surface of platelets, resulting in their rapid elimination by phagocytosis, mostly in the spleen. Because the spleen is also a major source of these antibodies a remarkable improvement or cure of ITP can be achieved by splenectomy. As in other forms of thrombocytopenia, the major manifestations of this disease are related to bleeding in various body sites.

Coagulation Mechanisms

The coagulation system seems increasingly complex as we learn more about it.

One good way to look at the coagulation system is that it is a part of the host's general response to injury. Many of the enzymatic relationships in coagulation are essential parts of the inflammatory response to injury, and involve kinins, complement, and the fibrinolytic systems. Coagulation mechanisms can be viewed as having two main functions: to form fibrin, which mechanically blocks the flow of blood through ruptured vessels, and to produce thrombin, which stabilizes the platelet plug. Incidentally, thrombin also converts fibrinogen to fibrin. A number of proenzymes and proteins, called coagulation factors, participate in coagulation in addition to platelets and calcium. The simplest scheme of coagulation, which dates from 1928, is seen in Figure 23–6. This scheme anticipates the relationship of inactive substances to the activation of circulating plasma proteins. One can view the coagulation process as a series of limited

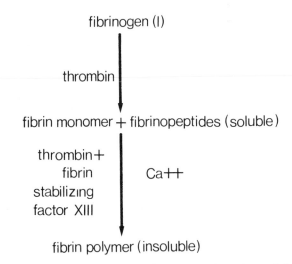

Fig. 23–6 This scheme shows the elementary, traditional **coagulation mechanism**, starting with fibrinogen at the top and ending with the insoluble polymers of fibrin at the bottom. Thrombin and calcium are shown as essential cofactors. (From Ratnoff, O.D.: Hemorrhagic disorders: coagulation defects. In *Cecil Textbook of Medicine*, 15th Ed. Edited by P. B. Beeson, W. McDermott, and J. B. Wyngaarden. Philadelphia, W. B. Saunders Co., 1979.)

cleavages of enzyme precursors. It is interesting that the cascade of reactions can also be viewed as a sequence of enzymatic conversions of substrate from an inactive state to an active one. Each conversion results in the production of a proteinase for the subsequent stage (Fig. 23–7). This process has the teleologic advantage of grading the response, so that it is not an all or none reaction, but it has the disadvantage of being complicated for study purposes.

The cascade of coagulation reactions can be divided into an intrinsic and an extrinsic pathway. These are defined by the fact that all coagulation factors necessary for the formation of a fibrin clot are present in the intravascular compartment in the intrinsic pathway, whereas the extrinsic pathway requires the addition

of a tissue factor (from thromboplastin) to make the clot. As the diagram shows, calcium is essential, as are phospholipid surfaces.

It is important to notice that coagulation can be triggered by extrinsic factors called thromboplastins which are released at sites of vascular damage. Coagulation also occurs optimally in contact with the phospholipids or the platelet surface. Finally, calcium is an important component of the process as it acts as a bridge between the various coagulation factors.

If we are to consider any of the factors involved in the clotting mechanism, we should start with fibrinogen. In order to simplify our consideration and to illustrate some of the principles outlined, we shall look at just three of the coagulation proteins: Factor I (fi-

COAGULATION FACTORS

FACTOR	NAME
I	Fibrinogen
II	Prothrombin
III	Tissue thromboplastin, thrombokinase
IV	Calcium
V	Proaccelerin, labile factor
VII	Proconvertin, stable factor
VIII	Antihemophilic A factor (AHF), antihemophilic globulin (AHG)
IX	Antihemophilic B factor (AHB), plasma thromboplastin component (PTC), Christmas factor
X	Stuart factor, Stuart-Prower factor
XI	Plasma thromboplastin antecedent (PTA)
XII	Hageman factor, contact factor
XIII	Fibrin stabilizing factor, fibrinase

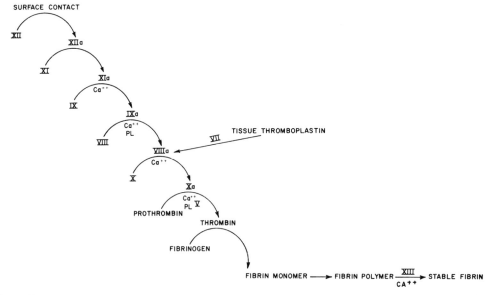

Fig. 23–7   This figure illustrates the **cascade of clotting** as we understand it today, including the intrinsic clotting mechanism, in which no extravascular components are necessary, and the extrinsic clotting mechanism, in which tissue factors play a role. (From Brown, B.: *Hematology: Principles and Procedures*, 2nd Ed. Philadelphia, Lea & Febiger, 1976.)

brinogen), Factor II (prothrombin), and Factor VIII (antihemophilic factor). In addition, we should write a few words about vitamin K, because of its importance in this scheme. The reader is referred to other sources for more detailed accounts of each of the known factors in the coagulation scheme and their interactions.

Fibrinogen (Factor I) is a large protein (340,000 MW) with a small proportion of carbohydrate (3 to 5%) synthesized by the liver cells, with a half-life of about 5 days. The structure of this molecule has recently been elucidated, and it has been shown to consist of two halves, each consisting of three paired subunits. How this molecule is cleaved, what happens to the subunits after cleavage, and how polymerization into the indeterminately long but insoluble strands of fibrin (Fig. 23–8) is accomplished has not yet been entirely deciphered and will be another chapter in molecular biology.

During conversion of fibrinogen to fibrin and its polymerization, an inactivating system precursor, of which there are many in normal blood, is incorporated into the growing clot. This substance, plasminogen, is normally kept in an inactive state by its own inhibitors, but in the clot it is sequestered or protected from these circulating inhibitory substances. Thus it comes to be activated to plasmin, which is a proteolytic enzyme. This substance, plasmin, is essential to the maintenance of the circulating system, rather as tow trucks are essential for the function of expressways, because plasmin degrades fibrin and other products of coagulation. It is safe to say that we are all constantly forming clots at sites of minor injury and are constantly breaking them down again. This process of clot lysis results in degradation products that can be detected in the circulating blood. These are called fibrin split products.

Prothrombin is a smaller (68,000 MW) proenzyme of interest, not only because on activation it becomes the highly active enzyme thrombin, but because the molecule has a calcium-binding region that is dependent on the presence of vitamin K. This molecule is also synthesized by liver cells and has a shorter half-life of about three days. We do not know whether the same liver cell produces prothrombin and fibrinogen, nor do we know precisely how these factors that regulate the production of essential coagulation proteins are controlled. Possibly, as for serum albumin, a decrease in the serum level of prothrombin stimulates liver cells to renewed synthesis of this protein.

The major importance of prothrombin lies in that it is a precursor of thrombin, which acts on fibrinogen. Normally, there is no thrombin in circulating blood. Thrombin can be produced either from the intrinsic source (prothrombin) or from the so-called extrinsic pathway, whose tissue components initiated its release. It is of relevance that blood may also coagulate when exposed to negatively charged surfaces, such as glass.

The third type of coagulation protein are molecules in excess of 1,000,000 MW. These molecules include at least two substances which are **antihemophilic globulins**. The absence of these substances results in serious, uncontrolled bleeding, i.e. hemophilia.

This brings us to the hereditary coagulation disorders. The most common are hemophilia due to deficiency or defects in Factors VIII or IX.

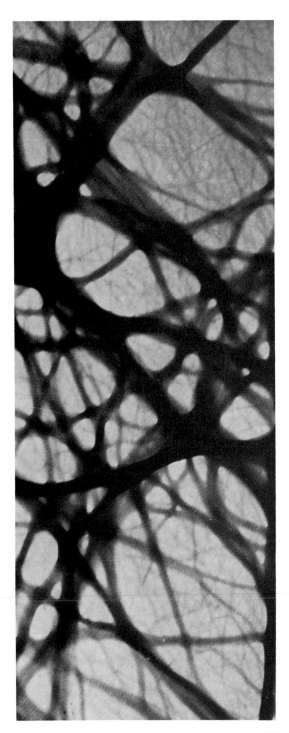

Fig. 23–8 This electron microphotograph shows the **network of fibrin** from a clot. This historic picture was taken by Dr. K. R. Porter in 1947 at the Rockefeller Laboratories.

The classic type of **hemophilia** is due to a deficiency of a normally functioning factor VIII. The hemophiliac's serum contains this factor, but it seems to be unable to act appropriately. This disorder occurs in 1 out of 10,000 of the world population, and it is transmitted in a sex-linked recessive pattern. Therefore, it appears in males but not in females. Males with the disorder transmit the gene to all their daughters but hemophilia is not manifest, and their sons are all normal. This diagnosis is suspected in families with the trait (see Fig. 4–10), but 30% of cases give no positive family history, suggesting this is a relatively frequent mutation. The most serious aspects of the bleeding tendency, apart from its life-threatening aspects following surgical operations or minor procedures (dental extraction), is bleeding into joints, which often results in destruction of the growing edges of bone and deformities of joints that do not heal. Before screening of blood products for the presence of HIV, a number of hemophiliacs became victims of AIDS. This problem has now been almost completely solved by appropriate HIV serology of the blood donors. Another significant advance has been the recent introduction of molecular biology tests detecting the disease in unborn fetuses.

A second hereditary disorder of the coagulation proteins is called **von Willebrand's disease,** and it is transmitted as an autosomal dominant. This, too, is caused by a Factor VIII abnormality. In addition, there is a defective serum protein necessary for normal platelet function. Thus such persons may have both disorders in platelet function and in their normal coagulation pattern. Transfusion of normal plasma has a markedly beneficial effect on these patients because normal serum replaces the missing components.

Vitamin K, as we have already described in Chapter

3, is essential for the normal biosynthesis of prothrombin and several coagulation factors (VII, IX and X). Recently, vitamin K has been shown to be involved in the biosynthesis of prothrombin by converting a precursor protein to active prothrombin.

Various tests to determine the presence or absence of the different factors have been used to separate one clinical disorder from another and to provide rational therapy for these hemorrhagic disorders. They are outlined in Table 23–7.

We can move on to consider another major category of diseases of the erythron, namely disorders of the white blood cell series: leukemias and lymphomas.

LEUKEMIA

This term was introduced by Virchow, and it literally means white blood. The term is applied to those disorders in which the normal growth and development of the white blood cells are no longer ordered and controlled (Table 23–8). This disorder is expressed in a rapid and excessive cellular proliferation of cells of the white blood series. The leukemic cells are present in bone marrow and peripheral blood and may infiltrate other organs such as the liver, spleen or kidney. Characteristically, the appearance of immature or "blast" forms of white blood cells in the peripheral blood indicates the loss of the normal controlling mechanisms (whatever they are) and confirms the diagnosis. The white blood cell count may rise to hundreds of thousands per mm^3 compared with a normal of 7 to 10,000 mm^3. The patient may have uncontrollable hemorrhages and anemia, because the bone marrow is replaced by the neoplastic proliferation, thereby precluding the orderly progression of maturation that maintains the normal populations of red blood cells, white blood cells, and platelets.

Experience has shown that leukemias can be sepa-

Table 23–7. Coagulation Tests

1. *Bleeding Time,* prolonged in patients with increased capillary fragility and/or inadequate platelet function. Examination of smear for platelets or direct platelet count is complementary information.

2. *Fibrinogen.* Circulating concentrations of fibrinogen greater than 100 mg/100 ml excludes fibrinogen deficiency as a cause of bleeding. Examples in which fibrinogen levels are decreased are disorders such as disseminated intravascular coagulation, thrombotic thrombocytopenic syndrome, and hemolytic-uremic syndrome. These disorders also have prolonged thrombin times.

3. *Thrombin Time.* Measurement of this time is required for fibrin clot formation when thrombin is added to plasma. Thrombin acts directly on fibrinogen. It is inhibited by fibrinogen degradation products and by heparin. Prolongation indicates either low fibrinogen content or presence of inhibitor.

4. *Prothrombin Time* is the time it takes fibrin to gel in plasma after calcium and complete thromboplastin have been added. The test involves VII, X, and V, prothrombin, and fibrinogen. Values are reported as percentage of control. Disorders in which it is prolonged are vitamin K deficiency and hepatobiliary disease.

5. *Partial Thromboplastin Time* (PTT) depends on glass activation of factor XII. This test will be prolonged in most bleeding disorders, but is particularly valuable in von Willebrand's disease when all the other tests (PT, thrombin, fibrinogen) are normal.

Table 23–8. Chromosomal Changes in Leukemias and Lymphomas

	NORMAL KARYOTYPES	CHROMOSOMAL CHANGES
Acute leukemia	40%	7,8,9 and 21
Chronic lymphocytic leukemia	75%	trisomy 9,17,21
Plasma cell leukemia	25%(?)	$14q^+$
Polycythemia vera	80%	$20q^-$; trisomy 8,9,21
Myeloproliferative disorder	10%	7,8,9
Burkitt's lymphoma	15%	t(8; 14)
Malignant lymphoma	?	isochromosome 17; $14q^+$; trisomy 7

rated into different groups because of their biologic behavior, morphology, and response to therapy. Leukemias with mature cells in the peripheral blood, rather than blast cells, tend to have a more benign course. There are a significant number of cases in which the number of cells in the peripheral blood is within normal limits, but immature forms are seen, indicating that the bone marrow examination will confirm the suspicion of leukemia. These cases are termed **aleukemic leukemia.** To make things more complicated, there are a few instances with excessively high white blood cell counts that turn out not to be leukemia at all, but rather a leukemia-like pattern (leukemoid reaction) in such other diseases as tuberculosis.

The etiology of leukemia (which can be considered another form of cancer) is of great interest because of a number of observations on leukemia in living forms other than man. To begin with, we should state that the etiology of human leukemias is not established. There are, however, three important associations with leukemia in man. In Down's syndrome (mongolism), in which there is an abnormal chromosome (trisomy 21), there is a remarkable increase over normal of acute leukemias. Radiologists and others exposed to radiation before significant protective measures were in use showed a tenfold increase in death from leukemia. Leukemia is increasingly apparent in persons treated with vigorous chemotherapy and immunosuppressive therapy for other disorders. None of these observations, put in the light of our ignorance of the etiologies of cancer in general, is overwhelming, but the data from observations on the incidence and transmission of leukemia in animals are more provocative.

Leukemias in such diverse species as chicken, mouse, cat, cow, monkey, and gibbon, are caused by RNA virus infection. Mice may transmit the virus vertically, that is, both parent and offspring may have leukemia, and, in some inbred strains, virtually every mouse develops leukemia. Whereas horizontal transmission, that is, passage from animal to animal, has been proved in several cases, this is not yet true for man. Although clusters of leukemia cases are reported in man, there are no clear-cut data to suggest either that leukemia is caused by a virus or that it is contagious.

We may divide the leukemias first into those types designated by the cell of origin. Thus there are leukemias that are acute and those which are chronic, involving granulocytic (granulocytes) or myelocytic (immature white blood cell) elements, and acute and chronic leukemias involving lymphocytes. The four general types we shall consider briefly are thus acute lymphocytic, chronic lymphocytic, acute myelocytic, and chronic myelocytic leukemias.

Acute Leukemias

The clinical pattern of the **acute leukemias** differs somewhat from that of the chronic leukemias. The most common catastrophic indication of acute leukemia is an episode of hemorrhage in an otherwise normal child or adult. Nose bleeds, bleeding from the gums, easy bruisability, and bleeding into the skin or gastrointestinal hemorrhage are common presenting findings. Failure to recover from an otherwise minor infection of the respiratory tract, urinary tract, or sinuses may be another prodromal episode, while the appearance of enlarged lymph nodes or splenomegaly are telltale signs of these blood dyscrasias. The crucial laboratory finding of blast cells on peripheral smear and an elevated white blood cell count confirm the clinical suspicion.

Acute leukemias, as the name implies, run a brief and hectic course. Persons so diagnosed seldom survive a year without treatment. Modern treatments, however, have altered this prognosis in many instances. The distinction between different subsets of acute leukemia is beyond the scope of this book, but we should differentiate the acute myelocytic types from the acute lymphocytic leukemias, because the treatment and prognosis are different.

Acute myelocytic leukemia occurs in the Western world at a constant rate from birth to age 55, fluctuating slightly between 10 and 15 cases per million. After 55, this disease rises slightly in frequency. In contrast, **acute lymphocytic leukemia** has an incidence of 50 per million between the ages of 2 and 4 years. This rate halves in the next 4 years, and halves again to 10 per million until age 65, when it rises once more to about 15 per million. This pattern suggests an infectious etiology with the greatest susceptibility in early years, compared with patterns for acute myelocytic leukemia that could be interpreted as supporting a cumulative risk. The important fact is that over 85% of children with acute leukemia have the lymphocytic type, whereas over 80% of adults with acute leukemia have the myelocytic variety. Specific chromosomal abnormalities are associated with subsets of acute leukemias and help to stratify them into categories having different prognoses.

Fortunately, modern therapies offer the possibility of cure for acute lymphocytic leukemia with the use of vincristine and prednisone, and 85% of patients have remissions. The schedules of treatment are changing quickly, and it is hoped that successful management may change the outlook from this disease's grim pattern in the recent past.

Chronic Myeloid Leukemia (Granulocytic, Myelocytic, Myelogenous)

This variant of leukemia is rare below the age of 20 and accounts for about one-fifth of all leukemias in North America. It becomes more common to about the age of 60 and occurs at the rate of about 15 cases per million. The classic chief complaint may consist of such nonspecific symptoms as anorexia and weight loss with easy fatigability. Occasionally, an incidental blood count may turn up the diagnosis by revealing counts as high as 500,000 cells per mm^3. On physical examination, there may be a significantly enlarged spleen. The largest spleens in any disease occur in chronic myelocytic leukemia; it is not rare to find a spleen weighing 5 kg, and infarcts in these enlarged spleens may be the patient's original complaint (pain in the left flank) which alerts the physician to the diagnosis.

The etiology of chronic myelocytic leukemia is unknown, but two relationships are apparent. One is to known carcinogens such as ionizing radiation and benzene, and the other is to the presence of an abnormal chromosome. Eighty to 90% of patients with chronic myelocytic leukemia show an abnormality designated as a Philadelphia chromosome, which is an exchange, called reciprocal translocation, between the long arms of chromosomes 9 and 22.

During the chronic stage, anemia is the principal finding, and in remission, patients may be asymptomatic. One complication of this disease is the elevated uric acid and elevated uric acid excretion, which reflects the turnover of nucleic acids from the greatly increased number of white blood cells that are dying. With treatment and destruction of huge numbers of white blood cells, these uric acid levels may skyrocket, occasionally leading to uric acid precipitates in the tubules of the kidney and complete renal shutdown. Patients with chronic myelocytic leukemia usually enter a phase called blast crisis, which is indistinguishable from acute leukemia. One can anticipate a median survival of three years, with a range from 1 to 10 years. The survival time has not changed significantly in decades. The discovery that normal cells can repopulate the bone marrow and can replace the cells that possess the Philadelphia chromosome offers hope that newer methods of treatment may change these statistics.

Chronic Lymphocytic Leukemia (Chronic Lymphatic Leukemia)

This type of leukemia, characterized by the appearance of small lymphocytes in the peripheral blood, lymph nodes, and bone marrow, is compatible with a much better survival rate (median survival 6 years), and many individuals live much longer, sometimes a quarter of a century. Often it is only the laboratory diagnosis that reveals the presence of increased circulating lymphocytes in a patient who is receiving a routine examination for some other reason. Vague or nonspecific symptoms are typical, and sometimes enlarged lymph nodes or spleen suggest the diagnosis. Chronic lymphocytic leukemia accounts for 30% of leukemias and is unusual below age 45, but is nearly twice as common in men. There is no epidemiologic or other evidence to incriminate any of the agents we have mentioned earlier in the etiology of chronic lymphocytic leukemia. Ionizing radiation, carcinogens, and oncogenic viruses have not been shown to play any role in this disorder.

One might regard chronic lymphocytic leukemia as the leukemic form of a well-differentiated lymphocytic lymphoma. Histologically, lymph nodes from patients with abnormal peripheral blood counts and smears cannot be distinguished from lymph nodes of lymphocytic lymphoma patients who have no peripheral blood abnormalities. Other organs, such as the liver and spleen, may be infiltrated, but massive splenomegaly is not characteristic. Immunologic abnormalities are a routine part of these disorders, and hypogammaglobulinemia is typical. This condition predisposes the patient to infections, which are a common and often terminal complication of chronic lymphocytic leukemia. Modern treatment is aimed at reducing the large numbers of lymphocytes.

The four common forms of leukemia are compared in Figure 23–9.

Neutropenia—Agranulocytosis

As the name suggests, this is a remarkable disappearance of the granulocytic series of leukocytes from the blood, with an accompanying drop in the total white cell count. Significant problems occur when neutrophils fall below $1000/mm^3$. The association of leukopenia with gangrenous lesions of the mouth is known as agranulocytic angina, the word "angina" in this sense meaning an acute inflammation of the throat.

There are many different causes and mechanisms of neutropenia, targeting on either defective production of neutrophils in the bone marrow, or their increased destruction in the peripheral blood or organs. To be practical, one encounters neutropenia most often in association with the therapeutic use of chemotherapeutic drugs used to treat malignant disorders or severe inflammatory disorders. Also, a long list of otherwise well-tolerated drugs cause idiosyncratic

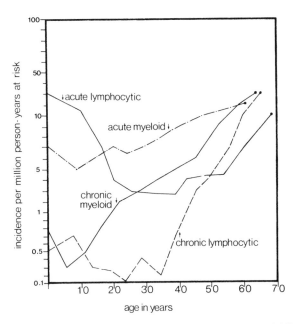

Fig. 23–9 This graph shows the frequency of the incidence of different types of leukemia in different age groups in cases per million person years. Acute lymphocytic **leukemia** has 2 peaks, 1 before the age of 20 and 1 after the age of 60. The incidence of chronic lymphocytic leukemia and of chronic myeloid leukemia both rise gradually toward the end of life. (From Upton, A.C.: Comparative aspects of carcinogenesis in ionizing radiation. Natl. Cancer Inst. Monogr., 14:221, 1964.)

neutropenic reactions in some patients. As predicted, neutropenia exposes the patients to fulminant bacterial or fungal infections.

Two groups of cases can be distinguished: (1) those occurring in persons who have been taking too much of some of the pain-killing drugs, particularly amidopyrine and the barbiturate series, i.e., chemicals containing the benzene ring; (2) cases in which no obvious cause can be discovered, although many industrial household agents have been incriminated. The two factors, diminished leukocyte count and severe mouth infections, probably assist each other.

The disease often begins with the extraction of teeth. It is marked by fever, increasing weakness and fatigue, and sore throat. There may be extensive destruction of the gums and even the jaw, so that the teeth may fall out. Unfortunately, the victim, on account of the pain of the mouth lesions, may continue to take even larger doses of the drug. Such cases cannot fail to go on to a fatal termination, as the leukocytes diminish in number to the vanishing point.

It is important to discontinue the use of any drugs that the patient may have been taking. The use of antibiotics has prevented the occurrence of serious infections in these cases, so that the patient's bone marrow will have a better chance of recovery from the damage done by the toxic drug.

DISORDERS OF THE LYMPH NODES AND RETICULOENDOTHELIAL SYSTEM

Lymphadenopathy or enlargement of a single lymph node or a localized group of nodes, such as along the side of the neck or in the axilla, is a frequent occurrence. Anyone with an infected tooth or a sore throat may have had the occasion to feel a mass where normally it was difficult to palpate any lymph nodes. The causes of local or generalized lymphadenopathy form the final section of this chapter. A consideration of the normal structure and function of the lymphatic system has been outlined in Chapter 6, on the immune system. This section will go on to consider one or two inflammatory causes of lymphadenopathy, and will then offer a consideration of tumors of the lymphoreticular system, such as Hodgkin's lymphoma and lymphocytic lymphomas. We have considered Burkitt's lymphoma elsewhere, and the rarer diseases such as eosinophilic granuloma need not concern us in this text.

Infectious Mononucleosis

This is a self-limited disease of the lymphoreticular system characterized by sore throat, fever, swollen lymph nodes, generalized lassitude, and, sometimes, enlargement of the spleen. The diagnosis is established by examination of the peripheral blood smear, the demonstration of atypical lymphocytes, and the laboratory demonstration of heterophile antibodies (serum that will clump together sheep's red blood cells in high dilution). This is the Paul-Bunnell test. The total white blood count may be elevated and the percentage of lymphocytes or mononuclear cells may be increased over normal. The absence of anemia and a normal platelet count are valuable suggestions that the lymph node enlargement is not due to leukemic infiltrate or malignant lymphoma.

Infectious mononucleosis is common among high school and college-age students; its incidence in the United States is more than 1,000 cases per 100,000 students per school year, indicating that one has a 1:100 chance of acquiring the disease. Figure 23–10 shows the attack rate by sex and academic class at 14 colleges, and Table 23–9 shows the incidence of infectious mononucleosis during the 1969 to 1970 school year in these colleges.

The Epstein-Barr virus is the causative agent of infectious mononucleosis. There is epidemiologic data suggesting that infectious mononucleosis occurs with increased social contact, and in fact may be spread by intimate contact. It has been called the "kissing disease."

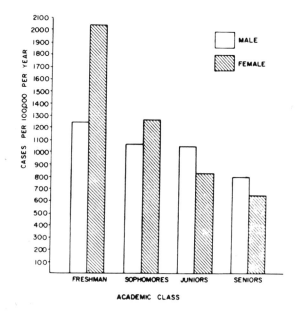

Fig. 23–10 **Infectious mononucleosis** attack rates, by sex and academic class, at 14 colleges, academic year 1969 to 1970. (From Brodsky, A.L., and Heath, C.W.: Infectious mononucleosis: epidemiologic patterns at United States colleges and universities. Am. J. Epidemiol. 96:87, 1972.)

Sarcoidosis

This disease was first described more than 100 years ago, and yet we are still completely ignorant of its cause. The microscopic lesions are granulomatous in character, closely resembling those of tuberculosis, yet the nature of the condition remains obscure. The disease is endemic in regions of pine forests, such as the Scandinavian countries and the New England region of the United States, so that it has been suggested that pine pollen may be at least one etiologic agent that can excite the reaction characteristic of sarcoidosis.

The lesions are remarkable for the diversity of their distribution, the chief tissues involved being the lymph nodes, both superficial and deep, but the skin, spleen, liver, lungs, and many other organs may be affected. The disease lasts for months or years, with a tendency to fibrosis and healing. Usually there is an astonishing absence of symptoms. The microscopic appearance is that of circumscribed masses resembling miliary tubercles, and easily is mistaken for these lesions.

Malignant Lymphomas

These are neoplasms of the lymphoreticular system. By lymphoreticular system we mean the lymph nodes and the spleen.

It is also important to include the lymphoid cells which are present in large numbers along the gastrointestinal tract.

Lymphomas, in spite of their ambiguous suffix, are always malignant. However, they have markedly different grades of malignancy and this is why it is important to classify them. Sorting out these different categories of lymphomas, and making sure that they are indeed lymphomas, not benign, reactive, proliferations of lymphoid tissue, is now much easier. This is due to a better knowledge of basic immunology that led to the individualization of the different types of lymphocytes and other mononuclear cells on the basis of surface markers and specific functions. Even more recently, molecular biology techniques have been introduced to detect and type very small clones of malignant lymphocytes. The reader is referred to the immunology section of this book for a more detailed account of lymphocyte differentiation.

An important consideration in the discussion of lymphomas is their multifocal manifestation with almost simultaneous enlargement of several adjacent or

Table 23–9. **Incidence of Infectious Mononucleosis at 7 Colleges and Universities by Race During the Academic Year 1969 to 1970**

SCHOOL	NUMBER OF CASES			UNDERGRADUATE POPULATION		RATES/100,000/SCHOOL YEAR	
	WHITE	NONWHITE	UNKNOWN	WHITE	NONWHITE	WHITE	NONWHITE
Alaska	9			1,288	214	699	
Bryn Mawr	5	1		689	54	726	1,852
Emory	48		2	2,275	46	2,110	
Harvard	103	3	1	5,642	370	1,826	811
Oklahoma State	151	3		14,660	291	1,030	1,031
Purdue	248	3		14,612	4,404	1,697	68
Yale	67		7	4,295	195	1,257	
Total	631	10	10	43,461	5,574	1,452	179

(From Brodsky, A.L., and Heath, C.W.: Infectious mononucleosis: epidemiologic patterns at United States colleges and universities. Am. J. Epidemiol., 96:87, 1972.)

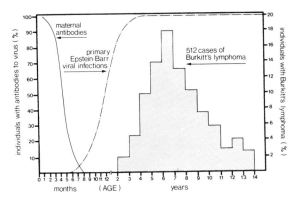

Fig. 23–11 This chart shows the relationship between the presence of maternal antibodies and infection with Epstein-Barr virus. The cases of Burkitt's lymphoma are shown in the bar graph. This indicates the latency between the primary infection and suggests a relationship between the Burkitt's lymphoma and previous Epstein-Barr infections. (From Henle, W., et al.: The Epstein-Barr virus. Sci. Am., 241:48, 1979.)

Fig. 23–12 **Hodgkin's disease**, showing enlarged glands in the neck.

distant lymph nodes. No genetic or environmental factor can be implicated in the overwhelming majority of lymphomas. Notable exceptions are Burkitt's lymphoma and nasopharyngeal carcinomas which are associated with Epstein Barr virus (Fig. 23–11). How directly causal this association is remains to be established. These two conditions are discussed in the neoplasia chapter.

There are two broad categories of lymphomas: Hodgkin's disease and non-Hodgkin's lymphomas.

Hodgkin's Disease

This disease of unknown etiology appears in young adults (20 to 40 years). In the Western world, there are an estimated 35 cases per million for white males and 25 cases per million for white females, with an annual death rate of 23 and 13 per million respectively, although we may expect these figures to decrease, since new methods of treatment are having significant success. The disease has two incidence peaks, one between ages 15 and 34, and the other after age 50. The disease announces its presence as a nonspecific malaise characterized by fever, anorexia, and enlargement of lymph nodes, and sometimes, the spleen and the liver (Fig. 23–12). Itching of the skin and bone pain following the intake of alcohol may be clinical clues to the correct diagnosis, which is established by histologic examination of the firm, rubbery lymph nodes. Sometimes, these lymph nodes are seen only on x-ray film or CT scan of the mediastinum or are discovered at laparotomy in the abdomen, along the aortic chain.

When lymph nodes of Hodgkin's disease are examined under the microscope, various types of changes are seen which significantly correlate with various

prognoses (Table 23–10). The diagnosis rests on the demonstration of large, bi-nucleated cells with prominent nucleoli, surrounded by halo, called Reed-Sternberg cells. In addition, the lymph nodes contain an heterogenous collection of lymphocytes, plasma cells, histiocytes, eosinophils, and neutrophils. The relative properties of these cells and the presence or absence of sclerosis helps to classify the various forms listed in Table 23–10.

Hodgkin's disease can present at various stages of extension, as summarized in Table 23–11.

The prognosis has improved remarkably with the introduction of type- and stage-adjusted chemotherapy and radiotherapy (Fig. 23–13). Cure rates of 50% to 100% can now be achieved.

Non-Hodgkin's Lymphomas

As seen by the heading of this section, these neoplasms may be an assortment. However, they have in common their origin in cells of the immune system. They are not rare; an estimated 15,000 new cases were diagnosed in 1977 in the United States; this represents 2% of all cancer diagnoses in that country. They may occur at all ages and in both sexes; their etiology is not known. However, patients with genetic or acquired disorders of immune deficiency are clearly predisposed to these malignant neoplasms, and such patients include those who receive immunosuppressive treatment for kidney grafted organs.

They are also found in AIDS patients, notably in their brain. In this form of lymphoma no Reed Sternberg cells are seen. Several types of classification have been used and, fortunately, the one that seems to be

Table 23–10. Histoplastic Classification of Hodgkin's Disease

TYPE	FEATURE	RELATIVE PROGNOSIS
Lymphocyte predominance	Abundant lymphocytic stroma; sparse Sternberg-Reed (S-R) cells	Most favorable
Nodular sclerosis	Nodules of lymphoid tissue of varying size, separated by bands of collagen and containing ''lacunar'' cell variants of S-R cells	Favorable
Mixed cellularity	More numerous S-R cells in pleomorphic stroma rich in eosinophils, plasma cells, fibroblasts, and lymphocytes	Guarded
Lymphocyte depletion	Paucity of lymphocytes; diffuse, irregular fibrosis in some instances; bizarre, anaplastic S-R cells usually numerous	Least favorable

Table 23–11. Staging of Hodgkin's Disease

Stage 0	No detectable disease.
Stage I	Disease limited to 1 anatomic region, or 2 contiguous regions on 1 side of the diaphragm (single lymph node or group).
Stage II	Disease in more than 2 anatomic regions, or in 2 noncontiguous regions on the same side of the diaphragm.
Stage III	Disease on both sides of the diaphragm, not involving more than the lymph nodes and spleen.
Stage IV	Involvement of any tissue or organ other than lymph nodes or spleen (e.g., bone, GI tract, lungs).

A: indicates the absence of generalized symptoms
B: Indicates the presence of generalized symptoms such as fever, pruritus, bone pain.

the most useful is based on the clinical outcome, i.e., it has a prognostic relevance. There are three main groups with increasingly worse prognoses: low grade, intermediate grade, and high grade. They are distinguished on the basis of histological features.

Well-differentiated lymphomas appear most commonly after the fifth decade and are slowly progressive. The neoplasm is best viewed as the tissue component of chronic lymphocytic leukemia, and its histologic pattern is identical, being a diffuse infiltration of homogeneous, small, well-differentiated lymphocytes. The patient's bone marrow is usually involved.

The clinical manifestations of this and other lymphomas are the presence of one or more enlarged lymph nodes, which may have been noticed for some time and might involve deep organs (Fig. 23–14). Fever and weight loss are not necessarily a prominent part of the pattern, but their presence alone may herald the development of these neoplasms. Involvement of the spleen, liver, and gastrointestinal tract (either stomach or small bowel) may cause the chief complaint. A high index of suspicion and a willingness to keep these tumors in mind in the differential diagnosis is often the only way a biopsy can be done early in the search for the cause of the general malaise

Fig. 23–13 These graphs show the **survival of patients with Hodgkin's disease** of all stages in 3 different therapeutic eras. The 62% 10-year survival of 1,009 cases treated with the linear accelerator x-ray and/or drug therapy can be compared with 754 cases treated with no specific therapy. (From Kaplan, H.S.: Hodgkin's disease: multidisciplinary contributions to the conquest of a neoplasm. Radiology, 123:551, 1978.)

Fig. 23–14 **Lymphoma**. Great enlargement of lymph nodes along abdominal aorta with involvement of both kidneys.

in a given patient. Staging procedures, such as those used for Hodgkin's disease, have been useful in some cases, but in others their significance is debated.

A complication of these lymphomas is anemia, as more than half the patients become severely anemic from involvement of their bone marrow, from hemorrhage, and from the response to therapy. Involvement of other systems, such as the central nervous system and the liver and occasionally organs adjacent to the lymphadenopathy (mediastinal structures), may be life-threatening because of mechanical interference, but infections, often of an unusual type such as fungal and viruses (herpes), frequently complicate the clinical course or cause death.

The short-term outlook for patients with non-Hodgkin's lymphomas has significantly improved during the last 10 years because of better use of various chemotherapeutic agents and radiotherapy, tools which have been used with much greater precision.

Multiple myeloma is a neoplasm of plasma cells and could be considered here. However, we discuss it in Chapter 25, to which the reader is referred.

SYNOPSIS

The common disorders of the hematopoietic system can be identified broadly as increased destruction, decreased production, or inherited disorders of the red blood cells (hereditary anemias) and proliferations of the white blood cells (leukemias). Less commonly, there are cases of increased production of red blood cells (polycythemias), or of decreased production of white blood cells and/or platelets (agranulocytosis, thrombocytopenia, aplastic anemia).

Laboratory examination (hematocrit, hemoglobin, red blood cell, white blood cell, and differential counts, and examination of the smear) generally reflects the function of the hematopoietic system.

Anemias may be regarded as due to inherited disorders, hemolytic disorders, as arising from increased blood loss (e.g., ulcers) or from decreased production (deficiencies of iron, folic acid, bone marrow depression). The symptoms are nonspecific; correct diagnosis depends on laboratory procedures.

Hemorrhagic disorders may have their origin in general depression of the bone marrow (leukemias, thrombocytopenia) or in disorders of clotting mechanisms (e.g., hepatic disease), and they may be inherited (hemophilia), acquired, or iatrogenic.

Leukemias can best be considered to be neoplasms of the white blood cell series, characterized by the presence of immature cells in the peripheral blood.

Diseases of lymph nodes and the reticuloendothelial system commonly include inflammations, infections, and neoplasms (lymphomas).

There are two main categories of lymphomas: Hodgkin's disease and non-Hodgkin's lymphomas.

Terms

Erythrocytes	*Megakaryocyte*	*Purpura*
Reticulocytes	*Platelets*	*Leukemia*
Hemoglobin	*Hemolysis*	*Neutropenia*
Hematocrit	*Anemia*	*Thrombocytopenia*
Leukocytes	*Polycythemia*	*Infectious mononucleosis*
Myeloblasts	*Hemophilia*	*Lymphoma*
		Hodgkin's disease

FURTHER READING

Bastuji-Garin, S., Richardson, S., and Zittoun, R.: Acute leukaemia in workers exposed to electromagnetic fields. Cancer, 26:1119, 1990.

Beck, W.S.: Diagnosis of megaloblastic anemia. Ann. Rev. Med., 42:311, 1991.

Bessis, M., and Delpech, G.: Sickle cell shape and structure: Images and concepts (1840–1980). Blood Cells, 8:359, 1982.

Bodey, G.P.: Fungal infections complicating acute leukemia. J. Chronic Dis., 19:667, 1966.

Bowman, J.M., and Chown, B.: Prevention of Rh immunization after massive Rh-positive transfusion. Can. Med. Assoc. J., 99:385, 1968.

Brodsky, A.L., and Heath, C.W.: Infectious mononucleosis; epidemiologic patterns at United States colleges and universities. Am. J. Epidemiol., 96:87, 1972.

Cazzola, M., and Beguin, Y.: New tools for clinical evaluation of erythron function in man. Brit. J. Hematol., 80:278, 1992.

Colby, T.V., Hoppe, R.T., and Warnke, R.A.: Hodgkin's disease: a clinicopathologic study of 659 cases. Cancer, 49:1848, 1982.

Da Prada, M., Lorez, H.P., and Richards, J.G.: Platelet granules. In *The Secretory Granule*. Edited by Poisner and Trifaro. New York, Elsevier Biomedical Press, 1982, p. 279.

Desforges, J.F., et al.: Hodgkin's disease. N. Engl. J. Med., 301:1212, 1979.

Green, D.: General considerations of coagulation proteins. Ann. Clin. Lab. Sci., 8:95, 1978.

Grufferman, S., et al.: Hodgkin's disease in siblings. N. Engl. J. Med., 296:248, 1977.

Gutensohn, N., and Cole, P.: Childhood social environment and Hodgkin's disease. N. Engl. J. Med., 304:135, 1981.

Harris, J.W.: *The Red Cell*. Cambridge, Harvard University Press, 1970.

Herrick, J.B.: Sickle cell disease. Arch. Intern. Med., 6:517, 1910.

Judson, H.: *The Eighth Day of Creation*. New York, Simon and Schuster, 1979.

Kaplan, H.S.: Hodgkin's disease: biology, treatment, prognosis. Blood, 57:813, 1981.

Lukes, R.J., and Butler, J.J.: The pathology and nomenclature of Hodgkin's disease. Cancer Res., 26:1063, 1966.

McIntyre, D.R.: Current concepts in cancer: multiple myeloma. N. Engl. J. Med., 301:193, 1979.

Moroz, L.A.: Normal blood fibrinolytic activity: its mandatory existence and role in intravascular homeostasis. Thrombosis Res., 18:585, 1980.

Narod, S.A.: Radiation, genetics and childhood leukaemia. Cancer, 26:661, 1990.

Open Forum: Etiology of childhood leukemia: A possible alternative to the Greaves hypothesis. Leukemia, Res., 14:937, 1990.

Owen, W.G.: The control of hemostasis. Role of endothelium in the regulation of inhibitory and catabolic pathways. Arch. Pathol. Lab. Med., 106:209, 1982.

Ratnoff, O.D., and Bennett, B: The genetics of hereditary disorders of blood coagulation. Science, 179:1291, 1973.

Reed, D.: On the pathologic changes in Hodgkin's disease with special reference to its relation to tuberculosis. Johns Hopkins Hosp. Rep., 10:133, 1902.

Seegers, W.H.: A personal perspective on hemostasis and thrombosis (1937–1981). In *Seminars in Thrombosis and Hemostasis*. Vol. VII, Nos. 3–4. Edited by E.F. Mammen. New York, Thieme-Stratton Inc. December, 1981.

Seufert, W., and Seufert, W.D.: The recognition of leukemia as a systemic disease. J. Hist. Med. Allied Sci., 37:34, 1982.

Suttie, J.W., and Jackson, C.M.: Prothrombin structure, activation, and biosynthesis. Physiol. Rev., 57:1, 1977.

Urba, W.J., and Longo, D.L.: Hodgkin's disease. N. Engl. J. Med., 326:678, 1992.

Wintrobe, M.M., et al.: *Clinical Hematology*, 8th Ed. Philadelphia, Lea & Febiger, 1981.

24

CENTRAL NERVOUS SYSTEM

The brain allows man to escape from the laws of evolution, since his body no longer has to keep adapting to environment to survive.—L. EISELEY

The nervous system may be arbitrarily divided into a central part, consisting of the brain and spinal cord, and a peripheral part, consisting of the nerves that carry motor messages from the brain and cord to the muscles and those that carry sensory messages from the skin and other parts of the body to the cord and brain. This chapter considers the central nervous system in the general context of those parts that are frequently involved by disease. For more details on the normal structure and function, and for information on the rarer diseases, the reader is referred to other sources. For notes on structure and function see the Appendix, p. 541.

While this text is not an encyclopedia of disease, it would be appropriate in the opinion of this writer to spend a few paragraphs on the serious problem of distinguishing diseases of the central nervous system for which we have reasonable explanations from those disorders of function for which the explanations are more difficult to determine.

It is important to recognize that disorders of function may range from gross disturbances such as coma to much more subtle derangements, which may be discovered only by careful neurologic assessment, by visual field testing, or by perceiving the changes in the personality over a long period. Mercifully, in many cases, the patient may be unaware of the changes that are occurring; disorders of the brain frequently provide their own anesthesia. However, for someone who is not a neurologist or psychiatrist, the most baffling problem may be to decide whether the impairment of function, such as a loss of recent memory, disorientation, lack of drive, difficulty in making decisions, impairment of judgment, and change in personality, is due to some treatable illness, or whether it is an irreversible disorder. In any case, the problem of how to manage the patient, who is often elderly, is difficult because depression, for example,

may have a radically different prognosis and treatment from senile dementia. To clarify this area, it is worthwhile enumerating a few of the classic, organic brain syndromes and saying a word or so about each (Table 24–1).

For practical purposes, the term **neuroses** can be defined as including all those mental disorders that have no demonstrable organic basis, and in which the patient may have considerable insight and unimpaired reality testing. He does not usually confuse his morbid, subjective experiences and fantasies with external realities. The patient's behavior may be greatly affected, although usually remaining within socially acceptable limits, but the personality is not disorganized. The principal manifestations of neuroses are excessive anxiety, hysterical symptoms, phobias, obsessional and compulsive symptoms, and depression. It is characteristic of many people that they may have episodes of decompensation, although they may have relatively adequate mental function. It

Table 24–1. Simplified Classification of Mental Disorders

ORGANIC BRAIN SYNDROMES	FUNCTIONAL DISORDERS
Cerebral arteriosclerosis	Psychoses
Alzheimer's disease	Schizophrenia
Korsakoff's psychosis	Manic-depressive psychosis
Wernicke's psychosis	Neuroses
Senile dementia	Anxiety
Delirium tremens	Depression
General paresis of the insane	Phobia
Toxic psychoses from	Hysteria
Alcohol	Hypochondriasis
Drugs	Personality disorders
Heavy metals	
Slow virus diseases	
Kuru	

is also characteristic that these persons respond inappropriately to stress. The age in which most neuroses are clinically apparent is between 25 and 45 years. There is no obvious difference between men and women, and over 80% of all patients with neuroses are both anxious and depressed.

Someone with a **psychosis** manifests a major disturbance of thinking, mood, and behavior to such a degree that he loses contact with reality. This interferes with the function of sleeping and eating, with work habits, and with interpersonal relations. A neurosis, on the other hand, has been defined as "a benign episode of disordered mental function, with an exaggeration of the individual's personality."

A third category of functional disorder comprises those situations that have been called **personality disorders,** in which there is a long-term maladaptation of behavior that suggests an arrest or distortion of the development of personality. Such persons tend to blame others and seem to have little capacity for insight into reasons for their behavior. A final group of disorders without organic brain disease are those transient **situational disturbances,** e.g., a depressive reaction to grief.

In concluding this rapid survey of functional disturbances, one might include those psychophysiologic disorders that at one time were called psychosomatic disorders, such as peptic ulcers, migraine, asthma, hypertension, and diseases such as ulcerative colitis, in which psychologic factors have been repeatedly seen to affect the patient.

A word or two may be devoted to schizophrenia in this discussion of the pathologic physiology of the brain, for it is a principal cause of chronic mental illness, and it is said to be responsible for more grave disability than any other illness in the whole of medicine. More than one half of the beds for chronic disease in our hospitals are devoted to mental disorder. The frontier of the mind and its diseases remains one of the last to be pushed back in this day of incredible medical advances.

The word **schizophrenia** is derived from the Greek, meaning a divided mind, and it connotes a disconnection between thoughts and feelings on the one hand, and actions on the other. It manifests itself most often between the ages of 15 and 25 years (hence the older name of *dementia praecox*), first by a gradual social withdrawal, followed by the development of all sorts of bizarre hallucinations. It has a prevalence of 1% of the population. It involves a fragmentation, a breaking-up, of all the processes of thought and feeling that enable a healthy person to remain in touch with the world; it might be regarded as a cancer of the mind, gnawing into the very soul of the patient. What inter-

ests us in the present discussion is that similar hallucinations can be induced in a normal person by means of the so-called hallucinogenic drugs, as a result of which the volunteer subject may experience marked distortions of reality. The significance of these observations is that they suggest that a chemical abnormality in a brain that is structurally normal may result in a condition of temporary insanity.

Evidence to support this hypothesis has recently accumulated from two sources. First, a small group of schizophrenics has been given hemodialysis which exchanges retained molecules that are excreted normally. Hemodialysis is usually given to patients with renal failure. Through serendipity, a schizophrenic patient in renal failure was found to be markedly improved after hemodialysis, and attempts to repeat this observation in other patients have shown surprisingly good results. However, a more recent study has failed to confirm the observation. The implication of this discovery is that there may be a biochemical substance exchangeable by dialysis that directly affects the ordered functioning of the central nervous system. Second, biochemical studies on a group of schizophrenics have shown that the amount of serotonin present in platelets is significantly different from the platelet serotonin in normal persons.

With the drugs now available, many victims of mental illness need not be sent to mental hospitals. Psychotherapy in the shape of psychoanalysis has proved its great value, but we should not let this exclude therapy with the aid of chemical agents. In our consideration of mental disease, it would appear that we must bring back the soma as well as the psyche, just as we saw that in our study of physical disease we must not concentrate too much on the soma to the exclusion of the psyche.

SYMPTOMS OF DISORDERS OF THE CENTRAL NERVOUS SYSTEM

Disorders of consciousness, or perception, and of response are the signposts of disorders of the nervous system, and a vocabulary of considerable size has evolved to specify particular dysfunctions. Since this is not a text for neurologic disorders, we shall limit the introduction of new terms and refer the reader to other sources.

Consciousness, the most obvious benefit of the nervous system, can be equated with responsiveness, and its pathologic alterations can be divided into several levels. **Lethargy** is a state of torpor or drowsiness that can have many causes, ranging from hypothyroidism and toxic states to an intracranial hemorrhage, which is simply pressing on the cerebral hemispheres. **Stupor** is a further step, in which the person is asleep, but can be aroused by appropriate stimuli, usually painful. However, he will return to the somnolent state after withdrawal of the stimulus. This state is an exaggeration of the previous level and suggests progression. More toxins, such as barbiturates, or increasing damage, such as extension of a hemorrhage or progression of an infection, are the classic causes of stupor. **Coma** is the state in which the patient is unresponsive except to the most painful stimuli, and in which the responses are limited to a reflex withdrawal. It has been defined as "sleeplike unresponsiveness without evidence of awareness of the self or environment, a state from which patients could not be aroused." The higher cortical functions are absent in coma, which again may be due to trauma, metabolic disorders such as unmanaged diabetes mellitus, or toxic agents. **Convulsions** and seizures are another symptom of disorder in the central nervous system.

Brain death is the final and, currently, a most controversial level of damage to the central nervous system because of its legal, moral, and ethical implications. As we outlined earlier in this book, it is difficult to define death, and we have leaned heavily on the concept of irreversible change in cells and in tissues in earlier considerations, but most were directed at tissues and did not imply the death of the thinking being.

The Harvard criteria for defining irreversible coma or brain death include several points:

1. The inability to respond to or to perceive any type of stimuli indicating loss of the higher centers, the cortex, and the thalamus.
2. No spontaneous respiration or movement after three minutes off a respirator.
3. Absence of postural reflexes with fixed, dilated pupils and absence of swallowing, yawning, and vocalization.
4. Flat electroencephalogram for at least 10 minutes.
5. Repeat testing within 24 hours showing no change.
6. No evidence of hypothermia or of central nervous system depression.

To put these technical matters in another way, several states have enacted laws, one of which reads as follows: "A person will be considered dead if, in the announced opinion of a physician, based on ordinary standards of medicine in a community, there is the irreversible cessation of spontaneous respirations and circulatory functions. If artificial means of support preclude a determination that these functions have ceased, a person will be considered dead if, in the announced opinion of a physician based on ordinary standards of medical practice in the community, there is the irreversible cessation of spontaneous brain function."

It is unwise to separate, for the purpose of this chapter, many varieties of disorders because the list becomes unnecessarily long. However, it is important to understand that some central nervous system disorders are developmental or congenital, that is, **childhood disorders.** Anencephaly, which is incompatible with life, and hydrocephalus, together with spina bifida and limb defects, can be listed here.

The most serious disorders of the nervous system may, however, be those in which the intellectual endowment is less than desirable. Attempts to catalog mental retardation are always controversial. A person with an IQ of less than 20 used to be referred to as an idiot, 20 to 50 an imbecile, 50 to 70 a moron, and over 70 but under 100 has many names. Other severe disabilities such as autism and major epilepsy, or inborn errors of metabolism that go unrecognized, cannot be discussed here.

VASCULAR DISEASE OF THE CENTRAL NERVOUS SYSTEM

For every 100 persons with any form of cerebrovascular disease, 50 will be permanently disabled and 10 will be institutionalized.

The most frequent diseases of the brain are the result of vascular disturbances. The prevalence of these diseases is found to be about 500/100,000 population in the western world. The word apoplexy comes from the Greek meaning a striking down, i.e., a seizure or stroke. It is an old term, for the condition was described by Hippocrates. To Galen it was "a sudden loss of feeling and of movement of the whole body, with the exception of respiration." The victim was believed to be struck down by some external force, as by the act of one of the gods. The word apoplexy is now seldom used in medical practice, rather the term stroke is used, particularly when the cause of the loss of sensation and motor function is not known. What are known as minor strokes, "little strokes" or "strokelets", are characterized by fleeting attacks of faintness, localized paralysis, aphasia (loss of speech), and visual disturbance. The attacks are so temporary that they are accompanied by no structural damage, and are apparently a manifestation of temporary cerebral anoxia, due to a combination of cardiac failure and cerebrovascular narrowing. They are spoken of as transient ischemic attacks, abbreviated as TIA.

A great change has taken place in our thinking regarding vascular disease in the central nervous system. The term "stroke" used to be synonymous with cerebral hemorrhage, and certainly a massive hemorrhage gives a classic picture. We realize, however, that the general term "stroke" cloaks our ignorance, and that the causes of loss of consciousness may be due to either ischemia (thrombosis) or hemorrhage. The term stroke is sometimes used interchangeably with "cerebrovascular accident," which hides an equal degree of ignorance. In developed countries, stroke is the third most common cause of death after cancer and myocardial infarction. There was a decrease in its incidence from 104 cases/100,000 population in the 1950s to 94/100,000 in the 1970s. This is in spite of greater access to medical facilities and better diagnostic techniques (CT scans). There is a general feeling that we see fewer massive strokes today and more small events. New studies suggest that prophylactic antiplatelet drugs (aspirin) on a regular basis reduce both the severity of the events and their frequency, as is true for myocardial infarction.

The major risk factors, we might repeat here, are hypertension, diabetes mellitus, other cardiovascular disease, elevated blood lipids, obesity and cigarette smoking. A recent review attributes 57% of strokes to systemic arteriosclerosis, 16% to embolism, 4% to intracerebral vascular disease, 10% to subarachnoid hemorrhage and 3% to other causes. Fifty per cent of people with strokes die within three days.

Ischemia most commonly is due to thrombosis, but it may also be due to embolism. The main arteries carrying blood to the cranial cavity are (1) the internal carotids in the neck, and (2) the vertebral arteries that arise from the subclavian at the root of the neck and pass upward in the vertebral canal. Revolutionary changes in the medical and surgical treatment of strokes demand accurate localization of the cause of the ischemia by means of cerebral angiography, using radiopaque material or other radiographic techniques.

The clinical picture of "cerebrovascular accident" varies within the widest limits. It may take the form of a violent assault, in which the patient collapses as if felled by an axe and is deprived of sense and motion. However, the most frequent type involves only a slight defect of speech, thought, motion, sensation, or vision; consciousness is not lost, and some degree of recovery is nearly invariable. It is obvious that the former type is likely to be caused by massive cerebral hemorrhage, the latter type by thrombosis. Ischemia is at least four times as common as hemorrhage, and carries with it a much graver prognosis.

Cerebral Hemorrhage. With advancing years, the arteries in the brain tend to narrow and become brittle

(Fig. 24–1). If at the same time the blood pressure is raised, there is danger that one of the brittle arteries will burst. Even in the absence of hypertension, massive hemorrhage may occur in an area of softening produced by vascular occlusion. The effect will naturally depend on the site of the hemorrhage and also on the extent. The most common position is, unfortunately, that part of the brain where the motor nerves to the body are gathered together into a comparatively small space before passing down the spinal cord. Here, hemorrhage easily destroys these nerves, the motor impulses are cut off from the muscles, and the side of the body (face, arm, and leg) supplied by the side of the brain affected is paralyzed, a condition known as hemiplegia. Should the patient survive, the paralyzed arm and leg gradually become flexed and assume a characteristic appearance. As the motor nerves from one side of the brain cross to the opposite side before passing down the cord, it follows that hemorrhage on the right side of the brain will be followed by a left-sided hemiplegia, and vice versa. The speech center in right-handed persons is on the left side of the brain, so that hemorrhage on the left side will produce a condition of speechlessness or aphasia, in addition to a right-sided hemiplegia.

Cerebrovascular accidents seldom produce sudden or instantaneous death, because the part of the brain in which they most often occur contains no vital centers. "Sudden" death is nearly always due to sudden heart failure or to pulmonary embolism. But if the hemorrhage is large and close to the ventricles, it may rupture into those cavities in the course of a day or so, a complication that is sure to prove fatal (Fig. 24–2). On the other hand, if the hemorrhage is small, the amount of damage to the brain is correspondingly limited, and only the arm or the leg may be affected. The blood of the hemorrhage is gradually absorbed, and the patient may make a good recovery, with only a slight disability in the affected limb. The signs of intracerebral hemorrhage—headache, vomiting, hemiparalysis, decreasing consciousness, and rapid respirations—are normally not preceded by warning signs, as in ischemic attacks. In 15 to 20% of patients who survive the first few days with no progression, attempts to prevent further loss of function may restore the patient to a useful life. Recently it has become clear that some of our older views of the irreversible nature of the adaptability of the central nervous system are in error. It has been convincingly shown that even in the adult, after significant brain injury, relearning can take place. But it is extremely important that the relearning take place immediately after the injury as the plastic nature of the central nervous system is soon lost when healing supervenes without

Fig. 24–1 At the base of the brain the vertebral basilar arteries and internal carotids can all be seen to be markedly distorted by **atherosclerosis.** (McGill University, Department of Pathology Museum.)

demands which take into consideration the short-lived but great potential for adaptation even in the CNS. In the jargon of the physiologist even the brain of a 68-year-old is not "hard wired."

One might mention the difference between intracerebral (see Figs. 24–2 and 24–3) and cerebellar hemorrhage, because the latter carries with it a vastly different prognosis, and strong indications for intervention are present in the case of any cerebellar hemorrhage.

Of course, there is always the danger of another hemorrhage later, a danger that hangs suspended over the patient's head like the sword of Damocles, but may never fall. The thought faculties are not necessarily interfered with. Pasteur did some of his best work after a small cerebrovascular accident.

Thrombosis. This is the most common cause of cerebral ischemia, comprising probably 50% of all cases.

Atherosclerosis is the primary lesion; it causes narrowing of the lumen, the occluding thrombus being added at a late stage to produce ischemia. The main site of obstruction is not in the brain, but in the extracerebral vessels, often in extracranial vessels, more particularly the internal carotid in the neck and the vertebral artery. Diagnosis of occlusion, and in particular the exact site of the occlusion, can be established with certainty by cerebral angiography (Figs. 24–4 and 24–5). Excision of the occluded segment of the artery and anastomosis or insertion of an arterial or synthetic graft may yield gratifying results in selected cases. This development would have been impossible to imagine only a few years ago. The lesions are infarcts followed by cerebral softening with eventual liquefaction or the formation of a cyst.

The clinical picture varies with the site of the vessel

Fig. 24—2   This section through the cerebral hemispheres of an adult brain shows **intracerebral and intraventricular hemorrhage** extending from the right lateral ventricle as far as the fourth ventricle (shown in the section through the cerebellum in the lower portion of the picture). Such a destructive hemorrhage will cause death, usually by compression of the brain stem due to the increase in intracerebral pressure. (McGill University, Department of Pathology Museum.)

Fig. 24—3   This CT scan shows the presence of a **dense mass in the left cerebral hemisphere**. Note that the pineal gland has shifted to the right, the ventricular system on the left is obscured, and the right ventricular system is moved to the right because of the space-occupying lesion.

myocardial infarct. The embolus usually passes into the left carotid artery and is most likely to lodge in the middle cerebral artery. The accompanying paralysis may be extensive. Cerebral embolism is distinguished from other vascular accidents by the extreme suddenness of the onset of symptoms, with complete development in 10 to 30 seconds and a total absence of warning.

occluded and with the size of the area of brain affected. It would be fruitless to give a detailed description here. Neurologic symptoms may take several days to develop. Compare this with the cerebral hemorrhage, in which the period is measured in minutes or at most in hours, or with cerebral embolism, in which the period is so short that it cannot be measured. There is a tendency for the occlusion to develop while the patient is asleep or within an hour of arising; a hemorrhage is likely to develop during waking hours of activity. The occlusion that is due to embolism may, of course, occur at any time.

Cerebral Embolism.   The third cause of cerebrovascular accidents is embolism to the smaller cerebral vessels within the brain. The embolus most often arises from the left side of the heart, either from a vegetation on the mitral or aortic valve or from a thrombus in the appendix of the left atrium, or from a mural thrombus that has formed in the left ventricle at the site of a

Fig. 24—4   This **cerebral angiogram** shows the lateral view of filling of the left carotid and its branches.

Fig. 24–5   This **cerebral angiogram** shows the anterior view of the distribution of the branches of the cerebral arterial tree.

Intracranial Hemorrhage

Hemorrhage is described in relation to the meninges, and may be extradural, subdural, or subarachnoid, or it may occur within the substance of the brain (Fig. 24–7).

Extradural hemorrhage is a condition in which blood pours out between the skull and the dura mater. It is commonly caused by bleeding from the middle meningeal artery. This artery lies in contact with the inside surface of the skull in the region of the temple, and is liable to be torn by a hairline fracture of the skull in this region. The condition is readily diagnosed because the patient is first stunned by a blow to the skull; he then recovers consciousness and appears to be all right for a few hours—this is known as the "lucid interval;" at the end of that time the patient becomes dull, drowsy, and finally loses consciousness again, owing to the increasing pressure of the blood that is accumulating between the skull and the brain outside the dura mater. The condition must be diagnosed, for by immediate operation the collection of blood can be removed, the bleeding vessel tied, and the life of the patient saved. There is no blood in the cerebrospinal fluid at lumbar puncture, because

the thick dura mater intervenes between the bleeding vessel and the cerebrospinal fluid.

Subdural hemorrhage is most frequently venous in origin, not arterial, and in this respect it differs fundamentally from extradural and subarachnoid hemorrhage. The condition is much more common than extradural hemorrhage, and it is of great importance because the life of the patient depends on a correct diagnosis, which is easily missed. The cause may be a blow in the frontal or occipital region (e.g., knocking the head against a shelf or door in the dark) that injures the cerebral veins passing into the subdural space. The blood clot so formed is converted into a kind of cyst, which may increase in volume. There is thus a continually increasing pressure on the underlying brain with the production of symptoms similar to those of a brain tumor. The confusing feature is that weeks may intervene between the relatively slight injury to the head and the development of cerebral symptoms, so that the injury may have been forgotten.

Intracranial hemorrhage of the newborn, a common cause of death, is a variety of subdural hemorrhage. The hemorrhage is due to injury during delivery that tears the cerebral veins crossing the subdural space to

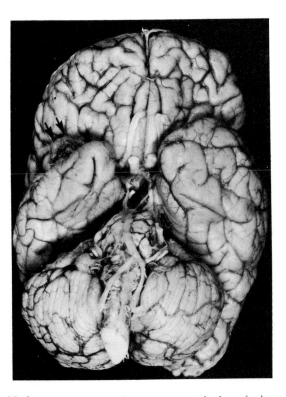

Fig. 24–6   This photograph shows (at arrows) the loss of substance of the right temporal lobe. Such **ischemic necrosis** and atrophy are common. They are symptomatic when functional areas of the brain are involved. (McGill University, Department of Pathology Museum.)

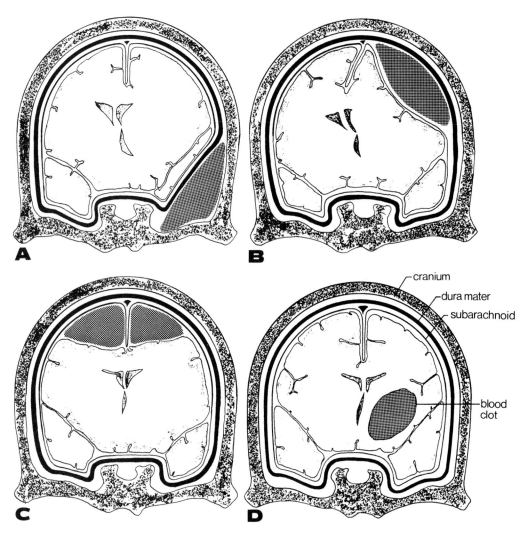

Fig. 24-7 These drawings show the distribution of hemorrhages into the various spaces of the brain. *A* shows an **extradural** hemorrhage. Note the presence of the skull and the displacement of the dura. *B* shows a **subdural** hematoma. Note the displacement of the brain substance. *C* shows a **subarachnoid** hemorrhage. *D* shows an **intracerebral** hemorrhage. (From Gilbert, E.F., and Huntington, R.W.: *An Introduction to Pathology.* New York, Oxford University Press, 1978.)

enter the longitudinal sinus. Death may occur in a few hours or in the course of a day or so. If the child survives, paralytic and other symptoms may develop later.

Subarachnoid hemorrhage is hemorrhage into the subarachnoid space between the arachnoid and the pia mater (Fig. 24–8A). Blood in large amount will be found in the cerebrospinal fluid at lumbar puncture. Such hemorrhage occurs when the surface of the brain is torn by a fracture of the skull, or it may be due to rupture of an aneurysm of an artery that lies beneath the arachnoid at the base of the brain (Fig. 24–8B). This condition, which is not uncommon in young people, was usually fatal in the past, but modern neurosurgery has made it possible to deal with the aneu-

rysm and to arrest the hemorrhage. Perhaps it is well to note that hypertension is the most important common predisposing cause of hemorrhage in the central nervous system, regardless of its location.

Today, the availability of computer tomography and magnetic resonance imaging (Fig. 24–9) for intracranial disease has made the diagnosis and management of vascular disease infinitely safer for the patient and easier for the neurologist and neurosurgeon.

Trauma

This subject may be considered in connection with cerebral hemorrhage, because the essential danger of this condition is laceration of the surface of the brain

Fig. 24—8 *A,* This photograph of the base of the brain shows the staining of the surface of the inferior aspect of the cerebellum, brain stem, and the cerebral hemispheres by fresh blood. This is a **subarachnoid hemorrhage** which commonly results from the rupture of an aneurysm. (McGill University, Department of Pathology Museum.) *B,* **Aneurysm of circle of Willis.** The aneurysm, which is of unusually large size and still unruptured, arises from the internal carotid artery. The location adjacent to a bifurcation is characteristic. (University of Alabama Medical School.)

Fig. 24—9 This CT scan shows the presence of dense material over the surfaces of the frontal poles (arrows). This is interpreted as the CT scan appearance of a **subarachnoid hemorrhage.**

with accompanying hemorrhage. The fracture may involve the upper part of the skull, or vault, or the base of the skull. The latter is by far the more serious, and is apt to prove fatal, if not properly treated. The fracture itself is of little moment, although it may open into the ear or nose, causing bleeding from those organs. There is nearly always an accompanying laceration of the base of the brain, with rapidly developing edema of the structure. Some of the most important vital nerve centers essential for life, those for the heart and for respiration, are situated in this part of the brain, and the increasing pressure on these centers caused by the edema may prove fatal. At the same time, there is an accumulation of cerebrospinal fluid in this region that increases the pressure further. It is evident that the most urgent need is to reduce the pressure inside the skull before the vital centers become paralyzed, and this is done most rapidly and effectively by creating burr holes (trephining, just as the ancients used to do). Since this method of treatment has been introduced, the mortality in cases of fracture of the base of the skull has been greatly reduced.

INFECTIOUS DISEASE OF THE CENTRAL NERVOUS SYSTEM

Inflammatory disease in the central nervous system is generally due to infectious agents and, fortunately, is much less common today than in yesteryear. One may look on infectious diseases of the central nervous system as diffuse or localized, or classify them according to their etiology (bacterial, fungal, viral, or protozoal). We shall consider local infection first, then meningeal disease, and, finally, viral and spirochetal infections.

Abscess of the Brain

The microorganisms that cause abscess of the brain may come from a focus of infection in the skull or may be carried by the blood stream from a distance, but by far the most common local source used to be infections of the middle ear or mastoid sinus. Antibiotic therapy has now given us control of this condition. The infection spreads inward and causes abscess formation in the adjacent part of the brain. Another source of danger is infection in the frontal and other air sinuses that communicate with the nose. Here the abscess is likely to be in the frontal part of the brain. If the infecting organisms come from a distance, the most common source is an abscess or other septic process in the lung. Indeed, a danger of abscess of the lung is the formation of a secondary abscess in the brain. Figure 24–10 shows a CT scan image of multiple abscesses in the brain of a 50-year-old patient with bronchiectasis. The diagnosis was not made until too late for effective treatment.

Clinical Pattern. The symptoms of abscess of the brain are apt to be misleading. It might be imagined that a collection of pus in so delicate a piece of machinery as the brain would cause a violent disturbance, but the reverse is the case. Many parts of the brain are what are called silent areas, that is to say, a lesion of that part produces no characteristic symptoms, and this is particularly true of those parts in which an abscess is likely to occur. Moreover, the inflammation is usually of a quiet rather than a violent character. For these reasons, the abscess may give rise neither to "localizing symptoms" nor even to those indicating infection. Instead, the clinical picture will be that of gradually increasing intracranial pressure, which may suggest a tumor instead of an abscess. Suspicion, however, will be aroused by the coexistence of middle-ear and mastoid infections, inflammation in the frontal sinus, or lung abscess.

Remarkably good results may follow the drainage of a brain abscess, provided the operation is performed by a surgeon who knows what he or she is

Fig. 24–10 This CT scan shows the appearance of 2 dense, small areas in the left posterior cerebral hemisphere. This is compatible with a diagnosis of **cerebral abscess**.

doing, but there is always danger of the infection reaching the meninges, with the production of a fatal meningitis. This complication may now be avoided by the use of antibiotics.

Meningitis

We have already seen that the brain and spinal cord are covered by membranes or meninges, inflammation of which is called meningitis. Many organisms may cause meningitis, but the common ones are meningococcus, streptococcus, pneumococcus, and tubercle bacillus. The first three organisms are pyogenic or pus-forming bacteria, so that the diseases they produce are acute in type; the tubercle bacillus is less violent in action and more difficult to diagnose.

The streptococcus and pneumococcus reach the meninges from the middle ear or the frontal sinus, but they may be carried by the blood stream from distant parts, especially the lung. The meningococcus comes from the cavity of the nose or throat. Meningitis may assume an epidemic form, with many cases developing in a single locality or in many places throughout the country. Such epidemic meningitis is always due to the meningococcus. The infection is spread by carriers, who harbor the organisms in their throat, but who do not themselves develop infection of the meninges. The term cerebrospinal meningitis is often applied to the meningococcal type, but the other forms of the disease are also cerebrospinal, in the sense that the meninges of both the brain and the spinal cord are inflamed.

Tuberculous meningitis is in a class by itself. It has none of the acuteness of the other forms of meningitis and used to be the most uniformly fatal, with a mortality of 100%. The hopeless outlook has dramatically changed by the use of antibiotics.

At autopsy, in a fatal case of meningitis, the subarachnoid space is filled with an acute inflammatory exudate in the meningococcal, streptococcal, and pneumococcal forms (Fig. 24–11), so that the brain and cord are covered with yellow pus. In tuberculous meningitis, however, there is only a thick, milky-white layer in which tubercles may be distinguished with difficulty.

Examination of the cerebrospinal fluid obtained by lumbar puncture usually establishes the diagnosis, including the type of bacterial infection. When normal cerebrospinal fluid is removed, it is as clear as water, and the pressure is so low that it flows out drop by drop. In meningitis, owing to the pyogenic bacteria, the fluid is turbid, because in reality it is thin pus. When the fluid is examined under the microscope, it is found to be crowded with polymorphonuclear leukocytes (pus cells) and to contain varying numbers of the bacteria responsible for the infection. In tuberculous meningitis, the spinal fluid is only slightly milky or may be almost clear, for as the inflammation is less acute, the cells are much fewer in number and are for the most part lymphocytes. The level of protein is increased, the sugar level is decreased and sometimes disappears, and the level of chloride is low. This last is the most valuable of all the chemical tests, for no other condition gives a really low chloride reading. The demonstration of tubercle bacilli is the conclusive proof of the etiology of the meningitis.

Syphilis of the Nervous System

Among the most tragic manifestations of syphilis are those due to infection of the central nervous system in cases untreated by penicillin. A peculiarity of these lesions is that they do not develop for many years after the original infection; it may be 10, 15, or even 20 years later. The patient may have been without symptoms for years, even may have almost forgotten that he ever had syphilis. Various parts of the nervous system may be attacked, so that the symp-

A　**B**

Fig. 24–11 *A,* This photograph of the superior aspect of the cerebral hemispheres of the brain of a young child shows the purulent exudate that is typical of **purulent meningitis,** caused by a variety of bacteria. This pus may occlude the circulation of the cerebrospinal fluid and lead to hydrocephalus. (McGill University, Department of Pathology Museum.) *B,* This photograph of the inferior aspect of the brain shows the disposition of an inflammatory exudate around the brain stem, pons, and cerebellum that is typical of **tuberculous meningitis.** (McGill University, Department of Pathology Museum.)

toms may be varied, but only two clear-cut clinical pictures or diseases will be described here. The first of these is general paresis or general paralysis of the insane, the second is tabes dorsalis or locomotor ataxia. Together they are referred to as neurosyphilis. In the period 1974–78 the incidence in Copenhagen was found to be 0.3/100,000 inhabitants per year for the 5-year period. This represented 23 patients in that area.

General Paresis. The name is descriptive, for it implies not only a weakness of the muscles, but also a general weakening of all the faculties of the mind. The even more sinister "general paralysis of the insane" describes the final state of the patient. The spirochetes of syphilis are scattered widely throughout the brain and produce multiple areas of inflammation, together with destruction of the nerve cells and nerve fibers. As a result of this destruction, the brain atrophies and wastes away, becoming much smaller than normal. This wasting particularly affects the cerebral cortex, that is to say, the part of the brain concerned with the highest functions of the mind. The areas concerned with muscular movements and with sensation are also involved.

Clinical Pattern. The symptoms of the disease are as diverse as the lesions are widely disseminated. The first indication that all is not well is a deterioration of the higher qualities of the mind. The moral sense is impaired, and there is a weakening of the faculties of judgment, reason, and self-control. Delusions of grandeur lead to domestic and financial difficulties, for if a man believes that he is worth millions and orders automobiles, aeroplanes, and grand pianos in corresponding amounts, it is not conducive to domestic happiness. The structure of the mind crumbles, and the final stage is that of childishness and complete dementia. All these changes are due to destruction of the nerve cells in the cerebral cortex. Tremors are highly characteristic; they involve the face, lips, and tongue, so that the speech becomes thick and indistinct, and the hands are tremulous. These tremors are due to lesions in the motor centers. The sensory centers are also involved, so that sensibility is dulled and pain may hardly be felt. The pupil of the eye no longer contracts when exposed to bright light, although it still does so when the eye looks at a nearby object, a condition known as the Argyll Robertson pupil. Convulsive seizures followed by unconsciousness are common. The weakness of the muscles implied in the name of the disease becomes extreme. In the end, the patient is not only mindless but helpless.

The cerebrospinal fluid shows changes that are of great importance, because they allow the physician to make an early diagnosis at a time when treatment may arrest the progress of the disease. The cells of the fluid, particularly lymphocytes, are increased in number, especially at the beginning of the malady. The protein level is increased, but far more significant is that the Wassermann test on the fluid is positive, showing that the patient is suffering from syphilis of the central nervous system.

Tabes Dorsalis. The word tabes means a wasting away, and as the lesion in this syphilitic disease of the spinal cord is a wasting of the posterior or dorsal part of the cord, the condition is called tabes dorsalis. In the dorsal columns of the cord run the nerves that carry the sensations of position, called muscle sense and joint sense. When these are lost, the patient is no longer certain of the position of his legs, so that he becomes unsteady or ataxic in his locomotion.

Anyone wishing to read a description of the onset of the symptoms of tabes by a master of literature should look up Kipling's wonderful little story, "Love o' Women." There is no muscular weakness, for the lesion is confined to the sensory nerves, but the power of muscular coordination is gradually lost, so that the patient is unable to make his legs do what he wants them to do. Things are not so bad as long as the patient has the assistance of sight, but in the dark he is completely at sea. The ordinary person walks by faith (without watching the ground), but the tabetic walks by sight. He walks with legs wide apart to increase stability, and is unable to stand with feet together and eyes closed without swaying or falling (Romberg's sign). To the trained eye, the tabetic can be recognized at once as he walks down the street, by his peculiar wide-based gait and by the way he throws his feet out and brings them down with a slap.

Other sensory disturbances are sudden, severe shooting pains passing down the legs, known as lightning pains, and occasional attacks of abdominal pain and vomiting, called gastric crises, which may be mistaken for acute appendicitis. There is loss of the knee-jerks, i.e., lack of response when the tendon below the knee-cap is tapped, loss of the normal contraction of the pupil to light (Argyll Robertson pupil), as in general paresis, and gradual wasting of the optic nerve, optic atrophy, with corresponding impairment of vision. The cerebrospinal fluid shows the same changes as in general paresis, so that its examination is of the greatest help in diagnosis. Again, in this form of central-nervous-system syphilitic infection, penicillin is the best method of treatment and may often arrest the progress of the condition and relieve many of the symptoms.

If the reader should ask why the *Treponema pallidum* attacks the brain in one patient and the spinal cord in another, there is no answer.

At any rate, tertiary syphilis of the central nervous system is much less prevalent today than it was 40 years ago.

Viral Diseases

Many viruses can attack the central nervous system, sometimes setting up an inapparent infection, not infrequently meningitis, less often encephalitis. Viruses with a special affinity for the nervous system are called neurotropic and cause some of the most serious diseases of that system, such as poliomyelitis and rabies. There is another group of common, febrile viral diseases (measles, chickenpox, smallpox, vaccinia), in which injury to the nervous system occurs on rare occasions.

Encephalitis is the characteristic pattern of disease caused by virus as contrasted with meningitis (caused by bacteria). Clinically, encephalitis appears as symptoms of headache and coma, whereas meningitis is normally recognized by the stiff neck and other signs of meningeal inflammation. **Viral encephalitis** constitutes a group of diseases, some of which are epidemic. Any detailed consideration of this group is beyond the scope of this book, but one or two members may be mentioned. Lethargic encephalitis, also called "sleeping sickness," appears in epidemic form at longer intervals and sweeps across the world. In an epidemic that William Boyd studied in Winnipeg in 1919, the patient was dull, lethargic, and somnolent. He would lie like a log in bed with drooping lids or closed eyes, sunk in a stupor that no external stimuli could penetrate, the dim rushlight of reason hardly flickering. About 20% of these cases subsequently develop some degree of postencephalitic paralysis agitans or parkinsonism, a condition of generalized rigidity of the face and body that is described later in relation to Parkinson's disease. **Equine encephalitis**, as its name indicates, is a viral disease of horses that appears in epidemic form. Farm workers may also fall victim to it. Human infection is probably due to mosquitoes, which convey the infection from horse to man. There have been new outbreaks in the United States in 1991 (Figs. 24–12 and 24–13). Secondary encephalitis may occur as a complication following one of the common viral fevers, usually measles, more rarely mumps and chickenpox. Finally, **postvaccinal encephalitis** must be mentioned, in which, in rare instances, a severe form of encephalitis follows vaccination for smallpox.

Poliomyelitis or infantile paralysis is an acute infectious disease of the spinal cord and brain caused by a filterable virus (poliovirus) and chiefly affecting children. Most of the infections are clinically inapparent

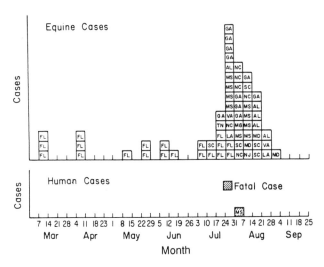

Fig. 24–12 Reported **eastern equine encephalitis** cases—United States, 1989. (From Centers for Disease Control, Morbidity and Mortality Weekly Report, 38(36):619, 1989.)

and go unrecognized. Today, we have a vaccine, and the disease has virtually disappeared from North America (Figs. 24–14 and 24–15).

There is no more dramatic and deadly example of viral infection than **rabies**. Its practical significance is that when a person has been bitten by a dog suspected of being rabid, microscopic examination of the animal's brain will show whether or not the fingerprint of rabies, the Negri body, is present in the nerve cells, and preventive lifesaving inoculation can be begun at once, if necessary. Finally, as in poliomyelitis, we are now beginning to practice preventive vaccination, yet this practice was introduced by Pasteur with complete

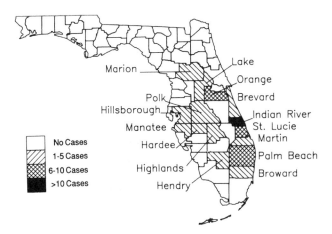

Fig. 24–13 Confirmed and presumptive cases of **St. Louis encephalitis**, by county—Florida, as of October 17, 1990. (From Centers for Disease Control, Morbidity and Mortality Weekly Report, 39(42):757, 1990.)

† Excludes Brazil, Cuba, Mexico and Paraguay, which use only 2 doses.

Fig. 24–14   **Oral polio vaccine** coverage in children one year of age and rate per 100,000 population of **reported paralytic poliomyelitis**, by year—the Americas, 1969–1989. (From Centers for Disease Control, Morbidity and Mortality Weekly Report, 39(33):558, 1990.)

success for the prevention of rabies more than 100 years ago.

Herpes is a viral disease characterized by the formation of small vesicles. The name is derived from the Greek word meaning to creep. There are two distinct forms: (1) herpes zoster or shingles, in which the vesicles follow or creep along the distribution of a sensory nerve, and (2) herpes simplex, in which there is no such distribution. An attack of the former is followed by lasting immunity, but in the case of the latter, there is no immunity. A puzzling feature is that the erup-

tion is always unilateral, running in a zone (zoster) as far as the middle line, being preceded by neuralgic pains, which in old people may be persistent and severe. The virus appears to be identical to that causing chickenpox, the spread in the latter case being by the blood stream, whereas in zoster it is along the nerves. Herpes simplex is the common form of herpes, usually on the lips as a complication of infective fevers, pneumonia, and even the common cold, so that it is best known as a "cold sore." This virus seems to be carried in cells of the epidermis and only becomes evident when such stimuli as sunlight or fever call it out to create lesions.

There is, in addition, a group of "degenerative" or chronic neurologic diseases that have been suspected of having a viral etiology, but of a different kind from the acute viral disease already discussed.

A **"slow" viral infection** is that in which the virus fails to cause acute disease, the host fails to clear the virus, and the result of the virus-host interaction evolves slowly, producing clinical signs and pathologic changes. The term was introduced in 1954 from studies on disease in Icelandic sheep. Slow viral infections differ from latent infections in that the virus may be isolated in a "slow" infection.

The concept of an infectious etiology for a group of diseases that have in common (1) infection in a single

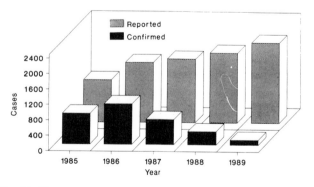

Fig. 24–15   **Reported and confirmed polio cases**, by year—the Americas, 1985–1989. (From Centers for Disease Control, Morbidity and Mortality Weekly Report, 39(33):558, 1990.)

species, (2) a long period of latency (months or years) between the possible infection and manifestation of this disease, (3) slow progression of the disease, and (4) limitation of the disease to a particular part of the nervous system, has been developed clearly during the last two decades, largely from studies on a disease of New Guinea cannibals (kuru), who relished eating brains and suffered the consequences. A model of this "slow virus" disease has been found in sheep in Scotland and Iceland, and human diseases of the nervous system have been transmitted to chimpanzees. There are also reports of transmission of a rare disease (Jakob-Creutzfeldt) from one patient to three others by electrodes contaminated with slow virus. This process is mentioned here not only because of its particular interest (the number of cases of kuru, Jakob-Creutzfeldt disease, and multifocal leukoencephalopathy is small), but also because of the concept that there can be such an agent and such a different type of response to an infectious agent. The strong evidence in favor of the existence of "slow virus disease" now draws attention to other diseases of unknown etiology and should direct your thinking to reconsider some of the processes that seem so mysterious in tissues other than the nervous system.

Recently there has been much attention given in the press to "Mad Cow" disease and its resemblance to some human diseases of uncertain etiology. Briefly, there has been an epidemic in Great Britain of chronic illness in milk and beef herds where the animals develop dementia. This epidemic, determined to originate about 1986, coincides with the practice of adding feed supplements rich in animal protein (derived from the processing of slaughter house offal). The rendering practices in Great Britain were changed about that time to conserve costs by eliminating the use of solvents and high temperature processing. Because the disease in cows resembled **scrapie** in sheep, clinically and pathologically, and because the cows were being fed sheep-derived offal, it was theorized that Mad Cow disease was indeed scrapie of cows. Since the agent of scrapie is not a conventional agent of disease (neither virus or bacteria, nor fungus or protozoa) and has not been isolated as a nucleic-acid-containing self-replicating or cell-dependent agent, its mode of dissemination is widely argued. The term **prion** has been put forward as a new term to identify its characteristics, and much work is currently in progress to define the possible modes of disease transmission for the scrapie agent. Meanwhile, the issue of trans-species transmission of unconventional agents of disease continues to perplex epidemiologists and students of disease.

DISEASE OF UNCERTAIN ETIOLOGY

It is easy to group many of the diseases of the central nervous system under such headings as traumatic, vascular, and infectious. In these instances, we have a good idea of the etiologic agent involved and of the meaning of the pathologic changes. Unfortunately, there remains a heterogeneous collection of conditions of unknown etiology, referred to vaguely as degenerative diseases of the nervous system. From this collection it seems justifiable to consider at least one group, known as the demyelinating diseases.

The essential feature of a demyelinating disease is destruction of the myelin sheaths and relative sparing of the axons, nerve cells, and neuroglia. Although we are ignorant as to the etiology and pathogenesis of the demyelinating diseases, several explanatory hypotheses have been put forward. Some of these diseases are genetically determined, and the myelin is abnormally formed. Others of these disorders are acquired, and the myelin is probably normal. The latter group comprises mostly adult diseases and is more prevalent than the former.

Multiple Sclerosis

This disease is the most common of these disorders and affects 250,000 people in the United States, and if we spend more time on it, it is because of its fascinating epidemiology and current attempts to discover its etiology. First, we shall describe the disease. The condition is also known as disseminated sclerosis. It is a chronic disease of the nervous system characterized by remissions and relapses and by the presence of patches of demyelination associated with sclerosis or hardening, scattered diffusely throughout the gray and white matter of the brain stem and spinal cord. Nerve fibers in the white matter degenerate and are replaced by glial scar tissue (Fig. 24–16). The disease runs a fluctuating, but usually progressive, course that affects various portions of the nervous system at different times. The plaques we have described show dead glial cells and loss of myelin that may have occurred at widely differing times.

Clinical Pattern. The disease, common among young adults in the western world, occurs usually at about age 30. In those instances in which the signs and symptoms suggest the diagnosis in a patient who is a child, or who is over 50 years old, the diagnosis is probably not correct. The disease is most frequent in the high latitudes, occurring in western Europe, the northern United States, southern Canada, New Zealand, and southern Australia. Five per cent of the cases are familial, usually occurring in siblings. Cases

Fig. 24–16 Multiple sclerosis. There are irregular asymmetrical patches of degeneration in the posterior and lateral columns. (Weigert's myelin stain.) (× 8.)

occurring in husbands and wives have also been reported. Epidemiologic studies of migrant populations show that those persons carry a low susceptibility from a low susceptible area when they move into an area of higher frequency. One study done in Israel indicated that persons immigrating there before their fifteenth year had the same liability for the disease as native Israelis, but those immigrating after 15 years of age had the same propensity for the disease as people in their country of origin. The incidence of the disease in northern areas ranges from 50 to 80 per 100,000 population.

The patient is often a young man, who sees a physician because of sudden onset of impaired vision that may progress to complete blindness in one eye, followed by partial or complete restoration of vision. Permanent blindness may come on again months later. Tingling or numbness in the extremities and transient urinary incontinence or frequency are also important hallmarks of the disease. Intention tremor, a stiff gait, jerky eye movements, and a peculiar, staccato speech always suggest involvement of the central nervous system by this disorder. The most important general criteria are the evidence of multiple signs in different parts of the central nervous system and their recurrence at different times. Considering the nature of the disease, it has often been noted that the patient seems inappropriately cheerful. The prognosis is guarded, because it is well recognized that the patient may live for many years despite the insidious progression of the disease.

The lesions of glial proliferation and demyelination are often bilateral, but not symmetrical, always central and never peripheral, and the explanation for the remissions and relapses are the presence of edema that resolves and the compensatory plasticity of alternate neurologic pathways. It is also likely that demyelinated axons may still conduct, or that remyelination may occur.

Examination of the cerebral spinal fluid may show no abnormality, although in many cases there is a mild lym-

phocytosis and an increase in protein. These changes may be absent in the advanced stage of the disease.

The etiology of multiple sclerosis remains unclear. Because gamma globulin is present in plaques, it has been suggested that the disease may be of immune origin; because patients with multiple sclerosis and their relatives belong most frequently to HLA groups 3 and 7, a hereditary etiology is spoken of; because coastal-dwelling fish eaters have a lower incidence of the disease than animal eaters at the same latitude, diet has been implicated; and because antibodies to measles virus are present in most patients, an infectious etiology has frequently been suggested.

A most interesting study was reported from the Faroe Islands, which lie between Norway and Iceland at latitude 62 north and longitude 7 west. They are a semi-independent unit of the Kingdom of Denmark, with a population of 41,000 in 1976.

As shown in Figure 24–17, there was an epidemic of multiple sclerosis on these islands in which new cases appeared in 1943 and disappeared, with one exception, by 1960. The explanation for this epidemic lies in that British troops occupied these islands from 1940 to 1945. The number of soldiers was as great as 8,000, bringing the ratio of outlanders to islanders to one in three. The diet of the Faroese seemed generally unchanged during the war, and possible explanations for the epidemic may be sought in classic causes such as the introduction of toxins or infectious diseases. The hypothesis is put forward that the epidemic is due to an infectious disease. It is of great interest that during this same period, the chief veterinarian of the islands reported that canine distemper was pandemic during the war and absent before the British occupation. Since 1956 or 1957, there has been no further distemper among dogs on these islands. The concurrence of the two epidemics suggests a relationship. Whether the virus of canine distemper can indeed lead in susceptible populations to multiple sclerosis is an unproven but provocative idea. The notion that such an infectious agent requires time to induce its effects, and that not all persons exposed will respond with a clinically apparent manifestation of disease, is important. It is of interest that other relationships of rare neurologic disorders to viral infections are being proven, as we have discussed in the section on slow virus, and as is apparent in sclerosing subacute panencephalitis syndrome, in the high proportion of antimeasles antibodies in such individuals.

Parkinson's Disease

Also known as "the shaking palsy," this disease is a chronic, nonkilling, but profoundly disabling de-

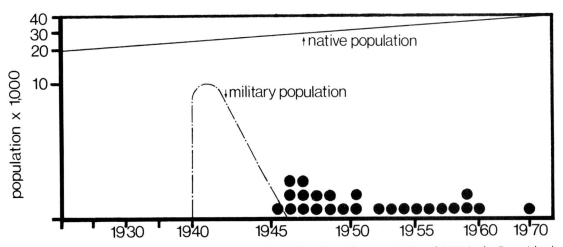

Fig. 24–17   This graph shows the presence (black dots) of cases of **multiple sclerosis** between 1945 and 1970 in the Faroe Islands. Each dot represents a single case. The native population rose during the period of 1920 to 1970 from 20,000 to 40,000, as shown on the top line. The military population resident on the islands arrived in 1940, with approximately 10,000 soldiers, and decreased over the next 5 years. Note the temporal relationship between the multiple sclerosis epidemic and the visit of the army to the islands. (From Kurtzke, J.F., and Hyllested, K.: Multiple sclerosis in the Faroe Islands: I. Clinical and epidemiological features. Ann. Neurol., 5:6, 1978.)

generation of the brain. The clinical picture was drawn in 1817 by Parkinson with the hand of a master. The classic triad of symptoms is rigidity, tremor, and an attitude of flexion. The rigidity involves all the voluntary muscles, until, in an extreme case, the unhappy sufferer becomes as rigid as a block of marble. This rigidity gives the face the familiar "Parkinsonian mask." The tremor affects the fingers and hands, giving a pill-rolling movement. Curiously enough, it is present when the part is at rest, disappearing for a few moments with movement, thus justifying the term "shaking palsy," and differing from the "intention tremor" of multiple sclerosis. The whole attitude is that of flexion. The head is flexed on the chest, the body is bowed, the arms and wrists are flexed, the knees are bent, and the forward-leaning posture enforces steps that are short and almost running, so that an advanced case of the disease can be diagnosed at a glance (Fig. 24–18).

In most cases, major changes are found in the nerve cells of the corpus striatum, consisting of the globus pallidus and substantia nigra in the midbrain. In the primary form, there is marked disappearance of the large, pale motor cells of the globus pallidus, whereas in the secondary form, the degenerative changes are in the substantia nigra, with loss of melanin in the pigmented cells and also of the neurohormonal transmitter dopamine, of which dopa is a precursor. The dopamine stores in the basal ganglia are depleted. There is a correspondingly low content of dopa in the urine. The essence of the condition seems to be an enzyme defect. A recent method of treatment is the daily intramuscular injection of dopa in the form of L-

dopa, a derivative. This has been extended by attempts to transplant adrenal tissue to the brain. This treatment results in a dramatic improvement in both the appearance and the behavior of the patient through reversal of the crippling effects of the disease. The disease used to be a rarity, but since around 1920 it has become much more common. This increased

Fig. 24–18   **Parkinsonism.** (Grinker's *Neurology*, Charles C Thomas.)

incidence may be because the viral agent of the encephalitis epidemic damaged the subthalamic cells, but not to a sufficient degree to produce clinical symptoms. The passage of the years or possibly some kind of delayed-fuse action brought the submerged disturbance to the surface. If this idea is correct, Parkinson's disease will, happily, soon become a rarity once more.

Alzheimer's Disease

The insidious loss of memory for recent events in someone about 50 years old with unpredictable or new changes in behavior suggest the diagnosis of presenile dementia, an entity which was first described in 1907. Disorders of thought, changes in mood, and other evidence of disturbances in mentation are characteristic of this disorder. The progression, from a few years up to a decade, to the loss of all perceptual, responsive, and motor ability is the usual outcome. Alzheimer's disease may occur late in life (at least the same pathological and clinical changes are found often in people over 80 years of age), but it is incorrect to assume it is characteristic of the aged since many nonagenarians are entirely lucid and mentally acute. Alzheimer's disease, characterized by diffuse cortical atrophy, can be identified with modern CAT scans or PET scans, and is confirmed histologically by the finding of neurofibrillary tangles, and the presence of neuritic plaques composed of a material called amyloid.

The significant lesion is the loss of cortical neurons and it is not clear whether this is programmed cell death (there are well-documented families with an autosomal dominant pattern of inheritance) or whether the deposition of the filamentous and amyloid material contributes to death of the neurons. One clue to the genesis of the disorder may be the finding that in Down's syndrome (Trisomy 21) individuals characteristically develop Alzheimer's lesions after 40 years of age.

There is no contemporary evidence to support the idea that Alzheimer's disease can be transmitted by any conventional agent of disease (virus, bacteria, protozoa).

It is essential that other causes of dementia be considered before making the diagnosis of Alzheimer's disease. In one instance known to me, an elderly physician was considered to have this disease, but a wise consultant discovered that the combination of sedative drugs (given for depression) and alcohol (taken privately) had caused the marked, rapid and debilitating change in his mentation and acuity.

TUMORS OF THE CENTRAL NERVOUS SYSTEM

We have already seen that the brain is composed of two types of cells, the nerve cells and the neuroglial cells. Tumors of the brain only arise from and are composed of neuroglial cells and therefore are called gliomas. Not uncommonly, a tumor grows from the meninges, which cover the brain, and is therefore called a meningioma (Fig. 24–19). There is a fundamental difference between these two types of tumor, for the meningioma is a benign tumor that is encapsulated and merely presses on the brain, whereas the glioma is a malignant tumor that infiltrates the brain and is not demarcated from it in any way. Table 24–2 lists the incidence of intracranial and intraspinal tumors in a given period.

Two points might be added to this brief summary. (1) It is evident that intracranial tumor may be intracerebral or extracerebral. The intracerebral tumors are the gliomas and metastatic carcinoma, as well as a few rarities that will not be mentioned. The extracerebral tumors are the meningiomas, tumors of the acoustic nerve, pituitary tumors, and craniopharyngiomas, which arise from the remnants of the epithelial tract from which the pituitary is formed. (2) The reason that intracerebral tumors are gliomas rather than nerve cell tumors is that glial cells, particularly astrocytes, are capable of unlimited mitotic division, whereas the adult nerve cells live on, but are usually incapable of multiplying. Cells that are not capable of division cannot give rise to tumors.

Fig. 24–19 This CT scan shows the presence of **2 meningiomas** impinging on the frontal lobes.

Table 24–2. Incidence of Intracranial and Intraspinal Tumors at Boston City Hospital, 1900 to 1930

Total no. of autopsies	10,592
Total no. of tumors	1,458
Tumors of other organs	1,270
Intracranial and intraspinal tumors	188 (12.7%)
Gliomas	81 (43.1%)
Pituitary adenomas	6 (3.2%)
Sheath tumors	22 (11.7%)
Meningioma	18
Acoustic neuroma	4
Metastatic tumors	29 (15.4%)
Blood vessel tumors	6 (3.0%)
Congenital tumors	8 (4.3%)
Granulomas	19 (10.1%)
Spinal cord tumors	4 (2.1%)
Unclassified	13 (7.1%)

From Wintrobe, M., et al.: *Harrison's Principles of Internal Medicine,* 7th Ed. New York, McGraw-Hill, 1974.

Fig. 24–20 This CT shows a large cystic space in the posterior cerebral hemisphere of the right side. Notice the slight displacement of the ventricular system. This is interpreted as **cerebral tumor**.

Although **gliomas** are malignant by virtue of their infiltrative power, they vary greatly in their degree of malignancy, and although some are rapidly growing and kill the patient in a few months, others grow slowly, and the patient may live for many years, especially if he receives skilful surgical treatment. Moreover, gliomas do not form metastases or secondary growths in other parts of the body as most malignant tumors do, probably because the tumor cells fail to escape from the interior of the skull.

There are many different kinds of glioma, but only four will be described. Of these four, two occur principally in the adult, namely, glioblastoma multiforme and astrocytoma; two occur in children, namely, medulloblastoma and ependymoma. The glioblastoma multiforme is a highly malignant tumor occurring in middle life and is usually found in one of the cerebral hemispheres (Fig. 24–20). Its margin is ill defined, so that the surgeon may have great difficulty in knowing where the tumor ends and the normal brain begins (Fig. 24–21). It is highly invasive and is likely to kill the patient in the course of a few months. The astrocytoma is much less malignant, and the average time of survival after operation is 6 years. It may occur in any part of the brain, but in children the common site is the cerebellum. The cerebellar tumor in children is usually completely benign. The medulloblastoma is a highly malignant and rapidly growing tumor in the roof of the fourth ventricle in the midline of the cerebellum (Fig. 24–22). The prognosis of this tumor of children is therefore the very opposite of that of astrocytoma. The ependymoma is the rarest of the four. It usually occurs in children and in the same location as the medulloblastoma. It is, however, much less malignant than that tumor.

A nearly always benign tumor arising from the meninges covering the brain, a **meningioma** is a common form of intracranial neoplasm. Although benign, it may obviously kill the patient in due time by virtue of its intracranial position and by the pressure it exerts on the brain, unless the tumor is removed. The meningioma is usually much firmer than the glioma, and it is adherent externally to the dura. As it presses on the brain from the outside, it forms a deep bed for itself, from which it can readily be lifted out. In the operating room, there is danger of severe or even fatal hemorrhage from large vessels that pass between the highly vascular overlying bone and the tumor. Local changes in the skull may be of great help in diagnosis. In about 25% of cases, there is bony thickening of the skull over the tumor that can be detected radiographically and sometimes even by physical examination.

Acoustic nerve tumor is another intracranial tumor that is much more closely related to meningioma than to the gliomas. It grows from the eighth cranial nerve at the angle between the pons and the cerebellum and forms a firm, round, well-encapsulated tumor. It presses on the nerve supplying the muscles of the face as well as on the acoustic or auditory nerve. The principal symptoms are therefore facial paralysis and deafness on one side. It is important to realize that the tumor is benign, so that, when removed surgi-

Fig. 24–21   **Glioblastoma multiforme**, showing massive infiltration of right and left frontal lobes. (University of Alabama Medical School.)

cally, there is no chance of its return. Peripheral nerve tumors also occur. One of the more common is a neurofibroma, illustrated in Figure A12–5.

One additional tumor worth mentioning is a congenital tumor, called a craniopharyngioma, that may remain clinically silent until middle or old age. Visual field loss at any age should suggest the presence of this growth, which is frequently calcified (98% in children) and is visible on x-rays (Fig. 24–23). Symptoms of increased intracranial pressure, headaches (86%),

and vomiting (74%), and such eye signs as papilledema, optic atrophy, and strabismus, all are classic findings. Surgical excision has become technically easier and carries the best chance of recovery for the patient.

When a diagnosis is made of tumor of the brain, the doctor has to bear in mind the possibility that the tumor may be a metastatic carcinoma (Fig. 24–24). In such cases, by far the most common tumor that metastasizes to the brain is bronchogenic carcinoma, constituting 30 to 40%; 15% come from cancer of the breast, kidney, and gastrointestinal tract (colon, rectum). The tumors are usually multiple rather than single, and on this account the clinical picture may be perplexing. To add to the confusion, the signs and symptoms may be entirely cerebral, with the primary tumor remaining silent. This situation is particularly likely in the case of bronchogenic carcinoma.

Clinical Pattern. The symptoms of a brain tumor may be divided into two groups, the first general and the second localizing. The general symptoms are due to the increased intracranial pressure produced by the mass of new tissue inside the skull and are more or less the same in whichever part of the brain the tumor is situated. The chief of these symptoms is headache, which may become excruciating in intensity. The cerebrospinal fluid pressure is greatly increased. Vomiting may be marked in the later stages, but is often absent. The pressure on the optic nerves produces

Fig. 24–22   This section through the fourth ventricle shows the cerebellum and whitish material that protrudes into the lumen of the ventricle. This is a **medulloblastoma.** (McGill University, Department of Pathology Museum.)

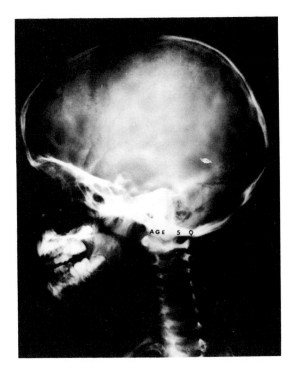

Fig. 24–23 This skull film shows the presence of calcification in and around the base of the skull. This is the classic sign of the presence of **craniopharyngioma**.

swelling of the termination of these nerves in the eye, a condition called optic neuritis, followed by optic atrophy, which can be recognized when the retina of the eye is viewed with the ophthalmoscope.

The localizing symptoms are naturally varied, because they depend on the site of the tumor in the brain. If the motor centers are involved, there will be weakness of the muscles of the face, arm, or leg. If the sensory centers are affected, there will be corresponding disturbance of sensation. Involvement of the special senses, such as sight or hearing, will point to the areas concerned with these functions (Fig. 24–25). It is for this reason that these symptoms are known as localizing, because, by a careful analysis of these disturbances, the physician is able to determine the exact location of the tumor, and the surgeon is then able to open the skull at the correct spot, where he will have access to the lesion. Modern radiologic techniques have greatly facilitated the localization of intracranial lesions.

The radiologist provides invaluable information in the diagnosis and localization of intracranial tumors. Gases that are radiolucent when introduced into the subarachnoid space, and thus into the cerebral ventricles, outline the ventricles and indicate the site of a tumor that may distort that outline. The use of radio-

paque oil in the spinal canal also localizes protruded intervertebral discs (Fig. 24–26), tumors, and obstructions to the free flow of fluids. This study is called myelography. Angiography, which consists of injecting a radiopaque solution into the cerebrospinal fluid, used to be used frequently. By this means, the outline of the tumor may be indicated even in those lesions that do not distort the ventricles. The procedure is of special importance in the case of intracranial aneurysms and other vascular anomalies (Table 24–3). However, these methods have now largely been supplanted by the use of computerized tomography, PET scans and nuclear magnetic resonance. These vastly expensive tools have revolutionized diagnosis of CNS lesions.

If the reader would like to get a vivid idea of what it is like to be a patient with a brain tumor, he should read *A Journey Round My Skull*, by the distinguished Hungarian novelist, Frigyes Karinthy, who himself was the patient. The rather terrifying description of the operation under a local anesthetic is perhaps somewhat highly colored.

Fig. 24–24 This section through the cerebral hemispheres shows a round discolored nodule that has caused a shift of the midline structures from the left to the right and an increase in the size of the left cerebral hemisphere. This space-occupying lesion is typical of a **metastatic tumor to the brain**. Such metastases commonly come from lung, breast, or kidney carcinomas. (McGill University, Department of Pathology Museum.)

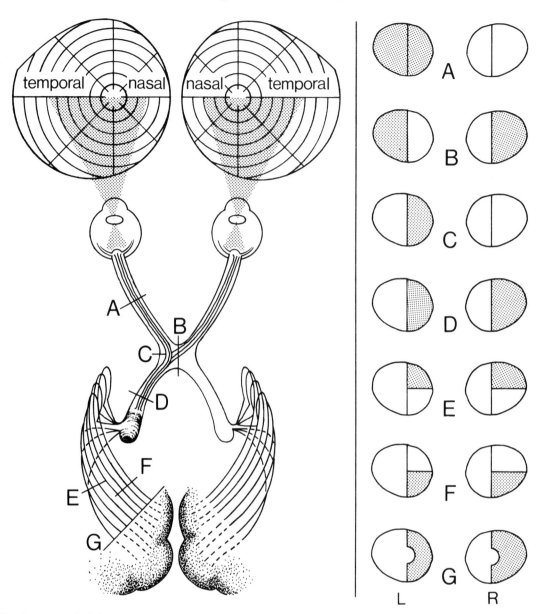

Fig. 24–25 The drawing on the left illustrates the **radiation of the visual fields** through the optic nerves at the decussation to the posterior lobes of the cerebral hemispheres. Lesions A, B, C, D, E, F, and G cause the abnormalities of vision shown on the right. Lesion A, for example, shows complete blindness in the left eye. (From Thorn, G.W., et al. (Eds.): *Harrison's Principles of Internal Medicine*, 8th Ed. New York, McGraw-Hill, 1977.)

The treatment of brain tumors is discouraging, but by no means hopeless. If the tumor can be located, much or all of it may be removed. In the case of meningioma, a complete cure may be expected. With the gliomas, it is much more difficult for the surgeon to know whether he has removed all the tumor, so that there is great danger that some of it may be left behind and that the growth will recur. But even if a cure cannot be assured, several years of comfort and comparative health may be added to the patient's life. Perhaps the most important advice for the patient with a brain tumor is to choose the right surgeon.

INCREASED INTRACRANIAL PRESSURE

Regardless of the cause, which ranges from the presence of hematoma, abscess, tumor in the closed box of the skull, to the effects of poisons such as lead or barbiturates, or metabolites, as in hepatic coma, to the serious problem of anoxia, the swelling of the brain may lead quickly to irreversible damage or death by compression of venous return, or by herniation and ischemic necrosis of the brain stem.

Headache, visual disturbances, slowing of the heart rate, and progressive loss of consciousness all suggest

Fig. 24–26   These **myelograms** show the presence in the radiopaque dye of a deformity, caused by a protruded disc, seen in both the anteroposterior (A) and lateral (B) views.

that there is increasing intracranial pressure. One great dilemma in these cases is whether to establish the diagnosis by direct measurement of the cerebrospinal fluid pressure with the cerebrospinal tap (thereby running the risk of precipitating herniation of the brain) or to use the physical signs such as papilledema or protrusion of the optic nerve and to institute therapy directed towards reducing the swelling. Such therapy will include the use of mannitol, anti-

inflammatory agents such as cortisone, hypothermia, and decompressive surgical procedures.

CEREBROSPINAL FLUID IN DISEASE

The normal spinal fluid is as clear as water, contains sugar and chlorides, no proteins, less than 5 lymphocytes per cubic millimeter, and no polymorphonuclear leukocytes. In acute meningitis (see Table

Table 24–3. Neurologic Imaging Techniques

PROCEDURE	IMAGE OF BRAIN THAT RESULTS
Neurologic consult	Imaginary construct of possible pathology
EEG	Surface electrical activity below 80 Hz
Skull films	Distribution of crystallized calcium in head
Ultrasound	Position of third ventricle
Isotope scan	Distribution of blood-brain barrier
Pneumoencephalogram	Locaton of CSF compartment
Cerebral angiogram	Location of blood compartment
Computerized tomogram	Distribution of tissue radio-density

(From Oldendorf, W.H.: The quest for an image of brain: A brief historical and technical review of brain imaging techniques. Neurology, 28:517, 1978.)

A24–1), the vessels in the inflamed meninges allow the constituents of the blood to pour into the fluid, so that it contains much protein and great numbers of polymorphonuclear leukocytes. The fluid is therefore purulent and turbid. The bacteria feed on and use up the glucose, so that it is reduced in amount. Bacteria are found in smears of the pus and in culture. Tuberculous meningitis, which is much less acute, gives a different pattern in the spinal fluid. The fluid is clear or only slightly milky, as it usually contains less than 100 cells per cubic millimeter, most of which are lymphocytes. The CSF protein is only moderately increased, and the glucose is diminished. The most characteristic findings are a marked diminution in the chloride level and the presence of tubercle bacilli in the smears.

In suspected brain tumor, the spinal fluid may be examined for tumor cells. These are much more likely to be found in secondary carcinoma than in glioma, although in the latter condition there may be a marked increase in the lymphocyte count. The use of the millepore membrane filter gives better results than the conventional sedimentation methods. In spinal cord tumors, which resemble intracranial tumors and are not considered here, the spinal fluid may show the "compression syndrome" if the canal is blocked. Below the obstruction, the characters of the fluid are as follows: (1) massive spontaneous coagulation, (2) xanthochromia or yellow coloration of the fluid, (3) marked increase in the protein, (4) no corresponding increase in the cells. The exact site of a spinal cord tumor may sometimes be determined by the intraspinal injection of Lipiodol followed by radiography (Fig. 24–26). It is evident that lumbar puncture can be of value in the diagnosis of suspected spinal cord tumors and is of particular value in establishing the presence of infection in the CNS.

SYNOPSIS

In considering diseases of the central nervous system we include: the skull, the meninges, the blood supply, the ventricular system, as well as the anatomic subdivisions of the cerebrum, cerebellum, and brain stem.

Obstructions to circulation of the cerebrospinal fluid may be due to congenital, inflammatory, or neoplastic disease.

Cerebrovascular disease may be due to rupture and hemorrhage of branches of the arterial tree or to thrombosis and occlusion of the arterial or venous system. Embolization may also cause infarction, but much less frequently.

Hemorrhage inside the skull most commonly results from trauma, hypertension, or rupture of an aneurysm. It may be localized to the extradural, subdural, or subarachnoid space, or it may occur within the substance of the brain or in the ventricular system.

Infections of the central nervous system are most commonly caused by pyogenic bacteria, tuberculosis, syphilis, or viruses. They may be localized (abscesses) or generalized (meningitis, encephalitis).

Demyelinating diseases (e.g., multiple sclerosis) are of unknown etiology, but recent evidence points towards "slow viruses" as an etiologic factor.

Tumors of the central nervous system are most commonly metastatic from the lung or other organs. Primary tumors arise from glial cells or from the meninges.

Terms

Hydrocephalus	*Subarachnoid hemorrhage*	*Demyelinating disease*
Hemiplegia	*Intracerebral hemorrhage*	*Gliomas*
Extradural hemorrhage	*Meningitis*	*Meningioma*
Subdural hemorrhage	*Encephalitis*	

FURTHER READING

Aldrich, M.S.: Current concepts: Narcolepsy. N. Engl. J. Med., 323:389, 1990.

Ban, T.A., and Lehmann, H.E.: Myths, theories and treatment of schizophrenia. Dis. Nervous System, p. 665, September 1977.

Black, P.M.: Medical progress: Brain tumors (first of two parts). N. Engl. J. Med., 324:1471, 1991.

Black, P.M.: Medical progress: Brain tumors (second of two parts). N. Engl. J. Med., 324:1555, 1991.

Blackwood, W., and Corsellis, J.A.N. (Eds.): *Greenfield's Neuropathology*, 3rd Ed. London, Edward Arnold, 1976.

Bradley, W.G.: A new hypothesis of the etiology of amyotrophic lateral sclerosis. The DNA hypothesis. Arch. Neurol., 39:677, 1982.

Bredt, D.S., and Snyder, S.H.: Nitric oxide, a novel neuronal messenger. Neuron, 8:3, 1992.

Brody, J.A.: An epidemiologist views senile dementia—facts and fragments. Am. J. Epidemiol., 115:155, 1982.

Brown, P., et al.: Diagnosis of Creutzfeldt-Jakob disease by western blot identification of marker protein in human brain tissue. N. Engl. J. Med., 314:547, 1986.

Brown, P., Cathala, F., et al. The epidemiology of Creutzfeld-Jakob disease: Conclusion of a 15 year investigation in France and review of the world literature. Neurol. 37:895, 1987.

Carpenter, W.T., et al.: The therapeutic efficacy of hemodialysis in schizophrenia. N. Engl. J. Med., 308:669, 1983.

Chan, B.S.H., and Dorsch, N.W.C.: Delayed diagnosis in subarachnoid haemorrhage. Med. J. Australia, 154:509, 1991.

Christie, D.: Prevalence of stroke and its sequelae. Med. J. Aust., 2:182, 1981.

Clausen, N., Garwics, S., Glomstein, A., et al.: Medulloblastoma in Nordic children. I. Acta Pediatr. Scand. Suppl. 371:5, 1990.

Collee, J.G.: Bovine spongiform encephalopathy. Lancet, November 24, 1990, pp. 1300–1303.

Constantinides, P.: Pathogenesis of cerebral artery thrombosis. Arch. Pathol., 83:422, 1967.

Dohrman, P.J., and Elrick, W.L.: Observations on brain abscess. Review of 28 cases. Med. J. Aust., 2:81, 1982.

Dorsch, N.W.C.: Subarachnoid haemorrhage. Med. J. Australia, 154:505, 1991.

Eaton, W.W.: Update on the epidemiology of schizophrenia. Epidemiol. Rev., 13:320, 1991.

Edelman, G.M., and Mountcastle, V.B.: *The Mindful Brain: Cortical Organization and the Group-Selective Theory of Higher Brain Function*. Cambridge, M.I.T. Press, 1978.

Finkbeiner, A.: A new role for gases: neurotransmission. Science, 252:1788, 1991.

Gajdusek, D.C.: Slow infections with unconventional viruses. Harvey Lect., 72, 1978.

Glenner, G.G. On primal causes in Alzheimer's disease. Neurobiol. Aging 7:506, 1986.

Guillemin, R.: New endocrinology of the brain. Perspect. Biol. Med., 22:S74, 1979.

Hebb, D.O. Consider mind as a biological problem. Neuroscience, 6:2419, 1981.

Hubel, D.H.: Evolution of ideas on the primary visual cortex, 1955–1978: a biased historical account. Bioscience Rep., 2:453, 1982.

Jaeckle, K.A.: Neuroimaging for central nervous system tumors. Sem. Oncology, 18:150, 1991.

Jennett, H.B., and Plum, F.: Persistent vegetative state after brain damage. Lancet, 1:734, 1972.

Katzman, R.: Alzheimer's disease. N. Engl. J. Med., 314:964, 1986.

Kety, S.S.: The biological roots of mental illness: their ramifications through cerebral metabolism, synaptic activity, genetics, and the environment. Harvey Lect., 71, 1978.

Kurtzke, J.F., and Hyllested, K.: Multiple sclerosis in the Faroe Islands: I. Clinical and epidemiological features. Ann. Neurol., 5:6, 1979.

Logigian, E.L., Kaplan, R.F., and Steere, A.C.: Chronic neurologic manifestations of Lyme disease. N. Engl. J. Med., 323:1438, 1990.

Martin, J.B.: Genetic linkage in neurologic diseases. N. Engl. J. Med., 316:1018, 1987.

Maugh, T.H.: Multiple sclerosis: two or more viruses may be involved. Science, 195:768, 1977.

Mazziotta, J.C., et al.: Reduced cerebral glucose metabolism in asymptomatic subjects at risk for Huntington's disease. N. Engl. J. Med., 316:357, 1987.

Munsat, T.L.: Poliomyelitis—new problems with an old disease. N. Engl. J. Med., 324:1206, 1991.

Murrell, T.G.C., Harbige, L.S., and Robinson, I.C.: A review of the aetiology of multiple sclerosis: an ecological approach. Ann. Hum. Biol., 18:95, 1991.

Musher, D.M.: Syphilis, neurosyphilis, penicillin, and AIDS. J. Infect. Dis., 163:1201, 1991.

Nelson, K.B., and Ellenberg, J.H.: Antecedents of cerebral palsy: multivariate analysis of risk. N. Engl. J. Med., 315:81, 1986.

Olson, G.A., Olseon, R.D., and Kastin, A.J.: Endogenous opiates: 1989. In: *Peptides*, Vol 11, Pergamon Press, 1990, p. 1277.

Perlow, M.J. Brain grafting as a treatment for Parkinson's disease. Neuros. 20:335, 1987.

Petersen, P., and Boysen, G.: Ischaemic stroke—prevention and treatment. J. Int. Med., 231:103, 1992.

Porter, R.: Exploring brain functional anatomy with positron tomography—introduction. In: *Exploring Brain Functional Anatomy with Positron Tomography,* Edited by D.J. Chadwick, J. Whelan. Chichester, John Wiley & Sons Ltd., 1991.

Poser, C.M.: Mulitple sclerosis—observations and reflections—a personal memoir. J. Neurol. Sci., 107:127, 1992.

Potter, H.: Review and hypothesis: Alzheimer disease and Down syndrome—chromosome 21. Nondisjunction may underlie both disorders. Am. J. Hum. Genet., 48:1192, 1991.

Prusiner, S.B.: Novel structure and genetics of prions causing neurodegeneration in humans and animals. Biologicals, 18:247, 1990.

Riise, T., Grønning M., Klauber, M.R., et al.: Clustering of residence of multiple sclerosis patients at age 13 to 20 years in Hordaland, Norway. Am. J. Epidemiol., 133:932, 1991.

Sabin, T.D.: The differential diagnosis of coma. N. Engl. J. Med., 290:1062, 1974.

Sacco, R.L., et al.: One-year outcome after cerebral infarction in whites, blacks, and hispanics. Stroke, 22:305, 1991.

Schoenberg, B.S. Epidemiology of Alzheimer's disease and other dementing illnesses. J. Chron. Dis. 39:1095, 1986.

Selkoe, D.J.: The molecular pathology of Alzheimer's disease. Neuron, 6:487, 1991.

Seligman, S.J.: The rapid differential diagnosis of meningitis. Med. Clin. North Am., 57:1417, 1973.

Snyder, S.H.: Opiate receptors in the brain. N. Engl. J. Med., 296:266, 1977.

Terry, R.D.: Dementia: a brief and selective review. Arch. Neurol., 33:1, 1976.

Vonarbin, M., Britton, M., and Defaire, U.: Mortality and recurrences during eight years following stroke. J. Int. Med., 23:43, 1992.

Welch, K.M.A., Levine, S.R., and Ewing, J.R. Viewing stroke pathophysiology—an analysis of contemporary methods. Stroke 17:1071, 1986.

Whitley, R.J.: Medical progress: viral encephalitis. N. Engl. J. Med., 323:242, 1990.

APPENDIX

Structure and Function of the Central Nervous System

The central nervous system altogether can best be considered as including: the skull and overlying skin, which are often subject to trauma; the coverings of the brain (the meninges), which are often involved by inflammation or hem-

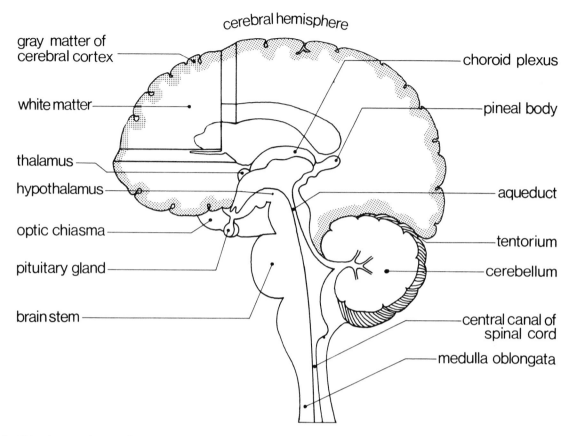

Fig. A24–1   This schematic drawing illustrates the **anatomic relationships** of the various parts of the central nervous system. The cerebral hemisphere is partly removed to show gray and white matter; the adjacent ventricular space is shown. The cerebellum and brain stem and pituitary gland are all shown in proportional sizes. (Redrawn and adapted from Ham, A.W.: *Histology*, 7th Ed. Philadelphia, J. B. Lippincott Co., 1974.)

orrhage; the blood supply to the brain (the arterial supply and venous drainage); the cerebrospinal fluid, which may be likened to the lymphatic circulation in the rest of the body; and the gray and white matter of the brain proper. Some disease processes are reflected particularly in one or another of these compartments, and it is wise to realize that each of these anatomic areas is subject to particular or peculiar diseases.

The brain proper consists of the cerebrum (right and left cerebral hemispheres), the brain stem, which connects the cerebrum with the spinal cord, and the cerebellum or little brain (Fig. A24–1). The cerebrum initiates motor impulses that pass to the muscles, receives sensory impulses from the periphery, and is the seat of thought and reason. The brain stem is composed of the midbrain, the pons, and the medulla, which is continued into the spinal cord. Through the brain stem pass the innumerable motor and sensory nerves; it also houses the groups of nerve cells from which arise the cranial nerves that pass to the eye, ear, face, and mouth. The cerebellum is concerned principally with coordination and with equilibrium, so that cerebellar disease is marked by incoordination and loss of equilibrium (ataxia).

The spinal cord is traversed by all the nerves going to and coming from the body. Those passing to the arm leave the cord in the upper or cervical region; those passing to the leg leave in the lower or lumbar region. The motor fibers from the brain terminate around nerve cells in the gray matter, which occupies the center of the cord, and from these motor cells a second set of fibers carries the motor messages to the muscles. The upper relay is called the upper motor neuron and is often injured in cerebral hemorrhage; the lower relay is called the lower motor neuron and is injured in poliomyelitis. Complete paralysis may be produced by destruction of either neuron, and by injury to the nerve cell or the nerve fiber that arises from it.

The central nervous system is composed of neurons and neuroglia (Figs. A24–2 and A24–3). **Neurons** are nerve cells, and nerve fibers that arise from them, which pass, sometimes for a long distance, through the brain and spinal cord (Fig. A24–4). The motor nerve fibers (efferent) arise from nerve cells in the gray matter of the spinal cord and leave the cord by the anterior nerve roots to become the peripheral motor nerves. These nerve cells and their fibers are called lower motor neurons; they receive and respond to impulses coming from upper motor neurons (the motor cells in the brain and their descending fibers). Sensory impulses of various kinds are carried by the sensory nerve fibers (afferent), which enter the cord in the posterior nerve roots and pass up to appropriate centers in the brain. Here messages, on reaching our consciousness, give information concerning the outside world.

Nerve cells, of which there are some 10,000,000,000, have certain peculiarities that distinguish them from all other cells. Two of their most striking characteristics are their lon-

Outer molecular layer

Granular layer

Purkinje cells

Molecular layer

White matter

White matter

A

B

Fig. A24–2 *A* and *B*, The **histologic section** shows an area of the cerebellum prepared with two different stains. Neurons of the cerebellum are called Purkinje cells. (Courtesy of P. Bailey.)

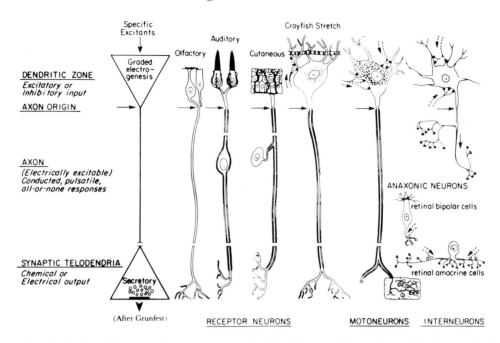

Fig. A24–3 The traditional selection of the mammalian motoneuron as the **"typical neuron"** has led to a misleading emphasis on the cell body as the focal point for analysis of neuron structure in functional terms—it being commonly assumed that dendrites must conduct toward and axons away from the cell body. The diagram presented here illustrates several variations in the position of the cell body in a number of receptor and effector neurons. A more important consideration in terms of function is the site of origin of the impulse. The location of the perikaryon in the neuron is not critical for the electrochemical functions of response generation, conduction, and synaptic transmission. The neuroplasm in the interior of the perikaryon is concerned primarily with the outgrowth and maintenance of the axon and dendrites and with metabolic functions other than membrane activity. (After D. Bodian.) (From Bloom, W., and Fawcett, D.W.: *A Textbook of Histology,* 10th Ed. Philadelphia, W. B. Saunders Co., 1975.)

gevity and their great susceptibility to metabolic disturbances, most particularly susceptibility to loss of oxygen or glucose. Nerve cells can live 100 years (compare this with the short life of the polymorph), but they pay a heavy price for their relative immortality, because they cannot be replaced when they are destroyed. They have great metabolic activity, but on that account they require a constant, large supply of oxygen and glucose, so that the cells of the cerebral cortex cannot survive 10 minutes of anoxia at normal body temperature. A marked fall in blood sugar level also results in loss of consciousness.

Nerve fibers in the central nervous system consist of two elements: the axon, which conducts the nervous impulses, and the myelin sheath, which surrounds it (Fig. A24–5). In the peripheral nerves a nucleated sheath, the neurilemma, is added. The myelin sheath is made of many layers of insulation created by a special cell (Schwann's cell), which wraps itself around the axon. When a peripheral nerve is cut, the myelin breaks up into fine droplets, which eventually disappear as the material is phagocytosed (Fig. A24–6). This process is called demyelination and it is of particular significance in the central nervous system, where it constitutes the principal feature of a group of so-called demyelinating diseases, of which multiple sclerosis is of special importance. When injury of this kind takes place, there is a response in the cell body of the neuron. This response can be seen with the light microscope and appears as a change in

staining quality of the cytoplasm. The nucleus of this neuron may also be shifted to one side. This shift is called chromatolysis and is shown in Figure A24–7.

The nerve cells that send out motor impulses along nerve fibers and those that receive sensory impulses along corresponding fibers are situated in the gray matter of the brain, which is spread for the most part as a thin layer over the surface, to form the cerebral cortex. These cells are collected in groups known as centers or nuclei. The various centers are linked by bundles of fibers known as association fibers. In the performance of an action, many centers are associated, and when this is repeated many times, the nervous impulse appears to flow along the corresponding association paths with increasing ease. Some such mechanism may form the physical basis of habit. Every act, indeed every thought, serves to make these paths more open and easily traversed. Every smallest stroke of virtue or of vice leaves its little scar. Nothing we ever do, in strict scientific literalness, is wiped out, but the tracks that are left are invisible to our current technology.

The interstitial tissue of the central nervous system has long been known as the **neuroglia.** Glia means glue in Greek, and the neuroglia was regarded as a kind of putty that served the humble purpose of holding together the more noble neurons. With ordinary stains, the interstitial elements appear for the most part as naked nuclei, but with gold and silver impregnation, the cells are seen to be provided with a forest of fibers. By the aid of these methods, it is possible to distinguish 3 types of cells in the interstitial tissue: (1) astroglia, (2) oligodendroglia, and (3) microglia.

The astrocytes, the cells of the astroglia, have peculiar processes called sucker feet, which are attached to the capillaries. For this reason, the astroglia is believed to be involved in the transport of water and electrolytes between the capillaries and the nerve cells. The repair of wounds in the brain is due entirely to the activity of the astrocytes, and the gliosis seen in general paresis and other chronic inflammations of the brain consists of astrocytes and their fibers. Finally, it is from the astroglia that the glioma, the common brain tumor, takes its origin. The oligodendroglia is the largest group of the interstitial cells, but their function is still unknown, perhaps to the relief of the reader. The cells are smaller than the astrocytes, and they possess a

Terminal branches of dendrite near surface of brain

Ascending dendrite

A

Collateral branches of axon

Axon

White substance

Fig. A24–4   The ramifications of a **neuron's axon and dendrites** are shown in this figure from a drawing done by the great Spanish neurocytologist, Cajal. (From Bloom, W., and Fawcett, D.W.: *A Textbook of Histology,* 10th Ed. Philadelphia, W. B. Saunders Co., 1975.)

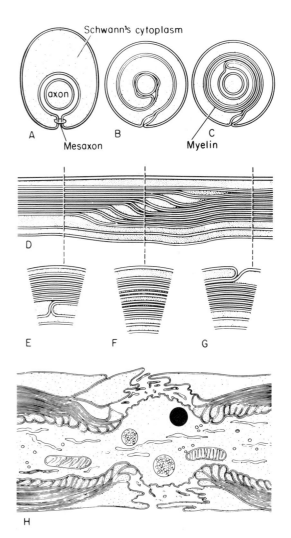

Fig. A24–5   This drawing shows the relationship between the **axon of the nerve and the Schwann's cell cytoplasm**, which is wrapped about the axon and which constitutes myelin. (From Bloom, W., and Fawcett, D.W.: *A Textbook of Histology,* 9th Ed. Philadelphia, W. B. Saunders Co., 1968.)

Fig. A24–6 This electron microphotograph shows the response of the myelin sheath to injury. This change is called **Wallerian degeneration**. The myelin sheath (my) which surrounds the nerve axon (ax) is the product of Schwann cell processes (S.p.), which have been wrapped around the axon as insulation. The outermost limit is the basement membrane (b.m.). After injury these lamellae of myelin break up into micelles of lipoprotein, as shown in the lower illustration. (From Thomas, P.K., and Sheldon, H.: Changes in the Fine Structures of Myelin During Wallerian Degeneration of Peripheral Nerve. J. Cell Biol., 22:715, 1964.)

small number of processes (Greek *oligos*, few). The microglial cells are tiny (hence the name) and are provided with numerous fine branching processes. These cells are the phagocytes or scavengers of the central nervous system, and, when called on to perform this function, they become greatly swollen, their processes are withdrawn into the cell, and the cytoplasm is filled with droplets of disintegrating myelin, which they carry away and discharge into the nearest vessel.

The normal physiology of the brain may be altered by disease that affects principally the motor or sensory functions, or that affects intellect and behavior, or some combination of these. It is customary to speak of (1) "organic" disorders in which gross or microscopic lesions can be demonstrated, associated with interference with the supply of oxygen or carbohydrate to the brain or with abnormalities of cerebral enzyme activity, and of (2) "functional" disorders in which no such changes can be shown. It is becoming more and more probable that this distinction is due to inadequacy in our techniques for studying the brain. What in the past we have called mental disease and have stigmatized as insanity or madness is probably in most cases a biochemical disturbance of nerve cells that will be corrected in the future by pharmacologic means. Most of the popular tranquilizers act on the biochemical interactions between nerve cells.

Memory is the ability to receive a sensory impression, to retain it, and to recall it at the appropriate moment. Learn-ing and memory are intertwined, and both may be lost because of disease and age.

We can now pass on to some other considerations.

The brain and spinal cord are enclosed in two bony cases that are continuous with each other, namely, the skull and the spinal column. They are therefore unable to expand when they become swollen with blood or as the result of inflammation, and the increased tension causes headache, that most common symptom. There is an ingenious mechanism that serves to take up some of the temporary increases of pressure that may occur inside the skull. The mechanism is the **cerebrospinal fluid,** which bathes the brain and in which the organ is suspended as in a water bath. This fluid not only covers the brain, but also passes down the spinal canal outside the spinal cord. There is far more spare space in the canal than in the cranial cavity, so that when the brain becomes swollen, the fluid flows out into the spinal canal, providing a much-needed safety valve. Cerebrospinal fluid is produced in a series of cavities in the interior of the brain known as the cerebral ventricles (Fig. A24–8).

From one of these (the fourth ventricle) it escapes by tiny openings in the roof of the ventricle to reach the exterior of the brain, the subarachnoid space, through the walls of which it is absorbed into the blood stream. The subarachnoid space with its contained fluid passes down outside the spinal cord to the third portion of the sacrum, whereas the cord ends at the level of the first lumbar vertebra; in its

Fig. A24–7 **Normal neurons** in the upper drawing are to be compared with the lower drawing of neurons that show large pale areas rather than the stippled blue material known as the Nissl substance in the cytoplasm. This accumulation of eosinophilic material and shift of the nucleus to one side is called **chromatolysis** and is a morphologic sign of injury. (From Bloom, W. and Fawcett, D.W.: *A Textbook of Histology*, 10th Ed. Philadelphia, W. B. Saunders Co., 1975.)

lowest portion, the sac contains only fluid. That is the site used to obtain samples of this fluid for study (lumbar puncture). There is a constant flow out of the ventricles into the subarachnoid space. Should the openings in the roof of the fourth ventricle become blocked, the fluid accumulates and distends the ventricles, pressing the brain against the skull

with serious results, a condition called hydrocephalus (Figs. A24–9 and A24–10).

The spinal fluid can be withdrawn by the simple procedure of lumbar puncture; a hollow needle is passed into the spinal canal between two contiguous vertebrae in the lumbar region, below the point where the spinal cord ends,

Table A24–1.   Examination of Cerebrospinal Fluid

TESTS	NORMAL	BACTERIAL MENINGITIS	TUBERCULOUS MENINGITIS	VIRAL MENINGITIS	NEOPLASTIC MENINGITIS	PRIMARY CEREBRAL NEOPLASM
Microscopic examination	No cells	Many polymorphonuclear leukocytes early in course	Moderate increase in lymphocytes	Moderate increase in lymphocytes	Increased mononuclear leukocytes	Normal, or a few extra lymphocytes
Smear	No bacteria	Often bacteria are seen on Gram stain	With prolonged search, acid-fast bacilli are often found	Negative	Malignant cells may be seen on cytology examination	Negative
Protein	15 to 45 mg/100 ml	Very high	Very high, may form "pellicle"	Elevated, usually not very high	Similar to tuberculosis	Normal or slightly high (very high with acoustic neuroma)
Glucose	About 20 mg less than blood	Very low	Moderately low	Normal or increased	Usually low	Normal
Chloride	120 mEq/L	Low	Very low	Normal	A little reduced	Normal

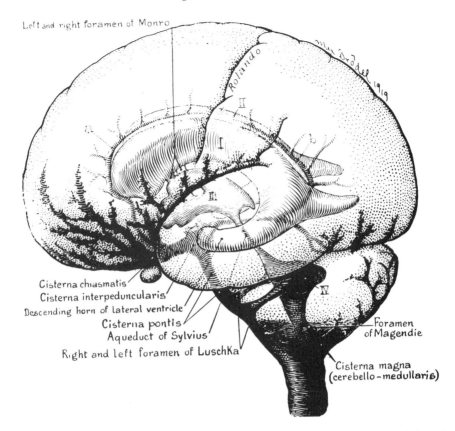

Fig. A24–8 In this schematic the relationship of the **ventricular system** to the central nervous system is shown in darker ink. This ventricular system receives fluid that is elaborated and circulated slowly from the different chambers and liberated onto the surface of the brain. The cerebrospinal fluid acts as a hydraulic cushion and also provides a second circulation similar to the lymphatic system.

Fig. A24–9 This photograph shows a young child with **hydrocephalus** at the turn of the century. The increased girth of the skull is due to the increased accumulation of fluid within the ventricular system. Frequently, this is due to a blockage in the cerebrospinal fluid circulation, which does not absorb the fluid that is secreted and leads to the thinning and atrophy of the substance of the brain. (The Evans Collection, Osler Library, McGill University.)

Fig. A24–10 This CT scan shows a remarkable increase in the size of the cerebral ventricles. This increase is typical of **hydrocephalus**.

and the fluid that escapes is collected. This procedure is a valuable means of diagnosis in diseases of the nervous system, for the fluid is a mirror in which are reflected many of the changes that may be affecting the brain and spinal cord (Table A24–1).

One structure still remains to be described, that is the membrane or rather membranes that cover the brain and cord, just as the pleura covers the lungs and the peritoneum the abdominal organs. These membranes are known as the meninges, of which there are 3, the dura mater, and arachnoid mater, and the pia mater. The dura is a tough membrane that lies in the cranial cavity and the spinal canal. The pia clothes the brain and cord like a glove, and the arachnoid like a mitt over the glove; there is, therefore, a space between these membranes, and that space, known as the subarachnoid space, is occupied by the cerebrospinal fluid.

It may be of interest to know that dura mater is derived from the Latin *durus*, hard, and *mater*, mother, while *pia* means soft. To the ancients the meninges were the "mother" membranes. Hence Shakespeare's phrase, "nourished in the womb of pia mater." The ancients were not aware of the existence of the arachnoid, which means spider-like.

25

MUSCULOSKELETAL SYSTEM

Parents are the bones on which children sharpen their teeth.—USTINOV

All our activities, except for the single act of thinking, depend on the integrity and interaction of elements of the locomotor system—muscles, bones, and joints—which have raised us from the primordial slime. This chapter is concerned with the structure, function, and common disorders of each of these elements.

BONE AND CARTILAGE

Normal Structure and Function

A bone is not a dead thing. It is true that it is impregnated with minerals, which gives it its rigidity, but the bone itself is just as much alive as the heart or the brain. It consists of cells surrounded by a modified fibrous tissue saturated with salts of calcium phosphate, in which there are spaces or interstices, which are particularly numerous at the ends of the bone. In the center of the shaft of the bone there is the medullary cavity, filled with bone marrow, which manufactures red blood cells and leukocytes (Fig. 25–1). This cavity is active in the long bones of young, growing people, but becomes replaced by fat after the age of 20. Lining the medullary cavity and interstices are cells called osteoblasts, whose function is to form new bone. In normal bone, there are also larger cells, giant cells, which contain several nuclei and are called osteoclasts. They are concerned with removal, instead of formation, of bone. There is evidence to support the idea that the osteoblasts are converted to osteoclasts under the stimulus of parathyroid hormone, as if these cells were the custodians of a bank of calcium and phosphate where they can function either as depositors or as withdrawers. There is also contradictory evidence that osteoclasts arise from monocytes.

During childhood and adolescence, bones grow in length. This they do entirely by virtue of a layer of cartilage at each end of the bone known as the epiphyseal apparatus (Fig. 25–2). When a child grows up, this cartilage becomes calcified and converted into bone, after which no more growth is possible. Bone responds to growth hormone secreted by the anterior pituitary. When this gland becomes overactive in early life as a result of a pituitary tumor, the growth of the epiphyseal cartilage is speeded up and the person becomes a giant. Gigantism is not possible once the cartilage has become converted into bone. Conversely, if the pituitary is insufficiently active, growth ceases and the individual remains a dwarf. However, whereas there is only one cause of gigantism, there are many causes of dwarfism (Fig. 25–3). Indeed the study of dwarfism is extensive; to discuss it here is out of place.

A bone must grow in thickness as well as in length. Increase in thickness is brought about by the periosteum (Fig. 25–4), a fibrous membrane that closely covers the bone and contains osteoblasts on its deep surface. It is through the periosteum that the superficial part of the bone receives its blood supply, so that anything that injures or removes the periosteum threatens the health and even the life of the bone.

We have said that epiphyseal cartilage is at the end of the bone, but this is not strictly true. It is separated from the actual end of the bone, i.e., the joint surface, by a small piece of bone known as the epiphysis. The epiphyseal cartilage therefore intervenes between the shaft of the bone and the epiphysis. Many of the most important diseases of bone (inflammation, tuberculosis, sarcoma) begin in this region of the bone on one or the other side of the epiphyseal cartilage.

Calcium is stored principally in bones, which contain 99% of the total body calcium as well as 90% of the phosphorus which is combined with calcium. In bone, the calcium phosphate crystals are deposited within the collagen fibril. One unanswered question is why bone collagen calcifies and other collagens normally do not.

The small amount of calcium that is not in the bones plays a vital role in most physiologic functions, for it affects enzyme activity, cell membrane permeability, cardiac rhythm, and neuromuscular excitability. A fall in the level of serum calcium may produce tetanic contractions and death. Serum calcium and phosphorus maintain a delicate inverse equilibrium with each other: when one goes up, the other goes down. A minor change in serum calcium results in a major

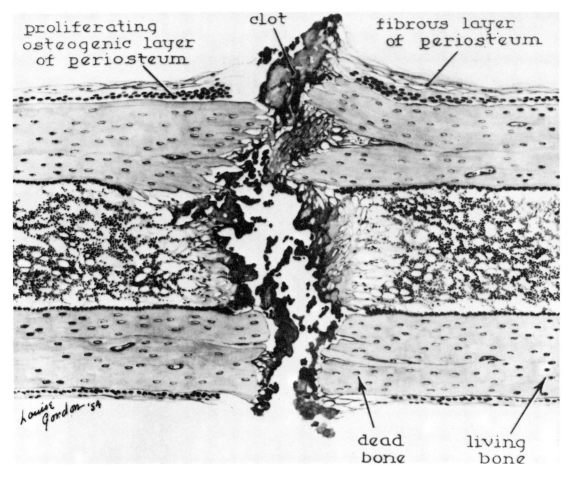

proliferating
osteogenic layer
of periosteum

clot

fibrous layer
of periosteum

dead
bone

living
bone

Louise Gordon '54

Fig. 25–1   This drawing shows a **fractured bone.** In the center of the bone is the marrow cavity. The drawing illustrates the relative proportions of the periosteum, living bone, marrow cavity, and hemorrhage in the area of fracture. (From Ham, A.W., and Harris, W.R.: In *Bourne's Biochemistry and Physiology of Bone.* New York, Academic Press.)

disturbance of health, but a change in phosphorus causes only a slight disturbance in metabolism.

The metabolism of calcium and phosphorus in relation to bone must be considered as a whole. When we speak of calcification, we mean of course the deposition of calcium phosphate and not merely calcium. Calcium and phosphorus metabolism is influenced by many different factors, such as parathormone (the hormone of the parathyroid glands); vitamin D (which controls absorption of calcium from the small intestine and absorption and excretion by the kidneys); and such hormones as estrogens, androgens, adrenal corticoids, thyroxin, and those of the anterior pituitary. When the complexity of the entire mechanism is considered, it becomes a matter of surprise that anyone has normal bones.

Osteoblasts, when multiplying rapidly, produce the enzyme alkaline phosphatase, which hydrolyses organic phosphate compounds, altering the local calcium-phosphate balance and resulting in the precipitation of calcium salts in the soft tissues. The phosphatase level of the serum may be raised either in excessive bone formation or in bone destruction, for in both of these phenomena, increased osteoblastic activity comes into play.

Metabolic Bone Disease

As with other systems, there are a variety of pathologic processes that may affect the tissue in question. Because bone is composed of three basic elements—the cells (osteocytes, osteoblasts, and osteoclasts), their product, the protein matrix (collagen), and the inorganic salts (hydroxyapatite), which impregnate the collagen—we can imagine several areas where lesions may occur. In theory, at least, there can be inadequate dietary intake of calcium and phosphate, there can be disorders of the collagen and its ability to initiate and to maintain calcification, and there may be disorders of the bone cells that result in decreased synthesis of collagen or other defects such as enzyme disorders. This, naturally, is not the entire list of possible problems, but it gives one a simple way of looking at metabolic bone disease.

The most common form of metabolic bone disease is called **osteoporosis,** or osteopenia, because the

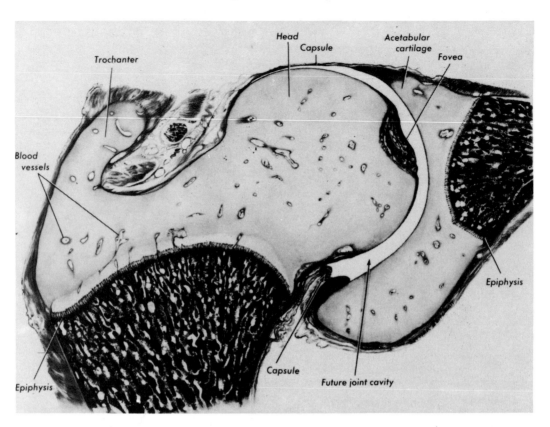

Fig. 25–2 Normal bone and cartilage. The epiphyseal apparatus and the head of the femur, its synovial space and capsule, and the acetabular cartilage of the hip. (From Bloom, W., and Fawcett, D. W.: *A Textbook of Histology,* 10th Ed. Philadelphia, W. B. Saunders, 1975.)

bones appear diminished in structure, as if the steel skeleton of a bridge or building had been heavily rusted and its mass severely decreased. However, osteoporotic bone is only diminished in amount. It is otherwise normal, having normal matrix and mineralization. This generalized disorder of the whole skeleton is seen commonly in those over 60; in fact, it is estimated that half the women over 60 in North America have osteoporosis, compared with the 35-year-old population. This diagnosis is most often made radiologically by comparison with bone of normal people. It is a quantitative, morphologic diagnosis, most easily seen in the vertebrae and pelvis, and is common in elderly persons or in those who have been bedridden for any length of time. It is to be expected in patients who have been given adrenal corticosteroids. The pathogenic mechanism common to all these processes is believed to be inhibition of normal collagen synthesis, although we acknowledge that the etiology of osteoporosis is unknown. Osteoporosis also occurs in the bones of a leg or an arm that has been placed in a cast, while the remainder of the skeleton continues to maintain a normal appearance. The stimuli to normal bone growth and development are both local and general, and so we can generalize that bone, like

all our other tissues, constantly adapts to the demands placed on it. The serum enzymes and ions related to bone integrity are all normal (alkaline phosphatase, calcium, phosphorus), a feature that distinguishes osteoporosis from osteomalacia.

In summary, osteoporosis or **osteopenia** may be due to: (1) senility or aging, for which the causes are related to protein metabolism; (2) atrophy of disuse, as in the single limb that is in a cast, or in the limbs of a paraplegic, or in the bedridden; (as an aside, one of the major biochemical problems of the astronauts was calcium loss—what role does gravity play in the maintenance of our skeletal system?); (3) gonadal deficiency; (4) adrenocortical hormone excess, whether endogenous or exogenous, as in patients with rheumatoid arthritis who are given steroid hormones or in those who have Cushing's disease.

The most common complications of osteoporosis are fractures of the femur or other weight-bearing bones such as the vertebrae. These fractures may be major or only visible with the most careful inspection. Management is often directed to improving protein metabolism, physiotherapy, and occasionally administering anabolic steroids.

The second generalized metabolic bone disease is

Fig. 25–3 This photograph shows a normal male on the right and three types of **dwarfism.** On the extreme left is a child who has failed to grow because of congenital absence of the thyroid gland (cretin). The next pair of dwarfs have entirely normal proportions but are half normal size. The next pair on the right show disproportionately short extremities but normal size trunk and head.

Fig. 25–4 Microscopic appearance of the periosteum, osteoblasts, osteocytes, and an area of new and old bone. (From Ham, A.W.: *Histology,* 7th Ed. Philadelphia and Toronto, J.B. Lippincott, 1974.)

that in which there are inadequate amounts of mineral in the bone. This is called **osteomalacia** in the adult and **rickets** in the child or person who is still growing. The name implies softening (*malakia*, Greek for soft). This can be due to an inadequate dietary intake during infancy or at any time, but the minimal requirement of the child is much more crucial than that of the adult, who has already built up a large store of calcium and phosphate. There are, however, other causes of rickets in addition to dietary deficiency. For example, there are rare cases of hereditary rickets, such as hypophosphatasia, and vitamin D-resistant rickets (inborn errors of metabolism), in addition to the better-known form caused by vitamin D deficiency.

We shall consider rickets more completely as it is an interesting and important disease, particularly for those in northern climates.

Rickets is a form of osteodystrophy completely different from those already considered, because it is a manifestation of a vitamin deficiency. We have already seen that the chief mineral constituents that impart rigidity to the bones are calcium and phosphorus, combined in the form of calcium phosphate. These substances are absorbed from the food and deposited in the bones. If they are not present in the food in sufficient amount, the bones remain soft and are easily bent.

Vitamin D is important to proper calcification. The ordinary food of a child usually contains a reasonable amount of calcium and phosphorus, but may be lacking in vitamin D. This vitamin is necessary for the proper absorption of calcium and phosphorus from the intestine, and in its absence, no matter how abundant the minerals may be in the food, the body is unable to use them, and rickets will result. Vitamin D is a fat-soluble vitamin, in contrast to some of the other vitamins that are water-soluble. It is therefore contained principally in fatty foods, although it is also found in certain vegetables.

The cause of rickets are deficiencies in some of the factors necessary for the proper calcification of bone. The fault may lie in the quality, not the quantity, of the food. A child may be starved and emaciated but show no signs of rickets, whereas a plump baby may show marked rickets. The disease is much more common in artificially-fed infants than in those who are breast-fed. Due to the absence of sunlight, rickets is more common in large, smoky cities and during the winter months. All the factors are included in the statement that rickets is a disease of the nutritionally disadvantaged in slums of large cities in countries that get little sunshine.

The symptoms are partly connected with bones, partly systemic. The disease is one of infancy and early childhood (6 months to 2 years), a period at which there is the greatest demand for calcium and phosphorus by the rapidly growing bones. The softened bones become deformed, especially those that bear the weight of the body (Fig. 25–5), and backward curvature of the spine develops (kyphosis). The head is large and square. The sternum is pushed forward (pigeon-breast) and a series of nodules develops at the anterior ends of the ribs called the rickety rosary. Nodular swellings are formed at the wrists, knees, and ankles. The most serious deformity is a narrowing of the inlet of the pelvis, which in the female may make normal delivery impossible in later life. Among the other signs and symptoms are sweating, restlessness, and flabbiness of the muscles, often giving the child a "pot belly." The serum phosphorus is markedly decreased.

Trauma

Trauma as a pathologic entity has already been considered in Chapter 3. However, a specific paragraph dealing with injury to bones is warranted, because of the frequency with which this occurs at all ages.

A fracture may occur without the skin's being torn; this is a simple fracture. If the broken ends of the bone project through the skin, the condition is a compound fracture. The great difference between the two types of fracture is that in the compound fracture there is danger of infection from the skin or air, which in the days before antisepsis and antibiotics often proved fatal. Compound fractures and battlefield wounds be-

Fig. 25–5 **Rickets**, showing large forehead, deformed chest, curvature of arms and legs, and pot belly.

fore the middle of the twentieth century were life-threatening. A greenstick fracture in children is a crack rather than a complete break of the pliable bone; it has been likened to the injury to a branch caused by bending a green twig. The relation of a pathologic fracture to some unrelated cause of weakening of the bone (carcinoma) has already been mentioned. Fractures of the skull are of particular importance, because even a minor crack may tear one of the numerous meningeal arteries that run in relation to the inner surface of the skull, with the possible development of a dangerous, or even fatal, hemorrhage.

The importance of fractures, generally speaking, is the extent to which the adjacent tissues are damaged or devitalized (hemorrhage), the extent of the systemic reaction (shock), the immediate complications (fat and other emboli), and the long-term complications (lack of union and loss of function). Naturally, the damage will depend on the areas of bone involved and on the nature of the injury. It is safe to say that current treatment emphasizes the use of immediate reduction and restoration of the patient to an ambulatory condition as soon as possible.

Infections of Bone

Although bone infections are much less common today, they require a few paragraphs.

The word **osteomyelitis** means inflammation of the bone (osteitis) and of the bone marrow (myelitis) (Fig. 25–6).

The inflammation is usually caused by gram-positive cocci, which gain access to the body through the skin, often causing a boil, and are then carried to the bone by the blood stream. The disease used to be one of children and adolescents in whom the bone is still growing, and it is three times as common in boys as in girls, probably because the former are more liable to trauma. As growth takes place only in the region of the epiphyseal cartilage, and as this is the part most abundantly supplied with blood vessels, it follows that the disease affects the end of the bone, usually on the side of the epiphyseal cartilage next to the shaft. Injury to bone is a common accessory factor, because this disease is apt to cause rupture of a small vessel, and the circulating staphylococci are able to settle down in the blood clot and grow rapidly. The

A

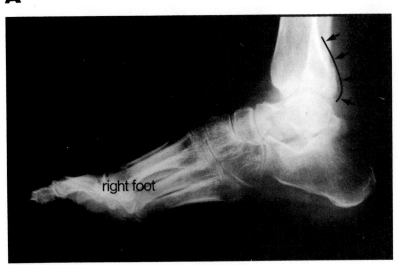

B

Fig. 25–6 *A*, This bone scan of the ankle in three views shows increased uptake (dark areas), which is consistent with **osteomyelitis**. A Gallium 67 scan would confirm that this case was due to inflammation. *B*, This conventional radiograph shows changes of periosteal elevation and inflammation at the arrows. This sign is typical of osteomyelitis.

injury may be a twist or a direct blow. The bones most frequently affected are the femur, tibia, and humerus.

The lesion begins as an abscess of the bone. As the result of acute inflammation, pus is produced and tends to spread down the medullary cavity and outward to the surface. When the pus reaches the surface, it raises the periosteum from the bone, and it may spread along the surface for a considerable distance. As it is from the periosteum that the bone receives a considerable proportion of its blood supply, it follows that a large area of the shaft may become devitalized and die. Such a piece of dead bone is called a sequestrum (Fig. 25–7), and in the course of time this becomes separated from the living bone by the action of the osteoclasts. The inflamed periosteum is stimulated to form a thick layer of new bone, which surrounds the sequestrum. In the new case, there are a number of openings through which purulent discharge escapes from the interior. One of the most serious results of the inflammation is thrombosis of the

Fig. 25–7 This radiograph shows diffuse destruction of bone with periosteal reaction and an area of decreased density surrounding a single, dense bony island. This island is a "sequestrum" of necrotic bone, seen within a focal area of destruction. This is typical of **osteomyelitis**.

vessels in the marrow. The thrombi become heavily infected with staphylococci, and they may break down and be carried by the blood to the lungs and other organs, where they set up multiple abscesses.

From what has been said, it is apparent that osteomyelitis tends to be both a local and a general infection; the symptoms are therefore both local and general. The local symptoms are pain and tenderness at the end of a long bone, often in the region of the knee, together with heat, redness, and swelling—in short, the classic signs of acute inflammation.

The general symptoms are those of any severe acute infection, i.e., high fever, chills, rapid pulse, marked leukocytosis, and the presence of bacteria in blood culture.

Fortunately, the entire picture of osteomyelitis has been changed since the introduction of antibiotic therapy. The only treatment for this disease used to be to open up the bone surgically, to allow the pus and the infecting organisms to escape. The condition is now treated by antibiotics, and if the diagnosis is made early and correct treatment is started at once, the widespread bacterial infection described in the preceding paragraphs will be prevented. It is evident also that if the patient is properly treated, there will be no development of a sequestrum or of sinuses.

Tuberculosis of bone, like osteomyelitis, is a chronic disease. Like the acute disease, it affects the ends of the bones, but begins in the epiphysis much more frequently than does osteomyelitis. The bones most often attacked are the long bones of the arms and legs, the bones of the wrist and ankle, and the vertebrae. As in the case of acute osteomyelitis, the region of the knee (lower end of femur and upper end of tibia) is a common site.

The lesion consists of a slow destruction of the end of the bone, not a wholesale destruction, but a nibbling here and there, giving the bone a worm-eaten appearance. If the disease begins in the shaft, the epiphyseal cartilage is gradually eaten away and the epiphysis is invaded. From the epiphysis, whether it is infected primarily or secondarily, the disease spreads to the articular cartilage, which is eroded bit by bit, until the articular surface comes to be formed by the diseased and roughened bone.

Tuberculosis of the spine, also known as **Pott's disease**, used to be a frequent occurrence in children, although it may also occur in the adult. The disease affects one or more vertebrae, which it slowly destroys, just as the ends of the long bones are destroyed. The pressure from above causes the softened vertebrae to collapse, with resulting deformity of the spine, so that the child develops a "humpback." It is possible that Quasimodo, the hunchback of Notre

Dame in Dumas's famous novel, had tuberculosis as a cause of his deformity (Figs. 25–8 and 25–9). A more serious result is pressure on the spinal cord, with the gradual production of paralysis of the legs. A tuberculous or cold abscess may develop, the peculiarity of which is that it tends to spread along the psoas muscle, which passes from the lumbar part of the spine to the upper end of the femur. This psoas abscess, as it is called, will therefore appear in the groin as a soft swelling which may easily be mistaken for a hernia.

Whichever joint is affected, be it the wrist, the knee, or the joints of the spine, the first symptoms will be limitation of movement. This is natural, because no one moves a diseased joint more than is absolutely necessary. If the disease starts in the bone, symptoms do not appear until the joint is also involved, unless there is a place where the periosteum is close to the surface, as in the tibia, or shin. The joint is swollen, owing to tuberculous swelling of the synovial membrane. The affected limb tends to be shorter than the normal one, partly because of the bone destruction, but mainly because the epiphyseal cartilage, which is responsible for growth in the length of the bone, is killed. When the articular cartilage is destroyed and the roughened ends of the bones come in contact, pain develops. There may be no pain during the day, because the muscles around the joint contract and prevent movement from occurring. But when the child falls asleep, the muscle watchdogs are no longer on guard, and the joint may be moved, causing intense pain, so that the child wakes with a start and a cry. These pains are therefore known as "starting pains" or "night pains." For a long time, the patient may show none of the general symptoms of tuberculosis such as fever or loss of weight.

It is hardly necessary to add that modern antibiotic therapy has completely altered this picture, but one should be aware that there has been a resurgence of tuberculosis in many persons who have received steroids or who have AIDS.

Legg-Perthes disease is the most common of a group of lesions known as aseptic or ischemic necrosis of bone. In Perthes disease, the lesion is confined to the head of the femur, but in other members of this group (known by other men's names), the epiphyses in a variety of bones are involved. The lesions are of clinical importance not because they cause any marked disability, but because they are so easily mistaken for bone tuberculosis. In all cases, the lesions represent a quiet necrosis of bone, aseptic and nonbacterial in character, and apparently due to ischemia, which develops for some unknown reason.

Perthes disease usually occurs in boys between the ages of 5 and 10 years. There is often a history of

Fig. 25–8 These drawings by Leonardo da Vinci show the normal lateral curves of the thoracic, lumbar, and sacral spine.

recent injury. The bone in the center of the epiphysis is fragmented, so that it may resemble fragments of mortar. As a result, the head of the femur becomes flattened and splayed. When healing occurs, the fragments coalesce and the bone regains some of its structure, but the flattening is permanent. The x-ray is absolutely characteristic, and it is by this means that a final diagnosis is made. The earliest symptom is a limp, accompanied by little or no discomfort. The condition must be distinguished from early tuberculosis in a child.

Fig. 25–9   This spine shows marked angulation, due to the presence of **tuberculosis (Pott's disease)**. (McGill University, Department of Pathology Museum.)

Syphilis of bone used to be a disease of great importance, but modern antibiotics have changed a common type of lesion into a rarity, so that we may dispose of the subject with welcome brevity. It differs from tuberculosis in the following respects: (1) it affects the shaft of the long bones rather than their ends, (2) the joint is seldom involved, and (3) osteosclerosis with new bone formation is much more prominent than osteoporosis or rarefaction. Destruction of the bones of the nose and hard palate used to be common, so that the bridge of the nose fell in at the root (saddlenose), and there might be a large perforation of the palate. It may avoid embarrassment to remember that not every saddle-nose is caused by syphilis.

Salmonella infections of bone in children are unusual; however, they seem to occur with some frequency in patients with sickle cell disease. The reason for this is unknown.

Tumors of Bone and Cartilage

We have already seen that bone is a complex structure composed of bone cells, periosteum, cartilage, marrow, and blood vessels. Tumors of various kinds may arise from any of these elements. For the purpose of this brief outline, however, bone tumors may be divided into primary and secondary, and the primary tumors may again be divided into benign and malignant.

Primary Tumors. These may be benign or malignant. The three chief benign tumors are osteoma, chondroma, and giant cell tumor. The osteoma and chondroma are similar, the former consisting of bone cells and the latter of cartilage. Both are hard tumors that usually arise at the end of a long bone, although they may occur in practically any bone in the body. Being benign, they are localized and usually remain small, but occasionally they grow to a great size. When removed, they show no tendency to recur.

Giant cell tumor develops in children and in young adults, usually before the age of 30 (Fig. 25–10). It occurs principally at the ends of long bones, and the common location is the knee. It is highly destructive locally, but does not cause metastases or kill the patient. It consists of a soft, red, hemorrhagic mass, which greatly distends the bone and almost completely destroys it. This gives the highly characteristic x-ray picture of large bubbles separated by thin strips of bone. The tumor gets its name from the many giant cells that are seen in the microscopic section.

The three chief primary malignant tumors of bone are osteogenic sarcoma, Ewing's tumor, and multiple myeloma.

Osteogenic sarcoma is the most common of the three tumors. It is a disease of young persons between the ages of 10 and 30 and is rarely seen after the age of 50. The location is similar to that of giant cell tumor, namely, at the ends of the long bones, usually in the region of the knee joint. The tumor expands the end of the bone, so as to give it a "leg of mutton" appearance (Fig. 25–11). The periosteum is lifted from the bone by the tumor, and spicules of new bone are laid down, which radiate outward from the central mass,

Fig. 25–10   Shown here are the large cystic spaces characteristic of **giant cell tumor** of bone. (McGill University, Department of Pathology Museum.)

Fig. 25–11 In the center of the upper field is a whitish mass replacing the normal marrow cavity. This is an **osteogenic sarcoma,** a primary malignant tumor of bone. Note the increase in size of the bone in this area. (McGill University, Department of Pathology Museum.)

the surface may present a laminated appearance in the film, like the layers of an onion. One of the most striking characteristics of the tumor is its response to radiation; it may melt away like a lymphosarcoma, only to return later.

Multiple myeloma, also known as plasma cell myeloma, is composed of plasma cells, but these cells are responsible for one of the most important characteristics of the tumor (Fig. 25–12). As the name myeloma

Fig. 25–12 Gross appearance of several vertebral bodies separated by intervertebral discs. The normal trabecular pattern has been replaced by currant-jelly reddish material, typical of **multiple myeloma.** (McGill University, Department of Pathology Museum.)

giving a characteristic "sun ray" effect in the x-ray film. Spread takes place by the blood stream, and metastases often appear first in the lungs. Secondary growths in other bones are rare; multiple bone tumors suggest Ewing's tumor in the young and multiple myeloma in the middle-aged.

Ewing's tumor occurs at an earlier age than does osteogenic sarcoma, usually between the ages of 5 and 15. It is rarely seen after the age of 30. It involves the bone much more diffusely than does osteogenic sarcoma, giving rise to a uniform thickening. The tumor does not begin at the end of a bone. One of the more striking features of the disease is that, as the tumor progresses, other growths become apparent in many widely distant bones, particularly the flat bones, such as the scapula, sternum, vertebrae, and skull. The x-ray shows diffuse involvement of the greater part of the shaft. There is a combination of bone formation and bone destruction; formation in the early stage, destruction later. The new bone on suggests, this is a tumor of bone marrow rather than of bone. It is usually multiple, and by the time the patient comes to the doctor, a large number of the flat bones may be involved (Fig. 25–13). The age incidence is in striking contrast to that of Ewing's tumor; 80% of the cases occur after the age of 40 years. Huge amounts of calcium may be freed from the bones, with

resulting high serum calcium levels and deposits of calcium in the kidneys, and pathologic fractures are common. Marrow aspiration shows tumor cells in the sternal marrow, even though there is no other evidence of a tumor. Recently, combined chemotherapy and radiation have dramatically extended the life span of patients in whom this diagnosis has been established.

Plasma cells normally produce gamma globulins, so it is only natural that a neoplasm of cells should produce these and related globulins in excess quantity. The total serum proteins are raised to 10 mg or higher, and there is a marked inversion of the normal albumin-globulin ratio, owing to the great overproduction of gamma globulin by the tumor cells. In addition, there may be a copious excretion in the urine of a unique protein, the **Bence Jones protein**, which was recognized in the urine over 100 years ago. It appears as a cloud when the urine is heated to 55°C disappears at 85°C or on boiling, but reappears on cooling. The reason it is found in the urine and not in the serum is that its molecular weight is only half that of albumin, so that it can readily escape from the blood into the urine through the glomerular filter. It must be noted that Bence Jones protein is present in the urine in less than 50% of cases of myeloma, so that its absence does not mean that the patient is not suffering from the disease. Renal failure may occur in the later stages, and may be so severe as to lead to uremia and death. This may be because large numbers of renal tubules may be blocked by casts of abnormal protein, and the calcification already alluded to cannot improve the functional capacity of the kidneys.

Treatment of malignant bone tumors consists in surgical removal at the earliest possible moment, in the hope that metastases may not yet have occurred. Radiologic examination of the lungs must first be made, because if secondary growths are found in these organs, no treatment is of any avail. Some forms of sarcoma respond well to x-ray treatment, and the tumor may disappear for a time, but the relief is only temporary, and sooner or later the tumor will recur. In general, as illustrated in Table 25–1, the prognosis for malignant tumors of bone is poor.

Secondary Tumors. Metastatic tumors of bone are carcinomas, the tumor cells coming from a cancer in some other organ. The most common forms of cancer that are likely to metastasize to bone are cancer of the breast, lung, prostate, and kidney (Fig. 25–14). The metastatic tumor destroys the bone, and the first indication of its presence may be the occurrence of a fracture from a trivial injury. Other evidence of the presence of a tumor in bone may be pain, of a constant and gnawing kind, or chemical evidence, such as the

Fig. 25–13 *A,* This routine lateral x-ray demonstrates the appearance of a **normal skull** in lateral projection. *B,* This film shows the multiple "punched-out" lytic lesions consistent with a diagnosis of **multiple myeloma or of metastatic tumor**.

Table 25–1. Estimated New Cases and Deaths From Some Cancers in 1974 (U.S.)

	NEW CASES	DEATHS
Sarcoma of bone	1,900	1,900
Thyroid carcinoma	7,900	1,150
Hodgkin's disease	7,100	3,500
Small intestine carcinoma	2,200	700
Lip carcinoma	4,000	225

Fig. 25–14 Shown in this gross specimen of vertebral bodies and intervertebral discs is the replacement of the vertebral body in the lower portion of the picture by a firm, white tissue characteristic of **metastatic carcinoma** from the prostate. (McGill University, Department of Pathology Museum.)

presence of elevated serum alkaline phosphatase or calcium. The bones commonly affected are the ribs, vertebrae, sternum, and skull (the flat bones), and the upper end of the femur and humerus. In all these bones, the marrow is of the red variety and is therefore well vascularized, and so it is natural that the blood-borne tumor cells will be arrested at these sites. It is evident from the nature of the condition that nothing in the way of treatment is of any avail.

Miscellaneous Bone Diseases

A condition known as **osteitis fibrosa cystica** (von Recklinghausen's disease) is characterized by highly porous and decalcified bones, which may be much deformed and curved, sometimes with the formation of bone cysts and spontaneous fractures of the rarefied bone. The decalcification is a manifestation of hyperparathyroidism, usually due to an adenoma, but occasionally to hyperplasia of the parathyroid glands, a condition that has already been described. The calcium removed from the bones appears in the blood, so that the serum calcium rises from 10 mg to 15 or 20 mg/100 ml, and the serum phosphorus is correspondingly low. The calcium may be deposited from the blood into the kidneys, giving shadows in the x-ray film, or it may form a single stone in the kidney.

Fibrous dysplasia of bone is readily confused clinically with osteitis fibrosa, but the pathogenesis of the two conditions is entirely different. Fibrous dysplasia is not related to hyperparathyroidism, but, as the name implies, is a congenital anomaly in the development of bone, with the formation of fibrous swellings that replace the bone and that give rise to deformities such as those of osteitis fibrosa. There is no disturbance in the serum calcium and phosphorus.

Paget's disease is otherwise called osteitis deformans; it is a common asymptomatic radiologic finding in elderly people, estimated to be present in 10% of all those over 60 years of age. It is twice as common in men as in women, and it is usually clinically recognized because of pain in the back, hips, or pelvis. The full-blown case of this disease of unknown etiology may have deafness, increasing head size (Fig. 25–15), headaches, neuromuscular signs and symptoms, and heart failure. The diagnosis is established by radiologic and serum alkaline phosphatase determinations. Urinary hydroxyproline determinations may be elevated as the disease progresses.

The explanation for these manifestations, although we do not know the cause of the disorder, is that there is an increase in bone cell activity, beginning perhaps with increased osteoclastic resorption, followed by

Fig. 25–15   This anteroposterior view of the skull shows a marked thickening of the cranial vault with densities typical of **Paget's disease** of the skull. This is called a leonine appearance.

the increased laying down of new bone (Fig. 25–16). This resorption and new bone formation proceeds rapidly with a change in the normal pattern of bone collagen and with the development of new vascular channels. The increased vascularity results in fistula formation, requires an increased cardiac output, and results in an increase in the temperature of the skin over the affected bones.

The complications of Paget's disease are structural deformities that may cause compression of spinal and cranial nerves and of the spinal cord, and the cardiovascular complications of heart failure following on the increased cardiac output, and finally, malignant change in the new bone. Osteogenic sarcomas are rare enough, but a patient with Paget's disease is at increased risk of developing this cancer.

JOINTS

Structure and Function

A joint is a structure of peculiar delicacy, and one that responds only too readily to injury. When we consider the amount of stress and strain, not to mention abuse in sports, to which the joints are subjected in a long life, it is little wonder that disease of the joints is among the most common of clinical disorders.

Man was not originally designed to stand upright, and so it is natural that the weight-bearing joints, in particular those of the lower limbs and vertebral column, should be among the principal sufferers.

A joint consists of two articular surfaces: a capsule or strong, fibrous structure, which joins the two ends of the bone together, and a synovial membrane, which lines the capsule and produces an oily fluid that lubricates the articular surfaces and ensures the smooth working of the mechanism. It now seems that the presence of lubricant and the health of the joint depend in some measure on the activity to which the joint is subject. Rather than having a totally destructive effect on joints, it seems more likely that moderate, regular exercise is beneficial, because it causes exchange of fluid between the underlying cartilage and the joint fluid. Any or all of these structures may be damaged by disease.

The Arthritides

Arthritis is a general term for inflammation of the joints, and we may arbitrarily divide all inflammations of joints into acute or chronic forms.

Pyogenic or suppurative arthritis used to be the most important form of acute arthritis; bacteria were introduced through a wound, or spread to the joint from a bone that was the seat of acute osteomyelitis. Antibiotic therapy has now pushed this complication into the background. Gonorrheal arthritis, formerly an occasional complication of acute gonorrhea affecting many joints, has also passed into the realm of the forgotten, as the result of the present adequate treatment of the infection with penicillin in the acute, stage of the disease. Rheumatic arthritis is the acute nonsuppurative arthritis of rheumatic fever. There is an acute synovitis with excess of turbid fluid in the joint. Extreme tenderness is characteristic of the swollen and acutely inflamed joint. The inflammation usually undergoes complete resolution, but some permanent stiffness occasionally may persist. Traumatic synovitis is a good example of acute nonsuppurative arthritis, the inflammation being confined to the synovial membrane (acute synovitis), with no destruction of tissue and therefore no permanent stiffness. The synovial membrane is swollen, juicy, and congested, while the synovial fluid is increased in amount and cloudy.

The chronic arthritides are more common and disabling and we shall mention several types. Tuberculous arthritis used to be more common than it is today.

Tuberculosis of the joints is a disease of children and is usually secondary to tuberculosis of the adjacent bone, a subject that has already been considered. When it occurs in an adult, it is more likely to be primary in the synovial membrane, the infection having been carried by the blood stream from some distant focus. The synovial membrane may be even

A   **B**

Fig. 25–16 *A,* This **nuclear medicine scan**, using technetium 99m methylene diphosphonate, which is a calcium-seeking agent that localizes in areas of active bone turnover, displays no skeletal abnormalities. The first scan of each pair shows the anterior bones, the second scan shows the posterior bones. *B,* The bone scan, using the same technique, shows increased uptake with areas of expansion of bone, particularly in the right lower limb and pelvis, typical of the appearance of Paget's disease.

thicker and more voluminous than in rheumatoid arthritis, so that it may fill the entire cavity. The fluid is usually scanty, but highly fibrinous, so that it contains flakes of fibrin that may develop into foreign bodies known as melon-seed bodies or rice bodies. The destruction of the articular surfaces that may develop and the resulting clinical picture already have been described in connection with tuberculosis of bone, and will not be discussed here.

Rheumatoid Arthritis. This widespread, tragic, and crippling disease is perhaps the second most common form of chronic arthritis. It is a chronic inflammatory condition that particularly affects the small joints of the hands and feet, although the larger joints may be affected later (Fig. 25–17). The condition usually occurs in women between 20 and 40 years of age. Rheumatoid arthritis is one of the greatest causes of disability in the north temperate zones, and it has been estimated that it is responsible for an annual loss

of $200,000,000 in the United States. This is perhaps not remarkable when we consider that there are an estimated 2,000,000 persons who suffer from the disease in Canada and the United States, and that 200,000 are totally disabled.

Etiology. An enormous amount has been written about the cause of rheumatoid arthritis, a sure indication that little is known about the subject. The most reasonable view appears to be that the arthritis is the result of a combination of minimal hematogenous bacterial infections with tissue hypersensitivity. The sensitization may be the result of a series of minor infections or a chronic focus that periodically discharges a few bacteria into the blood. At no time do the bacteria reach the joints in sufficient numbers to produce conventional lesions, but the tissues are constantly being sensitized, until finally one bacteremic episode culminates in a definite arthritis. Psychologic factors such as stress, operating perhaps through the adrenal cor-

Fig. 25–17   This conventional x-ray study of two hands shows narrowing of the metacarpophalangeal joints and of the proximal interphalangeal joints, with multiple erosions. This is consistent with the appearance of **rheumatoid arthritis**.

tex, seem to play a part. Marked and sometimes startling relief of the arthritis symptoms is common during the early months of pregnancy and is attributed to the increased availability of adrenal cortical hormones. This observation initiated the breakthrough in the late 1940s that resulted in the biosynthesis of cortisone.

Laboratory tests support the idea of an immunologic pathogenesis. A specific agglutination reaction occurs when the serum of the arthritic patient is added to a suspension of a variety of particles. At first, the red blood cells of sheep, coated with tannic acid and sensitized with human gamma globulin, were used, but more recently a suspension of latex particles mixed with gamma globulin has been used. Only a drop of serum is needed, a positive latex fixation test being indicated by an agglutination of the particles visible to the naked eye. The latex particles simply act as inert carriers of gamma globulin, and the same is true of the coated red blood cells. The reaction seems to be due to the presence of a rheumatoid factor in the blood, which has now been isolated and shown to be a macroglobulin antibody or antigen-antibody complex. By fluorescence microscopy, it has been demonstrated that the rheumatoid factor originates in the lymphocytes and plasma cells of the lymph nodes and the hypertrophied synovial membrane.

Lesions. The synovial membrane is primarily affected, so that the disease might be called synovioarthritis in contrast to osteoarthritis, the other great form of chronic arthritis. The pathologic changes resemble in certain respects those of joint tuberculosis, although it attacks many joints instead of one, and does not lead to destruction of the bone. There is the same swelling of the synovial membrane with the formation of pulpy masses or fringes and tags, which cause the joints to be enlarged, the same gradual destruction of the articular cartilage, the same interference with the function of the joint that finally results in complete disability and fusion of the joint surfaces. The most significant feature is the superabundance of lymphocytes and plasma cells, suggesting the immunologic character of the process. The periarticular soft parts share in the inflammatory swelling and edema. The ligaments become softened and absorbed, thus contributing to the deformities that form so distressing a feature of the end picture of the disease. Subcutaneous inflammatory nodules may be found in the neighborhood of the affected joints, particularly in the arms (Fig. 25–18). The course of the disease is marked by curious remissions and exacerbations, and at any stage the progress may be arrested. However, as in tuberculosis, the injury to the joint is permanent, and the hands and feet are twisted, gnarled, and crippled for life (Fig. 25–17). On this account, and because of its commonness, the disease is of great economic importance, since it is a disease of great morbidity but small mortality; it cripples, but does not kill.

Symptoms. The symptoms are pain and swelling of the joints, together with increasing stiffness and disability. In the later stages, the joints become distorted and deformed. During the exacerbations, the patient often suffers from mild fever, malaise, anemia, and sweating.

Treatment. During the acute phase of the rheumatoid arthritis, rest is of great importance, together with methods of physiotherapy that help to restore function and particularly to prevent crippling deformities. The maintenance of correct posture of the joints involved provides for the maximum of function when the acute process subsides. Relief of pain with mild analgesics is necessary in most cases. The use of corti-sone and ACTH in rheumatoid arthritis has proved beneficial in many cases. This treatment is accompanied by relief of pain, decrease in swelling, and increase in movement of affected joints. Unfortunately, in many instances this improvement is not maintained after the drug is stopped.

Ankylosing spondylitis may be a variant of rheumatoid arthritis; the name means stiffness of vertebral joints. Although rheumatoid in character, it differs from rheumatoid arthritis in that it has a high male sex incidence and a negative serologic reaction for the rheumatoid factor. The articular cartilage is destroyed, fibrous adhesions develop, and eventually bone fusion occurs with calcification of the intervertebral discs. The condition begins in the sacroiliac joints and spreads slowly upward, ending with extreme rigidity, which may justify the term poker back. In early cases, the x-ray film shows a fuzziness of the apposed surfaces of the bones, followed by calcification and later ossification of the vertebral ligaments (Fig. 25–19). In exceptional cases, there are lesions of the aortic valve and ascending aorta. It is a particularly tragic disease, because so often it affects young people.

Osteoarthritis. Probably the most common type of arthritis, osteoarthritis is the term applied to a degen-

Fig. 25–18 This photograph shows large nodules on the ulnar surfaces of both elbows. These are typical **rheumatoid nodules,** although in this instance they are somewhat larger than usual. (McGill University, Department of Pathology Museum.)

Fig. 25–19   *A,* This x-ray demonstrates a **normal cervical spine** in lateral projection. *B,* This demonstrates the bamboo spine appearance of **ankylosing spondylitis,** due to calcification in the anterior spinal ligaments and to fusion of the posterior joint spaces.

eration of articular cartilage and bone, so that it might well be called degenerative arthritis. In this it differs from rheumatoid arthritis, which is primarily an inflammation of synovial membrane, and indeed it differs from that condition in almost every respect. Thus it is as common in men as in women; it is a disease of the later period of life; there are no general symptoms; the large joints are commonly involved, often only one joint, particularly the hip; and there is no true ankylosis or fusion between the articular surfaces. The small joints of the hands and feet may also be involved, the knuckles becoming greatly swollen and knobby (Fig. 25–20).

The lesions are primarily atrophic, followed later by localized hypertrophy. The articular cartilage undergoes degeneration and softening, so that it is gradually worn away, until the underlying bone is exposed. There is atrophy of the central part of the bone, so that much of the head and neck of the femur may disappear. The peripheral part of the cartilage has a much better blood supply than the central area, and overgrowths of cartilage, which resemble candle drip-

pings, develop at the edge of the articular cartilage, a condition known as lipping of the joint. These cartilaginous excrescences tend to become ossified, so that the atrophied head of the bone is surrounded by a ring of bony excrescences, which may gravely limit movement and form a striking feature in the x-ray film. Thinning of the intervertebral discs is also a feature of diagnostic importance in the film.

The etiology of osteoarthritis is obscure. It is a degenerative condition in which the aging process, probably associated with local ischemia, plays a leading part. If a joint is continually exposed to trauma, as in a trade or in professional athletes, it may show the characteristic changes. The condition may indeed be described as "wear and tear" arthritis.

Lesions of the Intervertebral Discs

When we consider the important joints of the body, we are apt to forget the intervertebral discs (Fig. 25–21), and yet there is perhaps no part of the body in which strain and movement are so constant, and

Fig. 25–20 This routine x-ray study of the hands shows narrowing of the distal interphalangeal joints with multiple erosions and subarticular sclerosis. This is consistent with erosive **osteoarthritis.**

Endochondral ossification center   Nucleus pulposus   Endochondral ossification center

Fig. 25–21 This histologic preparation shows the appearance of the ossification center and the nucleus pulposus in sections of a **developing vertebral column**. (From Bloom, W., and Fawcett, D.W.: *A Textbook of Histology*, 10th Ed. Philadelphia, W.B. Saunders, 1975.)

in which impairment of movement, especially when associated with pain, so cripples the full enjoyment of life. Owing to man's upright position, the discs are subject to constant strain for which they were not originally intended, so that degeneration in later life is more common than in any other organ, with corresponding loss of the normal cushioning function.

The nucleus pulposus is the essential part of the disc, and plays the chief role in pathologic changes. It is a highly elastic, semifluid mass compressed like a spring between the vertebral surfaces. In youth, it presents a marked elastic turgor, depending on the fluid content of the tissue. With age, this turgor gradually diminishes, and it is completely lost in various degenerations.

An intervertebral disc may protrude or herniate into the vertebral canal and press on the spinal cord or stretch the nerves. This is the condition known popularly as "slipped disc." Protrusions occur at the sites of the maximum anterior spinal curvature, that is to say, the region between the fourth lumbar and first sacral, and between the fifth and seventh cervical vertebrae (Fig. 25–22). The cause of the protrusion varies.

Most common is trauma, either sudden, as in a fall from a height, or repetitious, as in heavy labor that involves lifting. The turgid nucleus pulposus is confined by a circular band of fibrous tissue, the anulus fibrosus. When this tissue is torn or degenerates, the disc is forced backward into the canal. In many cases, no cause can be suggested.

The chief symptoms are low back pain and sciatica or pain passing down the back of the leg along the course of the sciatic nerve, symptoms that carry little threat to life, but that may interfere greatly with living. In addition to the sensory disturbances, there may be severe spasm of the muscles of the back, causing marked disability. It is possible to localize the lesion accurately by clinical observations in over 75% of cases. Excision of the protruded disc is required in only a small proportion of cases.

TENDONS

The tendons in which the muscles terminate are nonvascular and therefore are relatively immune to inflammation, but the tendon sheath in which they

Fig. 25–22 *A,* Anteroposterior view of the spine following a myelogram. *B,* Lateral view. Here the myelogram demonstrates a protruded intervertebral disc.

move, especially at the wrist and ankle, is often in-flamed. Suppurative synovitis may result from spread of infection from a septic process in the fingers. Tuber-culous tenosynovitis is marked by the formation of tuberculous granulation tissue, which causes a "white swelling" such as that seen in tuberculosis of a joint. **Traumatic tenosynovitis** is the most common form, occurring in piano players, in typists, and in other persons whose tendons are subjected to excessive use. Fibrin is laid down on the surface of the tendon and the wall of the sheath, so that crackling is felt when the tendon is used.

Ganglion is a cystic swelling that develops in con-nection with a tendon sheath. The common site is the back of the wrist. It is attached to the outer surface of the tendon sheath and begins as a proliferation of the connective tissue of the sheath, which undergoes mu-coid degeneration, with the formation of numerous small cysts that eventually fuse to form a large cyst filled with soft mucoid material.

A bursa is a sac lined by synovial membrane, con-taining viscid fluid and situated at points where fric-tion would otherwise develop, usually close to a joint. Those with an interest in words may care to know that bursa is derived from the Latin word meaning a purse, from which comes our bursar, the man who holds the purse. Traumatic **bursitis** is usually caused by chronic and repeated irritation (housemaid's knee and student's elbow), but occasionally it is due to a blow. A common site is the region of the shoulder, involving the subdeltoid and subacromial bursae (subacromial bursitis), with pain most marked on mo-tion, so that the arm is not moved and a "frozen shoul-der" results. The bursa is distended with serous fluid (hydrops). Tuberculous bursitis usually takes the form of hydrops with melon-seed bodies, or the bursa may be filled with granulation tissue.

MUSCLE

Structure and Function

Muscle is the largest single kind of tissue in the human body (Fig. 25–23). It is a unique organ in that it is capable of converting chemical energy into me-chanical work; it can fine tune a violin or lift a thou-sand pounds. The elements of skeletal muscle are structural proteins that respond to a well-organized set of chemical pathways, arranged in neat packages. The unit of skeletal muscle is called the motor unit and consists of a single motor neuron located in the spinal cord with its axons distributed to the muscle fiber, where the connection is called the neuromuscu-lar junction, or motor end-plate (Fig. 25–24). Muscle

Fig. 25–23 Drawing by Leonardo da Vinci showing the major mus-cles of the back in man.

fibers are cylindrical, elongated cells that extend from points of attachment (tendons), usually bridging joints. Each muscle fiber has one or many nuclei, an intricate cytoplasmic membranous system (which provides a surface across which ions flux), mitochon-dria in large numbers that provide the ATP, and a system of myofibrils (Fig. 25–25).

Most skeletal muscle contains approximately equal amounts of two types of fibers arranged in a mosaic pattern, but each type belongs to one motor unit (Table 25–2). Until 1978, it was believed that the fiber types in a given muscle were genetically determined, and that marathon runners or sprinters were born, not made, because the proportion of red or white muscle fibers was fixed. Recent experiments have shown that fiber types in muscle can be shifted from white to red by physical training. It has been known for a longer time that muscles respond to demand by adapting to meet the demand; in skeletal muscles, this is more clearly seen in the response of the weight lifter's muscles, which show an increase in the num-

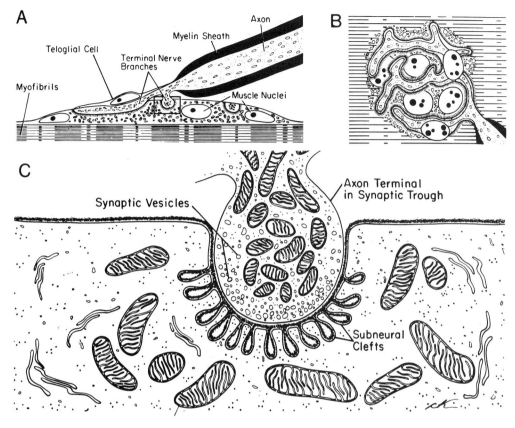

Fig. 25–24   These drawings show the appearance of a **neuromuscular junction**. (From Bloom, W., and Fawcett, D.W.: *A Textbook of Histology,* 10th Ed. Philadelphia, W.B. Saunders, 1975.)

bers of myofibrils. Endurance runners, on the other hand, show that their muscles adapt by increasing the number and size of mitochondria. A third type of adaptation is a change in the cytoplasmic enzyme systems with respect to their content of a variety of enzymes. A training program will enable muscles to use substrate more efficiently. Glycogen may be made more rapidly and calcium may be more easily transported. A fourth adaptation is the vascular supply to

skeletal muscle; there is considerable evidence that increased training creates a microvascular bed that enhances oxygenation to the muscle. And, finally, we know that just as bone loses its mass with disuse, muscle atrophies remarkably quickly if it is not used. There is no such biologic phenomenon as hoarding or saving your strength; the unused muscle wilts like a cut flower on a hot summer day.

Thus we have at least four different levels at which muscle may be affected by disease:

1. loss of motor neuron that leads to denervation atrophy;
2. interference with conduction or disuse that leads to atrophy;
3. interference with neuromuscular junction function that leads to loss of strength (myasthenia gravis);
4. primary disease of the muscle cell itself (storage disease or acquired disease, as in alcoholic myopathy).

A few additional points may be mentioned. Potassium affects muscle metabolism. Both too little potas-

Table 25–2.   Muscle Fiber Types

	SLOW (RED)	FAST (WHITE)
Mitochondrial enzymes (SDH)	High oxidative capability	Low oxidative capability
Creatinine phosphokinase mMoles/min/g protein	13.1	16.6
Lipids	High Content	Low Content
Glycogen enzymes (Phosphofructokinase) mMoles/min/kg	9.4	20.0
Capillary supply	+ + + +	+ + +

(Adapted from Saltin, B., et al.: Fiber types and metabolic potentials of skeletal muscles in sedentary man and endurance runners. Ann. N. Y. Acad. Sci., 301:3, 1977.)

SKELETAL MUSCLE

Fig. 25–25 This drawing illustrates the range of muscle from the gross appearance to the muscle fasciculus, to the muscle fiber, to the muscle myofibril, to the myofilaments, and, finally, to the myosin and actin molecules. The cross sections are shown in F, G, H, and I. (From Bloom, W., and Fawcett, D.W.: *A Textbook of Histology*, 10th Ed. Philadelphia, W.B. Saunders, 1975.)

sium (hypokalemia) and too much potassium (hyperkalemia) will cause paralysis of muscle. Transaminase (glutamic-oxaloacetic transaminase, abbreviated GOT) is an enzyme present in greatest concentration in cardiac and skeletal muscle. Destruction of this tissue results in a liberation of the enzyme into the serum, and an estimation of the transaminase serum level is a valuable test for determining the presence and extent of such injury, more particularly in myocardial infarction. Muscle is unusually adaptable to training. Nowhere is there better evidence of the general concept that many diseases are disorders of adaptation. Muscle responds to different stimuli by modifying its structure to meet the demand, provided the stimuli are within normal limits and recur sufficiently frequently to permit adaptation to take place. This is the basis for all sports training. It would be unwise for us to consider more than 1 or 2 of the many obscure diseases that may involve the muscles and tax the resources of the physiotherapist.

The general term **myopathy** is often applied to muscle disease. Unfortunately, this term is used casually, and it is not clear in many instances where the lesion lies, if indeed we know. This term may be applied to any disease or syndrome in which the patient's symptoms and/or physical signs can be attributed to pathologic, biochemical, or physical changes occurring in the muscle fibers or in the interstitial tissues of the voluntary musculature.

Hereditary myopathy, an example of which is **muscular dystrophy,** is a rare group of diseases of muscle characterized by progressive muscle wasting and weakness, accompanied, for a time at least, by a paradoxical increase in muscle size. Histologic features of muscle affected by these diseases include variations in fiber size, some fiber necrosis, and phagocytosis of muscle fibers with replacement by proliferating connective tissue and fat. Muscular dystrophy disease generally begins in childhood, shows a marked familial tendency, and attacks only males, but it is transmitted only by females. The large muscles of the hip and, later, the shoulder, are chiefly affected. In striking contrast to some other diseases of muscle, for example, myasthenia and myotonia, the dystrophies show change in muscle structure. The biochemical lesion of the muscular dystrophies seems to be a loss of storage of creatine by the affected muscle. It can be detected as an increased loss in the urine. The serum transaminase level is raised, especially when there is much pseudohypertrophy of the muscles. This observation suggests, then, that the disease is located in the cytoplasmic membranes of the muscle cell and is genetically determined.

For over 100 years, sporadic cases of episodic muscle weakness or paralysis, often occurring at night and improved by exercise, have been recognized and are called **periodic paralysis.** We now know that they may be traced to disorders of potassium, and there are at least 3 different types: 1 with high, 1 with low, and 1 with normal serum potassium levels. The familial cases appear to be inherited as an autosomal dominant with complete penetrance. Central core disease, another rare disorder characterized by muscle weakness, can be traced to a cellular disorder in which there is an absence of the normal sarcoplasmic reticulum in the muscle cells. However, both these disorders are so infrequent that it is exaggerating their importance even to mention them.

Inflammation of Muscle

When a young adult without previous training engages in strenuous athletic exercises such as running, jumping, or kicking a football, or in long marches, he or she may rapidly develop firm swelling, aching pain, and paralysis of the muscles in front of the tibia. In its milder form, this is known to athletes and their coaches as "shin splints." A more severe form, in which the affected muscles actually become necrotic, carries the more academic title of the **anterior tibial syndrome.** It is believed that the strenuous exercise of an untrained muscle liberates excess quantities of metabolites, which lead to swelling of the muscle, and that this swelling, in turn, causes pressure, first on the veins and later on the arteries, resulting in ischemic necrosis. It is now clear that such extraordinary work as running the marathon or skiing the 85 km Vasaloppet cross-country ski race may cause reversible metabolic injury to muscle that can be recorded in abnormalities of serum enzyme levels (e.g., creatine phosphokinase). The gradual increase in intensity and duration of such work (as with appropriate training, which cannot be done in days or weeks but only in months and years), to allow adaptive change to take place, decreases this risk.

Volkmann's contracture usually occurs in young persons and affects the muscles of the forearm. It is commonly associated with the pressure of splints or a tourniquet or with hemorrhage resulting from a fracture. Within a few hours of the injury, burning pain develops in the hand or forearm, followed by contracture of the fingers, which becomes fixed in the flexed position. This is an example of ischemic necrosis or infarction of the muscle, the ischemia being caused by arterial spasm resulting from injury to the vessel wall.

There are two kinds of ossifying myositis, or **myositis ossificans,** in which bone is formed in the muscle. Traumatic myositis ossificans is a common condition that may result from repeated injury to a muscle or from a single severe injury, especially when accompanied by hemorrhage. There is a danger that the lesion may be mistaken for an osteogenic sarcoma of bone invading the muscle. Progressive myositis ossificans is fortunately a rare progressive disease, which commences in childhood and slowly kills the patient. Soft swellings develop in the muscles, which are gradually converted into bone, until the body is finally enclosed in a bony sheath that makes breathing impossible.

There are other causes of inflammatory disease in muscles such as parasites and disorders of the immune system. **Trichinosis** is a relatively common muscle disease in the world, caused by the larvae of the round worm *Trichinella spiralis*, which is ingested in uncooked meat. The larvae have a predilection for muscle rich in cytochrome and seem to migrate selectively to the heart, extraocular muscles, and diaphragm, but they may be found in all muscles. These organs may also be the focus of our attention because they are crucial to our well-being. As with many diseases, the symptoms are directly related to the numbers of parasites, and muscle pain is the outstanding feature. The presence of large numbers of eosinophils in the peripheral blood, together with a history of eating raw pork, hamburger, or bear meat, will point to the correct diagnosis. Today, skin testing helps with the diagnosis, which should always be suspected when the eosinophil count is elevated.

Treatment is directed to alleviating the inflammatory response, and steroids are used. There is some evidence that at least one Arctic expedition foundered because the castaways all became severely infected with trichina after eating polar bear.

Dermatomyositis is a collagen vascular disease in which inflammatory muscle disease may be the principal clinical complaint, and, as are the others of this group, it is attributed to an autoimmune disorder.

Eosinophilia-Myalgia Syndrome

In 1989, a new clinical entity characterized by debilitating muscle pain, peripheral edema, and induration of the skin was reported in increasing numbers throughout North America. A uniform laboratory finding was a raised eosinophil count in the peripheral blood. By July 1990 a total of 1531 cases had been reported in the U.S. with 27 deaths, probably due to paralysis of the diaphragm. Figure 25–26 shows the distribution of these cases. Sixty-eight percent were white, non-Hispanic women aged 35 or older. The most frequent features of the illness, which came to be called the Eosinophilia-Myalgia Syndrome, were: arthralgia-myalgia 73%, rash 60%, cough or dyspnea 60%, edema 60%, elevation of aldolase and liver function tests 45%.

The outbreak was traced rapidly to a dietary supplement of Tryptophan, an essential amino acid used as an over-the-counter, self-medication in doses averaging 1.5 grams/day for complaints which ranged from insomnia and depression to pre-menstrual cramps.

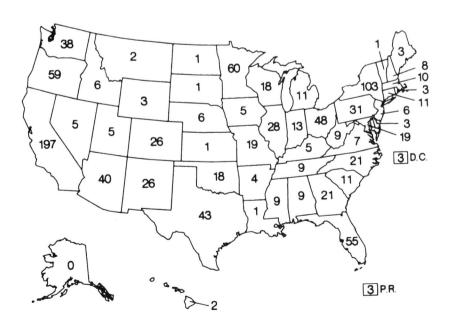

Fig. 25–26 **Eosinophilia-myalgia syndrome** cases, by area—United States, as of January 9, 1990. (From Centers for Disease Control, Morbidity and Mortality Weekly Report, 39(1):15, 1990.)

Ninety-one percent of the affected individuals identified the onset of symptoms as beginning after May 1989, and 97.9% reported taking Tryptophan. Since recall of the over-the-counter preparation in November 1989 there has been a rapid decrease in the number of reported cases (Fig. 25–27).

It is not clear yet whether the syndrome was caused by a contaminant of the tryptophan or because there is a long latency between taking the food supplement and the appearance of a fibrosing syndrome. One cannot escape the similarity of this entity to that described in 1975 by Shulman at NIH.

The mechanisms which may be postulated to operate in this disorder relate other metabolites or derivatives of tryptophan such as 5-hydroxytryptamine and methysergide, an antagonist of 5-hydroxytryptamine which are recognized agents which cause fibrosis. One may postulate that the involved pathways include cytokines, activation of fibroblasts and increased collagen production. It will be interesting to learn whether the individuals affected by the syndrome represent a population with idiosyncratic reactions to the agent and whether the tryptophan itself was responsible, or whether there was a contaminant.

Miscellaneous Muscle Disease

Myasthenia gravis, with its ominously descriptive name, is characterized by great weakness or rather fatigability, most marked in the muscles of the face, which is blank and expressionless, but shared to a lesser extent by all the voluntary muscles. After the muscle has been used a few times, it rapidly loses its power of contraction, only to regain it as rapidly with rest. In extreme cases, the limbs are so weak and easily fatigued (myasthenia) that they can hardly be lifted. This is not the same as paralysis.

The cause of the condition is the presence of antibodies which inhibit normal neuromuscular transmission (Fig. 25–24). No morphologic lesions to explain the astonishing weakness can be found in the motor nerve cells, the nerves, or the muscles they supply. Normally acetylcholine is released at the myoneural junction when impulses are passed across it; this stimulates the muscle fiber to contract. Cholinesterase is normally present and destroys whatever acetylcholine remains after the contraction is effected. It had been suggested earlier that in myasthenia gravis there is either an overabundance of cholinesterase or too little acetylcholine. Today we know that there are antibodies which block these normal reactions and thereby interfere with normal neuromuscular transmission. Treatment consists of the use of drugs antag-

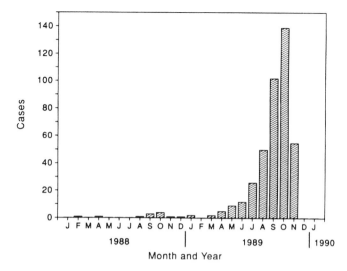

Fig. 25–27 Eosinophilia-myalgia syndrome cases, by month of onset—United States, January 1, 1988–January 9, 1990. (Six persons had EMS onset before 1988; one case each occurred in August 1982, March 1983, September 1986, and February, July and November 1987.) (From Centers for Disease Control, Morbidity and Mortality Weekly Report, 39(1):15, 1990.)

onistic to cholinesterase. Neostigmine is by far the most useful drug during acute attacks. In many cases, there is hyperplasia or a neoplasm of the thymus gland in the neck. What this association means is unknown, but in occasional cases, surgical removal of the thymus has been attended by dramatic improvement.

Passing reference may be made to the myotonias in spite of their rarity, because the condition is the reverse of myasthenia. As the name indicates, there is an increase of muscle tone, with the result that there is prolonged contraction of a muscle after cessation of the stimulus, the fibers being unable to relax. When a movement is repeated a number of times, the muscles warm up, and normal contraction and relaxation may then occur.

Muscle Tumors

Despite the fact that there are over 600 separate muscles in the human body and muscle tissue may account for more than 40% of the body mass, muscle tumors are extraordinarily rare. The only one worth mentioning is the **rhabdomyosarcoma,** and it occurs most frequently in the lower extremities. The diagnosis is made by the identification of cells with striations. The treatment is radical excision. The five-year survival rate is less than 10%; therefore these are tumors that we do not like to diagnose.

SYNOPSIS

Bone is composed of cells, matrix, and mineral. It depends on hormones, diet, and physical activity for its well-being.

Osteoporosis, osteomalacia, and rickets are important metabolic disorders of bone.

Osteomyelitis and tuberculosis are significant infectious diseases of bone.

Osteogenic sarcoma, giant cell sarcoma, multiple myeloma, and Ewing's tumor are important primary tumors of bone, but metastatic cancer from breast, prostate, and lung are more frequent.

Different types of arthritis (inflammatory, traumatic, degenerative) are an economically important cause of chronic disability.

Muscle diseases are of diverse etiologies, and, in comparison to the mass of muscle tissue in the body, these disorders are remarkably rare.

Terms

Osteoblast	*Rickets*	*Tenosynovitis*
Osteoclast	*Osteomyelitis*	*Muscular dystrophy*
Osteocyte	*Osteogenic sarcoma*	*Myasthenia gravis*
Osteoporosis	*Arthritis*	*Rhabdomyosarcoma*
Osteomalacia	*Osteoarthritis*	*Myopathy*

FURTHER READING

Adams, R.D., Denny-Brown, D., and Pearson, C.M.: *Diseases of Muscle*, 3rd Ed. Hagerstown, Md., Harper & Row, 1975.

Barker, D.J.P., et al.: Paget's disease of bone in fourteen British towns. Br. Med. J., 1:1181, 1977.

Carpenter, S., and Karpati, G.: The pathological diagnosis of specific inflammatory myopathies. Brain Pathol., 2:13, 1992.

Deighton, C.M., et al.: Contribution of inherited factors to rheumatoid arthritis. Ann. Rheumatic Dis., 51:182, 1992.

Deufel, T., and Gerbitz, K.D.: Biochemistry and molecular genetics of muscle diseases. Eur. J. Clin. Chem. Clin. Biochem., 29:13, 1991.

Drachman, D.B.: Present and future treatment of myasthenia gravis. N. Engl. J. Med., 316:743, 1987.

Duke-Cohan, J.S. The multifactorial nature of osteoporosis: the potential of corticosteroid-binding globulins as a unifying regulator. Med. Hypoth. 21:431, 1986.

Ferrell, P.B., and Tan, E.M.: Epstein-Barr (EB) virus antibodies in rheumatoid arthritis. Springer Semin. Immunopathol., 4:181, 1981.

Furukawa, T., and Peter, J.B.: The muscular dystrophies and related disorders. J.A.M.A., 239:1537, 1978.

Harris, J.B.: Muscular dystrophy and other inherited diseases of skeletal muscle in animals. Ann. N.Y. Acad. Sci., 317, 1979.

Hazenberg, M.P., et al.: Are intestinal bacteria involved in the etiology of rheumatoid arthritis? Acta Pathol. Microbiol. Scand., 100:1, 1992.

Hertzman, P.A., Blevins, W.L., Mayer, J., et al.: Association of the eosinophilia-myalgia syndrome with the ingestion of tryptophan. N. Engl. J. Med., 322:869, 1990.

Keiser, H., et al.: Clinical forms of gonococcal arthritis. N. Engl. J. Med., 279:234, 1968.

Lawrence, B., and Melton, L.J. III: Involutional osteoporosis. N. Engl. J. Med., 314:1676, 1986.

Lewkonia, R.M.: Myalgia and eosinophilia associated with ingestion of tryptophan. An intriguing new syndrome. Arch. Int. Med., 150:2005, 1990.

Macklem, P.T.: Muscular weakness and respiratory function. N. Engl. J. Med., 314:775, 1986.

Masi, A.T., and Medsger, T.A.: A new look at the epidemiology of ankylosing spondylitis and related syndromes. Clin. Ortho. Related Res., 143:15, 1979.

Nordin, B.E.C.: The definition and diagnosis of osteoporosis. Calc. Th. Intl., 40:57, 1987.

Orlander, J., et al.: Low intensity training, inactivity, and resumed training in sedentary men. Acta Physiol. Scand., 101:351, 1977.

O'Sullivan, J.B., and Cathcart, E.S.: The prevalence of rheumatoid arthritis. Ann. Intern. Med., 76:573, 1972.

Rasmussen, H.: The calcium messenger system (first of two parts). N. Engl. J. Med., 314:1094, 1986.

Rus, B., et al.: Does calcium supplementation prevent post-menopausal bone loss? A double-blind, controlled study. N. Engl. J. Med., 316:173, 1987.

Sinkovics, J.G., and Plager, C.: Bone sarcomas: clinical experience. Can. J. Surg., 20:542, 1977.

Siris, E.S., et al.: Paget's disease of bone. Bull. N.Y. Acad. Med., 56:285, 1980.

Swygert, L.A., Maes, E.F., Sewell, L.E., et al.: Eosinophilia-myalgia syndrome. Results of national surveillance. J.A.M.A., 264:1698, 1990.

Tilyard, M.W., et al.: Treatment of postmenopausal osteoporosis with calcitriol or calcium. N. Engl. J. Med., 326:357, 1992.

Waldvogel, F.A., and Vasey, H.: Osteomyelitis: the past decade. N. Engl. J. Med., 303:360, 1980.

Wheldon, G.D.: Osteoporosis. N. Engl. J. Med., 305:397, 1981.

26

CARE OF THE PATIENT

The real evil of old age is not the body's decline, but the soul's indifference.—A. MAUROIS

This text has thus far concerned itself with diseases and their causes. In this chapter, we digress slightly, in order to examine disease from the point of view of its effect on the individual, and talk about care of the patient. We look at disease from the point of view of the diseased person and his caretakers. This is a large subject; indeed, the care of the patient is the fundamental reason for the existence of the medical and paramedical professions. This care includes diagnosis and treatment of disease, preventative and palliative measures, hospitalization, home care, rehabilitation, and support of many kinds.

THE PATIENT

Each patient is unique, with a unique personality and past experiences. How he or she reacts to health professionals and how they in turn react to the patient will vary, depending on many different aspects such as age, the nature of the medical problem, his or her emotional resources, personality, and how the patient feels. Naturally, the characteristics of the caretakers, the institutions, and the patient's culture are very important in this relationship.

The patient may be more than one person. If a man recovering from an open heart operation needs counselling on when and how to resume his sex life, then he and his wife may become a "group" patient. If a child is dying, the whole family may become a patient. This concept is especially important in psychiatry, since family dynamics are often involved in a patient's disease. Not only the individual but all these persons require patience and understanding.

Many different health professionals are involved with most patients. Some are professionally trained physicians, nurses, physiotherapists, occupational therapists, pharmacists, speech therapists, social workers, clergymen, to name a few. Others are not licensed, but may nevertheless be even more closely involved; they are the relatives and friends of the patient. A recent study showed that the most important emotional support the patient received in hospital was from other patients, not from the medical staff.

AGING

In 1890 the life expectancy for women was 45 years and 47 years for men. This has nearly doubled in 100 years, but we cannot expect such an increase in the next one hundred. However, the increasing maximum life span for humans (Fig. 26–1), the rate of increase in life span potential (Fig. 26–2), and the gain in life expectancy if a particular cause were eliminated (Fig. 26–3), all underscore the importance of considering aging as a very significant part of human life. Above all, it appears that most of the serious illnesses which were addressed in the chapters of this text are diseases which appear in the latter half of an individual's life span. The number of elderly people in the world is increasing rapidly. This implies that there will be a rising cost for health care and an increasing number of cases of all diseases of the elderly.

It is worthwhile to consider here some aspects of aging from a biological point of view and some aspects from a human point of view. One might begin by considering what we mean by aging and what are the current theories to explain what we observe. With increasing age there is a decline in physiological function. In the most elementary way we do not expect the seventy year old to run as fast, jump as high or far, or lift the same weights as the twenty-four year old. In fact, physiological testing demonstrates a gradual decline in aerobic capacity, muscular strength, rapidity of reflex response, as well as acuity of vision and hearing. One might chronicle the age-related changes for each particular system such as changes with aging in the cardiovascular, pulmonary, endocrine, renal, reproductive, and sensory systems. The

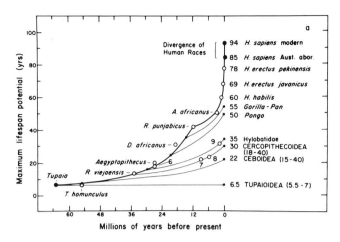

Fig. 26–1   Evolution of maximum life span potential for the Antropoidea. ○, fossil data; ●, living species. (From Cutler, R.G.: Evolution of longevity in primates. J. Human Evol., 5:169, 1976.)

appearance of disease in any part of the body indicates a change in the normal equilibrium between maintenance, repair, and loss of function.

There are two general theories to explain aging which are not incompatible. The first is the extension of the idea that to live to 100 it is necessary to have long lived parents. The implication that aging is genetically determined and is the product of multifactorial inheritance is most attractive and generally acceptable, but fails to explain the mechanism whereby the same systems operate for additional decades in some and fail to function in others. The cellular basis of aging is the modern equivalent of Ponce de Leon's search because of the implication that once we understand the molecular and cellular mechanism we may be able to anticipate, treat and modify tissues to alter the rush to senescence.

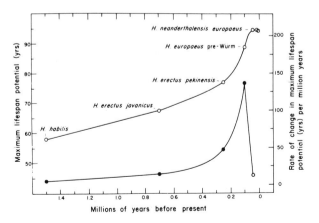

Fig. 26–2   Rate of increase in maximum life span potential along the hominid ancestral-descendant sequence leading to modern man. ○, MLSP; ●, rate of change in MLSP per million years. (From Cutler, R.G.: Evolution of longevity in primates. J. Human Evol., 5:169, 1976.)

CAUSE OF DEATH	GAIN IN EXPECTANCY OF LIFE (YRS) IF CAUSE WAS ELIMINATED	
	AT BIRTH	AT AGE 65
Major cardiovascular-renal	10.9	10.0
Heart disease	5.9	4.9
Vascular diseases affecting central nervous system	1.3	1.2
Malignant neoplasms	2.3	1.2
Accidents other than by motor vehicle	0.6	0.1
Motor vehicle accidents	0.6	0.1
Influenza and pneumonia	0.5	0.2
Infectious diseases (excluding tuberculosis)	0.2	0.1
Diabetes mellitus	0.2	0.2
Tuberculosis	0.1	0.0

Fig. 26–3   Gain in expectancy of life at birth and at age 65 due to elimination of various causes of death. (From "Some demographic aspects of aging in the United States," published by the National Center of Health Statistics, USPHS & U.S. Bureau of the Census, February 1973.)

The first theory to explain aging at the cellular level attributes the aging process to the accumulation of damage to molecules essential to cellular function. One route for the damage is the result of oxidation, a byproduct of metabolic activity. Evidence to support the idea that active oxygen species create toxic effects on cells is the observation that some antioxidants such as Vitamin E seem to have an anti-aging potential. Another observation which generally supports the idea is that the rate of aging is inversely proportional to the metabolic rate of a mammal. The observation that caloric restriction and a decreased nutritional intake prolong life are circumstantial findings which can be interpreted to function in such a manner.

On the other side there is more specific data in the area of genetic differences to support the idea that aging is genetically determined. One paper reports a significant decrease in the frequency of genetic markers HLA B40 and an increase of HLA DR5 in the oldest old people (over 85 years). This is in addition to the finding that in mice genes in the major histocompatibility complex are associated with a significant effect on life span.

BECOMING A PATIENT

When a patient arrives at the physician's office, the first step is taken in the patient's care, which is to attempt to establish a diagnosis. In order to do this, the physician employs at least three different disciplines of the science and art of medicine. These are:

(1) history taking, (2) physical examination, and (3) laboratory investigations.

History taking elicits the patient's description of what is presently wrong, and how the symptoms have changed or developed since he first realized that something was not normal. The history taker then asks questions that he considers to be relevant to the complaint, as well as questions about the patient's general health, past history, and family history.

The medical history serves two important functions: it describes the chronology of the patient's troubles and reveals the pattern of the disorder. It is said that a good physician can make the diagnosis from the history in more than half the cases seen. In addition, the clues given in the history will allow the examiner to focus on specific organ systems during the physical examination.

The history represents the patient's first contact with the health professional. It is during this initial meeting that a working relationship is established between the patient and the medical profession. The rapport, or lack of it, established in the initial interview often affects the subsequent relationship.

Taking a good history is a most difficult task (particularly if the patient is confused, delirious, vomiting, or unconscious). It demands all the skill, insight, and patience of the physician, and often it is the most valuable of all the examinations.

One oft-forgotten purpose of history taking is to establish confidence between the patient and physician that can permit subsequent examination of a more direct and intimate kind, and will permit the examination to be less threatening because of the confidence that has grown out of the dialogue during history taking. Some modern physicians are too harried and hasty, and they forget the great therapeutic value of the interview and its importance in securing the cooperation of the patient, since, after all, it is during this phase of the relationship that the patient reveals his troubles and in his own way describes the disease. Osler used to say, "Listen to the patient. He is telling you the diagnosis."

Physical examination means the employment of what used to be called the 5 senses, more particularly, sight (inspection), touch (palpation), and hearing (auscultation). Of these, inspection appears the easiest, yet it distinguishes the really skilled from the ordinary observer; palpation of the abdomen, breast, and other parts reveals much to the sensitive, educated fingers. Auscultation involves the use of a stethoscope. Smell also plays a role in diagnosis, but has often been superseded or ignored, as have these other perceptions, because of modern laboratory methods.

We might distinguish objective data from subjective impressions in the physical examination. It is customary to measure temperature (with a thermometer) rather than to estimate it, to measure the blood pressure (systolic and diastolic, usually in both arms), to count the pulse (for a minute to determine whether it is regular or irregular), and to count the respirations. These are called the **cardinal signs** and provide a most valuable guide to the general health or severity of illness of the patient. They frequently point the way to disorders of a specific system in the body.

Modern science has vastly extended the range of the unaided senses. A wide variety of fiberoptic scopes, radiologic techniques, and other machines have revolutionized diagnosis during the last 35 years. (Some of these have been described in detail in Chapter 3.) All of them represent extension and amplification (rather than replacement) of our special senses, by amplifying the sounds or the sights, by permitting us to look into otherwise hidden places, or by translating from one sense to another.

Laboratory examinations. It is in the field of laboratory examination of material from the patient that modern medicine has made the greatest leap forward, involving an incredible development of new methods, particularly those that are biochemical. Laboratory methods, which were first developed in connection with research, are quickly applied to the patient.

The explosive development of new methods of laboratory investigation during recent years is responsible for a natural tendency to place undue reliance on these techniques as opposed to the more traditional clinical methods outlined. It is well to recognize the limitations of laboratory procedures, as well as their considerable value. The data are compiled by fallible human beings, who are as liable to errors of technique and of interpretation as are all persons in every occupation. Mistakes may be made by those responsible for the collection and labeling of the material to be tested. Finally, it must be remembered that the normal figure for any given chemical value is variable from one person to another, just as height and weight vary. Moreover, we must recognize that even emotions can influence biochemical processes, although these processes are controlled by enzyme systems, ultimately under the direction of genes.

These modern diagnostic tools have been of invaluable assistance, but we must be careful not to rely too heavily on them for another reason; no diagnostic machine can yet replace the human nervous system. The unaided human senses can accomplish more than any machine. Richard Selzer provides a fascinating example of diagnosis using only the human senses in his book, *Mortal Lessons*. This procedure is described at the end of Chapter 3 and is worth reviewing.

From the pattern of the history, the physical examination, and the laboratory data emerge a set of possible explanations for the fever, or the pain, or the jaundice of the patient. This list of possibilities is called the **differential diagnosis** because a number of different disease processes may explain the patient's particular symptoms and signs. It is the responsibility of the physician to put on his thinking cap and to construct such a list, and then to decide which additional tests might make the diagnosis more certain, or which therapeutic trial he should embark on in managing the patient's discomfort.

THE HOSPITAL

The modern hospital is an institution that houses secondary and tertiary care facilities. (The initial contacts that a patient has with the health care system, family physician for example, are referred to as primary care; secondary care usually refers to specialties, e.g., surgery, and tertiary care is comprised of subspecialties, e.g., plastic or neurosurgery.) As specialties have developed from technologic advancements, the hospital, and in particular the university teaching hospital, has become an essential way of dispensing sophisticated diagnostic procedures and therapies. However, this process has created some disadvantages for the care of the patient. Often, the patient feels alienated from the medical staff because of the size of the institution. Much too often, the referring family physician (if the patient is lucky enough to have one) does not have admitting privileges to the institution and is made to feel an outsider or a nuisance by the house staff. The referring physician may have valuable information about the patient and his medical history and should be encouraged to visit the hospital to discuss the patient. This is particularly important if the patient's mental status was compromised on arrival at the hospital, casting doubt on the completeness and accuracy of the history obtained at that time. If the primary physician is not associated with the hospital, it is rare that he and his patient's new physicians meet. The patient's care, at worst, may become fragmented and discontinuous, and, at best, repetitive in the inquiry. This situation is unfortunate, but is not in itself serious. What is serious, however, is that often no member of the house staff fills the role of interpreter of medical care, which the primary physician has previously assumed. In fact, no member of the house staff assumes complete responsibility for the patient; he or she becomes the part-time patient of several physicians, and the full-time patient of none. Thus the patient is left without anyone in direct control, or responsible for his care,

with whom the patient can communicate his wishes and fears, and without a single person who communicates the results of diagnostic procedures and the prognosis of the disease.

The alienation that the patient experiences can corrode the touchstone of the medical profession—the physician-patient relationship. Without it, the modern advances of medicine cannot be used. Failure to keep appointments and the refusal to take prescribed medicine are common symptoms of this alienation. The most obvious symptom is the exponential rise in the number of malpractice suits, which in themselves further erode the physician-patient relationship.

When several physicians become involved in one case (as is frequent), another result is that the concept of the patient as a whole person disappears. The cardiologist is concerned with the patient's heart, the endocrinologist with the patient's hormones, the gastroenterologist with the gastrointestinal tract. The whole patient is lost in the mass of component parts, like the loose pieces of a jigsaw puzzle. This problem stretches beyond medicine and into the specialties of health care: physiotherapists, dietitians, pharmacists, and so on, each of whom is preoccupied with his own piece of the puzzle. The nursing staff may become the patient's most important contact under this circumstance, since nurses are with the patient 24 hours a day and are aware of all other professional contact and actions, medical and paramedical.

Teamwork and emphasis on team effort and collaboration represent an attempt to rectify this situation, to put the pieces of the puzzle together. In some psychiatric institutions, the psychiatrists, psychologists, social workers, and nurses meet regularly as a team to discuss the patients they all see. Together, they pool their information, create a total picture, and establish a team strategy for dealing with the patient's problems. At least one general hospital has tried the same approach, including doctors, nurses, physiotherapists, and pharmacists on their teams. One result has been a significant reduction in medication errors. However, whether they work as a team or not, all the professionals involved are concerned with the patient and do their utmost to promote his recovery.

Medicine certainly has changed from the cramped office occupied by the kindly, graying physician so often sketched by Norman Rockwell on the cover of the *Saturday Evening Post*. However, the patient still expects the concern for the individual captured in Rockwell's drawings, and it is still the goal of members of the health team. Today, the care of the patient must include the most up-to-date diagnostic and therapeutic regime suited to the situation, but the concern typified by the "old-fashioned M.D." cannot be replaced by modern technology, but rather, should remain the basis of care. (Fig. 26–4).

Nursing. When the patient is safely in bed, the nurse becomes the most important member of the team concerned with his care. There are endless services by which the nurse ministers to the patient's comfort and contributes to his eventual recovery. If he is to receive rest, both physical and mental, which we have already seen to be so essential, it is the nurse who is best qualified to provide it. The nurse must exercise keen observation of the patient, together with accurate recording of any changes in the symptoms and physical condition, including the function of the bowel and bladder. A broad cultural education with knowledge of past and current events, enabling the nurse to converse with and interest the patient, is a valuable asset. Together, the nurse and the physician form the core of the medical team. If the nurse fails to record and to communicate the details of the patient's function accurately, brilliant diagnosis and skill on the part of the attending physician can in no way make up the lack. The degree to which the nursing staff recognizes the needs of the individual patient is often reflected in the success and reputation of the hospital as a whole. In one particular neurologic institute, the quality of the nursing care alone materially increased the surgeons' success and decreased the postoperative complications. The physician and nurse must work together as a team with successful communication in both directions.

Mental Health. Being sick is rarely a pleasant experience, and being hospitalized is difficult and threatening for some persons. When a person becomes a patient, he is usually required to give up certain rights, such as privacy, dignity, self-destiny, and independence. Those who pride themselves on these values may find the transition to patienthood harrowing, and may even become management problems." A management problem is a two-way street—the patient behaves in a way that is inconvenient for the staff, and vice versa.

Treatment. Medical and paramedical treatments are far too numerous and complicated to be described here. However, a few general measures and the subject of drugs are worth our attention, because they apply to most patients. Two important measures taken to promote comfort and recovery are rest and diet. "The greatest physicians are Dr. Quiet, Dr. Diet and Dr. Merryman," said Jonathan swift.

Perhaps **rest** is the most important single therapeutic measure in combating disease. A sick animal does this by instinct, when it crawls into the bushes and lies low. It is difficult to explain on scientific grounds the exact manner in which rest helps the sick person. All infections are benefited by rest, whether they are general or local. An example of the value of local rest is afforded by immobilization of an infected hand by a splint or a sling. By this means, upward spread of the invading organisms along the lymphatics as a result of muscular movements may be reduced. Another example of local rest to an organ is the use of light diets for gastrointestinal disorders.

It is important, however, to remember that rest is not simply a state of inactivity, of freedom from toil.

Fig. 26–4   The doctor. (Luke Fildes)

There must be rest of the mind as well as of the body, relaxation and freedom from unnecessary worry. Mental fatigue is often more harmful than physical fatigue and more difficult to relieve. Sometimes the best way of resting a tired person is by changing from mental work to recreation through physical activity. The patient's worries and anxieties can often be relieved by an alert and concerned medical staff who are willing to spend time with the patient. Often the anxieties about a surgical procedure can be alleviated or ameliorated by a detailed explanation of what is to be expected. Too often, however, tranquilizers—the omnipotent Valium and Librium—are prescribed without first making efforts to discover the source of the anxiety. The patient may also have more nonmedical concerns and may need an opportunity to ventilate his or her concerns. We must remember that, in all probability, a patient's normal resources for communication are inaccessible now that he is in the hospital. Inconvenient visiting hours and lack of privacy may prevent the patient from using friends and relatives for this purpose. In these cases, it is important for the staff to be alert and available to listen. Often it does not matter who is the listener, whether nurse, doctor, clergyman, or the cleaning lady, so long as he knows how to listen.

Rest can be overdone, especially in the aged. When the octogenarian takes to bed for too long, he may never able to get out of it again. Prolonged disuse of an organ inevitably leads to deterioration of function, to be followed sooner or later by disintegration of structure. The dangers of prolonged rest in bed, particularly for the elderly, have been summarized as follows: "Look at the patient lying in bed. What a picture he makes with the blood clotting in his veins, the lime draining from his bones, the scybala stacking up in his colon, the flesh rotting from his seat, the urine leaking from his distended bladder, and the spirit evaporating from his soul." Prolonged bed rest has been much overprescribed.

Correct **diet** is assuming a position of ever increasing importance in the treatment of disease, as well as in the preservation of health. This illustrates the need for an expert dietitian in a well-organized hospital. Proteins are traditionally the principal source of material for the maintenance and repair of tissues. Such maintenance and repair may be specially needed in febrile and other diseases in which there is marked breakdown of tissue. Intravenous hyperalimentation is assuming a greater and greater role in the management of severely ill patients. Vitamins and minerals, such as zinc, calcium, and iron, are obviously vital in the treatment of dietary deficiency diseases. Low-protein diets are equally important in the treatment of liver and kidney disease, in which the diseased organs are unable to excrete harmful protein or metabolites properly. Low-sodium diets are frequently prescribed for certain types of cardiovascular disease (e.g., hypertension) and edema, associated with retention of sodium, which holds fluid in the tissues.

On the nurse rests the responsibility of seeing that the patient eats the prescribed diet; the nurse must report to the doctor if the patient does not do so. The regulation of fluids may be as important as the regulation of food. When there is much fluid loss, which may be due to vomiting or diarrhea, that loss must be made up. Conversely, when the tissues are waterlogged, as in heart or renal failure, the intake of fluid must be diminished.

Drugs. These agents have many different functions, and any specific drug may have several functions. Drugs put people to sleep, lower their blood pressure, and cure their bacterial infections. Human life from conception to death is influenced by drugs. Needless to say, they play a tremendous role in therapeutics, but, unfortunately, they are not without their side effects. They tend to be like the curly-haired girl in the nursery rhyme—when they are good, they are very, very good, but when they are bad, they are horrid. The side effects of drugs (or drug reactions) tend to fall into one of several categories.

Effects Due to the Drug Itself. Many drugs have well-known side effects, and these are considered before the drug is prescribed. For example, some of the antineoplastic agents result in temporary baldness. In the treatment of leukemia, this is obviously a minor consideration. The patient is forewarned and, though distressed, quickly warms his head with a wig or a hat.

An Idiosyncratic Drug Reaction. Many drug allergies fall into this category. These are reactions that are known to occur, but that occur rarely and unpredictably in any given person. Penicillin allergy is an example. The importance of any allergy is to inform the patient of its existence, so that the drug will not be administered again inadvertently.

Improper dosage can be caused by the patient or the physician, but most commonly by both. For example, if a depressed patient takes too many sleeping pills in a suicide attempt, the fault lies with the patient. However, the physician is not blameless; he prescribed either a large number of tablets or a drug known to be a potentially suicidal agent.

A prescription is often written but not explained fully to the patient, and improper dosages are taken through misunderstanding. Often, the "dose," though generally correct, is wrong for a given patient. For example, a drug excreted by the kidney must be reduced in a patient with impaired renal function. It is, therefore, obligatory for the physician to look for evidence of renal failure in a patient to whom he wishes to give the drug.

Drug Interaction. Often in any medical clinic a patient arrives carrying a large shopping bag filled with unlabeled syrups, pills, and suppositories, which are the legacy of several generations of physicians at several hospitals. The patient usually still takes a small percentage of the medication regularly, and often takes more as the condition worsens. Each drug alone might be of benefit (as it no doubt was when prescribed), but together the drugs may worsen the patient's medical problems or create new ones. As the saying goes, too many cooks spoil the broth.

Sometimes the problem is not the interaction per se, but rather, indiscriminate drug combinations. The classic case usually cited is antibiotic therapy. When a patient is hospitalized with septicemia, the patient's blood is cultured and he is given several antibiotics immediately. The culture results return in two days, and antibiotics are adjusted once the organism is isolated. However, sometimes the adjustment is not made, because cultures were not taken or because of faulty reasoning (the patient is getting better and no one wants to change the antibiotics). Organisms that are resistant to the prescribed antibiotics then grow, and the patient is left with unusual bacteria, fungi, or problems against which the usual antibiotics are obviously ineffective.

Placebo Effect. In many situations, nonspecific drugs are given for the purpose of helping the patient to have a night's sleep or to allay anxiety, and these drugs may in all honesty be directed at relieving the patient's symptoms. However, the mere action of giving a pill has a large positive effect on many patients because of our only too human trait of suggestibility. The readiness to believe is common. One professor sprayed water around a classroom and told the students to raise their hands as soon as they detected an odor. Seventy-three per cent of the class signified that they smelled the odorless water. In Latin, placebo means I shall please, and it is currently used in the medical context of a medicine given to suggest that treatment is being given, when the pill may in reality be of little or no benefit. Although placebos are used occasionally in clinical trials, one should not underestimate the important effect of faith in the practice of medicine. It is well recognized that inert medications and minor nostrums may provide relief to the patient, and this is testimony to the faith, confidence, and trust that the patient has in his caretakers.

Prevention. The most effective "treatment" of any disease clearly is its elimination through prevention. Immunization against bacterial and viral diseases is

the obvious example. Other preventive measures are just as important, though not as obvious. Prenatal classes and visits, diet counseling, screening for inborn errors of metabolism in newborns, and visual and auditory testing are other examples.

Basic research fits into the category of prevention, although its application is often not apparent until several years after discoveries have been made. In the late 1940s, a pragmatist might have argued that government funding should be channeled into portable iron lungs and special treatment centers for poliomyelitis victims. However, basic research in tissue culture paved the way for the isolation of the virus that caused polio and the development of a vaccine. In retrospect, the funding of the research has paid for itself many times over in actual money saved in the treatment of polio victims, let alone the saving in human suffering. The opportunities for basic undirected research must be maintained despite economic recession.

Modern theories of prevention include a popular notion that healthy habits can keep someone alive by avoiding the common causes of premature death—cancer, heart disease, and stroke. However, it should be kept in mind that we really do not understand the pathogenesis of all diseases, and thus our prevention rationale may not be as valid as we think. It is only theory, rising out of **association** of disease with life-style, not demonstrated causality. As Lewis Thomas has said in *On Magic in Medicine*:

"The popular acceptance of the notion of Seven Healthy Life Habits, as a way of staying alive, says something important about today's public attitudes, or at least the attitudes in the public mind, about disease and dying. People have always wanted causes that are simple and easy to comprehend, and about which the individual can *do* something. If you believe that you can ward off the common causes of premature death—cancer, heart disease, and stroke, diseases whose pathogenesis we really do not understand—by jogging, hoping, and eating and sleeping regularly, these are good things to believe even if not necessarily true. Medicine has survived other periods of unifying theory, constructed to explain all of human disease, not always as benign in their effects as this all is likely to be . . .

"Nobody can say an unfriendly word against the sheer goodness of keeping fit, but we should go carefully with the premises."

PREPARATION FOR DISCHARGE

At a certain point in the patient's progress, the patient, the physician, and the staff who have been active in his care begin to think about discharge from the hospital. Discharge-related questions arise: What is this patient's home like? What kind of situation will he return to? Will the family be able to care for the patient if he needs it, and cope with any problems that will arise? A patient, for example, may be left with an open wound; some operations on the bowel involve incisions that are not sewn up because of the danger of fecal contamination. Instead, the wound is packed with gauze that is changed and washed frequently, and the incision is allowed to heal from the bottom up (healing by second intention). This takes much more time, so that patient will take a large wound-care problem home. Who would help with this? In addition, any person who has experienced a major operation requires about 6 weeks before his energy level returns to its preoperative level.

Helping the patient and the family prepare for discharge can be an important part of care of the patient. We shall take the example of a young child who has just been hospitalized and is a newly diagnosed diabetic. Preparing this child's parents for homecoming involves many hours of teaching by physicians, nurses, and dietitians. The parents must learn how to care for their child at home, how to give injections, how to monitor their child's insulin requirements, how to recognize crises such as insulin shock, how to juggle the new diet and nutritional regime so that the child eats the right number of calories, and somebody must make sure that they understand and retain this information. This is additionally difficult because the parents are bound to be anxious, perhaps too anxious, to learn.

At first hospitalization for alcoholism-related problems affords another kind of discharge problem. When discharged, the patient may well be returning to a home situation that seems guaranteed to make him ill again. Here, social workers of the hospital become involved. If some attempt has been made by the staff to examine the patient's problem, rehabilitation and suitability for self-help groups such as Alcoholics Anonymous should be discussed. Alcoholism is a topic frequently avoided and regarded as hopeless by hospital staff. It certainly will be hopeless if no attempts to alter the situation are made. However, on the chance that this and other difficult psychosomatic problems have some solutions, it is the responsibility of the staff to investigate.

The patient may not be discharged to his home, but to a rehabilitation center. Rehabilitation may have already begun in the hospital through physiotherapy, occupational therapy, and related disciplines. These play a fundamental role in helping the patient to regain the use of a disabled or impaired body part, so that he can return to a former level of functioning as quickly as possible.

Finally, if the patient will require any home services, these should be arranged before discharge.

HOME CARE

Care of the patient has not finished when the patient leaves the hospital. Indeed, for many, it has only just begun. Professional concern, given on a regular basis, is of tremendous value to the patient and the family, who may know little about medicines, dressings, and peculiar new symptoms. Each new problem is likely to send them hurtling into chaos, unless they know someone they can trust and call on when necessary.

Caring for a sick person at home can be difficult for the family. One big problem is isolation; our health care system is simply not set up to care for patients at home, so patients and their families tend to become isolated from the medical community in many instances. Any elderly person who is disabled or weak, in pain, or unaccustomed to being awake for more than a half-hour obviously finds the task of coping impossible at times. The elderly desperately need physicians who make house calls. It is unfortunate that home care which is infinitely cheaper than institutional alternatives, is rendered so difficult by the present North American system. (It is also unfortunate for the physician that he does not visit the home, because this means that the patient can be far more easily depersonalized on arrival at the hospital.)

Home care of any bedridden patient can be a monumental job. The patient must be kept clean, as mobile as possible, guarded from pressure sores, fed, hydrated, medicated; urination and defecation must be closely monitored, and, most important, the patient must be kept comfortable. At home, there are no shift changes and no days off. There is no dietary staff to prepare special diets, there are no physiotherapists with expertise in exercise, no nurses constantly present to monitor medication and symptoms (unless at tremendous expense, which few can afford).

However, there are resources for patient care, and it is up to the family to locate these and to exploit them fully. Visiting nurses are invaluable and available in most communities; visiting physiotherapists are also available in some places. If the patient is lucky enough to have a family physician, he can always be reached by phone, though perhaps not for urgent problems. Many pharmacists are taking an active role in the use of medicines and are usually happy to discuss drugs and their uses and side effects. If there is a clergyman, he can also be a valuable resource. He may know much about what the community has to offer, and more important, he may be able to counsel both patient and family. In some communities, there are services that provide homemakers, "sitters," and then there are special organizations that provide information and help, such as the American Cancer Society, the National Hospice Association, and others, which can be found in the classified telephone directory under "Social Service Organizations."

TERMINAL CARE

Terminal care refers to the care that a patient receives while dying. It is a separate category because it has its own special problems, some of which represent the greatest challenges of medicine and life.

Before we deal with terminal care, we must define what we mean by terminally ill. How do we know when a patient is terminally ill? Obviously something is indicated from signs and symptoms, or from tissue diagnosis, which may fall into an identifiable pattern. The first question the physician must ask is: Do the patient's symptoms reflect the terminal phase of the disease, or do they result from a different, treatable condition? For example, a patient may be treated for colonic cancer and recuperate, and for several months have no symptoms. When he reappears at the hospital with abdominal pain, it will probably be assumed that cancer has recurred. If the patient goes into shock two days later, he may be assumed to be terminally ill, but it could be a ruptured appendix, an incarcerated inguinal hernia, or some other treatable condition. For this reason, it is crucial that the patient have a complete physical examination and history. It still happens occasionally that a patient who is assumed to be terminally ill dies or treatment is withheld for a condition that, on autopsy, is found to have been treatable (and unrelated to the assumed terminal disease).

The terminal patient has been defined as someone nearing death from progressive, unrelenting illness that cannot be arrested nor reversed in our present state of knowledge (or ignorance). The physician should investigate the symptoms to convince himself that this is indeed the case. Having reached this decision, several issues need to be dealt with, and some of these will be discussed here.

1. What does the patient know about the condition, and how does he feel about it? All staff members need to know the patient's state of mind, otherwise care becomes uncoordinated and based on the wrong assumptions. The easiest way to discern this information is for the physician to ask the patient what he understands about the illness. This provides the patient with the opportunity to tell the physician, directly or indirectly, how much he wants to know.

Usually he will ask questions, and these should be answered simply and truthfully.

It has often been noted that dying patients know that they are dying, even when told little or nothing about their condition. For most people, the truth dawns gradually, even when they do not ask and are not told. Some do not wish to discuss it, and we should respect their wishes. Even terminally ill children, who are frequently told nothing, come to know that they are dying. The various stages through which they learn this—through watching their distressed parents and relatives, frequent hospitalization, discussions with other sick children, and finally watching a fellow patient die of the same disease—have been outlined by Myra Bluebond Langner in her book *The Private Worlds of Dying Children*. This fact is a good reason for dealing with these patients truthfully; lying to them will only give rise to doubts, disbeliefs, and erosion of trust between staff and patient. This can be far more devastating than the truth.

Once the patient knows or suspects that he or she is dying, he may have any of several reactions, which have been well documented in recent years. Common emotional responses outlined by Kubler-Ross include denial, anger, bargaining, depression, and acceptance. An understanding of these responses will greatly help those professionals who deal with dying patients. Hinton has found that about one-quarter of patients in one study show acceptance and positive composure to their fate. They will comment that they are dying, and that they have had good lives. They speak positively of this feeling of consenting to life's ending. About one-quarter acknowledge that they are dying, with slight regret, but no distress. One-quarter are distressed, and one-quarter say little or nothing about it. Acceptance was found to be more common in the elderly, and those with young children were more likely to discuss the fact that they were dying.

2. How can the patient be made comfortable? There are some who consider that physical, mental, and spiritual comfort for those who are terminally ill can best be accomplished in the home or in a hospice, and adherents to this view are increasing. The term "hospice" once referred to a house or shelter, usually kept by a religious order, that provided rest for pilgrims and strangers. Today, however, it refers to a special kind of care for the dying. The hospice concept of care is to make the patients physically and mentally as comfortable as possible, with dignity and as much joy as possible. Hospice care may be given in a regular hospital, where some have installed palliative care units for this purpose, or in a special hospice care facility run by specially trained professionals.

Death is frequently associated with pain in the lay

mind, but this is not necessarily the case. Should the patient suffer pain, however, there is no reason why he should not be totally relieved of it. The cause of the pain must be ascertained, and treatment directed at the cause. The use of narcotics to treat intractable pain in the dying is commonplace today. At times, physicians and nurses are overconcerned about tolerance with these drugs, and out of caution provide less relief than is needed. Risk of tolerance is real, but that should not be a barrier to the use of narcotics in terminal care. Tolerance is far better than the alternative, whereby the patient becomes incapacitated with pain in his greatest hour of need.

Skilled nursing care can provide a great deal of comfort for the dying patient. Careful positioning and attention to hygiene and physiologic functions can prevent many uncomfortable complications. Attention to psychologic needs and flexibility on the part of the nurse can also bring great comfort. Above all, the patient should feel that the staff are doing their utmost and that they will not abandon him.

3. When should life-support or heroic measures be withdrawn? Efforts to preserve life become unethical at a certain point in the patient's progress, and outright useless toward the end; but exactly what constitutes a heroic measure, and when it should be withdrawn, and who sanctions the withdrawal, can become complicated issues.

Most persons feel that this should be the patient's decision, and, as a result, many states have enacted laws providing for "living wills"—legal documents that give patients their right to refuse heroic measures when in a terminal condition. The patient's autonomy has been thought to be the best way of insuring that any actions taken are strictly in the interest of the patient. Thus the patient decides, and the doctor carries out his wishes. However, it is not always so simple. Jackson and Younger have described 6 problems that can greatly complicate the heroic-measures decision.

(a) Ambivalence of the patient. The patient may oscillate between allowing life-supporting procedures and forbidding them. In this case, the staff does not know which of the patient's wishes to honor.

(b) Depression. The patient may refuse life-supporting therapy because he is depressed and has given up. However, if the depression lifts (for example, if temporary discomforting symptoms pass) he may request therapy.

(c) Refusal of life-support may, like an attempted suicide, be a plea for help and attention.

(d) The patient may refuse treatment out of fear, realistic or not, of the treatment.

(e) The wishes of the family and those of the patient may conflict. For example, the patient may state that

he wishes life-supporting therapy to continue, and then may lapse into a delirious state from which he cannot communicate. The family may wish at this point that no heroic measures be taken. Whose wishes should be honored?

(f) The staff may assume that a comatose patient with a terminal and painful condition would not want heroic treatment, when in fact this may not be the case.

Detailed examination of the patient's rationale for this decision, and discussion with the family at the time of the decision, may help to avoid some of these situations.

4. How is the patient's family coping? The family should be fully informed of the patient's progress. If they are kept in the dark, they may become anxious, and this anxiety may be manifested as hostility towards everyone and everything connected with their dying relative. They should also have opportunities to express their own feelings. Guilt, frustration, and fear are all intermingled with grief, and someone should let them know that these feelings are normal, and that the staff understands. Finally, they need to have some indication of the patient's life expectancy, but this should not be too specific, and they need to be forewarned about possible new developments in the patient's course.

In conclusion, it is not our purpose here to outline all aspects of care of the patient, but merely to put disease into the perspective of the patient and his caretakers. Disease does not appear in isolation; its diagnosis and treatment may be greatly compounded by the psychosocial circumstances of the sufferer. We talk frequently of such concepts as the compliance of the patient, the will to live, the difficult personality, and stress, all of which we suspect influence the development and outcome of disease. Health professionals who deal with disease must usually cope with far more than disordered structure and function of a particular organ. We would be remiss in not drawing to the attention of the reader that disease is not only an abstraction, but also that it exists in reality in the form of persons who need help.

FURTHER READING

Bordley, J., III, and Harvey, A.M.: *Two Centuries of American Medicine*. Philadelphia, W.B. Saunders Co., 1976.

Crichton, M.: *Five Patients, The Hospital Explained*. New York, Alfred Knopf, 1970.

Cutler, R.G.: Human longevity and aging: possible role of reactive oxygen species. Ann. N.Y. Acad. Sci., 621:1, 1991.

Dubos, R.J.: *The Mirage of Health: Utopia's Progress and Biological Change*. New York, Harper & Row, 1959.

Eisenberg, L.: What makes persons "patients" and patients "well?" Am. J. Med., 69:27, 1980.

Engel, G.L.: The care of the patient: art or science. Johns Hopkins Med. J., 140:222, 1977.

Fries, J.: Aging, natural death, and the compression of morbidity. N. Engl. J. Med., 303:130, 1980.

Gardner, J.J., and Ouimette, R.: A nurse-physician team approach in a private internal medicine practice. Arch. Intern. Med., 134:956, 1974.

Gillum, R.F., and Barsky, A.J.: Diagnosis and management of patient noncompliance. J.A.M.A., 228:1563, 1974.

Groves, J.E.: Taking care of the hateful patient. N. Engl. J. Med., 298:883, 1978.

Hinton, J.: *Dying*. New York, Penguin Books, 1972.

Ingelfinger, F.J.: Health: a matter of statistics or feeling? N. Engl. J. Med., 296:448, 1977.

Jackson, D.L., and Youngner, S.: Patient autonomy and "death with dignity." N. Engl. J. Med., 301:404, 1979.

Langner, Myra B.: *The Private Worlds of Dying Children*. Princeton, Princeton University Press, 1978.

Lantz, B., and Molander, A., and Nilsson, G.: Observations on biochemical and haematological parameters in healthy people above 80 years of age. Scand. J. Clin. Lab. Invest., 50:807, 1990.

Lasagna, L.: *The Doctor's Dilemmas*. New York, Harper & Bros., 1962.

Lee, R.V.: The generalist: a jaundiced view. I. The specialist veneer. Am. J. Med., 72:184, 1982.

Lee, R.V.: The generalist: a jaundiced view. VI. Playing doctor. Am. J. Med., 72:554, 1982.

Lee, R.V.: The generalist: a jaundiced view. XIII. The bedpan gap. Am. J. Med., 73:465, 1982.

Millstein, S.G., Adler, N.E., and Irwin, C.E.: Conceptions of illness in young adults. Pediatrics, 68:834, 1981.

Mount, B.M.: Palliative care of the terminally ill. Ann. Roy. Coll. Phys. Surg. Can., July 1978, p. 20.

Osmond, H.: God and the doctor. N. Engl. J. Med., 302:555, 1980.

Prado De Molina, M.: The confrontation with death. Am. J. Psychoanal., 36:261, 1976.

Rosenbaum, E.: *Living With Cancer*. New York, Praeger, 1975.

Smith, D.L.: *Medication Guide for Patient Counseling*. Philadelphia, Lea & Febiger, 1977.

Thomson, C.J.H.: Treatment of incompetent terminally ill patients. 2. Reflection on the American experience. Med. J. Aust., March 20, 1982, p. 246.

Torion, L.V., et al.: Decisions for and against resuscitation in an acute geriatric medicine unit serving the frail elderly. Archiv. Int. Med., 152:561, 1992.

Toynbee, P.: *Patient*. New York, Harcourt Brace Jovanovich, 1977.

Weed, L.L.: *Medical Records, Medical Education and Patient Care*. Cleveland, Case University Press, 1969.

PREFIXES AND SUFFIXES

An appreciation of the meaning of Latin and Greek prefixes and suffixes serves to make obscure and forbidding medical terms easy to understand and therefore far more interesting. Some of these more commonly used in the subjects we have been considering are given. To make the subject more living, the reader may care to put together the prefix and suffix in such words as hematemesis, pathogenesis, osteomalacia, dyspnea, and mennorrhagia.

PREFIXES

a- without or not: *achlorhydria,* absence of hydrochloric acid.

acro- extremity: *acromegaly,* large extremities.

adeno- gland: *adenitis,* inflammation of a gland.

an- without: *anuria,* suppression of urine.

ante- before: *antemortem,* before death.

anti- against: *antitoxin,* antagonistic to a toxin.

arthro- joint: *arthritis,* inflammation of a joint.

auto- self: *autolysis,* self-dissolution.

bio- life: *biology,* study of living things.

chol- bile: *cholecystitis,* inflammation of the gallbladder.

cyst- bladder: *cystitis,* inflammation of the bladder.

dia- through: *diarrhea,* a flowing through.

dys- difficult, bad: *dysmenorrhea,* difficult menstruation.

en- in, into: *encapsuled,* enclosed in a capsule.

endo- within: *endometrium,* lining of the uterus.

entero- intestine: *enteritis,* inflammation of the intestine.

epi- upon, outside: *epidermis,* outer layer of the true skin.

ex- out of: *exostosis,* bony growth from surface of bone.

hem-, hemo- blood: *hemoglobin,* coloring matter of red blood cells.

hetero- dissimilar: *heterophile* antibody, having affinity for antigen other than that for which it is specific.

homeo- similar: *homeostasis,* stability of normal body states.

hydro- water: *hydrothorax,* fluid in the pleural cavity.

hyper- above, excessive: *hyperacidity,* excessive acidity.

hypo- deficiency or beneath: *hypoacidity,* deficient acidity.

hyster- uterus: *hysterectomy,* excision of the uterus.

infra- below: *infraorbital,* beneath the orbit.

inter- between: *intercellular,* between cells.

intra- within: *intracellular,* within cells.

leuko- white: *leukocyte,* a white blood cell.

macro- large: *macrocyte,* an abnormally large red blood cell.

mal- bad: *malnutrition,* poor nutrition.

mast- breast: *mastitis,* inflammation of the breast.

mega- great: *megacolon,* enlargement of the colon.
melan- black: *melanin,* a black pigment.
men- month: *menses, menstruation,* monthly blood flow from uterus.
micro- small: *microcyte,* an undersized red blood cell.
myo- muscle: *myositis,* inflammation of muscle.
myx- mucus: *myxedema,* mucinous edema.
necro- death: *necrosis,* death of cells.
neo- new: *neoplasm,* a new growth or tumor.
nephr- kidney: *nephritis,* inflammation of kidney.
oligo- few: *oliguria,* scanty urination.
osteo- bone: *osteomyelitis,* inflammation of bone.
para- beside: *paramedical,* having a secondary relation to medicine.
peri- around: *pericardium,* the membrane around the heart.
phago- to eat, devour: *phagocyte,* a cell that devours bacteria.
phleb- vein: *phlebitis,* inflammation of a vein.
polio- gray: *poliomyelitis,* inflammation of gray matter of spinal cord.
poly- many: *polycythemia,* excess in number of red blood cells.
post- after: *postmortem,* after death.
pro- before: *prophylaxis,* measures taken to prevent disease.
pseudo- false: *pseudopodia,* false feet of astroglia.
pyo- pus: *pyosalpinx,* fallopian tube filled with pus.
syn- together with: *syndrome,* a constant complex of symptoms.
xantho- yellow: *xanthochromia,* yellow coloration of the cerebrospinal fluid.

SUFFIXES

-angio, vessel: *lymphangitis,* inflammation of a lymph vessel.
-algia, pain; *neuralgia,* pain involving nerves.
-ase, designating an enzyme: *amylase,* a starch-splitting enzyme.
-cele, a protrusion: *meningocele,* a hernial protrusion of the meninges.
-centesis, perforating or tapping: *thoracentesis,* aspirating fluid from the thorax.
-chole, bile: *acholic,* without bile.
-ectasis, dilate: *bronchiectasis,* dilatation of the bronchi.
-ectomy, excision: *tonsillectomy,* removal of a tonsil.
-emesis, vomit: *hematemesis,* vomiting blood.
-emia, blood: *anemia,* deficiency of red blood cells.
-esthesia, sensation: *anesthesia,* absence of sensation.
-genesis, generation of: *pathogenesis,* generation of disease.
-iasis, a process, especially a morbid one: *amebiasis,* state of being infected with amebae.
-itis, inflammation of the part named: *appendicitis,* inflammation of appendix.
-lith, stone: *phlebolith,* calcified body in a vein.
-lysis, to dissolve: *autolysis,* self-dissolution.
-malacia, softening: *osteomalacia,* softening of bone.
-megaly, large: *splenomegaly,* enlargement of spleen.
-odynia, pain: *pleurodynia,* pain in the region of the pleura.
-oid, like, resembling: *mucoid,* like mucus.
-oma, tumor: *osteoma,* a tumor of bone.
-osis, full of: *amyloidosis,* full of amyloid.
-ostomy, mouth: *gastrostomy,* to make an artificial opening into the stomach.
-otomy, cut: *gastrotomy,* to cut into the stomach.
-pathy, disease: *neuropathy,* any nervous disease.
-penia, poverty: *thrombocytopenia,* decrease in the thrombocytes or blood platelets.
-phila, affinity for: *eosinophil,* leukocyte staining with eosin.
-plasia, to form: *hyperplasia,* overgrowth of tissue.

-plegia, paralysis: *hemiplegia,* paralysis of one half (side) of the body.
-pnea, breath: *dyspnea,* difficult breathing.
-ptosis, falling: *visceroptosis,* falling of abdominal viscera.
-rhagia, bursting forth: *menorrhagia,* profuse menstruation.
-rhea, flow: *diarrhea,* abnormal flow from bowel.
-sclerosis, hardening: *arteriosclerosis,* hardening of the arteries.
-stasis, standing still: *hemostasis,* arrest of circulation.
-trophy, nourish: *atrophy,* wasting.
-uria, relating to urine: *anuria,* absence of urine.

Page numbers in **boldface** indicate illustrations; numbers followed by "t" indicate tables.